Cancer Pain Management

Cancer Pain Management

Michael J. Fisch, MD, MPH, FACP

Associate Professor

General Oncology

Division of Cancer Medicine

The University of Texas M. D. Anderson Cancer Center

Houston, Texas

Allen W. Burton, MD

Associate Professor of Anesthesiology and Pain Medicine

Chief of Cancer Pain Management

The University of Texas M. D. Anderson Cancer Center

Houston, Texas

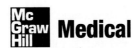

New York   Chicago   San Francisco   Lisbon   London   Madrid
Mexico City   Milan   New Delhi   San Juan   Seoul   Singapore   Sydney   Toronto

Cancer Pain Management

Copyright © 2007 by The McGraw-Hill Companies, Inc. All rights reserved. Printed in the United States of America. Except as permitted under the United States Copyright Act of 1976, no part of this publication may be reproduced or distributed in any form or by any means, or stored in a database or retrieval system, without the prior written permission of the publisher.

1 2 3 4 5 6 7 8 9 0   QPD/QPD   0 9 8 7 6

ISBN-13: 978-0-07-144535-1
ISBN-10: 0-07-144535-8

This book was set in Minion by International Typesetting and Composition, Inc.
The editors were Joe Rusko and Heather Cooper.
The production supervisor was Catherine Saggese.
Project management was provided by International Typesetting and Composition, Inc.
Cover design by Danielle Giacolone.
The indexer was Robert Swanson.
Quebecor World/Dubuque was printer and binder.

This book is printed on acid-free paper.

Photo Credit: Patrick McDonnell/Photo Researchers, Inc.
Photo Caption: Illustration of axons and dendrites of nerve cells meeting at synapses to transport nerve impulses.

Library of Congress Cataloging-in-Publication Data

Cancer pain management /[edited by] Michael J. Fisch, Allen W. Burton.
     p. ; cm.
  Includes index.
  ISBN 0-07-144535-8 (alk. paper)
  1. Cancer pain. 2. Cancer pain—Prevention. I. Fisch, Michael J. II. Burton, Allen W., 1964–
  [DNLM: 1. Neoplasms—complications. 2. Pain—therapy. 3. Palliative Care. QZ 200
  C21536355   2006]
  RC262.C3622   2006
  616.99′4—dc22
                                                  2006046616

In memory of my beloved parents, Linda & Monroe Fisch.
Michael J. Fisch

To Mom and Dad, and my dear Jo Anna and boys, Wade, Sam, and Jack.
Allen W. Burton

CONTENTS

CONTRIBUTORS

Joann Aaron, MA
Scientific Editor
The University of Texas M. D. Anderson Cancer Center
Community Clinical Oncology, Program Research Base
Houston, Texas

Madhuri Are, MD
Assistant Professor
Department of Anesthesiology and Pain Medicine
The University of Texas M. D. Anderson Cancer Center
Houston, Texas

Stefanía Ægisdóttir, PhD
Assistant Professor of Counseling Psychology
Ball State University
Department of Counseling Psychology
Teachers College
Muncie, Indiana

Ralph D. Beasley, MD
Assistant Professor of Anesthesiology
Dartmouth Medical School
Director
Medical Education
Pain Management Center
Dartmouth Hitchcock Medical Center
Lebanon, New Hampshire

William Breitbart, MD
Chief
Psychiatry Service
Department of Psychiatry
Memorial Sloan-Kettering Cancer Center
New York, New York

Allen W. Burton, MD
Associate Professor of Anesthesiology and Pain Medicine
Chief of Cancer Pain Management
The University of Texas M. D. Anderson Cancer Center
Houston, Texas

Juan P. Cata, MD
Resident
Division of Anesthesiology
Critical Care and Comprehensive Pain Management
Cleveland Clinic Foundation
Cleveland, Ohio

Victor T. Chang, MD
Associate Professor of Medicine
University of Medicine and Dentistry New Jersey Medical School
    (UMDNJ), Open Society, Institute Project on Death America
    (PDIA) Faculty Scholar
Section Hematology Oncology
VA New Jersey Health Care System
East Orange, New Jersey

Edward Chow, MBBS, MSc, FRCPC
Associate Professor
Radiation Oncology
University of Toronto
Toronto-Sunnybrook Regional Cancer Centre
Ontario, Canada

Charles Cleeland, PhD
Professor
Chair
Department of Symptom Research
The University of Texas M. D. Anderson Cancer Centre
Houston, Texas

Christopher Crane, MD
Associate Professor
Department of Radiation Oncology
The University of Texas M. D. Anderson Cancer Center
Houston, Texas

Ricardo A. Cruciani, MD, PhD
Vice-Chairman, Director
Research Division
Department of Pain Medicine and Palliative Care
Beth Israel Medical Center
New York, New York
Assistant Professor
Department of Neurology
Department of Anesthesiology
Albert Einstein College of Medicine
Bronx, New York

Eardie A. Curry III, PharmD, BCOP, MBA
Clinical Research Specialist
The University of Texas M. D. Anderson Cancer Center
Houston, Texas

Prajnan Das, MD, MPH
Assistant Professor
Department of Radiation Oncology
The University of Texas M. D. Anderson Cancer
    Center
Houston, Texas

Marc Delclos, MD
Associate Professor
Department of Radiation Oncology
The University of Texas M. D. Anderson Cancer Center
Houston, Texas

Egidio Del Fabbro, MD
Clinical Fellow
Department of Palliative Care and Rehabilitation
    Medicine
The University of Texas M. D. Anderson Cancer Center
Houston, Texas

Óscar A. de Leon-Casasola, MD
Professor of Anesthesiology
Vice-chair for Clinical Affairs
Department of Anesthesiology
State University of New York at Buffalo
Chief
Pain Medicine
Department of Anesthesiology and Pain
    Medicine
Roswell Park Cancer Institute
Buffalo, New York

Patrick M. Dougherty, PhD
Associate Professor
Department of Anesthesiology and Pain Medicine
The University of Texas M. D. Anderson Cancer
    Center
Houston, Texas

Alexandra M. Easson, MD, MSc
Assistant Professor of Surgery
University of Toronto
Toronto, Ontario, Canada

Ahmed Elsayem, MD
Assistant Professor
Department of Palliative Care and Rehabilitation
    Medicine
The University of Texas M. D. Anderson Cancer
    Center
Houston, Texas

Gilbert J. Fanciullo, MD, MS
Professor of Anesthesiology
Dartmouth Medical School
Director
Pain Management Center
Dartmouth Hitchcock Medical Center
Lebanon, New Hampshire

Christopher Fausel, PharmD, BCOP, BCPS
Clinical Pharmacist
Indiana University Hospital
Indianapolis, Indiana

Michael J. Fisch, MD, MPH, FACP
Associate Professor
Division of Cancer Medicine
The University of Texas M. D. Anderson Cancer Center
Houston, Texas

Anne Lederman Flamm, JD
Clinical Ethicist
The Clinical Ethics Service
Assistant Professor
Department of Critical Care
The University of Texas M. D. Anderson Cancer Center
Houston, Texas

Christopher Gibson, PhD
Research Coordinator
Department of Psychiatry
Memorial Sloan-Kettering Cancer Center
New York, New York

M. Spencer Gould, PA
Physician Assistant
Radiation Oncology Clinic
The University of Texas M. D. Anderson Cancer Center
Houston, Texas

Neil A. Hagen, MD, FRCPC
Professor and Head Canadian Province
Division of Palliative Medicine
Departments of Oncology, Clinical Neurosciences
    and Medicine
University of Calgary
Calgary Health Region Palliative and Hospice Care Service
Calgary, Canada

Kyle G. Halvorson, BA
Neurosystems Center and Departments of Diagnostic
    and Biological Sciences, Psychiatry, Neuroscience,
    and Cancer Center
University of Minnesota
Minneapolis, Minnesota

Albert Hwang
Associate Physician
Physical Medicine & Rehabilitation
Mercy Medical Group
Sacramento, California

Nora Janjan, MD, FACP, FACR
Professor
Department of Radiation Oncology
The University of Texas M. D. Anderson Cancer Center
Houston, Texas

David R. Jenkins, Rev.
Masters of Divinity
Director of Chaplaincy
The University of Texas M. D. Anderson Cancer Center
Houston, Texas

Tarun Jolly, MD
Department of Anesthesiology and Pain Medicine
The University of Texas M. D. Anderson Cancer Center
Houston, Texas

Fayez Kotob, MD
Fellow in Cancer Pain and Neuromodulation
Department of Anesthesiology
State University of New York at Buffalo
Pain Research Affiliate
Department of Anesthesiology and Pain Medicine
Roswell Park Cancer Institute
Buffalo, New York

Helena Knotkova, PhD
Research Scientist
Department of Pain Medicine and Palliative Care
Beth Israel Medical Center
New York, New York

Sunil Krishnan, MD
Assistant Professor
Department of Radiation Oncology
The University of Texas M. D. Anderson
    Cancer Center
Houston, Texas

Theresa Kruczek, PhD
Associate Professor of Counseling Psychology
Ball State University
Department of Counseling Psychology
Teachers College
Muncie, Indiana

Kathleen Larkin, MD
Assistant Professor of Anesthesiology
University of Washington
    School of Medicine
Department of Anesthesiology and Pain Medicine
Seattle Children's Hospital and Regional
    Medical Center
Seattle, Washington

Bianca B. Lee, PharmD
Pharmacy Clinical Specialist
Palliative Care
The University of Texas M. D. Anderson Cancer
    Center
Houston, Texas

Stephen T. Lutz, MD
Department of Radiation Oncology
Blanchard Valley Regional Cancer Center
Findlay, Ohio

Patrick W. Mantyh, PhD, JD
Professor
Department of Diagnostic and Biological Sciences
    Neuroscience, Psychiatry and Cancer Center
University of Minnesota, Minneapolis
Director of the Molecular Neurobiology Lab
VA Medical Center
Minneapolis, Minnesota

Cecelia C. Monge, MS, RN, CWOCN
Senior Wound Ostomy Continence Nurse
Department of Nursing, Nursing Professional Development
    and Education
The M. D. Anderson Cancer Center
Houston, Texas

Donald R. Nicholas, PhD
Professor of Counseling Psychology
Ball State University
Department of Counseling Psychology
Teachers College
Associate Director
Department of Psycho-Oncology
The Cancer Center of Ball Memorial Hospital
Muncie, Indiana

Steven D. Passik, PhD
Attending Psychologist
Department of Psychiatry
Memorial Sloan-Kettering Cancer Center
New York, New York

Phillip Phan, MD
Fellow
Department of Anesthesiology and Pain Medicine
The University of Texas M. D. Anderson Cancer Center
Houston, Texas

Peter W.T. Pisters, MD, FACS
Professor of Surgery
Department of Surgical Oncology
The University of Texas M. D. Anderson Cancer Center
Houston, Texas

Lois Ramondetta, MD
Associate Professor
Department of Gynecologic Oncology
The University of Texas M. D. Anderson Cancer Center
Houston, Texas

Maria L. Rotta
Research Associate
Department of Psychiatry
Memorial Sloan-Kettering Cancer Center
New York, New York

Ki Shin, MD
Associate Professor
Department of Palliative Care & Rehabilitation Medicine
The University of Texas M. D. Anderson Cancer Center
Houston, Texas

Debra Sivesind, RN, MSN, APRN-BC
Clinical Nurse Specialist
Psychiatry/Palliative Care
The University of Texas M. D. Anderson Cancer Center
Houston, Texas

Chad F. Slieper, JD
Clinical Ethicist
The Clinical Ethics Service
Instructor
Department of Critical Care
The University of Texas M. D. Anderson Cancer Center
Houston, Texas

Martin L. Smith, STD
Director of Clinical Ethics
Clinical Ethics Service
Professional Staff
Department of Bioethics
Cleveland Clinic
Cleveland, Ohio

Lucy J. Sullivan, BA
Neurosystems Center and Departments of Diagnostic and Biological
    Sciences, Psychiatry, Neuroscience, and Cancer Center
University of Minnesota
Minneapolis, Minnesota

Han-Rong Weng, MD, PhD
Assistant Professor
Department of Anesthesiology and Pain Medicine
The University of Texas M. D. Anderson Cancer Center
Houston, Texas

Joan Zampieri, PAC
Physician Assistant
Radiation Oncology Clinic
The University of Texas M. D. Anderson Cancer Center
Houston, Texas

More than 11 million individuals worldwide are diagnosed with cancer each year. By 2020, this number is expected to grow to 16 million. In the United States, cancer has eclipsed heart disease as the foremost cause of death. However, there has been encouraging progress in understanding the molecular biology of malignancy, and this advancement has presented new and exciting targets for treatment. In the United States, the cancer-related death rate has dropped by 1.1% per year from 1993 to 2002. The net effect of these trends and opportunities is a large and rapidly growing population of persons living as cancer survivors. One of the major imperatives of caring for cancer patients and survivors is dealing with pain due to cancer itself, cancer treatment, comorbid conditions, and interactions among these exigencies. Unfortunately, patients with cancer frequently receive care by physicians, nurses, and other health professionals who have only limited training and experience in pain management and palliative care. This conundrum is likely to continue in the future because of an increasing number of patients combined with reduced resources. Clinicians are able to recognize the most frequent clinical problems encountered in patients with specific primary tumors and the role of anticancer therapeutics in the care of these patients. However, the need to manage increasingly complex cancer pain problems and related symptoms is clearly evident.

Physicians generally turn to recent journals and professional meetings for up-to-date information about cancer care. However, the literature pertaining to cancer pain and symptom management is not confined to major oncology journals. The pertinent literature is diffused among innumerable journals. These range from general medical, surgical, and nursing journals to subspecialty journals that focus on palliative care, supportive oncology, neurology, anesthesiology, and pain. For this reason, oncology providers and nononcology health professionals and most students continue to turn to books for a more complete, interdisciplinary understanding of topics related to cancer care, cancer pain, and palliative care.

The target audience for this book is health professionals and students who are involved in caring for persons with cancer. The book is intended for specialists in oncology, but will also be relevant for primary care physicians, surgeons, nononcology subspecialists, physician assistants, nurse practitioners, nurses, physical therapists, pharmacists, speech pathologists, social workers, pastoral care providers, house officers, and undergraduates in medicine—each of who commonly play vital roles in the multidisciplinary care of cancer patients with pain and other difficult cancer-related symptoms.

This work provides comprehensive, yet practical, information about patient assessment, specific medications and procedures for pain management, and the biology and pathophysiology of pain. While important, these areas do not cover the totality of the care required by cancer patients and cancer survivors with pain. To understand the full scope of pain management and to optimize healthcare provider communication with this population, we found it important to also explore cultural aspects of patient care, the role of spirituality, the existence of different models of health, the role of complementary and alternative medicine in the menu of pain management options, the influence of the health system and specific healthcare settings, principles of biomedical ethics, and related problem areas such as psychosocial aspects of care, and dealing with substance abuse and addiction.

One challenge in assembling this work has been our goal of appealing and providing relevancy to a diverse audience in terms of both background discipline and knowledge base related to pain management. We have invited authors from various disciplines to address their topics in their own style, mindful of this diverse audience. Olympic ice-skating competitions combine a program of mandatory exercises with a freestyle program. As editors, we confronted a similar mandate, and our response was to allow the authors considerable flexibility in their approach to the topics of their expertise. This approach has allowed the authors to produce their creative best and has, we hope, satisfied the goal of making the content of the various chapters lively, practical, and understandable. Although there are guiding principles in pain management that are clearly reflected in this book, there is tremendous complexity in the care of patients with cancer pain and considerable variability in practice patterns. Rather than attempting to simplify this field and adopting a consistent viewpoint about all issues, we decided that an inclusive approach is more appropriate and reflects the authentic complexity (and controversies) in this realm. Another aspect of authenticity involves acknowledgement that there are individuals with expert points of view who are not strictly academic professionals. For example, clinical expertise and experience in wound care for cancer patients is found at our institution in our senior wound/ostomy nurses, and we have chosen to include this perspective too.

It has been exciting for us to see this work unfold, and it is our hope that this book will provoke interest in undertaking further research in this realm of clinical medicine and symptom science, and that it will provide inspiration for teachers as well as tangible information that can be applied to change the lives of cancer patients, survivors, and their caregivers.

ACKNOWLEDGEMENT

The authors would like to acknowledge the dedication, long hours, and great talent of Ms. Joann Aaron, MA.

PART 1

GENERAL PRINCIPLES IN CANCER PAIN MANAGEMENT

Assessment of Pain and Other Symptoms

CHAPTER

1

Victor T. Chang
Neil A. Hagen
Bianca B. Lee

INTRODUCTION

Symptoms have been an integral element of patient assessment since the beginning of the practice of medicine. Symptoms have been differentially interpreted within the context of prevailing pathologic paradigms, functioning as stepping stones to making a diagnosis. Confounding their usefulness within the medical model, symptoms are frequently transient, difficult for patients to describe, and their underlying basis is not always easily confirmed with objective tests. It is thus not surprising that symptom assessment has remained an area of interest and frustration to clinicians. This interest is deeply rooted in the history of medicine. In the first half of the nineteenth century, French physician Pierre-Charles-Alexandre Louis measured "the degree or violence of each symptom with as much accuracy as the case would admit" in his clinical studies.[1] In 1919, Graham Lusk quoted a letter from Theodore Janeway at the turn of the century of his desire to advance knowledge "that I may be able to persuade the students to regard symptomatology as the physiology of the 'sick life.'"[2]

Major methodologic advances in characterizing patients' subjective symptoms have developed during the past 150 years and collectively demonstrate that patient reports of symptoms can be reliably assessed by clinicians and followed over time. Many of these advances have occurred in clinical trials of symptom control medications.[3] Together, their findings offer great promise of facilitating the physician-patient encounter by empowering bedside assessment, thereby improving patient care.

The extent and severity of symptoms are often unrecognized and underestimated by clinicians. In a chart review of cancer patients seen by a palliative care service, a comparison of nursing records and concurrent symptom assessment forms completed by patients suggested that a substantial number of symptoms can be missed by caregivers.[4] Implementation of quantitative pain assessment in a private practice of medical and radiation oncology patients showed that 23% of the patients were experiencing significant pain.[5] Various studies have, in fact, shown that patients with cancer experience multiple symptoms, suggesting that unless clinicians employ systematic tools, patients will have unrecognized sources of distress. It has been recommended by a National Institutes of Health (NIH) Consensus Conference that symptom assessment should be regularly performed by clinicians.[6]

However, it can be time consuming to comprehensively evaluate patients for their symptoms. The time required to obtain a careful and comprehensive symptom assessment is justified by the following considerations:

Better communication. Patients and their families experience symptoms and their negative impact for long periods of time. A meticulous symptom assessment enables patients and caregivers to feel that they have been heard and that the healthcare professional with whom they interact really is interested in their well-being. Psychologically, this can be perceived as acknowledgement and validation of suffering, and as the first step in developing a therapeutic alliance with the patient.[7] The ability to explain how the disease creates symptoms and how treatments may relieve symptoms enhances patient and caregiver understanding and rapport. The patient history is a narrative, and there is increasing appreciation of the role of narrative as a means of patient communication.[8] Exploring the meaning of the symptom(s) for the patient may guide patient education and therapy.[9]

A better understanding of how to intervene. Knowledge of how the patient is affected by a symptom may suggest avenues of intervention (changing current therapy, starting a new therapy).

A better diagnosis. A detailed knowledge of the time course and aggravating and relieving factors may go a long way toward elucidating the underlying disease causing a symptom in frail patients who are not able to undergo extensive testing. One review of 276 consultations for cancer pain found a new underlying cause for pain in 64% of patients and a new neurologic diagnosis in 36% of patients.[10]

A springboard to discuss other areas. Often, a discussion of symptoms facilitates introducing a discussion of other sensitive issues, such as the patient's perception of his or her disease and prognosis, effect of the disease on the patient and caregiver, and patient's fears of what the future may hold.

Some Helpful Questions—General, Narrative Approach

Tell me how you have spent the last few days—Helpful for eliciting important but forgotten symptoms, and delineating interference of function by severity of symptoms.

Help the patient describe the symptom. Present a limited multiple choice question as well as a totally open-ended question. "Would you agree with the following statements about your symptom?"

Verify by summarizing "Let me make sure that I have heard you correctly. When you have the pain, it feels like a sharp knife over the front part of your thigh? Is there anything else you would like to add?"

What does the symptom make you think about?

GENERAL COMMENTS

Currently, the patients' description of their symptoms is given primacy over the report of their caregivers. One reason is that ratings of symptoms by caregivers, such as pain, often do not agree with the reports by patient, especially for patients with severe pain.[11] In this era of advanced technology, patient reports of symptoms may seem quaint. Nevertheless, symptoms are the products of an extraordinarily complex sensory apparatus—the nervous system.

Many discussions of symptom assessment tend to focus on the relationship between a symptom and pathophysiology. The goal of this chapter is to summarize a body of information accumulated over the decades that can inform and enrich the bedside assessment of a patient with symptoms, including pain. This field of study is growing rapidly; and as understanding of this information and what it means for patient care increases, symptom assessment will develop and improve.

▶ Psychophysics

Psychophysics studies the relationship between stimuli and psychological perceptions of those stimuli. It started as the study of the intensity of stimuli required to produce just noticeable differences. On a descriptive level, it has been applied to aid the design of lighting and sound systems. On an analytical level, it has been used to help infer mechanisms which underlie sensation. Psychophysics provides a way to understand and study patient ratings and is concerned with issues of sensory detection, discrimination, recognition, and scaling.[12]

Scales can be classified as nominal, ordinal, interval, and ratio scales. Nominal scales can be independent categories, such as respiratory symptoms, digestive symptoms, and others. Ordinal scales show a sequence such as ranging from "none" to "very much." In an interval scale the distance the points has meaning as well. In a ratio scale a zero point is a component of the scale. Psychophysics has been used in studies of hearing, vision, touch, taste, warmth, pain, dyspnea, and other sensations.

Magnitude estimation is an important psychophysical technique. The subject is asked to make direct numerical estimates of the sensory magnitude caused by various stimuli. What the subject reports is the psychological value for that stimulus. This practice has been successfully applied since the 1950s in many research settings, including pain.[13] In clinical practice with cancer patients, clinicians face the inverse problem—given a symptom rating, what stimulus could have led to this patient report?

▶ Psychometrics

Psychometrics is concerned with measuring psychological states through the design and analysis of questionnaires (tests or scales) from which inferences are deduced about the respondent's psychological state. A test is a sample of the behaviors, attitudes or feelings of the respondent that reflect the subject's psychological state. In more general terms, a psychological state is an example of a construct, or an intangible entity that can be observed in many ways. A test is made up of items, which can be a single question or a set of questions. A psychometrically sound set of items is an index.

Validity and reliability of scales

Validity refers to the extent to which the instrument measures the desired quantity. Content validity deals with the extent to which the items represent the concept under study. Criterion-related validity refers to the correlation between the scale and a criterion measure and to the predictive value of the scale in the future. Examples of criterion measures include "gold standard" instruments, and how the instruments perform in different populations. Construct validity examines the meaningfulness of the scale by comparing the scale to other scales for expected similar or dissimilar behavior.[14] Another form of validity is its responsiveness to change, for example, worsening scores as a patient's burden of disease progresses.

Reliability deals with measurement error—the more reliable the scale, the less the measurement error. Test-retest reliability examines responses at two times. Alternate form reliability compares responses to two alternative but equivalent versions of the test. Internal consistency is a measure of similarity to responses across items on the test, and is often summarized by the coefficient Cronbach's alpha.

Rating systems

Initial psychological scales were devised as descriptive ratings. The concept of a Visual Analog Scale (VAS) as a graphic rating scale was first proposed in 1920, with descriptive terms arrayed beneath the line. In contrast to other available methods, this method was thought to free raters from direct quantitative estimates, was easily scored, and required little motivation of the rater to complete the instrument. Studies were performed in industry and with college students.[15] In the 1970s, the VAS was studied as a way to measure moods, hunger, and pain. The VAS is a 10-cm-long line and the length of the mark made by the patient is thought to correspond to the magnitude of the symptom. The marks at each end should correspond to maximal descriptors. VAS markings have been considered to be ordinal, and can be compared within the same subject and between subjects, but are prone to clustering at the ends and in the middle. Populations for which the VAS may not be optimal include patients who are unable to think abstractly, are confused, and older patients.[16,17] For these patient groups, categorical scales may be more valid and reliable. Subsequently, verbal and numerical rating scales have been devised and their use has been contrasted to the advantages and disadvantages of VAS (Table 1-1).

Attributes and dimensions of symptom ratings

Historic aspects, such as temporal patterns, aggravating and relieving factors, and presence or absence of other pertinent symptoms are important for diagnostic purposes. Qualitative descriptive aspects of the symptoms may be important for certain symptoms, such as pain.

Symptom assessment has become more complex and interesting, with the concept that symptoms are not single entities, but are multidimensional and interactive, and that assessment is followed by symptom intervention and symptom outcomes.[18] A descriptive terminology has evolved. Symptom occurrence denotes the onset of the symptom. *Symptom recognition* is awareness by health professionals that the patient has experienced a symptom. Symptom dimensions include frequency, severity, and duration. Once the symptom is perceived, it may be assigned a meaning by the patient, who may possibly experience symptom distress and then respond to the symptom. The process of perceiving symptom dimensions and meanings has been called the *symptom experience*.[19] The symptom may then affect different aspects of function and quality of life for both the patient and the caregivers, and may itself influence the experience of other symptoms.

Common symptom attributes of interest are severity, frequency, distress, and interference. The first two are self-explanatory. *Symptom distress* has been defined as the degree of discomfort from the specific

Table 1-1

Advantages and Disadvantages of VAS

	Advantages	Disadvantages
Numerical Rating Scale	Simple and widely accepted for pain	Requires conceptual ability to correlate a sensation with numbers
Visual Analog Scale	Simple, universally used for many symptoms	Requires ability to conceptualize, and ability to see the line and draw
Verbal Rating (Categorical) Scale	Does not require ability to make correlations, more descriptive	Requires categorical techniques for statistical analysis
Descriptors	Easy to understand	Relationship between descriptors is unknown; may be culture-specific

symptom being experienced as perceived by the patient.[20] Symptom distress has become a major component of widely used symptom assessment instruments, such as the Rotterdam Symptom Checklist and the Memorial Symptom Assessment Scale. While intuitively appealing, it has been difficult to define more rigorously.[21,22] Since the original article, seven definitions of symptom distress have been proposed.[23]

The practical question is: how many aspects of a symptom does a clinician need to know for assessment purposes? Is severity alone enough? Some data suggest that for items such as appetite and fatigue, single questions may be as informative as multiple questions.[24,25] Single item assessments have the advantages of brevity and high completion rates, and for use with global constructs. Assessments of multiple attributes allow for more detailed assessments, more reliable instruments, and more complex analyses, but may be more burdensome for the patient and the caregiver. Patients are often quite willing to provide information about their symptoms. Clearly, the extent of symptom assessment depends on the question being asked.[26] As in other aspects of clinical care, a more comprehensive assessment may be important in the initial evaluation and for research purposes, and a more abbreviated assessment suitable for screening or follow-up. With further research into various dimensions of symptoms and their interconnectedness, it may become apparent that certain aspects are more relevant depending on the goal of the assessment. For example, symptom distress may be more relevant for quality of life, whereas symptom severity may be more useful for guiding therapy.

Symptom relief

Because symptom control is a key goal of palliative care, measurement of symptom relief is a standard dimension of patient evaluation.[27] Characterizing what exactly a patient means by relief varies depending on the symptom and a range of clinical factors. In addition to bedside evaluation, a practical application arises in clinical trials, where symptom instruments need to be responsive to clinical changes to allow for sample size calculations.

The underlying methodologic issue is the determination of a clinically significant difference.[28] Anchor-based patient ratings of change (e.g., much worse to much better, percent relief) are patient-rated, but include both the change and the patient's perception of change. As the patient's condition changes, his baseline also changes and may affect his perception of how much change has occurred. This is called a *response shift*. Statistically determined distribution-based changes rely upon a comparison of the size of the change in the instrument score to the standard deviation (SD), and represent a group norm. A variety of definitions have been proposed; a simple one is the effect size, based upon the SD of the measurement; a small effect size corresponds to 0.2 SD, medium 0.5 SD, and large 0.9 SD (Table 1-2).[29]

► Objective measures—behavioral aspects

While patients' self-report of their experience of subjective symptoms should be the gold standard, clinicians are still interested in objective ways to verify the presence of symptoms and document their impact. Behaviors and behavioral changes are often used by healthcare professionals in judging severity of symptoms. Behaviors are specific but not sensitive. Behaviors that can be described or quantified may strengthen the assessment of a symptom. For certain symptoms, behaviors are accepted and used as (insensitive) correlates of severity, acknowledging that behavior is also a modifiable response (Table 1-3).

Table 1-2

Use of Patient Ratings for Changes in Symptoms

	Advantages	Disadvantages
Patient-rated changes	Patient-rated information	Response shift
Statistical measures	Evidence that this is a universal type of measure	Which standard deviation to use? Relatively new for symptom measures

Table 1-3

Behaviors and Symptoms

Symptoms	Examples of Behavior
Nausea	Vomiting
Sadness	Crying
Pain	Inability to sleep Change in behavior Grimacing
Itch	Scratching
Constipation	Number of bowel movements, straining, need for disimpaction

▶ Psychological aspects

Psychological assessment of the patient may examine the coping mechanisms and associations that the patient makes with the symptom. These associations may be informed by the patient's experiences and the patient's cultural background, and are covered elsewhere in this book.

▶ New developments

Symptom clusters

Multiple surveys have established that cancer patients usually have many symptoms. A *symptom cluster* has been defined as three or more concurrent symptoms that are related to each other.[30] This concept has the potential to help simplify symptom assessment. Symptom clusters can arise from different etiologies, and lead to either synergistic or compensatory symptom interactions. For example, hiccups in a patient with painful bone metastases and poor appetite would represent a synergistic interaction. Drowsiness and fatigue in a patient with dyspnea might signify a compensatory interaction. Fatigue, weight loss, and lack of appetite may represent a cytokine-mediated sickness cluster.[31] The methodology and criteria for determining when symptoms are sufficiently related to form a cluster remains an area of investigation.[32] The use of multisymptom instruments may help identify symptom clusters.[33] Studies of symptom clusters have been undertaken in patients with lung cancer[34] and breast cancer.[35]

Electronic monitoring

New technologies currently used in clinical trials may make real-time symptom monitoring possible. A device called the actigraph can be worn on the wrist to capture patient movements. Computer screens have been found to be similar to pencil and paper questionnaires for quality of life and pain assessments.[36–38] Telephone interactive voice response technology provides another form of real-time monitoring.[39]

Functional magnetic resonance imaging

With the development of functional brain imaging has come the realization that multiple areas of the brain are activated by pain stimuli. These areas include the insula, which associates threat with nociception, the anterior cingulate cortex, which relates pain to unpleasantness, and the limbic system, which is associated with emotional response. This technique provides an anatomic correlate for the multidimensional (affective and cognitive) aspects of pain. Functional magnetic resonance imaging (fMRI) has been used to map activation of parts of the brain in response to stimuli, can provide further insight into the neurophysiology of symptoms, and form a basis for examining symptom clusters. However, as a research tool, fMRI is at an early stage of its development; and it must be remembered that "voxels are not neurons and increased blood flow is not the same as thought."[40]

APPROACHES TO SYMPTOM ASSESSMENT

▶ Patient interview and examination

The history and physical examination is historically accepted as the best way to start assessing a patient but, in fact, may often overlook symptoms. In one study, 24 family practitioners were asked to do a structured clinical examination on a cancer patient; performance was poorest in asking about previous pain history, temporal pattern of pain, and pain intensity. Performance on the pain assessment was best for eliciting pain location and pain-relieving factors.[41] A more integrated approach is to combine the history and physical examination, particularly in patients with pain. A directed physical examination based upon the history, as the history is being obtained, allows the clinician to test hypotheses and the patient clarify the history, in an iterative manner.

Another emerging approach is the structured interview, a research technique used in psychiatry to help standardize the diagnostic process. In a structured interview, various patient reports can be systematically reviewed and combined to form an assessment. A trial of this approach to elicit symptoms was reported in 69 patients, where two interviews were conducted for each patient, and patient VAS scores were obtained. The interview took 1 hour to administer, and there were good correlations with VAS scores and test-retest coefficients.[42]

▶ Proxy ratings

While it is accepted that the patient should be the primary source of information about symptoms, proxy ratings have become increasingly important in the setting of impaired patient communication. To understand a proxy rating, it is important to have an accurate characterization of the person who is doing the proxy rating. Studies to date have highlighted possible biases associated with demographic aspects of caregivers. In one study of 270 patients and their caregivers, younger caregivers were less likely to agree on the presence of pain, middle-aged caregivers on the presence of constipation, and older caregivers for nausea. Women caregivers were more likely to notice symptoms than men. Depressed caregivers were more likely to report symptoms, and optimistic caregivers to underreport symptoms.[43] In another study of caregiver pain ratings, the degree of pain overrating by the caregiver could be correlated with the caregiver's perception of patient distress, interpretation of the need for higher doses of analgesics, and caregiver distress caused by the patient's pain.[44] When the assessments of 98 home family caregivers of patients with advanced cancer were compared to patient responses, the investigators found good to excellent intraclass correlations for the physical symptoms, and fair correlations for the psychological symptoms.[45,46] In another study of 264 primary caregivers of patients with advanced cancer admitted to a hospice, caregivers significantly overestimated the three symptoms studied: pain, dyspnea, and constipation.[47] To a family member, any symptom distress will be interpreted as pain. A general theme that emerges is that proxy rating of physical symptoms is often closer to patient ratings than rating for psychological symptoms.

Health professionals are sometimes obligated to estimate symptoms. In one study, hospice providers rated symptoms in 348 home patients in a cross-sectional survey, and experienced difficulty rating psychological symptoms, similar to the difficulties reported by patient caregivers.[48]

One methodologic approach is suggested from a comparison of concurrent symptom assessments by the patient, nurse, and caregiver for 32 hospitalized advanced cancer patients with the Edmonton Symptom Assessment Scale. Generalizability theory was used to assess sources of measurement variability. Raters were consistent: rater effects did not contribute to the variability of assessment scores. By symptoms, anxiety, depression, nausea, well-being, and drowsiness showed substantial variation, with the highest variability for dyspnea. They concluded that having three raters on one occasion would provide more reliability than two raters on two occasions.[49]

▶ Symptom instruments

Symptom instruments have been developed for a wide variety of symptoms. These instruments can be observer-rated or patient-rated, and allow for some uniformity of assessment. The routine use of symptom assessment instruments has been recommended as part of regular symptom assessment in practice.[50] However, they may have been developed for a population different from the one you see, or may have been developed for a purpose different from the one you wish to pursue. In selecting an instrument for routine clinical practice, it may be helpful to see which instruments express questions the way you or your patients would. Piloting instruments with a small number of articulate, observant patients may help determine the acceptability of the instrument—"That was the most stupid question I have ever seen!" or "That's not how I talk with my doctor."

Symptom diaries are another way to help keep track of what the patient is experiencing and allow for more patient participation. Diaries have been used in clinical studies of pain management with good compliance.

BARRIERS TO SYMPTOM ASSESSMENT

▶ Being a healthcare professional

Physicians have been trained more to recognize the presence of severe symptoms than to make graded assessments of symptom severity. There is increasing evidence that physicians from diverse backgrounds consistently give lower pain ratings than their patients. These practitioners and settings include abdominal surgeons,[51] general practitioners,[52] family practice clinics,[53] oncology centers,[54] and emergency rooms,[55] and these discrepancies are greatest for patients with severe pain. This is a problem for other health professionals as well.[56]

▶ Linguistic

Are symptoms describable? Can symptoms be defined? Are definitions of symptoms an adequate basis for symptom questionnaires? The measured incidence of a symptom can vary with how a question is phrased.[57] The way symptoms are named and described may also vary with cultures. Even in English, patients may deny experiencing pain, but will acknowledge discomfort. In Spanish, patients may deny *dolor* (pain), but will agree to *molesta* (bother). In describing dental pain, Chinese- and English-speaking patients picked different descriptors.[58] In a study of dyspnea, African American and Caucasian patients with experimentally induced bronchoconstriction selected different descriptors.[59]

▶ Cultural aspects

Cultural competence may be critical for the assessment of symptoms. Time spent showing respect for the patient and family and their culture is repaid with more trust, a better history, and compliance with the diagnostic and treatment plan.

There is no convincing evidence of interracial differences in nociception or other neurophysiologic aspects of symptoms. However, it stands to reason that the ability to obtain a history and express findings in a manner compatible with the patient's culture will enhance the accuracy of the history and compliance by the patient. Culture can modify the expression of symptoms and the level of distress associated with symptoms.[60] How race and ethnicity affect the pain experience remains an area of investigation. The constructs of race and ethnicity are somewhat vaguely characterized within the published literature, especially in relation to the psychological and social aspects of pain behavior; many studies to date are primarily descriptive.[61] How that knowledge applies to assessment of symptoms of patients of different cultural backgrounds has not been described as clearly.

The expression of symptoms is a form of communication, and as such is regulated by the norms of the patient's culture. For patients from more traditional cultures (not North American), answers to yes/no questions may be governed by social considerations rather than factual content.[62] Whether a symptom is reported may be affected by the stigma attached to the symptom. For example, in a study of 87 hospice patients in the United Kingdom, psychological concerns and symptoms relating to anxiety and depression were frequently withheld by 60% of hospice patients when seen by a nurse.[63]

When the caregiver's culture is different from the patient's, misinterpretations can arise. One cultural continuum is the expressive/stoic axis of pain complaint behavior.[64] North Americans are considered to be more stoic, whereas people from the Mediterranean and South America are considered to be more expressive. However, the purpose of these mannerisms may also differ by culture. In one commentary on Mexican American patients, complaints and moans of pain were considered a report of pain by Mexican Americans, whereas it was interpreted as severe psychological distress by their North American nurses.[65] Arabs tend to understate their pain to staff, and family and friends are expected to be advocates for the patient when dealing with hospital staff.[66] The physician should encourage the patient to be as precise as possible about the pain. Education of the family about their role is important as the family may feel that the caregiver is shirking his responsibility by passing the work of providing care to the family.

Culture influences gender expressions of pain. In a study of Japanese and American patients, in both cultures, was considered acceptable for women to be expressive of their pain but not men, and American patients were more accepting of pain behavior than Japanese patients.[67]

In traditional cultures, not only the manner but the content of communication is affected by social relationships. In a study of pain in Northern India, younger women could complain of menstrual pain to each other, but not in the presence of men, or of senior women of the household.[68] Clinically relevant information may be suppressed depending on the context of the clinical conversation. As an authority figure, the medical professional may unconsciously influence the symptom history.

It has been recommended that time be spent on becoming familiar with the patient's culture and language and accompanying family members before embarking on the history and physical examinations.[69] Gentle behavior and patience may go a long way toward establishing trust. It may be helpful to find out how the patient describes common pains, such as a headache or a toothache, to better understand how the patient expresses pain or other symptoms, and to ask the patient to compare common pains to his or her pain. This approach has become the basis for a pain sensory scale.[70] Studies with the Brief Pain Inventory Short Form have shown that across different cultures, severities of pain ratings on a scale of 0–10 are comparable.[71] A similar study with the VAS, Memorial Pain Assessment Card,[72] and the Face Scale yielded similar results in a hospital population of Hispanics, African Americans, and European Americans.[73] Asking the patient what he or she believes caused the pain, why it started, and what it means may provide further insight into cultural interpretations of pain. Explanation of the treatment and what to expect will be even more important when patients are from a different background than their clinician. One study of Hispanic patients recommended incorporation of the patient's healthcare practices where possible, involvement of family members, and provision of pain literature in Spanish, as lack of understanding was the major cause of noncompliance.[74]

▶ Physical limitations

Patients with poor performance status may not have the stamina to answer more than a few questions at a time.

▶ Distrust of patient-reported outcomes and reliance upon objective measures

Ironically, subjectivity enters interpretations of radiographic and pathologic studies, two of the most objective measures we have of cancer. There are increasing data showing that changes in symptom scales such as pain are correlated with changes in quality of life, and in some cases with the objective measures of disease.

COGNITIVELY IMPAIRED PATIENTS

The term *cognitive impairment* refers to alterations in the ability to process and store information, and in a larger sense to "altered mental status." Cancer patients are at risk for cognitive impairment because of concurrent medications, comorbidities, underlying disease, organ dysfunction, and other causes. Domains of clinical interest include alertness (sedation), mood alterations (depression), memory and attention deficits, perceptual difficulties (e.g., delirium and hallucinations), and motor skills.

▶ Delirious patients

Patients with cancer are at high risk for delirium, and pain medications can also cause delirium, among other cognitive deficits.[75,76] However, little has been written on the assessment of pain in cancer patients who are delirious or become delirious. Delirium can magnify the patient's perceptions of pain and thereby affect its management.[77] One study found that verbal category rating scales were easier for confused patients to complete than numeric rating scales.[78]

▶ Demented patients

Assessment of pain in these patients is increasingly important as the population ages, and it remains an area of active investigation.

Older patients with none to mild dementia are able to answer questions about pain with different types of scales, but require more time and patience.[79,80] In one study, test-retest reliability was poor for cognitively impaired patients.[81] In noncommunicative patients, the concept of pain behaviors has proven useful. Based on an analogy with studies of infants in pain, the presence or absence of certain changes in behavior, together with known painful diagnoses, may lead to a determination of the presence of pain. These behaviors may include changes in facial expression, vocalizations, body movements, interpersonal interactions, activity patterns, and confusion or lability.[82] Other scales have been built on the presence of agitation, restriction of activity, grimacing, moaning, and lack of consolability.[83] As these patients cannot give direct verbal confirmation, the observation of these behaviors with known unpleasant stimuli (such as toileting), and their reduction with an empirical dose of analgesics, may be useful approaches to clinical assessment.[84,85] There is currently no ideal instrument for assessing pain in cognitively impaired older patients or for evaluating cancer pain.[86]

ASSESSMENT OF MULTIPLE SYMPTOMS

Patients with advanced cancer experience multiple symptoms. The number of symptoms alone may be informative, as the number of symptoms itself can correlate closely and inversely with quality of life.[87] Should patients with multiple symptoms complete multiple instruments, one for each symptom, or one instrument for multiple symptoms? And what should those symptoms be? Reviewing a number of multisymptom instruments that have been developed independently suggests that there may be a core set of symptoms that is of universal importance (Table 1-4).

Table 1-4

Assessment Scales

	Edmonton Symptom Assessment[88]	Rotterdam Symptom Checklist[89]	Symptom Distress Scale[90]	Condensed Memorial Symptom Assessment Scale[91]	MD Anderson, Symptom Inventory[92]
N	9	30	10	14	13
Concentration		+	+	+	
Pain	+		+	+	+
Lack of energy		+	+	+	+
Nervous	+	+		+	+
Dry mouth		+		+	+
Nausea	+	+	+	+	+
Drowsy	+			+	+
Sleeping		+	+	+	+
Sad	+	+		+	+
Worrying		+		+	+
Lack of appetite	+	+	+		+
Weight loss				+	
Dyspnea		+		+	+
Difficulty remembering					+

Preliminary work suggests that these scales may be responsive to changes in individual patients over time. In longitudinal studies of palliative care cancer patients, the Edmonton Symptom Assessment Scale, the Symptom Distress Scale, and the Memorial Symptom Assessment Scale Short Form[93,94] have shown changes over time. These scales also show differences after interventions to relieve symptoms.[95,96] The ability of these scales to combine symptoms into summary scales allows for exploration of the concept of symptom burden.[97]

SPECIFIC SYMPTOMS

▶ Pain

Pain assessment has progressed significantly over the last few decades. In this section, we summarize information that we consider to be useful in the assessment of cancer pain. Interested readers are directed to additional references for general discussions of pain assessment.[98–100]

▶ Psychophysics

In 1947, Hardy et al. reported on the amount of radiant heat from a lamp required to cause pain after a period of 3 seconds. He found that there were 21 different settings that could produce a just-noticeable difference in pain ratings. He defined the *dol* as the unit of pain, and equal to two just-noticeable differences.[101] This laid the basis for the 0–10 scale of pain measurement.

Validity of severity ratings

In a multinational study of 323 patients receiving cytotoxic chemotherapy preparatory to bone marrow transplantation, patients were followed for mouth pain, stomatitis, and dysphagia three times a week with 92% of assessments completed through day 22. Oral pain peaked on days 14–16, and worst mouth pain coincided within 1 week of peak stomatitis and dysphagia.[102]

Esophageal, rectal, or bladder distention has been used to measure visceral pain, and thermal stimulation of the skin has been used to measure cutaneous pain.

▶ Psychometrics

From a psychometric standpoint, the pain rating by the patient can be considered the psychological value of the pain for the patient.[103]

Pain severity has been measured with numerical rating scales, verbal rating scales, Likert scales, VAS, and other methods. More than 100 pain scales were found in the course of a literature review.[104] Nevertheless, most of these scales are equally effective in rating pain severity.[105]

For the VAS scale, pain greater than 30 mm out of 100 mm is generally clinically significant.[106] For the 0–10 scale, where 10 is anchored as "worst pain imaginable," the amount of interference associated with numerical pain ratings has been used to separate categories of pain severity. Based on this approach, the transition from mild to moderate pain occurs at 4 or 5 out of 10, and to severe pain at 6 or 7 out of 10.[107,108] Whether worst or average pain is more clinically meaningful remains a matter of debate, although worst pain correlates slightly more closely with quality of life scores. On a Likert scale, even a little bit of distress from pain may correspond to a 4 out of 10 pain severity rating (Table 1-5).[109]

Table 1-5

Numerical Rating Scale vs. VAS

	Severity Cut Point	Clinically Significant Change
0–10 Numerical Scale	>4 out of 10	2 points
Visual Analog Scale	30 mm	If VAS <34, change of 13 mm
		If VAS >68, change of 28 mm

▶ Assessment of pain relief

What constitutes a clinically significant change in pain level? Studies of breakthrough pain in cancer patients suggest that a change of 2 points, using a 10-point scale, in worst pain represents a minimally significant change in pain.[110] Similar results have been reported in studies of patients with nonmalignant pain.[111] A comprehensive review selected a 20-mm difference in VAS or a 30% decline in pain intensity as clinically significant.[112] Duration of pain relief is important in determining the optimal dose of pharmacologic agents. It is easy to be content with a relief rating of 80% without the knowledge that the relief lasts for only 1 hour. The adage of "Follow-up, Follow-up, Follow-up" is especially relevant to cancer pain assessment.

Different aspects of pain may be important for different outcomes. In one pilot study, pain relief was related to satisfaction with pain management, whereas pain interference was more related to quality of life.[113]

Other pain attributes

Other pain attributes include frequency, distress, and interference. *Frequency* is helpful for recognizing and assessing breakthrough pain. *Distress* can identify meaning-related and quality of life issues. *Interference* with function can help with interpreting a rating of pain severity, and provide diagnostic clues missed in the routine history and physical. The history is easy to obtain, and improving function can help define goals of pain management.

Descriptors

One result of studies with the McGill Pain Inventory was the finding that syndromes could be distinguished based upon profiles of pain descriptors endorsed by patients. This has led to interest in whether pain descriptors represent specific types of pain. The concept of inferring mechanisms of pain from clinical assessments to guide therapy continues to generate research interest.[114]

▶ Special issues with pain assessment

Pain subtypes

An important conceptual distinction is made between nociceptive and neuropathic pain. Nociceptive pain is related to pain from tissue damage and inflammation, whereas neuropathic pain is related to nerve injury or other dysfunction of the nervous system. A diagnostic assignment remains a clinical impression based upon the history, physical examination, and ancillary findings.

Pain descriptors associated with neuropathic pain include burning, electrical, shooting, tingling, cold, numb, and stabbing pains. These kinds of descriptors have formed the basis for recent research instruments to evaluate neuropathic pain.[115–117] Further work needs to be done to establish correspondences between these descriptions and underlying mechanisms.[118] In one review of therapy for neuropathic pain, the mechanism by which medications were known to work (provide greater than 50% relief) was not clearly related to the mechanism associated with a neuropathic pain condition.[119] Reasons for the limited correspondence may be that different mechanisms can lead to the same kind of pain descriptor, and conversely, that more than one mechanism can be present in a given pain syndrome.[120]

The detection of sensory abnormalities on physical examination is helpful in evaluating the presence of neuropathic pain. Two main categories of sensory findings can be present—loss of function (numbness) and impaired or distorted function (increased sensitivity or alteration in sensation).

Cancer pain syndromes represent another level of pain assessment and have been well described and summarized.[121–124] Identification of a pain syndrome often requires a synthesis of history, physical examination findings, and imaging studies. Organization of pain syndromes by region can aid in generating a differential diagnosis and workup (Table 1-6).

▶ Less common pain syndromes

Uncommon pain syndromes seen in cancer patients include myofascial pain, complex regional pain syndrome, and sympathetically maintained pain. Patients with intractable pain often come to the attention of consultation services.

Myofascial pain

Myofascial pain is defined as diffuse musculoskeletal aching and pain with multiple predictable tender points[125] called trigger points. Myofascial pain has been reported in patients with head and neck cancers. Patients present with complaints of localized aching or crampy sensations. On musculoskeletal examination, trigger points are found in the muscles that reproduce the pain. The *trigger point* is a tender tautness of the muscle associated with decreased range of motion. Training is required for reproducibility in the identification of trigger points. There is no consensus on diagnostic criteria.

Complex regional pain syndrome

Complex regional pain syndrome (CRPS) is uncommon in the cancer population. CRPS may be a paraneoplastic complication seen in patients with apical lung cancer, brain tumors on phenobarbital, lymphoma, breast cancer, pancreatic cancer, and malignancies of the sympathetic nervous system.[126] The hallmarks of CRPS are a constellation of symptoms, including disproportionately severe pain, which does not correspond to the distribution of a nerve, edema, abnormal sweating, change in temperature, and trophic changes. There is no specific test for CRPS or distinctive clinical finding; CRPS is a diagnosis of exclusion. The differential diagnosis includes CRPS type II, vasospasm, cellulitis, Raynaud's disease, Buerger's disease, thrombosis, neuropathy, palmar fasciitis, and erythromelalgia. Findings on examination may include allodynia, hyperalgesia, edema, and abnormal sweating at the site of pain.[127] The underlying mechanisms remain an area of research.[128]

Sympathetically maintained pain

Sympathetically maintained pain is a form of neuropathic pain relieved by blockade of the sympathetic system, and should be considered in patients with cancer pain in the extremities or face. Nociceptors are activated by norepinephrine released by the efferent sympathetic system.[129] It has also been associated with neuralgias, complex regional pain syndrome, phantom pain, herpes zoster, and metabolic neuropathies. It is important to recognize that sympathetically mediated pain is not an opioid responsive pain. Hyperalgesia with cooling (cold allodynia) is a sensitive, but not specific, marker for sympathetically mediated pain. Relief by a chemical (phentolamine infusion) or regional sympathetic block is diagnostic.

Intractable pain

Approximately 10%–15% of the population does not experience satisfactory pain control, as determined in surveys of cancer and hospice patients.[130,131]

An *intractable symptom* has been defined as a symptom that cannot be adequately controlled despite aggressive measures that do not compromise consciousness. Further interventions are deemed unlikely to provide adequate or timely relief, and are associated with intolerable morbidity.[132] Intractable pain is a feared complication of cancer.[133] When faced with this problem, a number of possibilities should be considered. These include

1. *Poor compliance with the medication regimen.* Noncompliance with pain medications is common.[134] The patient (and family) may not have been compliant for various reasons such as previous experience with side effects or misunderstandings about how to take (or administer) the medication.[135] For inpatients, pain medications could have been automatically discontinued for a hospital inpatient without anyone being aware. This could be part of a hospital pharmacy policy, or for an acute event which occurred after pain medications had been started, requiring these medications to be discontinued. Transfers between healthcare settings (e.g., between hospital wards or between institutions) represent other occasions during which pain medications and dosages can be inadvertently reduced.

2. *An incomplete or inaccurate pain diagnosis.* The original diagnosis may be wrong.[136] There may be components of myofascial pain, complex regional pain syndrome, or spiritual pain. Patients may state how much of the pain is spiritual. Somatization is more commonly seen in patients with concurrent depression. A multidisciplinary approach may be helpful for characterizing such complex situations.[137–139]

3. *Opioid side effects are severe and dose limiting.* A variety of strategies have been summarized by Mercadante et al.[140–142] Invasive approaches such as neurolytic block or intrathecal analgesia should be considered when systemic analgesics have failed with dose-limiting toxicity.

4. *Delirium.* In patients with delirium, pain may seem magnified.[143] If delirium is suspected, the patient should be reevaluated, medications should be reduced or discontinued, neuroleptics should be started, and underlying concurrent factors such as hypercalcemia or dehydration should be addressed as part of the overall management strategy.

5. *Progression of underlying disease.* If demonstrated, this may help provide meaning to the pain, and allow for consideration of another anticancer-directed therapy. In patients with a compressive neuropathy, pain may climax and then resolve once the nerve is severed by the mass.

6. A missed psychological or psychiatric diagnosis.

7. Inability of the patient to comprehend the question. When all else fails, be sure that the patient understands what you mean by 0 and 10.

Table 1-6

Table of Pain Syndromes by Region

	Nociceptive Somatic	Nociceptive Visceral	Neuropathic	Mixed/Other
Head and neck	**Disease** Locally invasive tumor Abscess Skull metastasis **Treatment** Radiation mucositis Chemotherapy mucositis	**Disease** Headaches (brain metastasis) **Treatment** Headache	**Disease** Base of skull Otalgia Glossopharyngeal neuralgia Referred pain from lung cancer **Treatment** RND syndrome **Other** Trigeminal neuralgia	**Disease** Myofascial pain **Benign** Cervical spondylosis/stenosis
Chest	**Disease** Chest wall syndrome Bone metastases **Treatment** Chest tube placement Gynecomastia Esophagitis	**Disease** Mediastinal pain referred to shoulder	**Disease** Carcinomatous brachial plexopathy Leptomeningeal disease **Treatment** Radiation brachial plexopathy Postmastectomy Postthoracotomy	**Disease** Pancoast tumor
Abdomen	**Disease** Psoas syndrome RPLN	**Disease** Hepatic distention Bowel obstruction Ureteral obstruction Adrenal distention Splenomegaly **Treatment** Constipation Radiation enteritis	**Disease** Celiac plexopathy Leptomeningeal disease Radiculopathy	
Back	**Disease** Bone metastases Pathologic vertebral body collapse	**Disease** Retroperitoneal infiltration or adenopathy	**Disease** Herpes zoster Epidural cord compression Leptomeningeal disease Radiculopathy **Treatment** Radiation myelopathy	**Disease** Vertebral body collapse **Benign** Osteoporotic collapse Myofascial pain
Pelvis	**Disease** Wound pain Acetabular syndrome Abscess **Treatment** Radiation proctitis Radiation cystitis	**Disease** Bladder spasm Rectal spasm Scrotal edema Penile pain **Treatment** Phantom bladder Radiation cystitis	**Disease** Lumbar plexopathy Sacral plexopathy Perineal syndrome **Treatment** Pelvic insufficiency fracture Phantom pain	
Limbs	**Disease** Pathologic fracture Erythromelalgia **Treatment** Avascular necrosis **Benign** Gout Osteoarthritis		**Disease** Pancoast tumor Leptomeningeal disease Carcinomatous plexopathy Cauda equina syndrome **Treatment** Phantom pain Radiculopathy Radiation Plexopathy Chemotherapy Neuropathy	**Disease** CRPS Bone pain Edema Ischemia Erythromelalgia Hypertrophic pulmonary osteoarthropathy **Treatment** Palmar plantar erythrodysesthesia Lymphedema

Symptoms associated with pain

In one survey of 593 patients with cancer pain treated by a cancer pain service, the most frequent symptoms were impaired activity (76%), anorexia (36%), mood changes (54%), insomnia (31%), constipation (27%), nausea (27%), and dyspnea (21%).[144] In another study of 240 veteran patients, those without pain were at increased risk for experiencing nausea (relative risk [RR] 3.38), dry mouth (RR 3.05), dyspnea (RR 2.59), lack of appetite (RR 2.33), fatigue (RR 2.32), and constipation (RR 2.24) compared to patients without moderately intense pain.[145]

PHYSICAL EXAMINATION

Introduction

The physical examination of a palliative patient with pain differs in several significant ways from the pain history. As outlined earlier, the various components of the pain history have been the focus of intensive study for many decades. The validity, reliability, predicative value, and cut points of a whole range of assessment tools have been characterized along with psychophysics and several other important attributes. Dimensions of the pain experience and their interrelatedness with suffering have also been explored, and the affective value of specific words has been quantified. The pharmacokinetics of analgesic medications and their relationship to relief of pain over time (pharmacodynamics) is grounded upon a broad area of evidence-based knowledge within the clinical pharmacology literature. There are validated ways of inquiry regarding substance abuse in palliative patients.[146] These are but a few examples of the many aspects of history-taking techniques in pain patients that have been intensely studied and have greatly informed clinical practice.

All of this acumen that supports the clinician in obtaining a comprehensive pain history stands in stark contrast to what is known about the physical examination of the patient in pain. Most textbooks on pain provide only modest guidance to the student on how to approach the physical examination. The reason for this is clear: the area has not been extensively studied.

A great deal is, however, known about specific disease entities and their manifestations on physical examination, from the presentation of the acute abdomen to bedside manifestations of pulmonary embolism and specific findings such as those in inflammatory arthropathies. If one pieces this material together, a picture begins to emerge of a more generic approach to the physical examination of a pain patient in a way that both complements the pain history and leaves the physician open to discovering unanticipated but clinically relevant findings.

In general, there are three basic steps in the physical examination of the palliative patient with pain.

▶ First, characterize underlying systemic illnesses and the extent of the disease by performing a general physical examination.

▶ Second, perform a regional pain examination. Palpate, perform range of motion testing and through other bedside techniques, gently reproduce the pain that brought the patient to the clinic in order to identify the pain-sensitive structure(s) and characterize each component of the pain experience.

▶ Third, as you perform the regional pain examination, based on the findings, generate and test hypotheses about the possible mechanism(s) of pain as somatic, visceral, neuropathic, or mixed. If there is more than one mechanism of pain present in the same region of body, hypothesize regarding their interconnectedness.

An example of this latter phenomenon is the presence of muscle spasm that can greatly contribute to overall pain within a region adjacent to an area of a painful bone metastasis.

Based on the extent of underlying illness, the identified pain-sensitive structure(s), and the inferred mechanism of pain, the clinician will be equipped to construct an overall analgesic strategy involving both pharmacologic and nonpharmacologic interventions.

Characterize the underlying systemic illness

If a patient who is known to have cancer develops a new and persistent pain, the new pain is most often due to cancer progression. It may be due to a new site of metastasis that has become symptomatic or may be arising in area of known disease that has become more clinically active. Predictably, certain clinical scenarios are more likely to occur at particular times along a disease trajectory. Consider, for example, a patient who has just undergone resection of an early stage melanoma, was found to have no evidence of regional nodal disease, and then develops a headache. He would be unlikely to have evidence of central nervous systems metastasis on physical examination. In contrast, a patient who is known to have disseminated melanoma with liver or lung metastases and then develops a headache, very likely has metastatic disease causing the headache: About 90% of patients who die from melanoma have central nervous system involvement found during autopsy. Therefore, identifying where the patient is along the disease trajectory can alert you to the findings that you will want to be careful to look for.

Commonly, on physical examination patients have more advanced disease than was initially anticipated.

Several systemic illnesses are often seen in association with cancer, such as acquired immunodeficiency syndrome (AIDS), organ failure, and peripheral vascular disease, and careful attention to elucidating cancer and noncancer mechanisms of pain is a key function of the physical examination.

A significant minority of cancer patients who develop a new pain will eventually be found to have a cause of pain that is not due to cancer. Even patients who have advanced cancer are not immune from other ills that befall mankind and, in some ways, they may be more prone to them. For example, acute herpetic neuralgia (shingles) is more common in cancer patients than in age-matched controls, and is much more common in patients who have cancer-related immune deficiencies such as myeloma. A patient with new onset of pain in the buttock or leg should be evaluated for evidence of claudication, as vascular disease is a common comorbidity with certain kinds of cancer such as lung cancer because of an association with cigarette smoking. Even if there is no reason to suspect that a particular patient has a nonmalignant cause underlying his or her pain, the clinician should always be wary of this possibility. This is poignantly highlighted in a case series of patients with a presumed diagnosis of malignant epidural cord compression who were irradiated. Upon subsequent investigation, the patients were found to have active radiculopathy from herniated disk material.[147]

The general physical examination of the palliative patient consists of a Mini-Mental Status Examination, a general neurologic examination, and examination of all systems, including cardiovascular, respiratory, gastrointestinal (GI), extremities, and so on. The clinician may identify underlying abnormalities that help shape the analgesic strategy, such as evidence of delirium (if present can reduce tolerability of analgesic medications), oral thrush (difficulty swallowing medications), underlying respiratory disease (difficulty tolerating opioids), cardiovascular disease (both drug metabolism and drug clearance decline precipitously in patients who have congestive heart failure), and GI disease (look for constipation and perform a rectal examination; look for evidence of liver disease including jaundice and bulky liver metastases; if the patient has nausea, look for evidence of upper or lower GI disease and for the presence of ascitic fluid).

▶ A regional approach to the pain physical examination

For centuries, a disease systems approach has informed the physician's orientation toward the general physical examination. For example, if while taking a history the patient describes shortness of breath with exertion in association with retrosternal chest pain and sweating, the standard practice is for the physical examination to focus on a cardiovascular assessment. In the pain patient, a systems approach is also highly relevant, to the extent that pain is often a heralding manifestation of underlying systemic illness. However, pain can be due to factors other than systemic disorders. Pain is often *functional*, such as pain with movement. Pain with movement may be due to sensitivity of the skin (see discussion on allodynia later), reflex muscle spasm with movement, pain from a weight-bearing bone, and so on. Therefore, in addition to a general physical examination, palliative clinicians commonly adopt a regional approach to the pain physical examination.

In broad terms, there are fairly limited ways in which pain can present. One simple approach is to divide the body into six separate regions. This involves characterizing pain as being present in one or more discreet regions of the body—head and neck, shoulder and arm, chest and midback, abdomen and pelvis, back and buttock, buttock and leg—if a patient has a pain in one of these regions, he or she would be said to have a regional pain syndrome. The clinician then undertakes a comprehensive pain examination of that region of the body. A common example is a patient who reports headache. The patient may come to the office complaining of *migraine,* but the regional approach to the pain physical examination would encourage the clinician to think in terms of *head and neck pain*. The patient may or may not be accurate with a self-diagnosis of migraine. The reality is that patients who have migraine also commonly have concurrent regional myofascial pain. Identifying the presence of regional myofascial pain can broaden the scope of analgesic interventions that are available to the patient who reported migraine. Heat, cold, stretch, and massage are nonpharmacologic interventions that are helpful for addressing the myofascial component of a regional pain. The following case history illustrates the value of the regional approach to the pain examination.

▶ Case history: right orbital pain of uncertain origin

A 55-year-old nonsmoking, nondrinking woman presented to a neurologist's office with a 3-year history of steady, right-sided retro-orbital pain. She had been diagnosed with chronic cluster headache but her headache had not responded to trials of ergotamines, lithium, and other standard pharmacological interventions.

After obtaining a history and performing a general physical examination, a regional pain physical examination of the head and neck was performed. Pain-sensitive structures that could potentially result in pain being experienced in the retro-orbital area were systematically palpated. This included: very light touch over the left orbit and then the right orbit; palpation of the frontal sinuses, ethmoid sinuses and zygomatic arch; and examination for tenderness of the temporalis muscles, the occipital-nuchal junction, and myofascial trigger points in the neck. Range of motion on the neck was performed in six directions: flexion, extension, left lateral flexion, left lateral rotation, right lateral flexion, and right lateral rotation. Anterior neck structures were palpated. While palpating very gently over right common carotid artery, the patient exclaimed "Oh my right eye! That's the pain!" The maneuver was performed sufficiently gently so that the pain was not severe but the maneuver was nevertheless diagnostic.

On direct questioning, the patient agreed that this was the pain which she had for the past 3 years and that had brought her to the physician's office that day.

The remainder of the physical examination, including the neurovascular examination, was otherwise unremarkable. There was no evidence of a Horner's sign or neurologic deficit.

The clinical diagnosis was *carotidynia*, an idiopathic pain syndrome characterized by tenderness of a carotid artery. It is most commonly found in women and is often responsive to indomethacin. The patient was placed on indomethacin 25 mg three times a day. Her pain promptly disappeared. An earlier magnetic resonance imaging (MRI) scan had shown no evidence of carotid dissection and her sedimentation rate was normal.

▶ Performing a regional pain physical examination

This case highlights the pattern of thought that a pain clinician uses to approach the regional pain physical examination. After looking for evidence of systemic disease by performing a general physical examination, potentially pain-sensitive structures referable to the symptomatic region of the body are systematically manipulated or palpated to look for tenderness. One begins by asking the patient, "Show me where your pain is." As he or she points to where the pain is felt, ask if it is all right if you touch that area. Indicate that it may hurt a bit but it would be useful for you to be able to touch the pain. Patients are often willing to endure some pain as long as they are warned in advance. The goal of bedside provocative maneuvers is to find areas of local tenderness and perform provocative maneuvers that elucidate the underlying pain-sensitive structure. As you progress through the regional pain examination, you will be generating and testing hypotheses about the possible mechanism(s) of pain, being somatic, visceral, neuropathic, or mixed, and if there is more than one mechanism of pain present in the same region of body, hypothesize regarding their connectedness.

A detailed approach to the regional physical examination is as follows. First, touch the skin overlying the area of tenderness very gently or wave your hand over the skin in order to brush the skin with the wind generated from the motion of your hand. If this maneuver is unpleasant, the patient might have allodynia. *Allodynia* is a condition whereby a nonpainful stimulus to the skin is experienced as being painful. Examples include *mechanical allodynia*, such as wind or light touch of the skin provoking pain, and *thermal allodynia*, whereby cold is felt as painfully cold or heat is felt as painfully hot. Often allodynia is associated with *after-sensations,* whereby the evoked pain persists like an echo, and can last a minute or even longer. It can be one of the most striking findings of the pain physical examination and will alert the clinician to look for regional numbness, reflex changes, and other evidence of regional nervous system dysfunction.

Next, palpate very gently in the area of pain and ask the patient "Is it unpleasant because I am touching you?" This helps distinguish an area of referred pain (see discussion on referred pain later) from the one where there is local tenderness.

Continue to feel in the region of pain in a widening circle and then look systematically at nearby structures such as paraspinal muscles, bones, ligaments, joints, arteries, typical myofascial areas of tenderness, and other structures. Then feel the nearby organs, and finally have the patient undergo range of motion and other bedside provocative maneuvers of those body parts appropriate to that region.

Examine structures nearby the pain for evidence of cancer, infection, or other underlying illness.

If at any point there is tenderness, ask the patient if it reproduces pain or part of the pain that they have been experiencing. Ask them to describe in words what the pain feels like (burning, sharp, dull, and so on). If there is a report of burning pain, consider whether there is evidence of muscle spasm or soft tissue damage, common causes of burning pain. A report of burning pain is not itself sufficient to diagnose neuropathic pain. To make a case for neuropathic pain, there ought to be a pattern of numbness, weakness, tingling, change of reflexes, or other evidence of regional nervous system disease on physical examination. Also, ask where the patient feels the pain: is it only where you are pushing or is it referred to somewhere else?

Referred pains

Most clinicians are familiar with pain that is referred down the leg in a radicular (dermatomal) pattern, such as L5 radiculopathy caused by a herniated disk, and that is reproduced on physical examination by a straight leg raise maneuver. Textbooks of pain have outlined *dermatomal body maps*.[148,149] Other parts of the nervous system can be responsible for referred neuropathic regional pain. One would, therefore, want to distinguish between a radicular pattern of leg pain and a peripheral nerve pattern such as that caused by a lateral peroneal neuroma, or a central pattern of neuropathic leg pain such as the clinical scenario of spinal injury pain. Different parts of the nervous system have fairly characteristic referral patterns, such as the brainstem pattern of neuropathic pain and numbness, described by Dejarine and Roussie.[150]

Less well-known, nonneurologic structures can also cause pain to be experienced in adjacent or distant parts of the body. Pain arising in soft tissues, such as ligaments and joints, can refer to other parts of the body, called *sclerotomal pain*. The pattern of referral may superficially be similar to a radicular pattern. Textbooks of pain have outlined *sclerotomal body maps*.[148,149] For example, in the presence of sacroiliitis, pushing over the ipsilateral SI joint with the thumb can result in pain being experienced down the ipsilateral leg into the lateral ankle. The pattern of referred pain can be difficult to distinguish from S1 nerve root radicular pain; to complicate the situation even further, patients who have chronic active lumbosacral radiculopathy commonly also develop sacroiliitis as an epiphenomenon, presumably related to biomechanical stress from an antalgic gait. The pain clinician then becomes a sleuth, teasing out the various components of the regional pain, which together form a tapestry of the patient's overall pain experience. Simply reproducing part of the pain that brought the patient to the office does not complete the physical examination; one must look for other potential pain-sensitive structures to see whether they are involved or not.

A third kind of referred pain is *myotomal pain*. Pain from muscle spasm or muscle disorders can be referred to other parts of the body within the same region. Myotomal pain is referred to body parts also innervated by the same myotome.[148,149] Myotomal pain can be difficult to distinguish from either sclerotomal pain or dermatomal pain, and commonly occurs concurrently with sclerotomal or dermatomal pain. Pushing over tender muscles, stretching muscles, or stimulating myofascial tender points can reproduce myotomal referred pain.

Finally, visceral pain is commonly experienced in a pattern of referral that is readily recognized by the clinician, such as cardiac pain felt going down the left arm, or liver pain experienced in the right shoulder.

Body maps outlining common patterns of referral of visceral pain are called *viscerotomes*.[144] In general, bedside provocative maneuvers using palpation only uncommonly result in visceral pain being felt in the area of referral described in the patient's history.

Specific bedside provocative maneuvers

Few bedside provocative maneuvers have been validated in pain patients. To illustrate further the diagnostic value of validated maneuvers, four bedside maneuvers that have been studied in some detail are summarized.

First is the straight leg raise maneuver, used to assess the presence of active nerve root compression from herniated disk material. If positive, it results in neuropathic pain felt below the knee with or without transient or persistent tingling or numbness in the same area. This bedside maneuver has been characterized and its validity, positive predictive value, and negative predictive value have been outlined in patients of several different age groups.[151]

Second is fibromyalgia. It is a prevalent condition that has been essentially defined by validated bedside provocative maneuvers. Eleven or more of eighteen tender points need to be present.[152,153] Each tender point has been carefully studied to distinguish *normal tenderness* from *pathologic tenderness* (anyone would hurt if pressed over a body part with sufficient force). A bedside pressure dolorimeter is a helpful tool used to quantify how hard the clinician is pressing. In general, most myofascial tender points usually don't hurt until about 4 kg of pressure per square centimeter are applied, whereas commonly in fibromyalgia, tender points are sore with less than 4 kg of pressure. For a tender point to be considered positive the patient must indicate that the palpation was painful; a finding of tenderness is not the same as a spontaneous report that it is painful.[154]

It has been described that the thumb commonly blanches when pressed to about 4 kg of pressure.[155] However, some physicians have found that thumbs can blanch with as little as 1 kg of pressure. Further, it takes a great deal of practice to reliably predict that one is pressing their thumb using 4 kg of pressure, and practice does not always result in a high level of reliability in performing this bedside provocative maneuver.[155] Imagine the convenience of a dolorimeter that you always have readily available with you at the bedside, wherever you go. A commercially manufactured pressure dolorimeter to guide the myofascial examination is a helpful tool to complement the bedside provocative diagnostic armamentarium.

A third validated bedside provocative maneuver is the Bruce Protocol, which characterizes the extent and severity of angina pectoris, and to a degree can predict the severity of underlying cardiovascular disease.[156]

A fourth, recently described bedside provocative maneuver for pain is a patient-assisted laparoscopic procedure whereby patients with endometriosis have chocolate cysts visualized and individually stimulated.[157] If a chocolate cyst is encountered that reproduces the patient's pain when stimulated, it is cauterized. Endometriosis commonly is blamed for idiopathic abdominal pain, and a patient-assisted laparoscopic procedure that stimulates individual chocolate cysts sheds a great deal of light on the mechanism of pain in a patient who may or may not have symptomatic endometriosis.

These four bedside provocative maneuvers have been well studied. Most others have not; yet the astute clinician can make useful inferences about the pain and its underlying mechanism by taking a systematic approach to the regional pain physical examination and finding ways to palpate, percuss, stretch, or otherwise evaluate the integrity of underlying structures. Above all else, obtain consent from the patient, explain ahead of time what you are planning to do, and be very gentle. You never know how tender an area might be, and need to be certain you cause no harm.

How to perform selected bedside provocative maneuvers

Spurling's maneuver is performed in patients with neuropathic arm pain. It provides evidence of active cervical radiculopathy. In patients with neuropathic arm pain, it can distinguish disease within the spinal canal from brachial plexopathy.[158] It is to the upper extremities what a straight leg maneuver is to the lower extremities. A positive Spurling's maneuver is present when the procedure results in neuropathic pain, numbness, weakness, or tingling that goes below the elbow, with or without ipsilateral transient or baseline tendon reflex changes. A positive Spurling's maneuver strongly suggests that there is a space-occupying lesion, or something behaving like a space-occupying lesion, pushing on the cervical thecal sac.

To perform this procedure, let us assume that the patient has a history of neuropathic pain in the right arm below the elbow. First, have the patient gently perform active neck range of motion in six directions as described below. It is extraordinarily uncommon that the patient will come to harm by doing voluntary neck range of motion, as pain will usually not allow a patient to move his or her neck in a way that it causes tissue damage such as cervical fracture. If the neck range of motion doesn't reproduce the patient's neck or arm pain, ask the patient to tilt the neck ipsilateral to the pain (in this case, toward the right), by instructing: "Put your right ear on your right shoulder." This should be sustained for at least 30 seconds and preferably for 1 minute. If it doesn't result in discomfort or other neurologic symptoms, have the patient continue to do the same maneuver but to also rotate the neck laterally to the right: "Throw your ear over your shoulder." Maintain this position for another 30 seconds. If this does not reproduce the pain, the patient should then laterally flex his or her neck contralateral to the side of the pain; in this instance, to the left and then laterally flex and laterally rotate the neck to the left. The Spurling's maneuver can be positive, either ipsilateral or contralateral to the side of the lesion. See Fig. 1-1.

Carnett's maneuver for abdominal pain is performed to provide bedside evidence of a somatic cause of left or right lower quadrant abdominal pain. Most often clinicians think of visceral causes of abdominal pain such as GI or liver disease. However, the *abdominal wall* is a common source of chronic abdominal pain, particularly the left lower or right lower abdomen, approximately in the vicinity of the medial insertion of the inguinal ligament. The actual pain-sensitive structure cannot usually be identified. Carnett's maneuver is often positive in chronic pain following hernia repair[159] but has also been described following a variety of abdominal procedures. It was initially described by Carnett as an idiopathic pain occurring without any clear antecedent cause.[160] It is rarely associated with peritoneal tumor or other serious diseases.[161] If Carnett's maneuver reproduces the abdominal pain and a computed tomography (CT) scan of the abdomen and pelvis is negative, the patient can generally be reassured and seen in follow-up. Opioids often reduce but do not eliminate somatic abdominal wall pain.

To perform this procedure, have the patient lay flat in bed. Gently palpate the area of left or right lower quadrant pain the patient has demonstrated to you. Gentle palpation should result in mild tenderness. Next, have the patient cross his or her arms over the chest so that the left hand is on the right shoulder and the right hand is on the left shoulder. As you gently press over the area of pain, have the patient lift the head and shoulders off the bed. A positive maneuver is when the pain increases concurrent with tensing of abdominal wall muscles. If, however, the pain-sensitive structure is visceral—within the peritoneal cavity—the tense abdominal muscles will often protect the pain-sensitive structure from the examiner's palpating hand and pain may actually decrease. If the pain decreases or does not change, the test for abdominal wall pain is negative. See Fig. 1-2.

A variation of Carnett's maneuver is: gently palpate over the area of pain in the left or right lower quadrant with the patient lying flat and the arms folded over the shoulders as described above. Have the patient lift both feet about 4 inches straight into the air (i.e., flex both hips and elevate both extended legs). The positive test reproduces the pain and an abdominal wall source of somatic pain is inferred; if the pain decreases with the maneuver, there may be an intra-abdominal cause of visceral pain; if there is no change in pain, the test is not diagnostic and is said to be negative.

The retroperitoneal stretch maneuver is performed to provide bedside evidence of a retroperitoneal process, including metastatic tumor

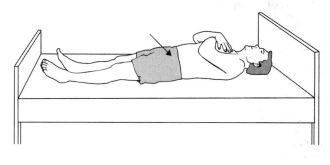

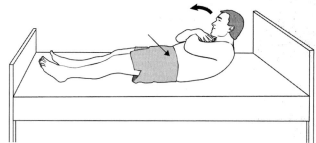

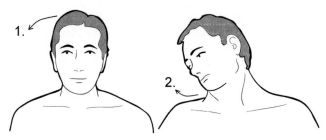

FIGURE 1-1 Spurling's Maneuver.
1. Ask the patient to laterally flex the neck: "Put your right ear on your right shoulder". This should be sustained for at least thirty seconds and preferably for a minute.
2. If it doesn't result in discomfort or other neurological symptoms, have the patient continue to do the same maneuver but to also rotate the neck laterally to the right: "Throw your ear over your shoulder." Maintain this position for another thirty seconds. If this does not reproduce the pain the patient should then laterally flex his or her neck contralateral to the side of the pain, in this instance to the left and then laterally flex and laterally rotate the neck to the left. The Spurling's maneuver can be positive either ipsilateral or contralateral to the side of the lesion.

FIGURE 1-2 Carnett's Maneuver for Abdominal Wall Pain.
Carnett's Maneuver helps distinguish somatic abdominal wall pain from other causes of chronic abdominal pain such as visceral pain from organ disease. While the examiner gently presses over the area of tenderness in the left or right lower quadrant (arrow), the patient folds the arms over the shoulders and lifts the shoulders off the bed.

or a primary retroperitoneal neoplasm such as pancreatic cancer. In cancer patients with back pain, it can help guide the clinician to look for visceral causes of pain rather than spinal metastases. A positive retroperitoneal stretch maneuver is present when the patient's back pain is reproduced by spine extension but not with spine percussion. The pain-sensitive structure that results in the positive sign is not known. While there is often evidence of lymph node metastases in patients who demonstrate the sign, there can also be other potential sources of pain such as adrenal metastasis, direct retroperitoneal invasion, or other concurrent sites of metastatic disease not seen on diagnostic imaging. The sign can disappear with a celiac plexus block and can diminish with effective doses of systemic opioids.

To perform this procedure, assume that the patient has a history of cancer and describes moderately severe midthoracic back pain that has been present for more than a month. This pain is sufficiently severe to interfere with function, resulting in sleep disruption. Note that such midthoracic back pain is almost always due to a serious process, unless there is evidence of a myofascial pain disorder or unequivocal evidence of advanced degenerative disease in the thoracic spine. On physical examination, the clinician will want to try to distinguish between bone metastases, paraspinal muscle spasm, retroperitoneal tumor, or other possible mechanisms of pain. First, examine the region of pain as pointed out by the patient. Include gentle percussion of each spinal level in the area of pain, palpation of each spinous process, and examination for evidence of paraspinal muscle spasm or tenderness on both the right and left side. If the above are negative, have the patient sit in a stretcher or bed with the head of the bed elevated to about 30°. Place a pillow in the small of the back so the thoracic and lumbar areas are partially extended, even though the patient's hips are flexed. The patient then lies down without a pillow for the head. *Gradually* lower the head of the bed with the patient remaining recumbent and fully relaxed. The positive maneuver is the recurrence of the pain the patient has been having, as the head of the bed is lowered. Often the bed cannot be made fully flat because of the development of pain. Some patients describe pain that only emerges and escalates after laying flat for several minutes. Patients with a positive retroperitoneal stretch maneuver will often report they cannot sleep supine in bed, but must instead sleep lying curled on their right side, left side, or in a reclining chair. See Fig. 1-3.

Observing pain-relieving maneuvers. Patients with a positive retroperitoneal stretch maneuver, as described above, are usually unable to lay flat for long. Therefore, when the clinician enters the examination room, such a patient will usually be found in a pain-relieving position, either lying in a bed with the head elevated or sitting upright. If the pain has been poorly controlled in the recent past, the patient may even be sitting with one or both knees brought up to the chest. Observing such spontaneous pain-relieving postures can be of diagnostic value. A description of pain-relieving positions may be obtained from the history, but may also be observed, or reproduced, on physical examination. There is a long list of such scenarios, and here are a few:

▶ The patient with a painful coccyx metastasis who stands in the physician's office because it hurts too much to sit;

▶ The patient with lumbar spine metastases and spinal stenosis from epidural tumor who cannot walk upright because of back pain and tingling of the legs, but can walk for a long time if leaning on a walker or shopping cart;

▶ The cluster headache patient who paces in comparison to the migrainous patient who lays perfectly still in a dark room;

▶ The patient with abdominal wall pain who pushes firmly over the area of pain to splint it in order to be able to move from a lying to a standing position;

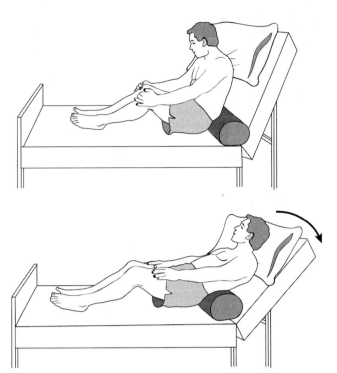

FIGURE 1-3 Retroperitoneal Stretch Maneuver.
The Retroperitoneal Stretch Maneuver helps distinguish pain from a retroperitoneal source such as pancreatic cancer from other causes of chronic back or flank pain such as metastatic bone disease. While the patient lays completely relaxed with the head of the bed elevated and the patient's lower back mildly lordotic, the head of the bed is slowly lowered by the examiner.

▶ The patient with active cervical radiculopathy from vertebral body metastasis who discovers partial relief of pain by keeping the neck perfectly straight and perfectly rigid, in comparison to the patient with active cervical radiculopathy from a lower cervical herniated disc who discovers relief of pain by laterally flexing the neck away from and laterally rotating the neck toward the side of pain.

▶ Drawing Conclusions

A widely held tenet of clinical medicine is that the most important contributor to a correct diagnosis is the patient's history. While this is legitimate advice, the physical examination of the palliative care patient with pain can result in findings that are unanticipated based on the patient's history alone. Organ or other systemic illness can be more advanced than expected and can warn the clinician about risks of toxicity of analgesic or oncologic interventions. Further, the identification of additional contributors to regional pain can characterize the tapestry of underlying mechanisms, such as severe muscle spasm in an area of bone metastasis, and thereby guide the construction of a comprehensive analgesic strategy that addresses each of the components of the pain.

This approach to the physical examination of the palliative pain patient has been evaluated. In a study of 50 consecutive patients with pain, the physical examination was modified to include provocative maneuvers to reproduce and assess the patient's pain complaint.[162] These maneuvers included palpation of nearby bone or spinal tenderness, palpable muscle spasms, myofascial tenderness, lymphadenopathy, Spurling's maneuver, Tinel's sign, and others. The 50 patients described a wide range of pains, and many patients had several pains and several mechanisms of those pains. Of the 89 pain complaints, 79 (89%) could be reproduced by physical examination, and one or more pain diagnoses could be made for 46 of the 50 patients, with new pain diagnoses for 34 of them. This approach was found to complement the pain history and contributed to the development of a comprehensive analgesic strategy, tailored to each patient's particular clinical situation (Table 1-7).

CONSTIPATION

▶ Definition

Many definitions of constipation exist, but there is no universally accepted definition. Constipation can be described as difficult evacuation of feces, straining, abdominal discomfort, hard stools, or decreased frequency of defecation.[163,164] Specific criteria for diagnosing functional constipation in adults have been defined in the Rome II classification system, which additionally includes a feeling of "incomplete evacuation" or "anorectal obstruction/blockade," manually removing feces, and less than three defecations in 1 week.[165]

Constipation is most often characterized by the frequency of defecation and the quality of stool. An older survey on constipation evaluated 1055 healthy adults on the number of bowel movements. The frequency of defecation was reported to range from three per day to three per week.[166] Another survey of patients with functional constipation rated straining and hard stools as the most bothersome symptoms.[167] These same symptoms were highly associated with constipation in a large study of older adults, while the feeling of incomplete evacuation, pain, and bloating were less associated.[168]

Stool hardness can be correlated with intestinal transit time.[169] Longer transit times correlate with harder stool, and opioids prolong transit time. Patients will complain that their stool "feels like a brick." Clinical trials have attempted to find a correlation between stool consistency and constipation. A texture analyzer using a probe was used to measure hardness of stool samples of constipated subjects

---

Table 1-7

Bedside Provocative Maneuvers for Pain Patients

Ask the patient: "Is it the pain, or is it any old pain?"
- ▶ If positive, the patient is happy (if the maneuver was gently done): the patient feels affirmed
- ▶ If positive, the physician is happy (it may be a diagnostic provocative maneuver)

General
- ▶ Lightly touch the skin over the painful part
- ▶ Push gently directly over the painful part
  - ▶ Superficial palpation
  - ▶ Deep palpation
- ▶ Systematically palpate nearby structures
- ▶ Evaluate for evidence of allodynia or other evidence of neurologic dysfunction
- ▶ First, palpate, percuss, and in other ways gently stress bone and joint structures, then perform range of motion
- ▶ Compare the normal side with the abnormal side
- ▶ If there may be neuropathic pain in the distribution of a nerve, look for Tinel's sign, first on the normal side then the abnormal side
- ▶ If pain is provoked by the patient moving, distinguish pain caused by muscle contraction (perform an isometric contraction maneuver) from pain caused by limb or joint movement (perform a range of motion maneuver while the patient actively relaxes all muscles)
- ▶ Have the patient perform other activities that the patient describes as reliably making the pain worse on history, and systematically observe

Head and neck region pain
- ▶ Palpate over bones such as the occipital condyle, cervical spinous processes, facial bones, sinuses
- ▶ Palpate myofascial areas such as the occipital nuchal junction, over the temporalis, facial, sternocleidomastoid, and other muscles as appropriate. Check for laxity of the jaw (pterygoids)
- ▶ Move the head: check neck range of motion in six directions: flexion, extension, left lateral flexion, left lateral rotation, right lateral flexion, and right lateral rotation
- ▶ Perform Spurling's maneuver: laterally flex and laterally rotate the neck ipsilateral to the shoulder or arm pain, then contralateral to it. Positive result: neuropathic arm pain or tingling, or decreased arm reflex
- ▶ Palpate the carotid artery
- ▶ Palpate potentially important soft tissue structures such as subcutaneous tissue, the orbits, salivary glands

Shoulder and arm region pain
- ▶ Palpate over bones, joints, ligaments, soft tissues, and axilla; then perform range of motion of shoulders and then elbows
- ▶ Systematically evaluate for the presence of myofascial tenderness, muscle spasm, or joint disease
- ▶ Perform a formal range of motion of the neck and perform a Spurling's maneuver
- ▶ Look for a Tinel's sign over Erb's point in the supraclavicular fossa

(Continued)

Table 1-7

Bedside Provocative Maneuvers for Pain Patients *(Continued)*

Chest and midback region pain

▶ Push over the chest wall, distinguishing if possible between ribs, muscle, skin, other

▶ Systematically palpate paraspinal muscles

▶ Perform range of motion of the thoracic spine (six directions)

Abdominal and pelvic pain

▶ Look for tender lymphedema by gently squeezing abdominal wall skin between your thumb and finger

▶ Perform a general abdominal examination to identify organ tenderness (liver, spleen, pancreas, colon, and so on). If indicated, perform a rectal examination, pelvic examination

▶ Abdominal wall examination: Carnett's test (1926)

▶ Examine for tenderness of superficial pelvic structures such as the pubic tubercle, subcutaneous tissue, insertion of adductor muscles, and so on

▶ Perform a neurologic examination of the abdominal wall looking for allodynia, numbness, weakness, and abnormal abdominal wall reflexes

▶ Perform range of motion of the hips (see below)

▶ If the spine is not tender, perform a retroperitoneal stretch maneuver:

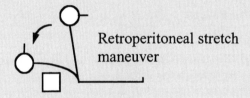

Retroperitoneal stretch maneuver

Low back

▶ Direct pressure over the vertebral bodies

▶ Paraspinal myofascial examination

▶ Spine range of motion, including six directions

▶ Evaluate for sacroiliac joint tenderness or disease

▶ Evaluate for coccygeal tenderness

▶ Perform a spine extension stress test looking for evidence of spinal stenosis

Buttocks and legs

▶ Check hips, pelvis (including S1 joint palpation), spine, and knees before the straight leg raise and reverse straight leg raise maneuvers

▶ Hips: palpate, including the trochanteric bursae and the anterior hip joint; perform a range of motion of the hips, including flexion, abduction, external rotation, and internal rotation

▶ Palpate groups of muscles systematically, such as gluteus, paraspinals, tensor fascia lata

▶ Perform a straight leg raise maneuver, and if indicated, a reverse straight leg raise maneuver

▶ Palpate the neurovascular bundle in the groin bilaterally

▶ Walk the patient and reexamine the patient when pain returns

and controls. No significant difference was found in stool consistency between the two groups.[170] The Bristol Stool Form Scale has been used as an objective measure in clinical trials, and may have some application in research. The 6-point scales range from hard lumps to mushy to describe stool consistency. The frequency of bowel movements and stool form is assessed by a patient or physician.[171]

A detailed medical history and physical examination are important in assessing constipation. Symptom diaries can also be useful in determining frequency of defecation and response to diet and/or laxatives.[172] The administration of anticholinergics, tricyclic antidepressants, opioids, calcium, or aluminum containing antacids, vinca alkaloids, iron, and anticonvulsants can contribute to constipation.[173]

Other factors include decreased dietary fiber and fluid intake, lack of privacy, hypercalcemia, decreased physical activity, older age, intestinal obstruction, and spinal cord compression.[174,175] Depression, physical abuse, and sexual abuse have been determined to be associated risk factors for constipation.[176]

The Constipation Assessment Scale (CAS) is a patient self-administered questionnaire consisting of eight characteristics. The CAS was validated by assessing constipation severity in 32 adults with cancer who were receiving vinca alkaloids or morphine and a control group of 32 adults. Test-retest reliability was assessed and found to have a high correlation.[177] In contrast, when the CAS was administered to caregivers to measure the accuracy between caregiver reporting and reporting by hospice patients, there was little agreement between the two groups. The caregivers significantly overestimated the severity of constipation, as well as the numeric rating scales of pain and dyspnea.[178]

Symptom questionnaires have been developed for evaluating constipation in other settings. There are few published studies evaluating the psychometric properties of instruments measuring the health-related quality of life in patients with constipation. The Patient Assessment of Constipation–Quality of Life (PAC-QOL) and Patient Assessment of Constipation–Symptom (PAC-SYM) questionnaires are both patient self-administered instruments. The PAC-QOL measures physical and psychosocial discomfort. The PAC-SYM measures abdominal, rectal, and stool symptoms such as frequency of defecation, straining, and stool size and consistency.[179] Another study demonstrated ease of use of the PAC questionnaire in older adults.[180] The results from a constipation scoring system evaluated in 232 patients with idiopathic constipation correlated well with the objective results from anorectal tests.[181] The bowel disease questionnaire developed at the Mayo Clinic has been used to diagnose functional or organic gastrointestinal disease.[182]

Physicians tend to use measures such as a combination of infrequent bowel movements with hard stool to define constipation, which can differ widely from patients' definitions of constipation, which can include hard stools alone.[183] The significance assigned to constipation by patients also differs; some patients associate severe constipation with impending death.[184]

▶ Objective findings

A digital rectal examination and/or radiologic assessment may be warranted to rule out fecal impaction.[185] Finding an empty vault on examination does not exclude constipation at a more proximal site. With a plain abdominal radiograph, the amount of stool in each of four quadrants is summed and quantified as the radiologic constipation score. Severe constipation is determined to be a score of 7 or more out of a total score of 12.[186] In a review of 122 patients admitted to a palliative care unit, the average score for patients was 7, with good correlation by two physicians. However, the investigators were unable to correlate this score with clinical constipation as chart documentation was poor.[187]

▶ Associated symptoms

Patients with constipation can experience related symptoms, such as abdominal distention or pain, decreased appetite, indigestion, and headache.[188] For patients on opioids, the term *opioid bowel dysfunction* encompasses a range of digestive symptoms, including increased gastrointestinal reflux, nausea and vomiting, bloating, abdominal distention, incomplete evacuation, constipation, and pseudo-obstruction.[189,190]

ACKNOWLEDGMENTS

Bianca Lee was supported in part by the Bronx, New Jersey VA Palliative Care Fellowship Program. The authors thank Dr. Basil Kasimis and Ms. Marian Gaballah for their helpful comments.

REFERENCES

1. Jackson J. Science at the bedside.In: Harvey AM, ed. *Clinical Research in American Medicine 1905–1945*. Baltimore: Johns Hopkins University Press; 1981:8.
2. Lusk G. Scientific medicine—yesterday and tomorrow. *JAMA*. 1919;73:181.
3. Portenoy RK, Bruera E, eds. *Issues in Palliative Care Research*. New York: Oxford University Press; 2003.
4. Stromgren AS, Groenvold M, Sorenson A, et al. Symptom recognition in advanced cancer. A comparison of nursing records against patient self rating. *Acta Anesthesiol Scand*. 2001;45:1080–1085.
5. Rhodes DJ, Koshy RC, Waterfield WC, et al. Feasibility of quantitative pain assessment in outpatient oncology practice. *J Clin Oncol*. 2001; 19:501–508.
6. Patrick DL, Ferketich SL, Frame PS, et al. National Institutes of Health State of the Science Panel. National Institutes of Health State-of-the-Science Conference Statement: Symptom Management in Cancer: Pain, Depression, and Fatigue, July 15–17, 2002. *J Natl Cancer Inst*. 2003;95:1110–1117.
7. Weiner JS, Cole SA. Three principles to improve clinician communication for advance care planning: overcoming emotional, cognitive, and skill barriers. *J Palliat Med*. 2004;7:817–829.
8. Carr DB, Loeser JD, Morris DB, eds. *Narrative, Pain and Suffering*. Progress in pain research and management, vol. 34. Seattle: IASP Press; 2005.
9. Cohen MZ, Williams L, Knight P, et al. Symptom masquerade: understanding the meaning of symptoms. *Support Care Cancer*. 2004;12: 184–190.
10. Gonzales GR, Elliott KJ, Portenoy RK, et al. The impact of a comprehensive evaluation in the management of cancer pain. *Pain*. 1991;47: 141–144.
11. Grossman SA, Sheidler VR, Swedeen K, et al. Correlation of patient and caregiver ratings of cancer pain. *J Pain Symptom Manage*. 1991;6:53–57.
12. Killian KJ. The objective measurement of breathlessness. *Chest*. 1985;88(Suppl. 2):84S–90S.
13. Gescheider GA. Psychophysical ratio scaling. In: Gescheider GA, ed. *Psychophysics. The Fundamentals*. 3rd ed. Mahwah: Lawrence Earlbaum Associates; 1997.
14. Tulsky DS. An introduction to test theory. In: Tchekmedyian NS, Cella DF, eds. *Quality of Life in Oncology Practice and Research*. Williston Park: Dominus Publishing Co.; 1991:19–24.
15. Freyd MT. The graphic rating scale. *J Educ Psychol*. 1923;14:83–102.
16. McCormack HM, Horne DJ, Sheather S. Clinical applications of visual analogue scales: a critical review. *Psychol Med*. 1988;18:1007–1019.
17. Wewers ME, Lowe NK. A critical review of visual analogue scales in the measurement of clinical phenomena. *Res Nurs Health*. 1990;13: 227–236.
18. Dodd M, Janson S, Facione N, et al. Advancing the science of symptom management. *J Adv Nurs*. 2001;33:668–676.
19. Armstrong TS. Symptom experience: a concept analysis. *Oncol Nurs Forum*. 2003;30:601–606.
20. McCorkle R, Young K. Development of a symptom distress scale. *Cancer Nurs*. 1978;1:373–378.
21. McClement SE, Woodgate RL, Degner L. Symptom distress in adult patients with cancer. *Cancer Nurs*. 1997;20:236–243.
22. Ridner SH. Psychological distress: concept analysis. *J Adv Nurs*. 2004;45:536–545.
23. Goodell TT, Nail LM. Operationalizing symptom distress in adults with cancer: a literature synthesis. *Oncol Nurs Forum*. 2005;32:E42–E47.
24. Hwang SS, Chang VT, Kasimis B. Comparison of three fatigue measures in a veteran cancer population. *Cancer Invest*. 2003;21:363–373.
25. Chang VT, Xia Q, Kasimis B. The Functional Assessment of Anorexia/Cachexia Therapy (FAACT) Appetite Scale in veteran cancer patients. *J Support Oncol*. 2005;3:377–382.
26. Sloan JA, Aaronson N, Cappelleri JC, et al. Clinical Significance Consensus Meeting Group. Assessing the clinical significance of single items relative to summated scores. *Mayo Clin Proc*. 2002;77:479–487.
27. Chang VT, Ingham J. Symptom Control. Review. *Cancer Invest*. 2003;21:564–578.
28. Sprangers MAG, Moinpour CM, Moynihan TJ, et al. Assessing meaningful change over time in quality of life: a user's guide for clinicians. *Mayo Clin Proc*. 2002;77:561–571.
29. Cohen J. *Statistical Power Analysis for the Behavioral Sciences*. 2nd ed. Hillsdale: Lawrence Erlbaum Associates; 1988:40.
30. Dodd MJ, Miaskowski C, Paul SM. Symptom clusters and their effect on the functional status of patients with cancer. *Oncol Nurs Forum*. 2001;28:465–470.
31. Cleeland CS, Bennett GJ, Dantzer R, et al. Are the symptoms of cancer and cancer treatment due to a shared biologic mechanism? A cytokine-immunologic model of cancer symptoms. *Cancer*. 2003;97:2919–2925.
32. Dodd MJ, Miaskowski C, Lee KA. Occurrence of symptom clusters. *J Natl Cancer Inst Monogr*. 2004;32:76–78.

33. Paice JA. Assessment of symptom clusters in people with cancer. *J Natl Cancer Inst Monogr.* 2004;32:98–102.

34. Gift AG, Stommel M, Jablonski A, et al. A cluster of symptoms over time in patients with lung cancer. *Nurs Res.* 2003;52:393–400.

35. Wilmoth MC, Coleman EA, Smith SC, et al. Fatigue, weight gain, and altered sexuality in patients with breast cancer: exploration of a symptom cluster. *Oncol Nurs Forum.* 2004;31:1069–1075.

36. Carlson LE, Speca M, Hagen N, et al. Computerized quality-of-life screening in a cancer pain clinic. *J Palliat Care.* 2001;17:46–52.

37. Chang CH, Cella D, Masters GA, et al. Real-time clinical application of quality-of-life assessment in advanced lung cancer. *Clin Lung Cancer.* 2002;4:104–109.

38. Berry DL, Trigg LJ, Lober WB, et al. Computerized symptom and quality of life assessment for patients with cancer. Part I: Development and pilot testing. *Oncol Nurs Forum.* 2004;31:E75–E83.

39. Cleeland CS. Cancer related symptoms. *Semin Radiat Oncol.* 2000;10:175–190.

40. Forensic Special Interest Group. American Pain Society Annual Scientific Meeting. 2005. Boston. MA.

41. Sloan PA, Donnelly MB, Vanderveer B, et al. Cancer pain among family physicians. *J Pain Symptom Manage.* 1997;14:74–81.

42. Wilson KG, Graham ID, Viola RA, et al. Structured interview assessment of symptoms and concerns in palliative care. *Can J Psychiatry.* 2004;49:350–358.

43. Kurtz ME, Kurtz JC, Given CC, et al. Concordance of cancer patient and caregiver symptom reports. *Cancer Practice.* 1996;4:185–190.

44. Redinbaugh EM, Baum A, DeMoss C, et al. Factors associated with the accuracy of caregiver estimates of patient pain. *J Pain Symptom Manage.* 2002;23:31–38.

45. Lobchuk MM. The Memorial Symptom Assessment Scale: modified for use in understanding family caregivers' perceptions of cancer patients' symptom experiences. *J Pain Symptom Manage.* 2003;26:644–654.

46. Lobchuk MM, Degner LF. Symptom experiences: perceptual accuracy between advanced-stage cancer patients and family caregivers in the home care setting. *J Clin Oncol.* 2002;20:3495–3507.

47. McMillan SC, Moody LE. Hospice patients and caregiver congruence in reporting patients' symptom intensity. *Cancer Nurs.* 2003;26:113–118.

48. Kutner JS, Kassner CT, Nowels DE. Symptom burden at the end of life: hospice providers' perceptions. *J Pain Symptom Manage.* 2001;21:473–480.

49. Nekolaichuk CL, Maguire TO, Suarez-Almazor M, et al. Assessing the reliability of patient, nurse, and family caregiver symptom ratings in hospitalized advanced cancer patients. *J Clin Oncol.* 1999;17:3621–3630.

50. Patrick DL, Ferketich SL, Frame PS, et al. National Institutes of Health State-of-the-Science Conference Statement: Symptom Management in Cancer: Pain, Depression, and Fatigue, July 15–17, 2002. *J Natl Cancer Inst.* 2003;95:1110–1117.

51. Forrest M, Hermann G, Andersen B. Assessment of pain: a comparison between patients and doctors. *Acta Anaesthesiol Scand.* 1989;33:255–256.

52. Mantyselka P, Kumpusalo E, Ahonen R, et al. Patients' versus general practitioners' assessment of pain intensity in primary care patients with non-cancer pain. *Br J Gen Pract.* 2001;51(473):995–997.

53. Sutherland JE, Welsey RM, Cole PM, et al. Differences and similarities between patient and physician perceptions of patient pain. *Fam Med.* 1988;20:343–346.

54. Grossman SA, Sheidler VR, Swedeen K, et al. Correlation of patient and caregiver ratings of cancer pain. *J Pain Symptom Manage.* 1991;6:53–57.

55. Marquie L, Raufaste E, Lauque E, et al. Pain rating by patients and physicians: evidence of systematic pain miscalibration. *Pain.* 2003;102:289–296.

56. Solomon P. Congruence between health professionals' and patients' pain ratings: a review of the literature. *Scand J Caring Sci.* 2001;15:174–180.

57. Ingham J, Portenoy RK. The measurement of pain and other symptoms. In: Doyle D, Hanks G, Cherny NI, Calman K, eds. *Oxford Textbook of Palliative Medicine.* 3rd ed. New York: Oxford University Press; 2004:167–184.

58. Moore R, Brodsgaard I, Miller ML, et al. Consensus analysis: reliability, validity and informant accuracy in use of American and Mandarin Chinese pain descriptors. *Ann Behav Med.* 1997;19:295–300.

59. Hardie GE, Janson S, Gold WM, et al. Ethnic differences: word descriptors used by African-American and White asthma patients during induced bronchoconstriction. *Chest.* 2000;117:935–943.

60. Koffman J, Higginson IJ, Donaldson N. Symptom severity in advanced cancer, assessed in two ethnic groups by interviews with bereaved family members and friends. *J R Soc Med.* 2004;96:10–16.

61. Edwards CL, Fillingim RB, Keefe F. Race, ethnicity, and pain. *Pain.* 2001;94:133–137.

62. *Cultural Competence in Cancer Care: A health care professional's passport.* Office of Minority Health, Health Resources and Services Administration. For copies, contact Baylor College of Medicine, Intercultural Cancer Council, http://www.iccnetwork.org.

63. Heaven CM, Maguire P. Disclosure of concerns by hospice patients and their identification by nurses. *Palliat Med.* 1997;11:283–290.

64. Lipton JA, Marbach JJ. Ethnicity and the pain experience. *Soc Sci Med.* 1984;19:1279–1298.

65. Calvillo ER, Flaskerud JH. Review of literature on culture and pain of adults with focus on Mexican Americans. *J Transcult Nurs.* 1991;2:16–23.

66. Reizian A, Meleis AI. Arab-Americans' perceptions of and responses to pain. *Crit Care Nurse.* 1986;6:30–37.

67. Hobara M. Beliefs about appropriate pain behavior: cross-cultural and sex differences between Japanese and Euro-American. *Eur J Pain.* 2005;9:389–393.

68. Pugh JF. The semantics of pain in Indian culture and medicine. *Cult Med Psychiatry.* 1991;15:19–43.

69. Palos G. Culture and pain assessment in Hispanic patients. In: Payne R, Patt RB, Hill CS, eds. *Assessment and Treatment of Cancer Pain.* Progress in pain research and management, vol. 12. Seattle: IASP Press; 1998.

70. Brattberg G, Thorslund M, Wikman A. The use of common pain experiences in designing a pain intensity scale for epidemiological purposes. *J Psychosom Res.* 1988;32:505–512.

71. Cleeland CS, Nakamura Y, Mendoza TR, et al. Dimensions of the impact of cancer pain in a four country sample: new information from multidimensional scaling. *Pain.* 1996;67:267–273.

72. Fishman B, Pasternak S, Wallenstein SL, et al. The Memorial Pain Assessment Card, a valid instrument for the evaluation of cancer pain. *Cancer.* 1987;60:1151–1158.

73. Ramer L, Richardson JL, Cohen M, et al. Multimeasure pain assessment in an ethnically diverse group of patients with cancer. *J Transcult Nurs.* 1999;10:94–101.

74. Juarez G, Ferrell B, Borneman T. Influence of culture on cancer pain management in Hispanic patients. *Cancer Pract.* 1998;6:262–269.

75. Lawlor PG. The panorama of opioid-related cognitive dysfunction in patients with cancer. A critical literature appraisal. *Cancer.* 2002;94:1836–1853.

76. Ersek M, Cherrier MM, Overman SS, et al. Cognitive effects of opioids. *Pain Manag Nurs.* 2004;5:75–93.

77. Coyle N, Breitbart W, Weaver S, et al. Delirium as a contributing factor to "crescendo" pain: three case reports. *J Pain Symptom Manage.* 1994; 94:44–47.

78. Radbruch L, Sabatowski R, Loick G, et al. Cognitive impairment and its influence on pain and symptom assessment in a palliative care unit: development of a Minimal Documentation System. *Palliat Med.* 2000;14:266–276.

79. Ferrell BA, Ferrell BR, Rivera L. Pain in cognitively impaired nursing home patients. *J Pain Symptom Manage.* 1995;10:591–598.

80. Closs SJ, Barr B, Briggs M, et al. A comparison of five pain assessment scales for nursing home residents with varying degrees of cognitive impairment. *J Pain Symptom Manage.* 2004;27:196–205.

81. Taylor LJ, Harris J, Epps CD, et al. Psychometric evaluation of selected pain intensity scales for use with cognitively impaired and cognitively intact older adults. *Rehabil Nurs.* 2005;30:55–61.

82. AGS Panel on Persistent Pain in Older Persons. The management of persistent pain in older persons. *J Am Geratr Soc.* 2002;50:S205–S224.

83. Warden V, Hurley AC, Volicer L. Development and psychometric evaluation of the Pain Assessment in Advanced Dementia scale. *J Am Dir Med Assoc.* 2003;4:9–15.

84. Herr K, Weiner D. Comprehensive interdisciplinary assessment and treatment planning: an integrative overview. In: Weiner D, Herr K, Rudy T, eds. *Persistent Pain in Older Adults: An Interdisciplinary Guide for Treatment.* New York, NY: Springer Publishing Company; 2002:18–57.

85. Villanueva MR, Smith TL, Erickson JS, et al. Pain Assessment for the Dementing Elderly (PADE): reliability and validity of a new measure. *J Am Dir Assoc.* 2003;4:1–8.

86. Stolee P, Hillier LM, Esbaugh J, et al. Instruments for the assessment of pain in older persons with cognitive impairment. *J Am Geriatr Soc.* 2005;53:319–326.

87. Chang VT, Hwang SS, Feuerman M, et al. Symptom and quality of life survey of medical oncology patients at a veterans' affairs medical center: a role for symptom assessment. *Cancer.* 2000;88:1175–1183.

88. Bruera E, Kuehn N, Miller MJ, et al. The Edmonton Symptom Assessment System (ESAS): a simple method for the assessment of palliative care patients. *J Palliative Care.* 1991;7(2):6–9.

89. De Haes JCJM, van Knippenburg FCE, Nejit JP. Measuring psychological and physical distress in cancer patients: structure and application of the Rotterdam Symptom Checklist. *Br J Cancer.* 1990;62:1034–1038.

90. McCorkle R, Young K. Development of a symptom distress scale. *Cancer Nurs.* 1978;1:373–378.

91. Chang VT, Hwang SS, Kasimis B, et al. Shorter symptom assessment instruments. The Condensed Memorial Symptom Assessment Scale (CMSAS). *Cancer Invest.* 2004;22:477–487.

92. Cleeland CS, Mendoza TR, Wang XS, et al. Assessing symptom distress in cancer patients: the MD Anderson Symptom Inventory. *Cancer.* 2000;89:1634–1646.

93. Hwang SS, Chang VT, Fairclough DF, et al. Longitudinal quality of life in advanced cancer patients: pilot study results from a VA medical cancer center. *J Pain Symptom Manage.* 2003;25:225–235.

94. Chang VT, Hwang SS, Alejandro Y, et al. Clinically significant differences (CSD) in the Memorial Symptom Assessment Scale Short Form (MSAS-SF). *Proc ASCO.* 2004;23:792, abstract 8269.

95. Cleeland C, Crawford J, Lubeck D, et al. Using the MD Anderson Symptom Inventory (MDASI) to assess symptom burden and interference: interim results of an open-label study of darbepoetin Alfa 200 mcg every 2 weeks (Q2W) for the treatment of chemotherapy-induced anemia (CIA). *Proc ASCO.* 2004;22(Suppl. 14), Abstract 8065.

96. Easson A, Bezjak A, Ross S, et al. Change in symptoms after paracentesis for symptomatic malignant ascites. *Proc ASCO.* 2005;23, Abstract 6071.

97. Cleeland CS, Reyes-Gibby CC. When is it justified to treat symptoms? Measuring symptom burden. *Oncology (Williston Park).* 2002;16 (9 Suppl. 10): 64–70.

98. Turk DC, Melzack R, eds. *Handbook of Pain Assessment.* 2nd ed. New York: The Guilford Press; 2001.

99. Cleeland C, Crawford J, Lubeck D, et al. Using the MD Anderson Symptom Inventory (MDASI) to assess symptom burden and interference: interim results of an open-label study of darbepoietin Alfa 200 mcg every 2 weeks (Q2W) for the treatment of chemotherapy-induced anemia (CIA). *Proc ASCO.* 2004;22(Suppl. 14); Abstract 8065.

100. Melzack R, Katz J. Pain measurement in persons in pain. In: Wall PD, Melzack R, eds. *Textbook of Pain.* 3rd ed. New York: Churchill Livingstone; 1994:337–351.

101. Hardy JD, Wolff HG, Goodell H. Studies on pain: discrimination of differences in pain as a basis of a scale of pain intensity. *J Clin Invest.* 1947;26:1152–1158.

102. Cella D, Pulliam J, Fuchs H, et al. Evaluation of pain associated with oral mucositis during the acute period after administration of high-dose chemotherapy. *Cancer.* 2003;98:406–412.

103. Backonja M. Personal communication.

104. Carr DB, Goudas LC, Balk EM, et al. Evidence report on the treatment of pain in cancer patients. *J Natl Cancer Inst Monogr.* 2004;32: 23–31.

105. Jensen MP. The validity and reliability of pain measures in adults with cancer. *J Pain.* 2003;4:2–21.

106. Collins SL, Moore RA, McQuay HJ. The visual analogue pain intensity scale: what is moderate pain in millimetres? *Pain.* 1997;72:95–97.

107. Serlin RC, Mendoza TR, Nakamura Y, et al. When is cancer pain mild, moderate or severe? Grading pain severity by its interference with function. *Pain.* 1995;61:277–284.

108. Paul SM, Zelman DC, Smith M, et al. Categorizing the severity of cancer pain: further exploration of the establishment of cut points. *Pain.* 2005; 113:37–44.

109. Chang VT, Hwang SS, Xia Q, et al. Pain distress in veteran cancer patients. American Pain Society, *J Pain.* 2005;6(Suppl. 1):S82; Abstract 897.

110. Farrar JT, Berlin JA, Strom BL. Clinically important changes in acute pain outcome measures: a validation study. *J Pain Symptom Manage.* 2003;25:406–411.

111. Farrar JT, Young JP, LaMoreaux L, et al. Clinical importance of changes in pain intensity measured on a 11-point numerical pain rating scale. *Pain.* 2001;94:149–158.

112. Carr DB, Goudas LC, Balk EM, et al. Evidence report on the treatment of pain in cancer patients. *J Natl Cancer Inst Monogr.* 2004;32:23–31.

113. Hwang SS, Chang VT, Kasimis B. Dynamic cancer pain management outcomes: the relationship between pain severity, pain relief, functional interference, satisfaction, and global quality of life over time *J Pain Symptom Manage.* 2002;23:190–200.

114. Woolf CJ. Pain: moving from symptom control toward mechanism-specific pharmacologic management. *Ann Intern Med.* 2004;140: 441–451.

115. Galer BS, Jensen MP. Development and preliminary validation of a pain measure specific to neuropathic pain: the Neuropathic Pain Scale. *Neurology.* 1997;48:332–336.

116. Bennett M. The LANSS pain scale: the Leeds assessment of neuropathic symptoms and signs. *Pain.* 2001;92:147–157.

117. Krause SJ, Backonja MM. Development of a Neuropathic Pain Questionnaire. *Clin J Pain.* 2003;19:306–314.

118. Jensen TS, Baron R. Translation of symptoms and signs into mechanisms in neuropathic pain. *Pain.* 2003;102:1–8.

119. Sindrup SH, Jensen TS. Efficacy of pharmacological treatments of neuropathic pain: an update and effect related to mechanism of action. *Pain.* 1999;83:389–400.

120. Hansson PT, Dickenson AH. Pharmacological treatment of peripheral neuropathic pain conditions based on shared commonalities despite multiple etiologies. Topical review. *Pain.* 2005;113:251–254.

121. Foley KM. Acute and chronic cancer pain syndromes. In: Doyle D, Hanks G, Cherny NI, Calman K, eds. *Oxford Textbook of Palliative Medicine,* 3rd ed. New York: Oxford University Press; 2004:298–316.

122. Cherny NI. Cancer pain: principles of assessment and syndromes. In: Berger AM, Portenoy RK, Weissman D, eds. *Principles and Practice of Palliative Care and Supportive Oncology.* 2nd ed. Philadelphia: Lippincott Williams and Wilkins; 2003:3–52.

123. Portenoy RK, Conn M. Cancer pain syndromes. In: Bruera E, Portenoy RK, eds. *Cancer Pain. Assessment and Management.* New York: Cambridge University Press; 2003:89–108.

124. Twycross R. Cancer pain syndromes. In: Sykes N, Fallon MT, Patt RB, eds. *Clinical Pain Management: Cancer Pain.* London: Arnold; 2003:3–20.

125. Merskey H, Bogduk N. *Classification of Chronic Pain.* 2nd ed. Seattle: IASP Press; 1994:45.

126. Mekhail N, Kapural L. Complex regional pain syndrome type I in cancer patients. *Curr Rev Pain.* 2000;4:227–233.

127. Merskey H, Bogduk N. *Classification of Chronic Pain.* 2nd ed. Seattle: IASP Press; 1994:41–43.

128. Baron R, Fields HL, Janig W, et al. National Institutes of Health Workshop: Reflex sympathetic dystrophy/complex regional pain syndromes—state-of-the-science. *Anesth Analg.* 2002;95:1812–1816.

129. Campbell JN. Complex regional pain syndrome and the sympathetic nervous system. Pain 1996—An Updated Review, Refresher Course Syllabus. Seattle: IASP Press; 1996:89–96.

130. Schug SA, Zech D, Dorr U. Cancer pain management according to WHO analgesic guidelines. *J Pain Symptom Manage.* 1990;5:27–32.

131. Hwang WS, Tsai YF, Chang HC, et al. A prospective study of pain treatment for patients with advanced cancer who receive hospice home care. *Zhonghua Yi Xue Za Zhi (Taipei).* 2002;65:331–335.

132. Cherny NI, Portenoy RK. Sedation in the management of refractory symptoms: guidelines for evaluation and treatment. *J Palliat Care.* 1994;10:31–38.

133. Kuuppelomaki M. Pain management problems in patients terminal phase as assessed by nurses in Finland. *J Adv Nurs.* 2002;40:701–709.

134. Miaskowski C, Dodd MJ, West C, et al. Lack of adherence with the analgesic regimen: a significant barrier to effective cancer pain management. *J Clin Oncol.* 2001;19:4275–4279.

135. Schumacher KL, West C, Dodd M, et al. Pain management autobiographies and reluctance to use opioids for cancer pain management. *Cancer Nurs.* 2002;25:125–133.

136. Terman GW, Loeser JD. A case of opiate-insensitive pain: malignant treatment of benign pain. *Clin J Pain.* 1992;8:255–259.

137. Fitzgibbon DR, Galer BS. The efficacy of opioids in cancer pain syndromes. *Pain.* 1994;58:429–431.

138. Lawlor P, Walker P, Bruera E, et al. Severe opioid toxicity and somatization of psychosocial distress in a cancer patient with a background of chemical dependence. *J Pain Symptom Manage.* 1997;13:356–361.

139. Al-Shahri MZ, Molina EH, Onschuk D. Medication-focused approach to total pain: poor symptom control, polypharmacy, and adverse reactions. *Am J Hosp Palliat Care.* 2003;20:307–310.

140. Mercadante S, Portenoy RK. Opioid poorly-responsive cancer pain. Part 1: Clinical considerations. *J Pain Symptom Manage.* 2001;21:144–150.

141. Mercadante S, Portenoy RK. Opioid poorly-responsive cancer pain. Part 2: Basic mechanisms that could shift dose response for analgesia. *J Pain Symptom Manage.* 2001;21:255–264.

142. Mercadante S, Portenoy RK. Opioid poorly-responsive cancer pain. Part 3: Clinical strategies to improve opioid responsiveness. *J Pain Symptom Manage.* 2001;21:338–354.

143. Coyle N, Breitbart W, Weaver S, Portenoy R. Delirium as a contributing factor to "crescendo" pain: three case reports. *J Pain Symptom Manage.* 1994;9:44–47.

144. Meuser T, Pietruck C, Radbruch L, et al. Symptoms during cancer pain treatment following WHO-guidelines: a longitudinal follow-up study of symptom prevalence, severity and etiology. *Pain.* 2001;93: 247–257.

145. Chang VT, Hwang S, Feuerman M, et al. Symptom and Quality of Life Survey of Medical Oncology Patients at a Veterans Affairs Medical Center. A Role for Symptom Assessment. *Cancer.* 2000:88: 1175–1183.

146. Passik SD, Kirsh SL. Managing pain in patients with aberrant drug-taking behaviors. *J Support Oncol.* 2005;3:83–86.

147. Goodkin R, Carr BI, Perrin RG. Herniated lumbar disc disease in patients with malignancy. *J Clin Oncol.* 1987;5:667–671.

148. Bonica JJ, Loeser JD. Applied anatomy relevant to pain. In: Butler C, Chapman C, Turk DC, eds. *Bonica's Management of Pain,* 3rd ed. Philadelphia: Lippincott Williams and Wilkins; 2001:196–209.

149. Coda BA, Bonica JJ. General considerations of acute pain. In: Butler C, Chapman C, Turk DC, eds. *Bonica's Management of Pain,* 3rd ed. Philadelphia: Lippincott Williams and Wilkins; 2001:225–235.

150. Dejerine J. *Seminologie des affectations du system nerveux.* Paris: Masson et Cie; 1914:831–839.

151. Wisneski RJ, Garfin SR, Rothman RH. Lumbar disc disease. In: Rothman RH, Simeone FA, eds. *The Spine,* 3rd ed. Philadelphia: WB Saunders; 1992:689–699.

152. Wolfe F, Cathey MA. The epidemiology of tender points: a prospective study of 1520 patients. *J Rheumatol.* 1985;12:1164–1168.

153. Wolfe F, Smythe HA, Yunus MB, et al. The American College of Rheumatology 1990 criteria for the classification of fibromyalgia: report of the multicenter criteria committee. *Arthritis Rheum.* 1990;33:160–172.

154. http://www.rheumatology.org/publications/classification/fibromyalgia/fibro.asp?aud=mem.

155. Smythe H. Examination for tenderness: learning to use 4 kg force. *J Rheumatol.* 1998;25:149–151.

156. Selwyn AP, Braunwald E. Ischemic heart disease. In: Fauci A, Braunwald E, Isselbacher KS, Lilson JD, Martin JB, Kasper DL, Hauser SL, Longo DL, eds. *Harrison's Textbook of Internal Medicine,* 14th ed. New York: McGraw-Hill; 1998:1367–1368.

157. Demco L. Mapping the source and character of pain due to endometriosis by patient-assisted laparoscopy. *J Am Assoc Gynecol Laparosc.* 1998; 5:241–245.

158. Yeung MC, Hagen NA. Cervical disc herniation presenting with chest wall pain. *Can J Neurol Sci.* 1993;20:59–61.

159. Cunningham J, Temple WJ, Mitchell P, et al. Cooperative hernia study: pain in the postrepair patient. *Ann Surgery.* 1996;224:598–602.

160. Abdominal wall tenderness test: could Carnett cut costs? *Lancet.* 1991;337:1134.

161. Hershfield NB. The abdominal wall: a frequently overlooked source of abdominal pain. *J Clin Gastroenterol.* 1992;14:199–202.

162. Hagen NA. Reproducing a cancer patient's pain on physical examination: bedside provocative maneuvers. *J Pain Symptom Manage.* 1999;18: 406–411.

163. Sandler RS, Drossman DA. Bowel habits in young adults not seeking health care. *Dig Dis Sci.* 1987;32:841–845.

164. Johanson JF, Sonnenberg A, Koch TR. Clinical epidemiology of chronic constipation. *J Clin Gasteroenterol.* 1989;11:525–536.

165. Thompson WG, Longstreth GF, Drossman DA, et al. Functional bowel disorders and functional abdominal pain. *Gut.* 1999;45(Suppl. II): II43–II47.

166. Connell AM, Hilton C, Irvine G. Variation of bowel habit in two population samples. *Br Med J.* 1965;2:1095–1099.

167. Glia A, Lindberg G. Quality of life in patients with different types of functional constipation. *Scand J Gasteroenterol.* 1997;32:1083–1089.

168. Harari D, Gurwitz JH, Avorn J, et al. How do older persons define constipation? Implications for therapeutic management. *J Gen Intern Med.* 1997;12:63–66.

169. Heaton KW, O'Donnell LJ. An office guide to whole-gut transit time. Patients' recollection of their stool form. *J Clin Gastroenterol.* 1994;19: 28–30.

170. Aichbichler BW, Wenzl HH, Santa Ana CA, et al. A comparison of stool characteristics from normal and constipated people. *Dig Dis Sci.* 1998;43:2353–2362.

171. Heaton KW, Radvan J, Cripps H, et al. Defecation frequency and timing, and stool form in the general population: a prospective study. *Gut.* 1992;33:818–824.

172. Diamant NE, Kamm MA, Wald A, et al. American Gastroenterological Association technical review on anorectal testing techniques. *Gastroenterology.* 1999;116:735–760.

173. Mancini I, Bruera E. Constipation in advanced cancer patients. *Support Care Cancer.* 1998;6:356–364.

174. McMillan SC. Assessing and managing narcotic-induced constipation in adults with cancer. *Cancer Control.* 1999;6:198–204.

175. Locke GR III, Pemberton JH, Phillips SF. AGA technical review on constipation. American Gastroenterological Association. *Gastroenterology.* 2000;119:1766–1778.

176. Leroi AM, Bernier C, Watier A, et al. Prevalence of sexual abuse among patients with functional disorders of the lower gastrointestinal tract. *Int J Colorectal Dis.* 1995;10:200–206.

177. McMillan SC, Williams FA. Validity and reliability of the Constipation Assessment Scale. *Cancer Nurs.* 1989;12(3):183–188.

178. McMillan S, Moody L. Hospice patient and caregiver congruence in reporting patients' symptom intensity. *Cancer Nurs.* 2003;26(2): 113–118.

179. Frank L, Kleinman L, Farup L, et al. Psychometric validation of a constipation symptom assessment questionnaire. *Scand J Gasteroenterol.* 1999;9:870–877.

180. Frank L, Flynn J, Rothman M. Use of a self-report constipation questionnaire with older adults in long-term care. *Gerontologist.* 2001;41:778–786.

181. Agachan F, Chen T, Pfeifer J, et al. A constipation scoring system to simplify evaluation and management of constipated patients. *Dis Colon Rectum.* 1996;39:681–685.

182. Talley NJ, Phillips SF, Wiltgen CM, .et al Assessment of functional gastrointestinal disease: the bowel disease questionnaire. *Mayo Clin Proc.* 1990;65:1456–1479.

183. Herz MJ, Kahan E, Zalevski S, et al. Constipation: a different entity for patients and doctors. *Fam Pract.* 1996;13:156–159.

184. Friedrichsen M, Erichsen E. The lived experience of constipation in cancer patients in palliative hospital-based home care. *Int J Palliat Nurs.* 2004;10:321–325.

185. Lembo A, Camilleri M. Chronic constipation. *New Engl J Med.* 2003;349:1360–1368.

186. Starreveld JS, Pols MA, Van Wijk HJ, et al. The plain abdominal radiograph in the assessment of constipation. *Z Gastroenterol.* 1990;28: 335–338.

187. Bruera E, Suarez-Almazor M, Velasco A, et al. The assessment of constipation in terminal cancer patients admitted to a palliative care unit: a retrospective review. *J Pain Symptom Manage.* 1994;9:515–519.

188. McShane RE, McLane AM. Constipation: consensual and empirical validation. *Nurs Clin North Am.* 1985;20:801–808.

189. Kurz A, Sessler DI. Opioid-induced bowel dysfunction. Pathophysiology and potential new therapies. *Drugs.* 2003;63: 649–671.

190. Pappagallo M. Incidence, prevalence and management of opioid bowel dysfunction. *Am J Surgery.* 2001;182(Suppl.):11S–18S.

Pharmacology of Opioids and Other Analgesics

Eardie A. Curry III
Christopher Fausel

INTRODUCTION AND BASIC PRINCIPLES

Pain in cancer patients is common, and may be multifactorial or have a primary source.[1] Cancer pain can originate when the primary or metastatic tumor invades soft tissues, organs, bone, or causes nerve injury. Pain may be iatrogenic: radiation-induced mucositis, chemotherapy-induced peripheral neuropathy, radiation fibrosis, chronic postsurgical incision pain, as well as caused by infections and multiple other sources.[2,3]

Unfortunately, even with advances in the treatment of pain, and publication of guidelines by the World Health Organization (WHO) and the National Cancer Center Network, among others, a high percentage of cancer patients still have pain.[4–10] The American Chronic Pain Association guidelines state that the primary goal in treating chronic pain patients with opioids is to increase their level of function rather than to provide only symptom relief, optimize function, and minimize suffering.[11] Chemotherapy, such as gemcitabine in pancreatic cancer, may be used to palliate pain in the setting of advanced cancer.[12] For patients who need analgesia, pain medicines must be appropriately utilized. The focus of this chapter is to outline the pharmacodynamic, pharmacokinetic, and toxicity profiles of the major classes of drugs used to treat patients with cancer pain.

NONOPIOID ANALGESICS

▶ Nonsteroidal anti-inflammatory agents

Nonsteroidal anti-inflammatory agents (NSAIDs) are frontline therapy for mild to moderate cancer pain.[4] NSAIDs are a diverse group of drugs that inhibit the cyclooxygenase (COX) enzyme, which exists as two isoforms. The constitutive isoform, COX-1, is needed for normal homeostasis, and is expressed in the endothelium, stomach, kidneys, and platelets. COX-2 is considered to be the inducible isoform, as it is expressed in the body during the inflammatory process. Known pharmacologic effects of NSAIDs include pain relief, antipyresis, and anti-inflammation.

Side effects include renal insufficiency, potential alterations in vascular tone, gastric irritation, platelet inhibition, hepatic dysfunction, sodium retention, hyponatremia, and central nervous system (CNS) effects such as dizziness, sedation, and confusion.

NSAIDs have a demonstrated ceiling effect. That is, beyond a certain dose, the risk of side effects increases while the analgesic benefit does not. This maximum effective dose varies among the NSAID agents. The response to various NSAIDs is widely variable. Due to their ceiling effect, NSAIDs are not recommended as the sole agent for treating moderate to severe pain. Dose titration within the therapeutic index, as well as rotation to another agent, are both reasonable ways to maximize the therapeutic benefit of the NSAID class. If one NSAID does not work, then rotation to another may benefit the patient.

NSAIDs have traditionally been used for both acute and chronic pain. Some of the chronic pain syndromes that NSAIDs are used for include headaches, low back pain, fibromyalgia, and cancer pain. For the purpose of discussion, the NSAIDs will be broken down into the following subclassifications based on chemical structure: salicylates, acetic acids, propionic acid derivatives, benzothiazine derivatives, alkanones, and COX-2-specific inhibitors. The drug names, the usual starting doses, and the recommended maximum daily doses are listed in Table 2-1.

Salicylates

The salicylates include aspirin, choline magnesium trisalicylate, and diflunisal. Aspirin is perhaps the most commonly used pain medicine. It is used for its anti-inflammatory as well as its cardioprotective antiplatelet effect. Aspirin irreversibly binds both COX isoforms, so platelet function can be impaired for as long as a week, and is reestablished only after new platelets are produced. Common side effects of aspirin include stomach upset, nausea, gastrointestinal (GI) ulceration and hemorrhage, as well as liver and kidney dysfunction.

Choline magnesium trisalicylate and diflunisal cause less GI irritability and less platelet inhibition than aspirin. They are both excellent anti-inflammatory and antianalgesic salicylates.

Acetic acids

Agents in the pyrrolacetic acid class include diclofenac and ketorolac. Besides GI difficulties, diclofenac requires periodic liver function tests with use beyond 8 weeks. Diclofenac is preferential to COX-2 over COX-1, and therefore seems to produce less GI toxicity. Ketorolac is an excellent analgesic, but its high toxicity profile (GI and renal) precludes its use beyond 5 days. Parenteral and oral forms are available, but the drug is mainly used postoperatively.[13] Indoleacetic acid derivatives include etodolac, indomethacin, and sulindac. Etodolac is the third agent in the class, but it appears to have a cleaner side-effect profile than both sulindac and indomethacin.[14] Indomethacin has been widely used, but its high incidence of GI toxicity, and other adverse events such as depression and fluid retention, limits its application in the management of cancer pain.

Table 2-1

Nonopioid Analgesics

Generic Names	Dosing Schedule	Recommended Starting Dose (mg/dose)	Maximum Daily Dose (mg)	Comment
Salicylates				
Aspirin	Q4-6H	325–650 PO	4000	Irreversibly binds platelets
Choline magnesium trisalicylate	Q12H	1500 X1, then 1000 Q12H	4000	–
Diflunisal	Q8-12H	1000 mg X1 PO, then 250–500 PO	1500	–
Acetic Acids				
Diclofenac	Q8-12H	50–75	200	Less GI events vs. ketorolac
Ketorolac tromethamine	Q6H	30 mg IM/IV X1, then 15 mg IM/IV/PO Q6H	120	Use ≤5 days. Lower dose for age >65, renal impairment, or weight <50 kg
Etodolac	Q6-8H	200–400	1200	–
Indomethacin	Q8-12H	25–50	200	Toxicity limits use
Sulindac	BID	150	400	Reversible hepatotoxicity
Propionic Acids				
Ibuprofen	Q4-6H	400 PO	3200	Widely used
Naproxen	Q12H	250	1250	More GI side effects than ibuprofen
Naproxen sodium	Q12H	275	1375	
Ketoprofen	Q6-8H	25–50	300	–
Oxaprozin	Q24H	600	1800	Single daily dosing
Benzothiazines				
Piroxicam	Q daily	20	40	Meloxicam has a better GI profile than piroxicam*,†
Meloxicam	Q24H	7.5	15	
Alkanones				
Nabumetone	Q daily	1000	2000	
Selective COX-2 Inhibitors				
Celecoxib	Q12-24H	100	400	Please see Table 2-2
Valdecoxib	Q24H	10	40	
p-Aminophenol Derivative				
Acetaminophen	Q4-6H	650–1000 PO 650 PR	4000	Use with caution in liver dysfunction
Corticosteroids				
Dexamethasone	BID-QID	2–8 mg PO/SC/IV	For pain: ~16	For CNS issues doses may be much higher‡

Note: Mefenamic acid, meclofenamic acid, and phenylbutazone are not recommended for cancer pain therapy.
*All medications are oral, unless otherwise specified.
†These medications can also be given rectally in suppository forms.
‡CNS issues: spinal cord compression, brain metastases, or herniation. Other corticosteroids may also be used.

Sulindac is less toxic than indomethacin, but it has been causally linked to reversible liver dysfunction.[15]

Propionic acids

This class of agents includes ibuprofen, naproxen, ketoprofen, and oxaprozin. Ibuprofen is available over the counter and by prescription, alone and in combination with other agents such as oxycodone and hydrocodone. Naproxen has more GI side effects than ibuprofen.[16] The National Institute on Aging halted a clinical trial studying naproxen in patients who were at risk of developing Alzheimer's disease when preliminary analysis showed evidence of increased risk of cardiovascular events compared to placebo.[17] Ketoprofen has also been linked to GI side effects.[18] The 55-hour half-life of oxaprozin allows this drug to be prescribed on a once-a-day schedule.[19] With regard to usage and experience, ibuprofen is the agent with the best combination of flexible dosing and side-effect profile in this class.

Benzothiazines

The two agents in this class are meloxicam and piroxicam. A small study (n = 44) in healthy volunteers, and a large trial in patients with osteoarthritis demonstrated the GI adverse effect profile superiority of meloxicam over piroxicam.[20,21] Meloxicam, due to its COX-2-selective reduced side-effect profile, is the agent of choice in this subclass of NSAIDs.

Alkanones

Nabumetone is a partially selective COX-2 inhibitor that is acceptable for use in cancer pain. It has a superior GI side-effect profile compared to other selected NSAIDs, such as piroxicam and sustained-release diclofenac.[22,23]

Selective COX-2 inhibitors

It is believed that COX-2 selectivity prevents GI toxicity, and three agents have been marketed as selective COX-2 inhibitors in the United States: celecoxib, rofecoxib, and valdecoxib. These agents are touted to relieve pain, while avoiding the negative side effects (such as dyspepsia) of nonselective NSAIDs.[24,25] However, there is ongoing debate about the efficacy and side effects of these agents. In head-to-head clinical trials, COX-2-specific agents do not always improve efficacy or lower the total adverse side-effect profile compared to traditional NSAIDs.[26,27] The recent withdrawal from the market of rofecoxib due to cardiac-related deaths has cast a veil of suspicion on the chronic use of COX-2-specific agents to treat cancer pain (Table 2-2).[28,29] Celecoxib and valdecoxib remain on the market and have utility in the treatment of cancer pain. However, a large randomized trial looking at celecoxib for colorectal adenoma prevention demonstrated a dose-related increase in the composite endpoint of death from cardiovascular causes, myocardial infarction, stroke, or heart failure.[30] Safety concerns about agents in this class illustrate the fact that additional studies are needed to determine the safety of COX-2 inhibitors in the chronic treatment of cancer pain.[31,32]

▶ Other Nonopioid analgesics

Acetaminophen

Acetaminophen is used for mild cancer pain. It is available orally, rectally, and in many combination products. It is metabolized in the liver to inactive metabolites, and its half-life is between 2 and 4 hours. Acetaminophen is an excellent adjuvant treatment for malignant pain and has been combined with many opioid and nonopioid pain analgesics.[33] The maximum adult dose of acetaminophen is 4000 mg/day, but caution should be used for patients who drink more than three alcoholic drinks every day, or have known liver disease. Side effects can include hypothermia, rash, GI bleeding, hepatotoxicity, and nephrotoxicity.

Corticosteroids

Corticosteroids are an excellent analgesic, alone or combined with opioids, especially where there is spinal cord compression, cancer-related brain complications (herniation, edema, or metastases), as well as malignant nerve and bone pain.[34–37] Due to their adverse event profile, they are recommended only for patients with advanced disease or for short-term use, particularly in the palliative care setting. The agent of choice for adjuvant pain control is usually dexamethasone dosed at 2–16 mg/day in 2–4 divided doses via oral, subcutaneous (SC), or intravenous routes (IV). Short-term side effects can include euphoria/depression, GI distress, hypertension, impaired skin healing, increased risk of infection, increased appetite, weight gain, and hyperglycemia.

OPIOID ANALGESICS

▶ Physiological effects of opioid agonists

Drugs that bind to opioid receptors (mu, kappa, and delta) to produce analgesia are classified as opioid agonists, and they are the backbone of cancer pain management in patients with moderate to severe pain. Opioid receptors are spread throughout the body, and as such, this class of agents, in addition to altering analgesia, can affect respiratory, cardiovascular, GI, and neuroendocrine function. Delta-receptor agonists are also potent analgesics in animals whose clinical development has been limited by their inability to cross the blood–brain barrier. Metkephamid, a relatively selective delta opioid receptor agonist, causes orthostatic hypotension in healthy volunteers, with an attenuated change in heart rate and no increase in noradrenalin concentration.[38] There are currently no pure delta-receptor agonists on the market or in clinical trials. Kappa (K)-receptor-selective agonists may produce less severe respiratory depression and miosis. K-receptor agonists engender dysphoria and psychotomimetic effects.[39] They are primarily being studied for use in visceral pain and irritable bowel syndrome.[40,41] Buprenorphine, a partial agonist at the mu-opioid receptor and an antagonist at the kappa-opioid receptor, is U.S. Food and Drug Administration (FDA)-approved for the management of opioid dependence.

Table 2-2

Cardiovascular Morbidity and COX-2-Specific Inhibitors

Author	Drug	Dose	No. of Patients	CV Death Rate (%) Treatment	CV Death Rate (%) Placebo
Bombardier[28]	Rofecoxib	50 mg daily	4047	0.2	0.2
Bresalier[32]	Rofecoxib	25 mg daily	1287	0.2	0.07
Solomon[30]	Celecoxib	400 vs. 800 mg daily	400 mg: 685	400 mg: 3.8	2.5
			800 mg: 671	800 mg: 4.6	
Nussmeier[31]	Valdecoxib (V) Parecoxib + valdecoxib (P/V)	(V): 40 mg daily (P/V): (P) 40 mg IV daily then (V) 40 mg daily	Both arms: 544	(P): 0.4 (P/V): 0.6	0

Abbreviation: CV = cardiovascular.

Transdermal buprenorphine has efficacy in the treatment of chronic pain, which may move buprenorphine into a more prominent role in treating cancer pain.[42] For now, buprenorphine use should be limited to clinical trials that will best determine its place in therapy.

Despite aggressive marketing of newer agents, morphine remains the gold standard opioid for moderate to severe cancer pain. Morphine, as do most other clinically relevant opioid agonists, wields its effects through interaction with mu-opioid receptors. However, there are multiple mechanisms of action among mu-opioid receptor subtypes, and the response to morphine is variable.[43] There appear to be differences in interindividual receptor mu-subtype expression. Individual variables, such as renal and hepatic function, oral tolerance, receptor polymorphisms, types of pain and others, affect analgesia relief with opioids. Due to this interindividual variability, if a patient fails to achieve relief with one opioid, rotation is a reasonable therapeutic option (Table 2-3).[44–47]

▶ Opioid analgesia for mild to moderate pain

Codeine

Codeine (methylmorphine) is the prototype of a weaker opioid analgesic. Codeine is given primarily via the oral route, with a 200-mg dose of codeine equal to a 30-mg oral dose of morphine. It has an oral bioavailability of approximately 60%. Codeine has a half-life of 2–4 hours, and is considered a prodrug, with approximately 10% of administered codeine being o-demethylated, by cytochrome P-450 enzyme (CYP450) CYP2D6, to form morphine, the active metabolite. Codeine is considered to be the standard centrally acting antitussive.[48] The antitussive action of codeine appears to involve specific receptors that bind codeine itself.[49] Codeine is often combined with other nonopioid agents, and constipation and nausea are its most common side effects. For patients who need mild pain control, but want to avoid NSAIDs, single agent codeine is an appropriate option.

Renal Dysfunction Caution is recommended in using codeine for patients with renal impairment.[50] Irwin et al. recommend the following dose reductions: for creatinine clearance (CrCl) greater than 50 mL/min—no dose adjustment, for CrCl between 10 and 50 mL/min—25% dose reduction, and for CrCl less than 10 mL/min—50% dose reduction.[51] The same caution used for dosing morphine in renal dysfunction should be applied to codeine.

Hepatic Dysfunction Codeine should be dosed with caution in the presence of hepatic dysfunction, as the duration of action of morphine will be prolonged and requires dose adjustment.

Hydrocodone

Hydrocodone is a semisynthetic, centrally acting narcotic analgesic and anticough agent that is chemically related to codeine.[49] Hydrocodone combination products that contain either acetaminophen or ibuprofen are available to treat pain. Both agents' daily usage is limited by the nonhydrocodone component. However, hydrocodone combination products have shown efficacy in clinical trials for chronic pain, exercise-induced muscle damage, postoperative pain, and acute low back pain.[52–56] While the hydrocodone-ibuprofen combination should be taken with food, and is FDA-approved for less than 10 days usage, acetaminophen-containing products do not have either restriction. Side effects include nausea, vomiting, skin rash, pruritus, respiratory depression, drowsiness, and constipation.

Renal Dysfunction The presence of renal failure may require dose reductions of hydrocodone, but data evaluating the kinetics of the drug in renal failure are lacking.

Hepatic Dysfunction The effects of liver disease on the pharmacokinetics of hydrocodone have not been studied. Obviously, most

Table 2-3

Opioid Analgesics

Opioid	Usual Starting dose	Maximum Daily Dose
Codeine (alone or with acetaminophen or aspirin)	PO/IM/SC: 15–30 of codeine Q3-4H	360 mg of codeine or 4000 mg of acetaminophen or aspirin
Hydrocodone (with acetaminophen, ibuprofen, or aspirin)	PO: 5–10 mg Q3-4H IV: NA	40 mg of hydrocodone or 4000 mg of acetaminophen or 3200 mg of ibuprofen
Oxycodone (alone or with acetaminophen)	PO: 5–10 mg Q3-4H IV: NA	4000 mg of acetaminophen
Tramadol (alone or with acetaminophen)	PO: 25 mg PO QID IV: NA	400 mg of tramadol or 4000 mg of acetaminophen
Morphine	PO: 5–10 mg Q3-4H IV/IM/SC: 5–10 mg Q3-4H	Maximum daily dose of these agents is limited only by toxicity. There is no analgesic "ceiling effect."
Oxycodone	PO: 5–10 mg Q3-4H	
Hydromorphone	PO: 2–4 mg Q3-4H IV/IM/SC: 1–2 mg Q3-4H PR: 3 mg Q6-8H	
Fentanyl	TOP: 25 μg/hpatch SL: 200 μg QID IV/SQ: 25–50 μg CIV	
Methadone	Starting dose: please see Table 2-5. Route: IV/SC/PR/PO/SL	

Abbreviations: PO = oral, IM = intramuscular, SC/SQ = subcutaneous, IV = intravenous, PR = rectal, SL = sublingual, TOP = topically, CIV = continuous intravenous infusion.

hydrocodone preparations contain acetaminophen, so caution should be used in dosing acetaminophen in the presence of known hepatic dysfunction.

Tramadol

Tramadol is FDA-approved for oral usage, but is used parenterally in non-U.S. markets. It has a 70% bioavailability, half-life = 1.7 hours, one active metabolite (M1) produced by CYP2D6, and is mainly excreted via the kidneys. Tramadol is a mild mu agonist, with additional nonopioid properties evidenced by its lack of naloxone reversibility. It also prohibits the neuronal reuptake of norepinephrine and serotonin.[57] Duration of analgesia is approximately 6 hours, and it has shown efficacy for both cancer and neuropathy pain.[58–61] Tramadol should be tried in patients in whom neuropathy contributes to their pain syndrome. Side effects include constipation, diarrhea, nausea, vomiting, dizziness, drowsiness, headache, pruritus, anaphylactic reactions, cognitive dysfunction, hallucinations, seizures, dyspnea (rare), orthostatic hypotension (rare), syncope (rare), and tachycardia (rare).

Renal Dysfunction In renal impairment (CrCl <30 mL/min), increase the dosing interval to 12 hours with a maximum of 200 mg/day.[62]

Hepatic Dysfunction The recommended dose for patients with cirrhosis is 50 mg every 12 hours.[62] Other researchers believe that alternative options should be exercised for patients with cirrhosis.[63]

Propoxyphene

Propoxyphene is a synthetic analgesic related to methadone, reportedly equipotent to codeine. The duration of its analgesic effect is 3–6 hours. However, the effect of propoxyphene's major metabolite, norpropoxyphene, is 30–36 hours, which is thought to be responsible for the drug's side effects: sedation, dizziness, light-headedness, nausea, vomiting, and constipation. Norpropoxyphene has proarrhythmic effects, and is considered inappropriate for patients older than 65 years. Patients with renal or hepatic dysfunction are more sensitive to its adverse effects. In addition to its side-effect profile, propoxyphene is no more effective than, and is perhaps inferior to, acetaminophen, aspirin, codeine, or ibuprofen.[64] Propoxyphene should not be used for cancer pain, especially in elderly patients.[5]

▶ Opioid analgesia for moderate to severe pain

Morphine

Morphine is the prototype strong opioid, and is the drug of choice for severe cancer pain.[4,5,65] Morphine may be administered through rectal, oral, and multiple parenteral routes, with a half-life of approximately 2 hours. Oral immediate-release products usually provide analgesia for 2–4 hours. Sustained-release formulations can be commenced after titration with the immediate-release or parenteral products, and can provide analgesia by dosing as infrequently as once daily.[66] Morphine is also available as an extended-release liposomal epidural injection.[67]

Morphine undergoes glucoronidation in the liver, mainly into two major metabolites: morphine-3-glucuronide (M3G) and morphine-6-glucuronide (M6G). M6G binds to mu receptors with a similar affinity as morphine, provides analgesia, and may account for the lowered ratio of parenteral to oral ration (3:1) observed with chronic morphine administration.[68] M3G does not provide analgesia, and

may actually contribute to the adverse reactions (allodynia, myoclonus, seizures, hyperanalgesia) to morphine.[69,70] Using in vitro models, Hemstapat et al. hypothesize that M3G's neuroexcitatory effects are mediated via indirect activation of *N*-methyl-*D*-aspartic acid receptors.[71] Both of these water-soluble metabolites are cleared by renal excretion, and their accumulation can lead to an increased incidence of side effects.[72] The serum concentrations of morphine, M6G, and M3G do not predict pain intensity, cognitive function, constipation, nausea, fatigue, treatment failure, or treatment success, so therapeutic drug monitoring of morphine and its two major metabolites has limited clinical value.[73,74] Morphine is excreted through glomerular filtration, primarily as M3G, with 90% of the total excretion occurring in the first day. The side effects of morphine include constipation, nausea, urinary retention, vomiting, dizziness, headache, light-headedness, sedation, weakness, allergic reaction, confusion, histamine release, hypotension, and respiratory depression.

Renal Dysfunction It has been recommended that patients with moderate renal failure (glomerular filtration rate [GFR] 10–50 mL/min) receive 75% of the normal dose at the usual intervals, and patients with severe renal failure (GFR less than 10 mL/min) receive half of the normal dose at the usual intervals; no dosage adjustment is necessary for patients with mild renal failure (GFR greater than 50 mL/min).[75] For patients who have rapidly changing renal function, or those with baseline renal insufficiency, caution should be used before dosing morphine.

Hepatic Dysfunction Studies of morphine in patients with cirrhosis and decompensated liver function demonstrate reduced morphine clearance and altered production of metabolites, as well as a doubling of morphine's half-life when compared to normal hepatic function.[76,77] The duration of action of morphine is prolonged in patients with hepatic insufficiency, and dosages should be adjusted. For cirrhotic patients, Mazoit et al. recommend increasing the dosing interval of morphine by 1.5–2 times that of a normal dose.[76]

Oxycodone

Oxycodone has received much negative media publicity for its abuse.[78–80] Due to the legal issues swirling around this product, the smallest number of pills needed to safely treat the patient should be dispensed, with monthly follow-up to reassess the patient's analgesia requirements. Similar to other opioids, but especially with oxycodone, healthcare providers should be mindful of patients who obtain (or attempt to obtain) early refills or patients who present prescriptions from several doctors for similar medications. In an attempt to avoid diversions and outright theft, some pharmacies in problem areas (such as the Appalachian states) are no longer stocking oxycodone on their shelves.

Oxycodone is a semisynthetic opioid with a high bioavailability (>50%) after oral dosing. The half-life is 2–3 hours, and its duration of action is 4–6 hours. Oxycodone has two main metabolites: noroxycodone and oxymorphone, the latter of which is an active metabolite formed through *O*-demethylation catalyzed by CYP2D6. Oxymorphone accounts for 10% of the oxycodone metabolites, and is considered to be 14 times more potent than oxycodone. However, oxycodone has two metabolites that are present in plasma in such low concentrations that they are thought not to contribute to the pharmacological effects of oxycodone.[81,82] When combined with either acetaminophen or aspirin, oxycodone is used for mild to moderate pain control. However, when used as a sole agent, oxycodone (in both the immediate and sustained-release formulation) should be considered a high potency opioid. Oxycodone can be used for around-the-clock as well as breakthrough dosing. There are no FDA-approved parenteral formulations. Parris and Kaplan each demonstrated that opioid-exposed cancer pain patients can be treated with either controlled-release oxycodone (CRO) administered every 12 hours or immediate-release oxycodone four times daily at the same total daily dose, with CRO offering the benefits of twice daily dosing.[83,84] Citron et al. used CRO tablets every 12 hours to successfully manage cancer pain over a 12-week period. Importantly, side effects diminished over time without a concomitant change in efficacy.[85] In a randomized, double-blind crossover study of controlled release morphine and oxycodone (median oxycodone:morphine ration of 1.5:1), no significant differences in adverse effects and similar efficacy and preference in the treatment of cancer pain were observed.[86] Side effects of oxycodone can include asthenia, dizziness, light-headedness, sedation, constipation, dry mouth, nausea, vomiting, pruritus, apnea, respiratory arrest, respiratory depression, and hypotension.

Renal Dysfunction As elimination half-life is increased by 1 hour, dose initiation of oxycodone in patients with CrCl less than 60 mL/min should be conservative with dosages adjusted according to the clinical situation.

Hepatic Dysfunction Oxycodone should be started at one-third to one-half of the usual dose in patients with hepatic impairment and dose titration should proceed carefully. The mean elimination half-life of oxycodone in end-stage liver disease is 13.9 hours. After liver transplant, half-life returns to 3.4 hours.[87] Therefore, care must be exercised when oxycodone is used in cirrhosis or end-stage liver disease, and it is necessary either to reduce doses or to extend dose intervals.

Hydromorphone

Hydromorphone is a hydrophilic semisynthetic opioid that is available for administration through the oral, parenteral, and rectal routes. For the patient who does not tolerate morphine, or for whom morphine does not provide adequate analgesia, hydromorphone is an excellent alternative. Hydromorphone has a bioavailability of ~50% (oral) and ~35% (rectal), with an oral:parenteral analgesic potency ratio of 5:1.[88,89] Its half-life is approximately 2 hours. Hydromorphone is primarily metabolized to hydromorphone-3-glucuronide (H3G) in the liver and excreted via the kidneys. In rats, infusions of H3G into the cerebrospinal fluid have been shown to cause agitation, myoclonus, and seizures in a dose-dependent manner.[90] Thwaites completed a retrospective study looking at three neuroexcitatory opioid symptoms: agitation, myoclonus, and seizures. These three symptoms appeared to be independently associated with the dose of hydromorphone and the number of days on treatment. The incidence of having one of these symptoms increased to greater than 50% if the continuous parenteral hydromorphone dose was greater than 20 mg/h and was used for more than 15 days. These findings suggest that continuous parenteral hydromorphone has few neuroexcitatory symptoms until hydromorphone accumulates past a neurotoxic threshold, at which point these symptoms manifest themselves. H3G concentrations accumulate with long-term dosing and renal insufficiency. Dying patients on elevated or extended doses of hydromorphone may be at an increased risk for H3G-induced neuroexcitatory symptoms because of the natural decline in renal function.[91] Side effects of hydromorphone include dizziness, drowsiness, sedation, weakness, loss of appetite, nausea, vomiting, respiratory depression, hypotension, confusion, myoclonus, and seizures.

Renal Dysfunction The role of hydromorphone in renal insufficiency is somewhat unclear, and it should be used with caution in renal impairment, as H3G may contribute to the side-effect profile. However, Lee et al. demonstrated the safety and efficacy of hydromorphone in the face of renal dysfunction.[92] Additional studies should elucidate the role of hydromorphone in renal dysfunction.

Hepatic Dysfunction Hydromorphone in moderate hepatic dysfunction (Child-Pugh score of 7–9) resulted in a 285% increase in the area under the curve (AUC) of drug.[93] Therefore, dosing reductions should be considered in patients with hepatic insufficiency, and patients must be closely monitored for toxicity.

Extended-release hydromorphone

In September 2004, the FDA approved an extended-release (ER) hydromorphone hydrochloride capsule for "the management of persistent, moderate to severe pain in patients requiring continuous, around-the-clock opioid analgesia with a high potency opioid for an extended period of time generally weeks to months or longer." Mean terminal half-life of hydromorphone in this compound, which contains individual controlled-release pellets of hydromorphone, is 18 hours. Hydromorphone ER should only be used in patients who are already receiving opioid therapy, who have demonstrated opioid tolerance, and who require a minimum total daily dose of opiate medication equivalent to 12 mg of oral hydromorphone. The manufacturer defines opioid tolerant as those patients who are taking at least 60 mg oral morphine/day, at least 30 mg oral oxycodone/day, at least 8 mg oral hydromorphone/day, or an equianalgesic dose of another opioid for a week or longer. Hydromorphone is dosed once daily, may not be chewed, crushed, or dissolved, and should never be used as a first-line opioid treatment.[94] Palangio et al. showed that hydromorphone ER could be titrated for efficacy in an outpatient setting for the treatment of chronic malignant and nonmalignant pain.[95] The best role of hydromorphone ER in the management of chronic pain is being defined, but along with methadone, morphine, oxycodone, and fentanyl, it provides a fifth option for using the same opioid for long-acting relief and breakthrough pain.

Hepatic Impairment Hydromorphone ER was not studied in patients with severe hepatic impairment and is not recommended for use in such patients. Care in initial dose selection and careful observation are recommended in patients with evidence of mild to moderate hepatic impairment.

Renal Impairment In patients with mild to moderate renal impairment, based on calculated CrCl, the concentrations of hydromorphone in plasma were slightly higher than in subjects with normal renal function. Dose should always be adjusted according to the clinical situation.

Fentanyl

Fentanyl is a potent, lipophilic, synthetic mu-opioid agonist. It is 80–100 times as potent as morphine.[65] The drug is metabolized primarily by *N*-dealkylation to norfentanyl and other inactive metabolites. Less than 10% of active drug is excreted unchanged in the urine. Fentanyl is metabolized by CYP3A4. Therefore, CYP3A4 inhibitors, such as macrolide antibiotics, may prolong the effect of fentanyl, and inducers, such as phenytoin, may decrease the effect of fentanyl. Time to peak analgesia after bolus intravenous fentanyl administration is ~5 minutes, but analgesia is quickly lost without further administration of drug. The short duration of effect (about 30 minutes) after the administration of a single dose of fentanyl is due to its rapid redistribution from the sites of action in the brain to storage sites (muscle and fat) and metabolism by the liver.[96] With repeated administration, continuous infusion, high doses, or application of a topical patch, accumulation in body tissue may lead to a prolonged duration of action.

In addition to parenteral administration, its lipophilic properties and potency allow it to be given through the transdermal and transmucosal routes. Terminal elimination half-life for transmucosal and parenteral fentanyl is about 3.5 hours, while the elimination half-life of transdermal fentanyl is 13–22 hours.[97,98] Side effects of fentanyl include asthenia, confusion, dizziness, sedation, constipation, dry mouth, nausea, vomiting, pruritus, sweating, urinary retention, arrhythmias and chest pain (1%–3%), hypertension, hypotension, apnea (3%–10%), hypoventilation, and respiratory depression.

Transmucosal Transmucosal fentanyl (TMF) is indicated only for the management of breakthrough cancer pain (BTP) in patients who are already receiving and are tolerant to opioid therapy for their underlying persistent cancer pain. The package insert defines opioid tolerant as patients who are taking at least 60 mg morphine/day, 50-μg transdermal fentanyl/hour, or an equianalgesic dose of another opioid for a week or longer. TMF must not be used in opioid naïve patients.[99] Lichtor et al. reported that the TMF:IV morphine equivalence was approximately 1:10.[100] However, the optimal dose of TMF needed to treat BTP requires titration, and is not predicted by the total daily dose of the fixed scheduled opioid.[101] In a randomized trial, Coluzzi et al. compared TMF to immediate-release morphine sulfate (MSIR) tablets. For all outcomes measured, TMF was superior to MSIR, and indicates that TMF is an effective option for the management of BTP in nonopioid naïve patients.[102] Burton and colleagues, in a retrospective chart review, observed success with TMF in the outpatient management of severe pain crises. For cancer pain patients taking at least 40 morphine equivalents per day, with a mean Visual Numeric Score (VNS) of 9, TMF was able to reduce the mean VNS to 3. Analgesia was provided while avoiding parenteral opioids and reducing hospitalizations (7.7% admissions), both of which reduce total healthcare costs.[103] In patients with grade 3 or 4 radiation-induced mucositis, 200 μg of TMF did not offer superior analgesia to placebo when administered 45 minutes before radiation treatment.[104] Further studies are needed to best define the role of TMF in the management of cancer-related pain syndromes.

Transdermal Transdermal fentanyl (TDF) is a long-acting analgesic. The time to onset is within 12–24 hours of applying the patch, and 16 hours after its removal ~50% of the drug is cleared from the body.[98] In randomized cancer pain trials, TDF has demonstrated efficacy for 66%–77% of patients.[105,106] TDF offers the option for an additional route of opioid administration for the patient who is unable to tolerate oral or parenteral routes. Due to its late onset of action, a short-acting rescue medication must be made available for patients who are started on TDF. Also, dosing sizes are fixed, and upper limits of the dosing range are limited by the availability of

skin onto which multiple patches can be applied. Transdermal administration of fentanyl through a rate-controlled patch can be altered by fever (40°C body temperature can increase absorption by one-third) or body fat, but provides equal absorption from the chest, abdomen, or thigh. Since cachexic or debilitated patients may have altered pharmacokinetic parameters due to poor fat stores, muscle wasting, or reduced clearance, caution is advised when using TDF for these patients. Serious life-threatening hypoventilation has been reported with TDF, particularly in the postoperative and opioid-naïve settings. Along with those contraindications, TDF should not be used for children under 12 years of age or patients under the age of 18 who weigh less than 50 kg (110 lb). Adverse reactions related to skin, such as rash and application site reactions, erythema, papules, itching, and edema, can occur at a rate of between 1% and 2%.[98]

Renal Dysfunction If a patient has a GFR of 10–50 mL/min, 75% of the normal fentanyl dose should be administered, and 50% of the dose should be administered if the GFR is less than 10 mL/min. An increase in sensitivity to the drug's effect is present in end-stage renal disease.

Hepatic Dysfunction Fentanyl is a high-extraction drug and its disposition is affected more by hepatic blood flow than by hepatocellular function. Fentanyl does not appear to be affected by liver cirrhosis, but should be used with caution in the known presence of impaired liver blood flow or liver failure.[96]

Methadone

Methadone is a synthetic mu-delta opioid agonist, which is structurally unrelated to the other opioid analgesics. First developed by German scientists during World War II because of a shortage of morphine, it was introduced into the United States in 1947 as an analgesic and gained popularity during the 1960s for the management of narcotic addicts.

Methadone is a basic, lipophilic drug that can be administered through the oral, rectal, and parenteral routes. Methadone has a mean bioavailability of about 75%, and a rectal bioavailability that is approximately the same.[107] It is primarily protein bound to alpha-1-acid-glycoprotein, and its lipophilic properties allow for its extensive distribution.[108] Methadone undergoes extensive *N*-demethylation in the liver by CYP3A4, and the inactive metabolites are excreted through the kidneys. The drug has biphasic elimination, with an analgesic half-life of 4–8 hours and a mean elimination half-life of 22 (range 5–130) hours.[107] This accounts for the short analgesic effect seen with single doses, and the tendency for drug to accumulate in the body with repeated doses. Methadone has the additional pharmacodynamic subtleties of being a potent noncompetitive antagonist of the *N*-methyl-*D*-aspartate (NMDA) receptor, and being able to inhibit the reuptake of norepinephrine and serotonin.[109] NMDA receptor antagonism lessens and reverses the development of morphine tolerance, as well as providing antihyperalgesia effects.[107,110] This may account for why the ratio of morphine to methadone increases as the morphine equivalent daily dose (MEDD) increases.[109,111] The side effects of methadone include constipation, nausea, vomiting, dizziness, drowsiness, weakness, cardiac arrest, circulatory depression, histamine release, respiratory arrest, respiratory depression, and shock.

Barriers to the use of methadone in the management of cancer pain include the stigma of its known use for heroin addicts, large interindividual variations in pharmacokinetics, and limited knowledge concerning the large amount of variability in the equianalgesic ratio of methadone to other opioids.

However, a large body of literature supports the use of methadone for cancer pain. Mercadante et al. in a prospective study showed that switching from oral morphine to methadone improved pain intensity and decreased side effects.[112] In 196 outpatients with advanced cancer who had moderate to severe pain, methadone treatment every 8 hours via an oral route produced appropriate pain relief. Thirteen (6.6%) patients withdrew due to methadone-related side effects, and 11.2% of patients withdrew from the study due to analgesic inefficacy.[113] In a randomized trial, methadone 7.5 mg by mouth (PO) every 12 hours (plus methadone for BTP), provided pain relief with reasonable side effects, but was not superior to morphine 15 mg PO every 12 hours (plus morphine for BTP) in the frontline treatment of cancer pain.[114]

Three possible hypotheses could account for large interindividual variability. First, the structure of methadone may result in a different type of binding to heterogeneous opioid receptors. Differential methadone-receptor binding could result in an incomplete tolerance to methadone. Second, NMDA, an excitatory amino acid, has demonstrated a role in the development of opioid tolerance, and NMDA receptor antagonism by d-methadone has been found to reverse opioid tolerance in rat models.[110,115] Methadone is a potent NMDA antagonist, and this activity may allow methadone to reverse previous opioid tolerance. Thirdly, methadone has no active metabolites, and by rotating away from drugs with active metabolites, such as M3G and H3G, a reduction in neuroexcitatory side effects may be seen.[116]

Renal Insufficiency Methadone, due to its lack of active metabolites, is considered safe to use in patients with renal disease. Because of high protein binding and extensive volume of distribution, methadone is not dialyzed.[50] Increasing the dosing interval and decreasing the dose are options used for utilizing methadone in a setting of renal dysfunction.

Hepatic Dysfunction Terminal half-life was prolonged in patients with severe cirrhosis, but no changes in methadone disposition were reported in patients with moderate cirrhosis or mild chronic liver disease (hepatitis, cholestasis, alcoholic hepatitis, and fatty infiltration).[117] These data suggest that methadone maintenance doses do not need to be changed in patients with stable chronic liver disease, specifically cirrhosis. For patients with severe or fluctuating liver dysfunction, or those with known or pending liver failure, dosing with methadone (as well as all opioids) should be undertaken with caution.

Meperidine

Meperidine is a less-potent opioid agonist than morphine. The half-life of meperidine is 3 hours, but that of its active metabolite, normeperidine, is 15–30 hours. Normeperidine accumulates in renal dysfunction and is known to cause multifocal myoclonus and grand mal seizures.[118] Meperidine should not be used for the management of cancer pain.[5]

▶ Opioid rotation

In the face of uncontrolled pain with a dose escalation, or unacceptable side effects, there are four different options: opiate rotation, lowering the opiate dose with increased use of adjuvant medications,

Table 2-4

Equianalgesic Opioid Chart

Analgesic	Oral/Rectal Dose	Parenteral Dose (mg)
Morphine	30	10
Hydromorphone	8	2
Oxycodone	20	(Not available)
Methadone	Please see Table 2-5	
Levorphanol	4	2
Fentanyl	Not available*	0.1 (100 mcg)
Fentanyl (transdermal)	100 mcg/h patch = 4 mg/h morphine IV	
Meperidine (not recommended)	300	75
Codeine (not recommended)	200	120
Hydrocodone	20	(Not available)
Propoxyphene	130	(Not available)

*Please see section in text on transmucosal fentanyl.

treating the unwanted symptoms, or improving clearance of the opiate. Rotating to a structurally different opiate is recommended at 25%–50% of the equivalent dose, and may allow a better balance between pain control and adverse effects. There is a diversity of opioid receptors that suggest that the cross-tolerance of all opioids is variable. Table 2-4 lists dose equivalents for the common opioids.

Nonmethadone opioid rotation

Indelicato and Portenoy provide an excellent road map for opioid rotation,[119] starting with calculating the equianalgesic dose of the new opioid based on the information given in Table 2-4. Consistent use of the same table, while monitoring outcomes to ensure efficacy, is a must. If switching to any opioid other than methadone or fentanyl, decrease the equianalgesic dose by 25%–50%. If switching to methadone, the information in Table 2-5 can be used. If switching to TDF, the equianalgesic dose should not be reduced, as the manufacturer's equianalgesic chart utilizes a safety factor. If the patient is elderly or has significant cardiopulmonary, hepatic, or renal disease, consider further dose reduction and carefully select the most appropriate opioid for the circumstances. If the patient has severe pain,

Table 2-5

Methadone Conversion Chart

Suggested Daily Dosing of Oral Methadone Based on Morphine-Equivalent Daily Dose (MEDD)	
Oral MEDD (mg/day)	Initial Dose Ratio (Oral Morphine: Oral Methadone)
<30	2:1
30–99	4:1
100–299	8:1
300–499	12:1
500–999	15:1
≥1000	≥20:1

consider a smaller dose reduction, or do not reduce at all. The rescue dose should be 10%–15% of the total daily baseline opioid dose, and the patient must have appropriate access to analgesia for BTP pain. Reassess the adequacy of the pain relief being given, and titrate the new opioids as needed. Tables will not work in all cases, but if outcomes are consistently unacceptable, clinical experience can guide the table to best fit the needs of the practice.

Opioid conversion to methadone

Opioid rotation is indicated for patients experiencing opioid-induced neurotoxicity, or in whom side effects are limiting efficacious dosing of opioids. Rotating to methadone is controversial, complex, and should only be done by a practitioner trained in its use. Several conversions are described in the literature.

British researchers started 33 patients on methadone at one-tenth (max 40 mg) of the previous 24-hour MEDD (mean: 480 mg, range 20–1200 mg), given at intervals of 3 hours or more. Dextromoramide was used for BTP, and after the methadone dose was stable, the previous 24-hour dosage of methadone was split into two doses and administered every 12 hours. Inpatient monitoring continued for 2 more days, and necessary adjustments were made. Thirty-three patients were treated, with 88% stabilized on a regular dose in 3 (range 2–18) days, with the median final dose being 80 (range 20–360) mg/24 h. Pain scores were significantly reduced, with 78% of patients identified as good responders, and 23 (70%) of patients safely discharged home. This trial demonstrates that methadone is an excellent analgesic for patients who cannot tolerate another opioid, and for inpatients, it presents a reasonable option for conversion.[120]

Two studies evaluated conversion to methadone from fentanyl. Eighteen cancer patients were rotated from patient-controlled analgesia (PCA) fentanyl to intravenous PCA methadone. Patients were stable on the fentanyl dose for at least 3 days, and were rotated due to uncontrolled pain and opioid-induced sedation or confusion. The conversion used was 25 μg/h of fentanyl to 0.1 mg/h of methadone (0.25 μg fentanyl:100 μg of methadone). PCA boluses of methadone were equal to 50%–100% of the hourly infusion rate every 20 minutes, and nurses could administer additional boluses of 100%–200% of the basal rate every 60 minutes. Within 4 days, 16 patients had satisfactory pain control without significant side effects. Based on their dose escalations, the authors concluded that their study conversion might be a bit low. They suggested a final conversion ratio of 25 μg/h of fentanyl to 0.125 mg/h of methadone with additional methadone available for BTP.[121]

TDF was rotated to oral methadone in 17 cancer patients. First, the oral morphine dose was calculated based on a 1:100 TDF to oral morphine ratio. Then, a ratio of morphine to methadone of 5:1 was used. A more conservative ratio of 10:1 was used for patients who (1) were receiving ≥400 μg/h TDF, (2) reported aggressive increasing fentanyl doses, and (3) were in delirium and unable to give a reasonable history of TDF usage. Rescue doses of morphine were not included in the methadone calculation. After TDF removal, scheduled methadone doses (every 8 hours) were initiated in the following fashion: a dose of TDF ≤100 μg/h—start oral methadone 8–12 hours later, for TDF between 100 and 300 μg/h—12–16 hours later, for TDF from 200 to 300 μg/h—16–18 hours later, and TDF greater than 300 μg/h—18–24 hours later. Rescue doses of methadone were 10% of the daily dose PO every 2 hours as needed, and starting doses of methadone were adjusted every 72 hours. Of patients with somatic pain, 80% were successfully treated. In two patients, neuropathic pain did not respond to methadone. Myoclonus disappeared from all patients within approximately 24–36 hours of stopping TDF, and delirium was reversed in 6 days for 80% of the patients. No patient had to stop methadone due to adverse effects.[122]

Mercadante reported using a rapid stop-and-go approach to switching patients with uncontrolled pain from oral morphine to oral methadone, with a ratio of 4:1 for a morphine dose less than 90 mg/day, 8:1 for 90–300 mg/day of morphine, and 12:1 for patients on greater than 300 mg/day. Methadone was administered every 8 hours, with one-sixth of the daily dose used for up to three rescue doses per day. Patients receiving less than 300 mg/day of morphine experienced a significant improvement in pain and side effects. For those receiving more than 300 mg/day of morphine, only two out of the three patients had acceptable pain relief. In this study, dose titration took 3–4 days, and methadone was increased in 50% of the patients. The small number of patients taking more than 300 mg/day of morphine (3) limits drawing conclusions about the appropriateness of the ratio used for that dose range.[112]

At the University of Texas M. D. Anderson Cancer Center, the algorithm for converting opioid analgesics to methadone that is in clinical use is found in Table 2-5.[111] For patients taking very high doses of opioids, conversion to methadone may be gradually completed over the course of several days to weeks. Methadone, with its ease of manufacture and low cost, should always be considered as an option for patients who require opioids but do not tolerate morphine. The best ratio to use for rotation is under investigation.

Conversion away from methadone

While methadone is an excellent option after other opioids, rotating away from methadone must be done with caution. Vigano et al. described a case of a patient with advanced renal carcinoma and neuropathic pain who was rotated from hydromorphone (MEDD 1050) to methadone (MEDD 36) over a period of 3 days. The patient's neuropathic pain was resolved, and the patient had stable pain for 3 months. Over the course of the fourth month, however, increasing pain led to increased methadone, which caused myoclonus, sedation, and mild delirium, with only fair pain control. The patient was rotated from methadone (MEDD 480) to parenteral hydromorphone (MEDD 3000–4950). After 4 weeks of hydromorphone (MEDD 2850), the patient developed nausea and drowsiness, and was rotated back to methadone (MEDD 24) and had less drowsiness. The exact mechanism that allows for a lower MEDD during the second rotation to methadone is unknown. The possibilities include intrapatient variability, changing opioid receptor sensitivity, or NMDA receptor activity.[123] Moryl et al. attempted rotation away from methadone in 13 cancer patients in response to the patients' sedation, pain, and the perception that methadone caused them to be viewed as drug addicts. Methadone was rotated to hydromorphone (6), morphine (1), fentanyl (4), and levorphanol (2). Eleven patients needed dose escalation due to increased pain within the first 24 hours. Dysphoria, confusion, and sedation were reasons cited for rotation back to methadone. Only one patient (on hydromorphone) did not rotate back to methadone. Due to rapid escalation of the second opioid, the authors could not establish an equianalgesic ratio for rotation away from methadone. This study demonstrates the lack of data and consensus on how to best perform the transition from methadone to other opioids.[124] Further delineation of the role of NMDA receptors in opioid tolerance, as well as a better understanding of opioid receptors and cross-sensitivity will help determine the best way to rotate away from methadone.

NEUROPATHIC PAIN

Neuropathic pain is defined as pain initiated or caused by a primary lesion or dysfunction of the nervous system.[125,126] The location of the nervous system lesion may be central, peripheral, or both. Common peripheral neuropathic pain syndromes associated with cancer patients include chemotherapy-induced polyneuropathy, iatrogenic neuralgias (e.g., postmastectomy pain, postthoracotomy pain), and postherpetic neuralgia. A central neuropathic pain syndrome in cancer patients includes postradiation myelopathy.[127] Neuropathic pain may present alone or in combination with somatic or visceral pain in cancer patients. Patients often report a sensation of pain as burning, shooting, or stabbing.[128] Neuropathic pain is typically unresponsive to commonly used analgesics such as acetaminophen, NSAIDs, or opioid agonists. Oncologists have had the greatest degree of success with classes of drugs that modulate nerve conduction, such as anticonvulsants and antidepressants.[129] A listing of these various agents by drug class with dosage and schedule information is found in Table 2-6.

▶ Anticonvulsants

Anticonvulsant agents encompass a diverse number of drug classes that are utilized alone or in combination to control various seizure disorders. Due to their ability to modulate neuronal conduction, these agents have been used to treat neuropathic pain.[130,131]

Carbamazepine

Carbamazepine is an iminostilbene derivative anticonvulsant, which is chemically related to the antidepressant imipramine and is FDA-approved for treating trigeminal neuralgia. The precise mechanism of action of carbamazepine in preventing seizures is unclear, but may involve reducing polysynaptic responses and blocking posttetanic potentiation. Carbamazepine putatively suppresses pain via central and peripheral mechanisms that involve blocking ion conductance. This allows carbamazepine to block Aδ and C fibers that are responsible for pain impulse transmission while preserving normal nerve conduction. Carbamazepine is hepatically metabolized by the CYP450 enzyme system and it is remarkable for its induction of CYP450 isoenzymes. Table 2-7 lists the major pharmacokinetics of drug interactions among the agents used in treating neuropathic pain. Common toxicities associated with carbamazepine include myelosuppression (also, aplastic anemia and agranulocytosis), hepatotoxicity, syndrome of inappropriate diuretic hormone (SIADH), and rash.

Gabapentin

Gabapentin is an amino acid that is structurally related to the inhibitory neurotransmitter γ-aminobutyric acid (GABA). However, gabapentin does not have any GABA-ergic action and does not affect GABA uptake or metabolism. The drug does not bind to GABA or benzodiazepine receptors. Modulation of α-2-δ calcium channels is one proposed mechanism for gabapentin's analgesic activity. Additionally, gabapentin has been shown to inhibit ectopic discharge activity from damaged peripheral nerves. Preliminary evidence demonstrates gabapentin-mediated antagonism at NMDA receptors for D-serine at the NMDA-glycine binding site. The net analgesic effect of gabapentin observed in animal models of analgesia was preventing allodynia and hyperanalgesia. Response to painful stimuli in neuropathic pain models and in peripheral inflammation models were blocked or decreased by gabapentin.[132,133] Gabapentin requires adjustment for renal insufficiency (Table 2-8) and it is approved for use in treatment of postherpetic neuralgia. Common toxicities of

Table 2-6

Treatment Dosing for Management of Neuropathic Pain

Generic Names	Dosing Schedule	Recommended Starting Dose (mg/dose)	Maximum Daily Dose (mg)
Carbamazepine	TID-QID	200–400 PO	1200
Clonazepam	TID	0.5–2 PO	20
Gabapentin	TID-QID	100–800 PO	3600
Lamotrigine	BID	25–350 PO	700
Phenytoin	TID	100–200 PO	600
Valproic acid	Q daily	500–1000 PO	1000
Amitriptyline	QHS	10–300 PO	300
Desipramine	QHS	25–300 PO	300
Duloxetine	QAM	60 PO	60
Fluoxetine	QAM	20–80 PO	80
Imipramine	QHS	30–300 PO	300
Nortriptyline	Q4-6H	30–100 PO	100
Paroxetine	QAM	10–50	50
Sertraline	QAM	50–200	200
Clonidine	Continuous infusion (epidural)	30–40 µg/h	40 µg/h
Clonidine	TID	0.1–0.6	2.4
Clonidine TTS	Qweek	0.1–0.3 released daily	0.3
Lidocaine 5% patch	Apply to affected area for 12 consecutive hours daily	As needed	Three patches
Ketamine	Start 0.5 mg/kg/day and titrate to sedation or effect. Clinical trials are encouraged.		

Table 2-7

Drugs to Treat Neuropathic Pain and Interactions with CYP450 Isoenzymes

Agent	Inhibitor	Inducer	Substrates
Amitriptyline			CYP2D6
Carbamazepine		CYP3A4,5	
Desipramine			CYP2D6
Fluoxetine	CYP2C19, CYP2D6		
Imipramine			CYP2D6
Methadone	CYP2D6		CYP3A4
Paroxetine	CYP2D6		
Phenytoin		CYP3A4,5	

gabapentin include somnolence, fatigue, dizziness, rash, low blood pressure, ataxia, and nystagmus.

Pregabalin

Pregabalin is a novel compound that binds to α-2-δ protein, an auxiliary subunit associated with voltage-gated calcium ion channels. Pregabalin has no activity at either GABA$_A$ or GABA$_B$ receptors, nor does it have GABA-mimetic activity. Agonist binding at this site diminishes calcium influx at nerve terminals, thereby preventing the release of neurotransmitters such as substance P, glutamate, and norepinephrine. Pregabalin has a toxicity profile notable for somnolence, dizziness, headache, blurry vision, dry mouth, and peripheral edema.[134–137]

Valproic acid

Valproic acid is a carboxylic acid-derivative anticonvulsant with a largely unknown mechanism of action. The drug appears to increase brain concentrations of GABA, which may contribute to its anticonvulsant and analgesic effects. Other proposed mechanisms include inhibition of the enzymes GABA transferase and succinic aldehyde, both of which mediate GABA catabolism. Increased potassium conductance may contribute to the inhibition of neuronal activity. Adverse effects of valproic acid include hepatotoxicity,

Table 2-8

Dose Modification for Gabapentin in Renal Insufficiency

Creatinine Clearance (mL/min)	Total Daily Dose Range (mg/day)	Dose Regimen (mg)
>60	900–3600	300 TID, 400 TID, 600 TID, 800 TID, 1200 TID
30–59	400–1400	200 BID, 300 BID, 400 BID, 500 BID, 700 BID
15–29	200–700	200 daily, 300 daily, 400 daily, 500 daily, 700 daily
15	100–400	100 daily, 125 daily, 150 daily, 200 daily, 300 daily
Hemodialysis		125 post HD, 150 post HD, 200 post HD, 250 post HD, 350 post HD

Abbreviation: Post HD = following hemodialysis.

thrombocytopenia, pancreatitis, sedation, tremor, ataxia, fatigue, dizziness, confusion, headache, weight gain, nausea, diarrhea, abdominal cramps, and rash.

Lamotrigine

Lamotrigine is a phenyltriazine derivative that is thought to inhibit glutamate release via blockade of voltage-dependent sodium channels. In animal models, lamotrigine diminishes the hyperalgesia observed in rodents with iatrogenic diabetes. Other pharmacodynamic effects of lamotrigine observed in rats include reduction of mechanical hyperalgesia and cold allodynia in the mononeuropathy model.[138] Adverse events associated with lamotrigine include ataxia, diplopia, dizziness, headache, somnolence, headache, blurred vision, nausea, vomiting, and rash.

Phenytoin

Phenytoin suppresses the repetitious firing of action potentials induced by seizure activity. This effect is likely to occur at the motor cortex. Standard doses of phenytoin slow the ability of voltage-activated sodium channels to recover from inactivity. Enhanced neuronal sodium efflux inhibits seizure activity. This stabilizes the threshold against hyperexcitability caused by excessive stimulation or environmental changes capable of reducing the membrane sodium gradient, including the reduction of posttetanic potentiation at synapses. Cortical seizure foci are prevented from loss of posttetanic potentiation from detonating adjacent cortical areas. Phenytoin reduces the maximal activity of brainstem centers responsible for the tonic phase of tonic-clonic seizures. Phenytoin appears to produce its effects by depressing the sodium action potential, "filtering out" sustained high frequency neuronal discharges and synaptic activity. Other proposed pharmacodynamic effects of phenytoin include inhibition of presynaptic glutamate release and suppression of spontaneous ectopic discharges. Phenytoin is a unique entity when one considers the Michaelis-Menten pharmacokinetics associated with the drug. Increasing dosages can saturate hepatic enzymes, precipitously increasing serum concentrations. Given the narrow therapeutic index for phenytoin (10–20 µg/mL), a sudden onset of dose-related toxicity, such as nystagmus, ataxia, and lethargy, can accompany dosage increases. Other toxicities include myelosuppression (agranulocytosis and aplastic anemia), hepatotoxicity, cardiac arrhythmias, gingival hyperplasia, choreoathetosis, acute interstitial nephritis, and rash. Phenytoin is highly protein bound, and the fraction of unbound phenytoin increases in the presence of either hypoalbuminemia or renal dysfunction. In patients with renal disease, the following equation has been used to relate the measured, or observed, phenytoin concentration to the phenytoin concentration one would expect to measure if there was normal protein binding:

$$C\ (normal) = \frac{C\ (observed)}{0.1 \times albumin + 0.1}$$

where C (normal) = normal serum phenytoin concentration in nonuremic patients and C (observed) = observed serum phenytoin concentration in uremic patients.

▶ Antidepressants

Antidepressants represent the general therapeutic class with the greatest amount of clinical experience in treating neuropathic pain.

Tricyclics

Tricyclic antidepressants (TCAs) have the most extensive clinical application. Their chief mechanism of action is the blockade of reuptake for both norepinephrine and serotonin at the presynaptic α-2 receptors at the terminal neuroaxonal junction, thus prolonging the effects of norepinephrine and serotonin. This increases the synaptic reservoir time for norepinephrine and serotonin, allowing for increased binding to postsynaptic α- and β- adrenergic receptors. Upon stimulation, β-adrenergic postsynaptic receptors stimulate G proteins to activate adenyl cyclase, which converts adenosine triphosphate (ATP) to cyclic adenosine monophosphate (AMP). Postreceptor α-1 receptors via G proteins activate phospholipase C, converting phosphatidylinositol bisphosphate to inositol triphosphate and diacylglycerol. As a consequence, intracellular calcium is liberated and protein kinases are modulated. This effects downstream synthesis and release of norepinephrine to propagate postsynaptic nerve conduction. Amitriptyline, desipramine, imipramine, and nortriptyline are the most commonly used tricyclic agents for neuropathic pain.

The broad use of the TCAs is limited by their considerable toxicity profile. Enhanced adrenergic tone yields significant anticholinergic side effects. Among them, urinary retention, constipation, xerostomia, mydriasis, cycloplegia, and hyperthermia are most common. TCAs have cardiovascular effects that require close monitoring, including postural hypotension, mild sinus tachycardia, and direct depression of the myocardium. Electrocardiogram (ECG) changes associated with TCAs include inversion or flattening of T waves, indicating the presence of global conduction abnormalities. This phenomenon occurs with supratherapeutic serum concentrations. Other toxicities well known to TCAs include sedation, weakness, fatigue, dizziness, edema, and muscle tremors.

Selective serotonin reuptake inhibitors

The selective serotonin reuptake inhibitors (SSRIs) are the most recent class of antidepressants used to manage neuropathic pain. These agents exert a pharmacodynamic effect that is similar to that from TCAs, except that they specifically block the reuptake of serotonin at the presynaptic terminal nerve axon, without blocking norepinephrine reuptake. Fluoxetine is the prototype "second-generation" antidepressant SSRI. Fluoxetine and other SSRIs are distinct molecular entities from TCAs, devoid of the tertiary tricyclic amine base. Fluoxetine is a 100-fold more potent reuptake inhibitor than norepinephrine and has negligible anticholinergic or adverse cardiac effects. Other SSRIs utilized for neuropathic pain include sertraline and paroxetine. Duloxetine, a newly approved selective serotonin and norepinephrine reuptake inhibitor, is indicated for peripheral neuropathic pain secondary to diabetes. The toxicity profile of SSRIs is remarkable for nausea, vomiting, anorexia, weight loss, sweating, sexual dysfunction, hypotension, anxiety, insomnia, anorexia, and suicidal ideation.

▶ Alpha-adrenergic agents

Clonidine

Clonidine is an α-2-selective adrenergic receptor agonist that provides an initial, brief vasoconstrictive effect, presumably from activation of postsynaptic α-2 receptors in smooth muscle. Paradoxically, the binding of α-2 receptors in the cardiovascular control centers in the CNS diminishes sympathetic tone and results in vasodilatation and a lowering of blood pressure. Animal models have demonstrated that clonidine has analgesic effects mediated by effects on muscarinic and nicotinic receptors.[139]

▶ Local anesthetics

Lidocaine

The first topically available dosage in the form of a patch has recently been FDA approved for treating neuropathic pain. The lidocaine 5% patch should be applied directly to the area of worst pain for 12 consecutive hours daily. It can be used as a frontline treatment for neuropathic pain. Three is the maximum number of patches that can be worn at one time, and 2 weeks are needed for an adequate trial. Side effects include mild skin reactions.[129,140]

▶ N-methyl-D-aspartate receptor antagonists

The development of chronic and intractable pain appears to be related, in part, to the instigation of NMDA receptors in the brain.

Ketamine

Ketamine is an NMDA receptor antagonist with analgesic and dissociative (general anesthesia without sedation) anesthetic properties. It has attracted use in the treatment of cancer pain because it is believed to provide pain relief via nonopioid mechanisms, and may have benefit in the treatment of neuropathic pain.[141] Ketamine is usually given with opioids as an adjuvant for pain, and may be administered through the oral, intramuscular, subcutaneous, intravenous, epidural, and intrathecal routes. Ketamine has demonstrated efficacy in the management of cancer pain.[142–144] The most common adverse effects of ketamine are hallucination and sedation. The appropriateness of subanesthetic use of adjuvant ketamine for opioid-refractory cancer pain is a matter of ongoing debate.[145] While promising, further clinical studies are necessary to define the optimal role of ketamine in the management of cancer pain.

REFERENCES

1. Higginson IJ, Hearn J. A multicenter evaluation of cancer pain control by palliative care teams. *J Pain Symptom Manage*. 1997;14:29–35.
2. Ballantyne JC. Chronic pain following treatment for cancer: the role of opioids. *Oncologist*. 2003;8:567–575.
3. Banning A, Sjogren P, Henriksen H. Treatment outcome in a multidisciplinary cancer pain clinic. *Pain*. 1991;47:129–134; discussion 127–128.
4. World Health Organization. Pain Relief Ladder. Available at: http://www.who.int/cancer/palliative/painladder/en. Accessed June 20, 2005.
5. National Cancer Center Network. Cancer Pain Guidelines v1.2004. Available at: http://www.nccn.org/professionals/physician_gls/PDF/pain.pdf. Accessed February 27, 2005.
6. Jadad AR, Browman GP. The WHO analgesic ladder for cancer pain management. Stepping up the quality of its evaluation. *JAMA*. 1995;274:1870–1873.
7. Butler LD, Koopman C, Cordova MJ, et al. Psychological distress and pain significantly increase before death in metastatic breast cancer patients. *Psychosom Med*. 2003;65:416–426.
8. Desbiens NA, Wu AW, Broste SK, et al. Pain and satisfaction with pain control in seriously ill hospitalized adults: findings from the SUPPORT research investigations. For the SUPPORT investigators. Study to Understand Prognoses and Preferences for Outcomes and Risks of Treatment. *Crit Care Med*. 1996;24:1953–1961.
9. Trowbridge R, Dugan W, Jay SJ, et al. Determining the effectiveness of a clinical-practice intervention in improving the control of pain in outpatients with cancer. *Acad Med*. 1997;72:798–800.

10. Elliott TE, Murray DM, Oken MM, et al. Improving cancer pain management in communities: main results from a randomized controlled trial. *J Pain Symptom Manage.* 1997;13:191–203.

11. American Chronic Pain Association. ACPA Medications & Chronic Pain Supplement 2005. Available at: http://www.theacpa.org/documents/ACPA%20Meds%202005%20SDSF.pdf. Accessed June 20, 2005.

12. Rothenberg ML, Moore MJ, Cripps MC, et al. A phase II trial of gemcitabine in patients with 5-FU-refractory pancreas cancer. *Ann Oncol.* 1996;7:347–353.

13. Toradol (ketorolac tromethamine) package insert. Available at: http://www.rocheusa.com/products/toradol/pi.pdf. Accessed February 28, 2005.

14. Brocks DR, Jamali F. Etodolac clinical pharmacokinetics. *Clin Pharmacokinet.* 1994;26:259–274.

15. van Stolk R, Stoner G, Hayton WL, et al. Phase I trial of exisulind (sulindac sulfone, FGN-1) as a chemopreventive agent in patients with familial adenomatous polyposis. *Clin Cancer Res.* 2000;6:78–89.

16. Kaufman DW, Kelly JP, Sheehan JE, et al. Nonsteroidal anti-inflammatory drug use in relation to major upper gastrointestinal bleeding. *Clin Pharmacol Ther.* 1993;53:485–494.

17. Federal Drug Administration. Available at: http://www.fda.gov/medwatch/SAFETY/2004/safety04.htm#Naproxen. Accessed June 20, 2005.

18. Lanza FL, Codispoti JR, Nelson EB. An endoscopic comparison of gastroduodenal injury with over-the-counter doses of ketoprofen and acetaminophen. *Am J Gastroenterol.* 1998;93:1051–1054.

19. Makarowski W, Weaver A, Rubin B, et al. The efficacy, tolerability, and safety of 1200 mg/d of oxaprozin and 1500 mg/d of nabumetone in the treatment of patients with osteoarthritis of the knee. *Clin Ther.* 1996;18:114–124.

20. Lipscomb GR, Wallis N, Armstrong G, Rees WD. Gastrointestinal tolerability of meloxicam and piroxicam: a double-blind placebo-controlled study. *Br J Clin Pharmacol.* 1998;46:133–137.

21. Dequeker J, Hawkey C, Kahan A, et al. Improvement in gastrointestinal tolerability of the selective cyclooxygenase (COX)-2 inhibitor, meloxicam, compared with piroxicam: results of the Safety and Efficacy Large-scale Evaluation of COX-inhibiting Therapies (SELECT) trial in osteoarthritis. *Br J Rheumatol.* 1998;37:946–951.

22. Scott DL, Palmer RH. Safety and efficacy of nabumetone in osteoarthritis: emphasis on gastrointestinal safety. *Aliment Pharmacol Ther.* 2000;14:443–452.

23. Morgan GJ, Jr, Kaine J, DeLapp R, Palmer R. Treatment of elderly patients with nabumetone or diclofenac: gastrointestinal safety profile. *J Clin Gastroenterol.* 2001;32:310–314.

24. Petrella R, Ekman EF, Schuller R, Fort JG. Efficacy of celecoxib, a COX-2-specific inhibitor, and naproxen in the management of acute ankle sprain: results of a double-blind, randomized controlled trial. *Clin J Sport Med.* 2004;14:225–231.

25. Simon LS, Weaver AL, Graham DY, et al. Anti-inflammatory and upper gastrointestinal effects of celecoxib in rheumatoid arthritis: a randomized controlled trial. *JAMA.* 1999;282:1921–1928.

26. Doyle G, Jayawardena S, Ashraf E, Cooper SA. Efficacy and tolerability of nonprescription ibuprofen versus celecoxib for dental pain. *J Clin Pharmacol.* 2002;42:912–919.

27. Silverstein FE, Faich G, Goldstein JL, et al. Gastrointestinal toxicity with celecoxib vs nonsteroidal anti-inflammatory drugs for osteoarthritis and rheumatoid arthritis: the CLASS study: a randomized controlled trial. Celecoxib Long-term Arthritis Safety Study. *JAMA.* 2000;284:1247–1255.

28. Bombardier C, Laine L, Reicin A, et al. VIGOR Study Group. Comparison of upper gastrointestinal toxicity of rofecoxib and naproxen in patients with rheumatoid arthritis. VIGOR Study Group. *N Engl J Med.* 2000;343:1520–1528, 2 p following 1528.

29. Merck Press Release. Available at: http://www.vioxx.com/rofecoxib/vioxx/consumer/index.jsp Accessed June 20, 2005.

30. Solomon SD, McMurray JJ, Pfeffer MA, et al. The Adenoma Prevention with Celecoxib (APC) Study Investigators. Cardiovascular Risk Associated with Celecoxib in a Clinical Trial for Colorectal Adenoma Prevention. *N Engl J Med.* 2005;352:1071–1080.

31. Nussmeier NA, Whelton AA, Brown MT, et al. Complications of the COX-2 Inhibitors Parecoxib and Valdecoxib after Cardiac Surgery. *N Engl J Med.* 2005;352:1081–1091.

32. Bresalier RS, Sandler RS, Quan H, et al. The Adenomatous Polyp Prevention on Vioxx (APPROVe) Trial Investigators. Cardiovascular Events Associated with Rofecoxib in a Colorectal Adenoma Chemoprevention Trial. *N Engl J Med.* 352;1092–1102.

33. Stockler M, Vardy J, Pillai A, Warr D. Acetaminophen (paracetamol) improves pain and well-being in people with advanced cancer already receiving a strong opioid regimen: a randomized, double-blind, placebo-controlled cross-over trial. *J Clin Oncol.* 2004;22:3389–3394.

34. Kaal EC, Vecht CJ. The management of brain edema in brain tumors. *Curr Opin Oncol.* 2004;16:593–600.

35. Nguyen T, Deangelis LM. Treatment of brain metastases. *J Support Oncol.* 2004;2:405–410; discussion 411–416.

36. Abrahm JL. Assessment and treatment of patients with malignant spinal cord compression. *J Support Oncol.* 2004;2:377–388, 391; discussion 391–393, 398, 401.

37. Cherny NI. The management of cancer pain. *CA Cancer J Clin.* 2000;50:70–116; quiz 117–120.

38. Pasanisi F, Sloan L, Rubin PC. Cardiovascular properties of metkephamid, a delta opioid receptor agonist, in man. *Clin Sci (Lond).* 1985;68:209–213.

39. Pfeiffer A, Knepel W, Braun S, et al. Effects of a kappa-opioid agonist on adrenocorticotropic and diuretic function in man. *Horm Metab Res.* 1986;18:842–848.

40. Delvaux M, Beck A, Jacob J, et al. Effect of asimadoline, a kappa opioid agonist, on pain induced by colonic distension in patients with irritable bowel syndrome. *Aliment Pharmacol Ther.* 2004;20:237–246.

41. Riviere PJ. Peripheral kappa-opioid agonists for visceral pain. *Br J Pharmacol.* 2004;141:1331–1334.

42. Sittl R, Griessinger N, Likar R. Analgesic efficacy and tolerability of transdermal buprenorphine in patients with inadequately controlled chronic pain related to cancer and other disorders: a multicenter, randomized, double-blind, placebo-controlled trial. *Clin Ther.* 2003;25:150–168.

43. Pasternak GW. Multiple opiate receptors: deja vu all over again. *Neuropharmacology.* 2004;47:312–323.

44. Quigley C. Opioid switching to improve pain relief and drug tolerability. *Cochrane Database Syst Rev.* 2004;CD004847.

45. Moryl N, Santiago-Palma J, Kornick C, et al. Pitfalls of opioid rotation: substituting another opioid for methadone in patients with cancer pain. *Pain.* 2002;96:325–328.

46. Mancini I, Lossignol DA, Body JJ. Opioid switch to oral methadone in cancer pain. *Curr Opin Oncol.* 2000;12:308–313.

47. Mercadante S. Opioid rotation for cancer pain: rationale and clinical aspects. *Cancer.* 1999;86:1656–1666.

48. Chung KF. Drugs to suppress cough. *Expert Opin Investig Drugs.* 2005;14:19–27.

49. Gutstein HB, Akil H. Opioid analgesics. In: Hardman JG, Limbird LE, Gilman AG, eds. *Goodman & Gilman's The Pharmacological Basis of Therapeutics.* New York: McGraw-Hill; 2001:589.

50. Dean M. Opioids in renal failure and dialysis patients. *J Pain Symptom Manage.* 2004;28:497–504.

51. Irwin RS, Curley FJ, Bennett FM. Appropriate use of antitussives and protussives. A practical review. *Drugs.* 1993;46:80–91.

52. Palangio M, Damask MJ, Morris E, et al. Combination hydrocodone and ibuprofen versus combination codeine and acetaminophen for the treatment of chronic pain. *Clin Ther.* 2000;22:879–892.

53. Allen GJ, Hartl TL, Duffany S, et al. Cognitive and motor function after administration of hydrocodone bitartrate plus ibuprofen, ibuprofen alone, or placebo in healthy subjects with exercise-induced muscle damage: a randomized, repeated-dose, placebo-controlled study. *Psychopharmacology (Berl).* 2003;166:228–233.

54. Fricke JR, Jr, Karim R, Jordan D, Rosenthal N. A double-blind, single-dose comparison of the analgesic efficacy of tramadol/acetaminophen combination tablets, hydrocodone/acetaminophen combination tablets, and placebo after oral surgery. *Clin Ther.* 2002;24:953–968.

55. Palangio M, Wideman GL, Keffer M, et al. Dose-response effect of combination hydrocodone with ibuprofen in patients with moderate to severe postoperative pain. *Clin Ther.* 2000;22:990–1002.

56. Palangio M, Morris E, Doyle RT, Jr, et al. Combination hydrocodone and ibuprofen versus combination oxycodone and acetaminophen in the treatment of moderate or severe acute low back pain. *Clin Ther.* 2002;24:87–99.

57. Scott LJ, Perry CM. Tramadol: a review of its use in perioperative pain. *Drugs.* 2000;60:139–176.

58. Sindrup SH, Andersen G, Madsen C, et al. Tramadol relieves pain and allodynia in polyneuropathy: a randomised, double-blind, controlled trial. *Pain.* 1999;83:85–90.

59. Harati Y, Gooch C, Swenson M, et al. Maintenance of the long-term effectiveness of tramadol in treatment of the pain of diabetic neuropathy. *J Diabetes Complications.* 2000;14:65–70.

60. Grond S, Radbruch L, Meuser T, et al. High-dose tramadol in comparison to low-dose morphine for cancer pain relief. *J Pain Symptom Manage.* 1999;18:174–179.

61. Wilder-Smith CH, Schimke J, Osterwalder B, Senn HJ. Oral tramadol, a mu-opioid agonist and monoamine reuptake-blocker, and morphine for strong cancer-related pain. *Ann Oncol.* 1994;5:141–146.

62. Ultram (tramadol) PI. Available at: http://www.ortho-mcneil.com/products/pi/pdfs/ultram.pdf. Accessed June 20, 2005.

63. Grond S, Sablotzki A. Clinical pharmacology of tramadol. *Clin Pharmacokinet.* 2004;43:879–923.

64. Kamal-Bahl SJ, Doshi JA, Stuart BC, Briesacher BA. Propoxyphene use by community-dwelling and institutionalized elderly Medicare beneficiaries. *J Am Geriatr Soc.* 2003;51:1099–1104.

65. Hanks GW, Conno F, Cherny N, et al. Expert Working Group of the Research Network of the European Association for Palliative Care. Morphine and alternative opioids in cancer pain: the EAPC recommendations. *Br J Cancer.* 2001;84:587–593.

66. Avinza (morphine sulfate extended-release capsules) PI. Available at: http://www.ligand.com/pdf/AVINZAPI.pdf. Accessed February 28, 2005.

67. Depodur (morphine sulfate extended-release liposome injection) PI. Available at: http://www.depodur.com/PDF/DepoDur_Package_Insert.pdf. Accessed February 28, 2005.

68. Pasternak GW, Bodnar RJ, Clark JA, Inturrisi CE. Morphine-6-glucuronide, a potent mu agonist. *Life Sci.* 1987;41:2845–2849.

69. Smith MT. Neuroexcitatory effects of morphine and hydromorphone: evidence implicating the 3-glucuronide metabolites. *Clin Exp Pharmacol Physiol.* 2000;27:524–528.

70. Andersen G, Christrup L, Sjogren P. Relationships among morphine metabolism, pain and side effects during long-term treatment: an update. *J Pain Symptom Manage.* 2003;25:74–91.

71. Hemstapat K, Monteith GR, Smith D, Smith MT. Morphine-3-glucuronide's neuro-excitatory effects are mediated via indirect activation of N-methyl-D-aspartic acid receptors: mechanistic studies in embryonic cultured hippocampal neurons. *Anesth Analg.* 2003;97:494–505.

72. Osborne R, Joel S, Grebenik K, et al. The pharmacokinetics of morphine and morphine glucuronides in kidney failure. *Clin Pharmacol Ther.* 1993;54:158–167.

73. Klepstad P, Borchgrevink PC, Dale O, et al. Routine drug monitoring of serum concentrations of morphine, morphine-3-glucuronide and morphine-6-glucuronide do not predict clinical observations in cancer patients. *Palliat Med.* 2003;17:679–687.

74. Quigley C, Joel S, Patel N, et al. Plasma concentrations of morphine, morphine-6-glucuronide and morphine-3-glucuronide and their relationship with analgesia and side effects in patients with cancer-related pain. *Palliat Med.* 2003;17:185–190.

75. Aronoff GR, Berns JS, Brier ME, et al., eds. *Drug Prescribing in Renal Failure: Dosing Guidelines for Adults.* Philadelphia, PA: American College of Physicians; 1999.

76. Mazoit JX, Sandouk P, Zetlaoui P, Scherrmann JM. Pharmacokinetics of unchanged morphine in normal and cirrhotic subjects. *Anesth Analg.* 1987;66:293–298.

77. Hasselstrom J, Eriksson S, Persson A, et al. The metabolism and bioavailability of morphine in patients with severe liver cirrhosis. *Br J Clin Pharmacol.* 1990;29:289–297.

78. Newsweek. Kentucky's Pain. Available at: http://www.msnbc.msn.com/id/5972112/site/newsweek/. Accessed June 20, 2005.

79. Government Accounting Office. Prescription Drugs: OxyContin Abuse and Diversion and Efforts to Address the Problem. Available at: http://www.gao.gov/new.items/d04110.pdf. Accessed June 20, 2005.

80. Hays LR. A profile of OxyContin addiction. *J Addict Dis.* 2004;23:1–9.

81. Heiskanen T, Olkkola KT, Kalso E. Effects of blocking CYP2D6 on the pharmacokinetics and pharmacodynamics of oxycodone. *Clin Pharmacol Ther.* 1998;64:603–611.

82. Poyhia R, Seppala T, Olkkola KT, Kalso E. The pharmacokinetics and metabolism of oxycodone after intramuscular and oral administration to healthy subjects. *Br J Clin Pharmacol.* 1992;33:617–621.

83. Parris WC, Johnson BW, Jr, Croghan MK, et al. The use of controlled-release oxycodone for the treatment of chronic cancer pain: a randomized, double-blind study. *J Pain Symptom Manage.* 1998;16:205–211.

84. Kaplan R, Parris WC, Citron ML, et al. Comparison of controlled-release and immediate-release oxycodone tablets in patients with cancer pain. *J Clin Oncol.* 1998;16:3230–3237.

85. Citron ML, Kaplan R, Parris WC, et al. Long-term administration of controlled-release oxycodone tablets for the treatment of cancer pain. *Cancer Invest.* 1998;16:562–571.

86. Bruera E, Belzile M, Pituskin E, et al. Randomized, double-blind, cross-over trial comparing safety and efficacy of oral controlled-release oxycodone with controlled-release morphine in patients with cancer pain. *J Clin Oncol.* 1998;16:3222–3229.

87. Tallgren M, Olkkola KT, Seppala T, et al. Pharmacokinetics and ventilatory effects of oxycodone before and after liver transplantation. *Clin Pharmacol Ther.* 1997;61:655–661.

88. Ritschel WA, Parab PV, Denson DD, et al. Absolute bioavailability of hydromorphone after peroral and rectal administration in humans: saliva/plasma ratio and clinical effects. *J Clin Pharmacol.* 1987; 27: 647–653.

89. Parab PV, Ritschel WA, Coyle DE, et al. Pharmacokinetics of hydromorphone after intravenous, peroral and rectal administration to human subjects. *Biopharm Drug Dispos.* 1988;9:187–199.

90. Wright AW, Mather LE, Smith MT. Hydromorphone-3-glucuronide: a more potent neuro-excitant than its structural analogue, morphine-3-glucuronide. *Life Sci.* 2001;69:409–420.

91. Thwaites D, McCann S, Broderick P. Hydromorphone neuroexcitation. *J Palliat Med.* 2004;7:545–550.

92. Lee MA, Leng ME, Tiernan EJ. Retrospective study of the use of hydromorphone in palliative care patients with normal and abnormal urea and creatinine. *Palliat Med.* 2001;15:26–34.

93. Durnin C, Hind ID, Ghani SP, et al. Pharmacokinetics of oral immediate-release hydromorphone (Dilaudid IR) in subjects with moderate hepatic impairment. *Proc West Pharmacol Soc.* 2001;44:83–84.

94. Palladone (hydromorphone hydrochloride extended-release capsules). Available at: http://www.fda.gov/cder/foi/label/2004/021044lbl.pdf. Accessed February 28, 2005.

95. Palangio M, Northfelt DW, Portenoy RK, et al. Dose conversion and titration with a novel, once-daily, OROS osmotic technology, extended-release hydromorphone formulation in the treatment of chronic malignant or nonmalignant pain. *J Pain Symptom Manage.* 2002;23: 355–368.

96. Tegeder I, Lotsch J, Geisslinger G. Pharmacokinetics of opioids in liver disease. *Clin Pharmacokinet.* 1999;37:17–40.

97. Egan TD, Sharma A, Ashburn MA, et al. Multiple dose pharmacokinetics of oral transmucosal fentanyl citrate in healthy volunteers. *Anesthesiology.* 2000;92:665–673.

98. Muijsers RB, Wagstaff AJ. Transdermal fentanyl: an updated review of its pharmacological properties and therapeutic efficacy in chronic cancer pain control. *Drugs.* 2001;61:2289–2307.

99. Actiq (oral transmucosal fentanyl citrate). Available at: http://www.actiq.com/physicians/aboutbtcp/default.asp. Accessed June 21, 2005.

100. Lichtor JL, Sevarino FB, Joshi GP, et al. The relative potency of oral transmucosal fentanyl citrate compared with intravenous morphine in the treatment of moderate to severe postoperative pain. *Anesth Analg.* 1999;89:732–738.

101. Portenoy RK, Payne R, Coluzzi P, et al. Oral transmucosal fentanyl citrate (OTFC) for the treatment of breakthrough pain in cancer patients: a controlled dose titration study. *Pain.* 1999;79:303–312.

102. Coluzzi PH, Schwartzberg L, Conroy JD, et al. Breakthrough cancer pain: a randomized trial comparing oral transmucosal fentanyl citrate (OTFC) and morphine sulfate immediate release (MSIR). *Pain.* 2001;91:123–130.

103. Burton AW, Driver LC, Mendoza TR, Syed G. Oral transmucosal fentanyl citrate in the outpatient management of severe cancer pain crises: a retrospective case series. *Clin J Pain.* 2004;20:195–197.

104. Shaiova L, Lapin J, Manco LS, et al. Tolerability and effects of two formulations of oral transmucosal fentanyl citrate (OTFC; ACTIQ) in

patients with radiation-induced oral mucositis. *Support Care Cancer.* 2004;12:268–273.

105. Ahmedzai S, Brooks D. Transdermal fentanyl versus sustained-release oral morphine in cancer pain: preference, efficacy, and quality of life. The TTS-Fentanyl Comparative Trial Group. *J Pain Symptom Manage.* 1997;13:254–261.

106. Kongsgaard UE, Poulain P. Transdermal fentanyl for pain control in adults with chronic cancer pain. *Eur J Pain.* 1998;2:53–62.

107. Eap CB, Buclin T, Baumann P. Interindividual variability of the clinical pharmacokinetics of methadone: implications for the treatment of opioid dependence. *Clin Pharmacokinet.* 2002;41:1153–1193.

108. Garrido MJ, Troconiz IF. Methadone: a review of its pharmacokinetic/pharmacodynamic properties. *J Pharmacol Toxicol Methods.* 1999;42:61–66.

109. Manfredi PL, Houde RW. Prescribing methadone, a unique analgesic. *J Support Oncol.* 2003;1:216–220.

110. Davis AM, Inturrisi CE. d-Methadone blocks morphine tolerance and N-methyl-D-aspartate-induced hyperalgesia. *J Pharmacol Exp Ther.* 1999;289:1048–1053.

111. Fisch MJ, Cleeland CS. Managing cancer pain. In: Skeel RT, ed. *Handbook of Cancer Chemotherapy.* Philadelphia, PA: Lippincott Williams & Wilkins; 2003:663.

112. Mercadante S, Casuccio A, Fulfaro F, et al. Switching from morphine to methadone to improve analgesia and tolerability in cancer patients: a prospective study. *J Clin Oncol.* 2001;19:2898–2904.

113. De Conno F, Groff L, Brunelli C, et al. Clinical experience with oral methadone administration in the treatment of pain in 196 advanced cancer patients. *J Clin Oncol.* 1996;14:2836–2842.

114. Bruera E, Palmer JL, Bosnjak S, et al. Methadone versus morphine as a first-line strong opioid for cancer pain: a randomized, double-blind study. *J Clin Oncol.* 2004;22:185–192.

115. Cady J. Understanding opioid tolerance in cancer pain. *Oncol Nurs Forum.* 2001;28:1561–1568; quiz 1569–1570.

116. Bruera E, Sweeney C. Methadone use in cancer patients with pain: a review. *J Palliat Med.* 2002;5:127–138.

117. Novick DM, Kreek MJ, Fanizza AM, et al. Methadone disposition in patients with chronic liver disease. *Clin Pharmacol Ther.* 1981; 30:353–362.

118. Todd M. Meperidine and the management of pain: what you need to know. *Lippincotts Case Manag.* 2004;9:241–242.

119. Indelicato RA, Portenoy RK. Opioid rotation in the management of refractory cancer pain. *J Clin Oncol.* 2003;21:87–91.

120. Scholes CF, Gonty N, Trotman IF. Methadone titration in opioid-resistant cancer pain. *Eur J Cancer Care (Engl).* 1999;8:26–29.

121. Santiago-Palma J, Khojainova N, Kornick C, et al. Intravenous methadone in the management of chronic cancer pain: safe and effective starting doses when substituting methadone for fentanyl. *Cancer.* 2001;92:1919–1925.

122. Benitez-Rosario MA, Feria M, Salinas-Martin A, et al. Opioid switching from transdermal fentanyl to oral methadone in patients with cancer pain. *Cancer.* 2004;101:2866–2873.

123. Vigano A, Fan D, Bruera E. Individualized use of methadone and opioid rotation in the comprehensive management of cancer pain associated with poor prognostic indicators. *Pain.* 1996;67:115–119.

124. Moryl N, Santiago-Palma J, Kornick C, et al. Pitfalls of opioid rotation: substituting another opioid for methadone in patients with cancer pain. *Pain.* 2002;96:325–328.

125. Mersky H, Bogduk N. *Classification of Chronic Pain: Descriptions of Chronic Pain Syndromes and Definitions of Pain Terms.* 2nd ed. Seattle, WA: IASP Press; 1994.

126. Woolf CJ, Mannion RJ. Neuropathic pain: aetiology, symptoms, mechanisms, and management. *Lancet.* 1999;353:1959–1964.

127. Bridges D, Thompson SW, Rice AS. Mechanisms of neuropathic pain. *Br J Anaesth.* 2001;87:12–26.

128. Dworkin RH. An overview of neuropathic pain: syndromes, symptoms, signs, and several mechanisms. *Clin J Pain.* 2002;18:343–349.

129. Dworkin RH, Backonja M, Rowbotham MC, et al. Advances in neuropathic pain. *Arch Neurol.* 2003;60:1524–1534.

130. Backonja MM. Use of anticonvulsants for treatment of neuropathic pain. *Neurology.* 2002;59:S14–S17.

131. Tremont-Lukats IW, Megeff C, Backonja MM. Anticonvulsants for neuropathic pain. *Drugs.* 2000;60:1029–1052.

132. Mellegers MA, Furlan AD, Mailis A. Gabapentin for neuropathic pain: systematic review of controlled and uncontrolled literature. *Clin J Pain.* 2001;17:284–295.

133. Rose MA, Kam PC. Gabapentin: pharmacology and its use in pain management. *Anaesthesia.* 2002;57:451–462.

134. Rosenstock J, Tuchman M, LaMoreaux L, Sharma U. Pregabalin for the treatment of painful diabetic peripheral neuropathy: a double-blind, placebo-controlled trial. *Pain.* 2004;110:628–638.

135. Feltner DE, Crockatt JG, Dubovsky SJ, et al. A randomized, double-blind, placebo-controlled, fixed-dose, multicenter study of pregabalin in patients with general anxiety disorder. *J Clin Psychopharmacol.* 2003;23:240–249.

136. Sabatowski R, Galvez R, Cherry DA, et al. 1008-045 Study Group. Pregabalin reduces pain and improves sleep and mood disturbances in patients with post-herpetic neuralgia: results of a randomized, placebo-controlled clinical trial. *Pain.* 2004;109:26–35.

137. Dworkin RH, Corbin AE, Young JP, Jr, et al. Pregabalin for the treatment of postherpetic neuralgia: a randomized placebo-controlled trial. *Neurology.* 2003;60:1274–1283.

138. McCleane GJ. Lamotrigine in the management of neuropathic pain: a review of the literature. *Clin J Pain.* 2000;16:312–316.

139. Pan HL, Chen SR, Eisenach JC. Intrathecal clonidine alleviates allodynia in neuropathic rats: interaction with spinal muscarinic and nicotinic receptors. *Anesthesiology.* 1999;90:509–514.

140. Davies PS, Galer BS. Review of lidocaine 5% patch studies in the treatment of postherpetic neuralgia. *Drugs.* 2004;64:937–947.

141. Bell RF, Eccleston C, Kalso E. Ketamine as adjuvant to opioids for cancer pain. A qualitative systematic review. *J Pain Symptom Manage.* 2003; 26:867–875.

142. Kotlinska-Lemieszek A, Luczak J. Subanesthetic ketamine: an essential adjuvant for intractable cancer pain. *J Pain Symptom Manage.* 2004;28:100–102.

143. Lossignol DA, Obiols-Portis M, Body JJ. Successful use of ketamine for intractable cancer pain. *Support Care Cancer.* 2004;13;188–193.

144. Mercadante S, Arcuri E, Tirelli W, Casuccio A. Analgesic effect of intravenous ketamine in cancer patients on morphine therapy: a randomized, controlled, double-blind, crossover, double-dose study. *J Pain Symptom Manage.* 2000;20:246–252.

145. Hocking G, Cousins MJ. Ketamine in chronic pain management: an evidence-based review. *Anesth Analg.* 2003;97:1730–1739.

Prevention and Treatment of Opioid Side Effects

CHAPTER

3

Egidio Del Fabbro
Ahmed Elsayem

INTRODUCTION

Significant progress has been made in treating cancer pain during the past 20 years, and as a result, opioid use has increased. Fear of addiction and the attitudes of physicians, nurses, and state medical legislators[1] still remain barriers to pain control. Addressing opiophobia and overcoming misconceptions about side effects require educating nurses, physicians, patients, and their caregivers. Fortunately, treatment is being initiated earlier and often at higher doses than in the past, but the increased use has revealed that clinically apparent side effects such as opioid-induced neurotoxicity[2] are more common than previously thought. In addition, side effects involving the endocrine and immune systems that were thought to be of questionable clinical significance are now recognized as emerging concerns.

The purpose of this chapter is to review the common and clinically important side effects of opioids used in the treatment of cancer pain and to elaborate on the prevention and treatment of these side effects.

GENERAL MEASURES

Effective opioid management requires anticipation of side effects, use of prophylactic measures to prevent common side effects, awareness of the risk factors for developing them, and regular assessment of patients for early signs and symptoms of opioid toxicity.

The prevalence of side effects depends on the type and stage of cancer, the dose and duration of opioid use, as well as the presence of comorbidities. Table 3-1 highlights the most important side effects. Patients develop tolerance over a period of days to some side effects, such as nausea, sedation, and respiratory depression. Other side effects are dose dependent and persist indefinitely. These include constipation, hormonal and immune effects, and the risk for neurotoxicity.

A reduction in the opioid dose and side effects can often be achieved by nonpharmacologic modalities such as radiation, neuroblocks, and adjuvant drugs such as corticosteroids, anticonvulsants, intravenous (IV) biphosphonates, nonsteroidal anti-inflammatory drugs (NSAIDs), and acetaminophen.

Prevention and early treatment of these side effects necessitates identifying patients who are at increased risk and regularly asking them about early symptoms such as myoclonus or hallucinations. The risk factors include high doses, prolonged exposure, advanced age, baseline dementia, concomitant use of other psychoactive drugs, and renal dysfunction. Since most opioids are predominately excreted by the kidneys, maintaining hydration is important to prevent accumulation of toxic metabolites. Patients who are unable to tolerate the oral route and have no IV access may be given a subcutaneous (SC) infusion (hypodermoclysis) of approximately 1 liter daily. Morphine's metabolites include morphine-3-glucuronide (M3G) and morphine-6-glucuronide (M6G), both of which are glucuronized in the liver, and normorphine. M3G does not bind to opioid receptors and can cause generalized hyperexcitability, myoclonus, and grand mal seizures in animals. Normorphine also causes central nervous hyperexcitability. M6G can accumulate and cause late opioid toxicity with oral and intraspinal administration. Furthermore, M6G is up to 45 times more potent than M3G in animal studies. Similarly, other opioids produce toxic metabolites; hydromorphone produces hydromorphone-3-glucuronide, oxycodone produces noroxycodone, and fentanyl produces the metabolite norfentanyl. Methadone produces no known active metabolites. Opioids such as meperidine and propoxyphene should be avoided entirely, since they are largely metabolized to their excitatory forms normeperidine and norpropoxyphene, which can accumulate in the presence of renal dysfunction and cause neurotoxicity.

Patients who may be at risk for dose escalation include those who have neuropathic pain, incident pain, that is, pain that worsens with maneuvers such as movement, or a history of somatization or addiction. Patients who somatize have an increased expression of pain and, despite dose escalation, report very little or no improvement. Physicians should acknowledge their underlying pain, but a multidisciplinary approach is suggested, with attention to alleviation of existential and psychological suffering that is expressed physically. Taking a collateral history is helpful since a patient who has coped in this manner in the past is likely to continue such behavior when faced with a serious illness. Counseling such patients about the difference between physical pain and psychological suffering can reduce the use of opioids and decrease the incidence of adverse effects. In many cases, antidepressants are indicated for depression and anxiety that accompanies somatization.

Screening for substance abuse and alcoholism (using the CAGE questionnaire) is important, because even a distant history of addiction presages maladaptive coping behavior during times of stress. The addicted brain and its reward circuit display permanent long-term physiologic changes[3] (brain plasticity), which remain well after the addictive drug has been discontinued. Opioids stimulate some of the same reward pathways, leading to increased use and dose escalation in patients with a history of addiction. Comorbid psychiatric conditions, including depression and anxiety, require treatment with medication

Table 3-1

Common Opioid Side Effects

Central Nervous System	Sedation
	Opioid-induced neurotoxicity:
	Hyperalgesia, allodynia
	Myoclonus
	Hallucination
	Delirium
	Seizure
Gastrointestinal	Nausea and vomiting
	Constipation
Cardiopulmonary	Respiratory depression
Others	Pruritus
	Urinary retention
	Endocrine abnormalities (e.g.,
	hypogonadism)
	Immune effects
	Drug interactions

or counseling. Opioids or illicit drugs may have been used to alleviate the symptoms of a preexisting psychiatric disorder. Treatment with 5-minute empathic counseling sessions that emphasize self-sufficiency, responsibility, and appropriate goals of either abstinence or reduction can result in decreased opioid use. By identifying patients at risk, treatment can be directed to relieve their suffering and prevent alienation from family and society.

CENTRAL NERVOUS SYSTEM SIDE EFFECTS

The central nervous system (CNS) can be affected by a broad spectrum of side effects, ranging from temporary mild sedation to opioid-induced neurotoxicity.

In the early stages of cancer, opioids can cause a subtle cognitive impairment that is largely related to initial dosing or dose increases.[4] In practice these psychomotor effects are not clinically significant, but it is prudent to advise patients to refrain from driving for 3–4 days until they become tolerant to an initial dose or following a dose escalation of 30% or more.

More severe side effects may be encountered in patients with advanced cancer. Opioid-induced neurotoxicity is a syndrome that includes some or all of the following symptoms: severe sedation, delirium, hallucinosis, myoclonus, seizures, hyperalgesia and allodynia, and cognitive impairment. A cognitively intact patient may be suffering from either visual or tactile hallucinations, but will not volunteer the information unless asked, for fear of being labeled with a psychiatric disorder.

▶ Sedation

Sedation is one of the most common side effects, particularly in opioid-naïve patients and those who receive rapid dose escalation. Mild to moderate sedation is not a symptom of neurotoxicity, and patients often improve over 4–7 days as tolerance develops. They may also be somnolent as a result of "catch-up" sleep if they have been in pain and plagued by insomnia.

Prevention and treatment

All drugs that exacerbate sedation should be discontinued or tapered, including benzodiazepines, antihistamines, antidepressants, and phenothiazines. Screening for delirium with an assessment tool based on DSM IV criteria is essential since changes in attention, perception, and cognition may not be readily apparent. In addition, constant reassessment is required to identify the possible contributory causes listed in Table 3-2, many of which are treatable, such as dehydration, infection, and hypercalcemia. Investigations such as a blood urea nitrogen test (BUN), calcium, sodium, creatinine, bilirubin, and chest x-ray may be appropriate. The potential of causing discomfort to a patient should be taken into account before ordering other tests, such as head computed tomography (CT) scans and lumbar punctures.

▶ Respiratory depression

Severe sedation and respiratory depression are uncommon events in cancer patients with chronic pain, even those whose opioid dose has been increased by 30% in response to inadequate pain control. Most opioid-naïve patients are able to tolerate morphine (15 mg sustained release q12h and 5 mg q4h as needed) or methadone (7.5 mg q12h and 5 mg q4h as needed) as starting doses without intolerable sedation.[5] Although rare, respiratory depression can occur with incorrect equianalgesic dosing during opioid rotation, particularly when rotating from other opioids to methadone.

Use of naloxone may precipitate a withdrawal syndrome,[6] arrhythmias, seizures, and severe pain, and should only be considered

Table 3-2

Causes of Delirium

Opioids
Other drugs:
  Chemotherapy (methotrexate, vincristine, ifosfamide, vinblastine, bleomycin, carmustine, procarbazine, and fluorouracil)
  Psychoactive (antidepressants, antiparkinsonian, benzodiazepine, metoclopramide, prochlorperazine, antihistamines)
  Corticosteroids, anticholinergics, H2-blockers, NSAIDs, anticonvulsants, theophylline, alcohol, quinolones, cephalosporins, cardiac glycosides
  Withdrawal syndromes: alcohol, corticosteroids, opioids, benzodiazepines
  Illicit drugs
Metabolic: dehydration and uremia
  Hypoxia, chronic obstructive pulmonary disease, congestive heart failure, anemia
  Liver failure
  Hyper/hyponatremia
  Hypercalcemia
  Hypoglycemia
  Adrenal failure
  Hyperthyroidism or hypothyroidism
Disseminated intravascular coagulation
Brain: metastases, leptomeningeal disease, cerebrovascular accident, intracranial hemorrhage, seizure disorders
Infection: CNS (meningitis or encephalitis) or systemic
Toxins: heavy metals, carbon monoxide
Nutritional deficiencies: vitamins B_1, B_3, B_{12}, folate

for patients with a respiratory rate of less than 6/min, and for those who are not arousable. The American Pain Society recommends placing an endotracheal tube in comatose patients prior to naloxone administration to prevent aspiration. There have been cases of pulmonary edema when opioid-induced hypoventilation has been reversed postoperatively with naloxone in young, otherwise healthy patients.[7] Some physical stimulation and close monitoring for at least 3 hours past the time of expected peak analgesic concentration is usually sufficient. If required, however, a dilute solution (0.4 mg ampul in 10 mL saline administered as 0.5 mL by IV push every 2 minutes) may be administered. It is important to remember that the duration of effect is relatively short (30 minutes) so that a continuous infusion may be required, which can be discontinued when pain recurs.

The general principles of managing typical opioid-induced sedation are to reduce the dose of opioids if pain is controlled, and then, if sedation persists, either to add a stimulant such as methylphenidate, dextroamphetamine, pemoline, or modafinil, or an acetylcholinesterase inhibitor. A dose reduction may be achieved by decreasing the dose between 2 and 6 AM, and increasing it around 6 PM, when opioid requirements are likely to be greater.

Methylphenidate is most commonly used and has been found to improve cognition[8] and also reduce sedation[9,10] in randomized crossover studies. Additional benefits are improved depression, fatigue, and pain control[11] in patients on opioids. Starting doses are usually 10 mg/day given in divided doses in the morning and at noon to avoid insomnia.

Modafinil's expense and lack of published studies in advanced cancer patients limit its use.

Pemoline is a seldom used secondline agent that requires monitoring of alanine aminotransferase (ALT) every 2 weeks.

Contraindications to the use of psychostimulants include a past psychiatric history, especially with paranoid ideation and hallucinations, and a history of addiction, weight loss, arrhythmias, or congestive heart failure. Psychostimulants lower the seizure threshold and, despite case reports showing improved hypoactive delirium, may precipitate agitation and confusion. These agents are thus best reserved for sedation in patients in whom there is no evidence of cognitive decline or perceptual disturbance.

Acetylcholinesterase inhibitors such as donepezil, galantamine, and rivastigmine have few drug interactions, a more favorable cardiovascular safety profile, and have been used successfully in Alzheimer's patients and may enhance the antinociceptive effect of opioids. A pilot study of donepezil in patients receiving opioids for cancer pain showed significant improvement in sedation, fatigue, anxiety, well-being, anorexia, depression, insomnia, and fatigue.[12] Side effects included nausea, vomiting, diarrhea, muscle and abdominal cramps, and anorexia, but overall the drug was well tolerated. A retrospective review[13] also demonstrated benefit in patients with delirium and myoclonus, and postulated a decreased likelihood of developing tolerance compared to psychostimulants.

If sedation is persistent and pain is under control, rotation to another opioid with a 30%–50% reduction in the equianalgesic dose is indicated because of incomplete cross-tolerance. Sedation accompanied by pain requires rotation without dose reduction. If sedation accompanied by pain persists after rotation and the MMSE is normal, the presence of psychological distress and suffering should be considered.

Myoclonus

Myoclonus is underrecognized as a complication of opioid treatment. It appears to be related to the metabolite M3G, which has no analgesic activity and accumulates more rapidly during renal impairment. It is characterized by brief asymmetrical jerks involving a whole muscle or it can be limited to the activity of a small number of fibers.[14] Patients may not complain early on if symptoms are not severe, and, therefore, must be screened frequently, particularly during dose escalation.

Prevention and treatment

The importance of myoclonus is that it may be a preseizure phenomenon, and treatment principles similar to those used for sedation may be followed: dose reduction if pain is controlled, reversal of factors such as dehydration and renal failure, and discontinuation of medications such as antidepressants, antipsychotics, and NSAIDs. Opioid rotation is frequently required when these measures fail. Benzodiazepines such as clonazepam, lorazepam, and midazolam may be effective in relieving myoclonus but will increase sedation and the likelihood of progression to delirium, and so should only be used as a last resort.

Delirium

Delirium is a common neuropsychiatric complication found in as many as 44% of advanced cancer patients admitted to medical institutions. It is reversible in approximately 50% of patients. Diagnosis using *Diagnostic and Statistical Manual of Mental Disorders, Fourth edition (DSM-IV)* criteria emphasizes an abrupt onset, fluctuating course, inattention, perceptual disturbance, and decreased cognitive function (Fig. 3-1). The causes are multifactorial, (Table 3-2) and a

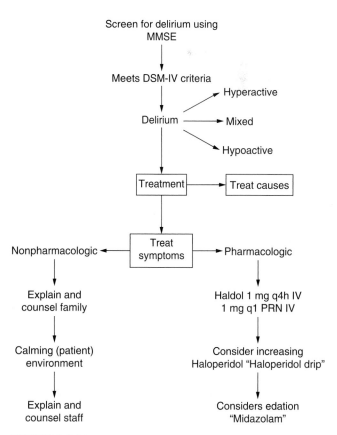

FIGURE 3-1 Delirium.

study of patients admitted to a palliative care unit revealed a median of three precipitating factors per episode.[15] There is increased recognition that prolonged opioid exposure, especially in high doses, places patients at high risk for developing delirium. Fortunately, along with dehydration it is also most commonly associated with delirium reversal.[15] Metabolic encephalopathies and hypoxia are not as responsive to treatment. Risk factors for opioid dose escalation and delirium are listed in Table 3-3.

The clinical manifestations of delirium range from slowed cognition and restlessness to severe agitation accompanied by hallucinations and delusions. Families and medical staff find these symptoms distressing, and there is a danger that overexpression of pain by a disinhibited delirious patient may result in inappropriate treatment with more opioids, thereby worsening delirium. The withdrawn hypoactive delirium that mimics depression may be less disturbing to families but poses a more challenging diagnosis, so a high index of suspicion and frequent assessment with a screening tool such as the MMSE are essential.

Prevention and treatment

Treatment should be initiated emergently with simultaneous management of symptoms and identification of causes. Throughout the episode it is important to reassure the patient, maintain a calming environment, and avoid unnecessary stimuli. Families, as well as nursing staff who are unfamiliar with advanced cancer patients, require explanation of the symptoms, particularly the risk of aggressive or unreasonable behavior.

Despite decreased fluid requirements in patients with advanced cancer, rehydration is always a worthwhile option for decreasing the accumulation and excretion of hydrosoluble opioid metabolites. In the patient with advanced cancer who is taking prolonged high doses of opioids, a reduction in dose alone is unlikely to improve delirium, and rotation with a 30% reduction in the equianalgesic dose is advisable.

Treatment both of agitated or hypoactive delirium with IV or SC haloperidol is effective. Although patients may initially exhibit features of only hypoactive or hyperactive delirium, if followed over time they will usually transition either completely or to fluctuate between the two states of delirium. Starting doses of haloperidol are usually 0.5 mg q6h with 0.5 mg q1h PRN for breakthrough symptoms. Although sedation has been a reported side effect, it is infrequent even with IV doses greater than 100 mg. Parenteral haloperidol can demonstrate an improved adverse effect profile with fewer patients prone to developing extrapyramidal symptoms (EPS).[16] An imbalance between

dopaminergic/acetylcholinergic systems may also protect against the development of EPS. If sedating drugs such as chlorpromazine or midazolam are required to control symptoms, opioids alone would be an unlikely cause of delirium and the patient may be experiencing terminal delirium.

The atypical antipsychotics have not demonstrated superiority in randomized controlled trials for the treatment of delirium, and in view of their expense should be regarded as secondline agents, except possibly in hypoactive patients who have a high risk for or history of EPS.

Finally, it should be noted that once a patient has developed opioid-induced neurotoxicity, the risk of developing further episodes is increased, so the intervals between opioid rotations may decrease.

GASTROINTESTINAL SIDE EFFECTS

Constipation and nausea are common side effects of opioid use in patients with advanced cancer (Fig. 3-2). Nausea typically lasts several days and then improves; however, tolerance to constipation does not develop and as many as 90% of patients suffer from this side effect.

▶ Constipation

Constipation is common in females, elderly patients, and those with intra-abdominal malignancies. Atypical presentations of constipation are frequently seen in patients with advanced cancer, and include nausea and vomiting, overflow diarrhea, incontinence, urinary retention, and confusion. Opioids are the most frequent cause of constipation that can, if untreated, lead to complete bowel obstruction or perforation. Other causes of constipation in advanced cancer patients include hypercalcemia, bowel obstruction by tumor, anorexia/cachexia, autonomic failure, or nerve plexus invasion.

The underlying mechanisms include decreased forward peristalsis, an increased transit time with increased absorption of water, and decreased biliary and gastrointestinal secretions, which result in desiccation of stool. Both intrathecal and systemic opioids induce constipation, although fentanyl and methadone may be less constipating than morphine or hydromorphone.

Prevention and treatment

Prevention of constipation should be a goal from the outset. Stimulant laxatives should be prescribed simultaneously with the first opioid. Other constipating medications such as iron, anticholinergics, calcium channel blockers, antihistamines, NSAIDs, diuretics, 5-HT$_3$ antagonists, tricyclic antidepressants, levodopa, and phenothiazines should be eliminated. Physical activity should be encouraged. Patients should be educated about the myth of anorexia causing decreased bowel movements, since constipation may well be the cause rather than the result.

Initial treatment should include both a stimulant laxative, which increases intestinal propulsion, and a stool softener. Senna and docusate can be titrated from one tablet daily up to four tablets QID if necessary. In refractory cases, an osmotic laxative such as milk of magnesia, sorbitol or, more commonly, lactulose may be added every 6 hours until a bowel movement occurs. The sweet taste of lactulose may precipitate nausea and occasionally cramping. There is also concern that long-term use of osmotic laxatives may cause fluid shifts and electrolyte imbalances.

Table 3-3
Risk Factors for Opioid-Induced Neurotoxicity
High opioid dose (increased risk with somatization, substance abuse, neuropathic, and incidental pain)
Prolonged opioid exposure
Preexisting borderline cognition
Dehydration
Renal failure
Advanced age
Opioids with mixed antagonist/agonist activity (e.g., pentazocine, butorphanol, nalbuphine)
Psychoactive drugs (benzodiazepines, tricyclic antidepressants)

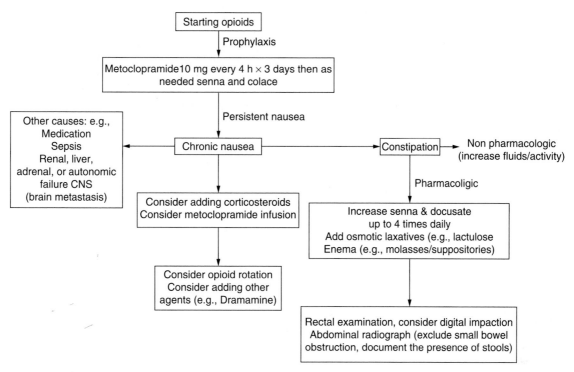

FIGURE 3-2 Nausea and constipation.

Polyethylene glycol (PEG) is used as a laxative prior to gastro-enterologic procedures and, because there is no metabolization or enzymatic breakdown, it has the theoretical advantage of no added gastrointestinal gas production. It hydrates stools and increases volume, which triggers peristalsis. Its initial effect is seen after 3 days. Patients must be able to take 125 mL of fluid with the sachet of PEG, and its tolerability and effectiveness may be preferable to lactulose, but this has not yet been firmly established in randomized trials. If 72 hours have passed and the patient has not had a bowel movement, bisacodyl suppositories or enemas are required. Milk and molasses may be used. The recipe for the milk and molasses enema: (1) 3 ounces powdered milk; water: 1 cup (175–200 cc), hot (37.8°C–40.6°C, 100°F–105°F) water—mix well; (2) 4 ounces molasses; (3) Pour half of the milk solution into the molasses container. Secure the lid and shake to mix. Combine the rest of the milk solution and the molasses mixture in an enema bag and mix evenly; (4) Repeat up to 4 times until fluid is clear.

Any change in symptoms, especially abdominal discomfort or poor response to medication, should prompt a rectal examination for diagnosis and treatment of a distal impaction. An empty rectum may indicate proximal impaction and magnesium citrate may be helpful. Decreased anal sphincter tone or sensation requires a magnetic resonance imaging (MRI) to exclude possible cord compression. Persistent constipation or cramping requires an abdominal x-ray, which may confirm the presence of large amounts of stool (ground glass appearance), or demonstrate air fluid levels suggestive of either ileus or obstruction. Air in the rectosigmoid suggests that complete obstruction is unlikely (unless the obstructive process is in its very early stages). A water-soluble contrast enema is rarely required in addition to the x-ray for confirmation. Opioid rotation to either methadone or fentanyl may be reasonable for patients with refractory constipation. Suspicion of complete obstruction may require an abdominal CT and discontinuation of laxatives or motility agents.

Psuedo-obstruction (or Ogilvie's syndrome) is a rare condition characterized by a large dilated cecum, which may respond to treatment with neostigmine.[17] Increased respiratory secretions and bradycardia are potential serious side effects resulting from this cholinergic agent.

In the past, opioid antagonists such as naloxone and naltrexone were used at low doses with some success, but unfortunately there is a risk of inducing a withdrawal syndrome.

Methylnaltrexone[18] is less lipid soluble, and in both oral and parenteral forms does not cross the blood–brain barrier and, therefore, does not reverse analgesia. Blocking the peripheral mu receptors in the gastrointestinal tract and elsewhere has the potential to be a major advance in the treatment of opioid side effects. Oral cecal transit time in chronic opioid users is significantly reduced; there is also a reversal of the delay in gastric emptying and patients often have an immediate laxation response. Other promising benefits of methylnaltrexone in preclinical studies include prevention of opioid-induced emesis, pruritus, and possibly urinary retention.

Another peripheral opioid antagonist, alvimopan, is orally administered, has high affinity for opioid receptors and poor systemic absorption, and has shown to be successful postoperatively in reducing ileus and shortening inhospital length of stay.[19]

Tegaserod is a 5-HT$_4$ agonist approved by the U.S. Food and Drug Administration (FDA) for constipation-predominant irritable bowel syndrome but it has not been evaluated for opioid-induced constipation.

Mineral oils, which soften and lubricate the stool, may be useful in the short term, but have potential deleterious side effects, including local irritation, malabsorption, and lipoid pneumonia (caused by an exogenous accumulation of fat in the lung). Prokinetic agents such as metoclopramide have occasionally been successful, as have NSAIDs, which are believed to reverse constipation by increasing the opioid-sparing effect and inhibiting prostaglandin synthesis.

Nausea and vomiting

Chronic nausea is common in patients with advanced cancer, and often has a multifactorial etiology. The altered gastrointestinal motility associated with cachexia, autonomic failure syndromes, and constipation is exacerbated by opioid use. Opioids may cause nausea through several pathways associated with these conditions, directly or indirectly. They stimulate receptors both in the chemoreceptor trigger zone (CTZ) and the true vomiting center, inducing peripheral effects that lead to gastroparesis and constipation. Ambulatory patients are more likely than bed-bound patients to complain of vertigo and nausea. Altered vestibular sensitivity or stimulation of the eighth cranial nerve may be the underlying causative mechanism of these complaints. Chronic nausea, however, differs from chemotherapy or radiation-induced nausea.

Prevention and treatment

Anticipatory, prophylactic treatment around the clock is important for all patients, especially those at high risk: age younger than 65, female gender, and stomach, breast, or gynecological cancer. Metoclopramide, the drug of choice, has proven efficacy, few side effects, and is inexpensive. It exerts a central antidopaminergic effect on the CTZ where opioids exert their emetic effect, and it acts peripherally to improve gastric motility.

When opioids are started, metoclopramide (10 mg q4h) should be given around the clock. In addition, breakthrough doses of 10 mg q2h, as needed, for nausea can be continued for 3 days, and then tapered as tolerance to opioids develops. A daily assessment of the intensity (using a 0–10 rating), onset, duration, frequency, quantity, and quality of the patient's nausea and emesis should be carried out. The number of bowel movements should be assessed daily, since nausea and vomiting may be presenting symptoms of constipation. Unlike other side effects, tolerance to constipation does not develop, so patients should remain on their laxative regimens indefinitely. Any medication that can contribute to nausea should be discontinued, if possible. These include iron, digoxin, cytotoxic agents, imidazoles, some antibiotics, tricyclic antidepressants, and NSAIDs.

If nausea worsens or persists despite treatment with metoclopramide, other possibilities should be entertained in the patient with advanced cancer, such as raised intracranial pressure, bowel obstruction (a promotility agent such as metoclopramide should be discontinued), ischemia, sepsis, and renal, adrenal, or autonomic failure. Should nausea persist, dexamethasone at a dose of 10 mg BID SC or IV may be added. It is a useful adjuvant therapy since it may also improve fatigue, pain, and appetite. Agitation and hallucinations are potential side effects, so the dose should be titrated downward depending on the improvement in nausea.

Corticosteroids have been used with success for chemotherapy- and radiation-induced emesis as well as for chronic nausea. A recent multicenter double-blind, parallel group comparative trial demonstrated that after 48 hours of metoclopramide treatment, dexamethasone produced a faster onset of antiemetic[20] effect but was not significantly better than placebo for improving the intensity of nausea over an 8-day period. Explanations include a significant placebo effect or a delayed response to metoclopramide requiring 1 week of treatment before its full benefit is achieved.

If nausea is still refractory, the dose of metoclopramide can be increased to 20 mg q4h around the clock or as an IV or SC infusion. Phenergan and prochlorperazine may be given as suppositories but are more prone to induce sedation. Metoclopramide also has the advantage of aiding gastrointestinal motility, and may continue to decrease the intensity of nausea for up to a week after initiation of therapy.

Prochlorperazine and metoclopramide can cause EPS, particularly in younger patients. EPS can be treated with clonazepam or benztropine; however, even at higher doses these side effects are rare. Akathisia (subjective feeling of restlessness characterized by increased movement and agitation) is often quite subtle at first and when suspected requires either a decrease in or cessation of the offending antiemetic.

Rotating opioids should be considered next, although this strategy does not appear to be as successful in reducing nausea as in reducing CNS side effects. A trial of haloperidol can be used in the event of metoclopramide failure. The atypical antipsychotic olanzapine and the antidepressant mirtazapine may be useful adjuvant treatments for nausea.[21] Like ondansetron, their mechanism of action appears to be via 5-HT$_3$ receptors. These drugs may be especially useful in patients with nausea who have delirium, anxiety, depression, or poor appetite. High cost and sedation are limitations of both drugs, though tolerance may develop with olanzapine and a higher dose of mirtazapine will be less sedating. The high cost of 5-HT$_3$ antagonists and their propensity for causing constipation make them unattractive for patients with advanced cancer. These agents should be reserved for patients undergoing chemotherapy for which they are the most effective.

IMMUNE SYSTEM SIDE EFFECTS

Immunosuppression by opioids has been documented both in animal and human studies. Animals treated with opioids have higher rates of infection, and in lipopolysaccharide-induced endotoxemia, opioids may have a synergistic effect that exacerbates sepsis.[22] Morphine also impairs the migration of neutrophils and increases susceptibility to *Streptococcus pneumoniae* lung infection.[23]

Opioid effects include inhibition of phagocytic activity, reduced capacity to generate antibodies, decreased natural killer cell activity, altered cytokine production, atrophy of thymus and spleen, and apoptosis of populations of immune cells.[24] If these changes are mediated directly through opiate receptors on immune cells, then a peripheral opioid antagonist may have a clinically applicable therapeutic role.[25] Other mechanisms of action include receptors in the CNS, which may activate the hypothalamic-pituitary axis.

Prevention and treatment

The clinical importance of the immune effects described for patients with advanced cancer are unknown; nevertheless, the development of new agents such as methylnaltrexone could attenuate opioid-induced immunosuppression without decreasing analgesia.

HORMONE ABNORMALITIES

Endocrine abnormalities can be associated with opioid usage, although few studies have explored the relationship between endocrine dysfunction and opioid use. Intrathecal opioids for chronic nonmalignant pain are known to cause hypogonadotropic hypogonadism in both males and females.[26,27] Hormone-level fluctuations appear to be clinically significant, with as many as 95% of males experiencing a sudden decrease in libido or potency after initiating opioid administration.[26] Approximately 15% develop hypocorticism and a similar number develop growth hormone deficiency. Case reports of patients taking oral opioids also demonstrated adrenal insufficiency, so the patient who has fatigue may well benefit from further investigation and hormonal supplementation.

Hypogonadism is common in men on sustained-action oral opioids for nonmalignant pain.[28] A case control study of male survivors of cancer who were taking oral opioids for longer than 1 year found that 90% demonstrated hypogonadism with low testosterone levels, sexual dysfunction, and elevated levels of fatigue and depression.[29] Although the underlying mechanism has not been elucidated, opioids are also believed to cause hyperprolactinemia, resulting in sexual dysfunction and hypogonadism.

▶ Prevention and treatment

Testosterone replacement can be used to treat these side effects and others such as chronic anemia, muscle atrophy, osteoporosis, and cognitive dysfunction associated with chronic hypogonadism. In hormone-dependent tumors, such as prostate cancer, testosterone is contraindicated.

Thyroid function tests are usually not affected by opioid use (slight elevation of T3 occasionally), and while there may be vasopressin release by intrathecal opioids resulting in edema, this effect may be attenuated in the long term.

DRUG INTERACTIONS

Awareness of the potential for drug interactions and individual variations in drug metabolism is important in preventing side effects. Pharmacokinetics (one drug affecting the disposition of another) and pharmacodynamics (interaction at the site of action) may each play a role.

Lowering the urinary pH may increase excretion of methadone, whereas fatty meals decrease the absorption of oxycodone. Sedating drugs should be avoided (Table 3-2) in general, but benzodiazepines may antagonize opioids at the receptor level, resulting in increased opioid requirements and increased sedation. NSAIDs and, occasionally, angiotensin-converting enzyme (ACE) inhibitors, can decrease renal function and increase the toxic effects of renally excreted metabolites of fentanyl hydromorphone and morphine.

Methadone has the advantage of hepatic excretion and no active metabolites, but has potential drug interactions, and along with fentanyl undergoes metabolism by the cytochrome P-450 system. Powerful 3A4 inducers such as dexamethasone may decrease the levels of methadone, while sertraline, grapefruit juice, aprepitant, and fluconazole may increase levels. Methadone also inhibits cytochrome P-450 2D6 and autoinduces its own metabolism. At high doses of 300–600 mg or more, methadone may cause torsades de pointes.[30,31] In clinical practice these high doses are seldom used (<0.6% of outpatients at the M. D. Anderson Cancer Center).[32] Caution is required with doses higher than 200 mg daily in a patient with a preexisting cardiac condition, severe hypokalemia, or hypomagnesemia, or in combination with drugs that are metabolized by the cytochrome P-450 system, and that may prolong the QT interval.[32]

Fluvoxamine can increase methadone levels significantly and cause drowsiness by inhibiting methadone metabolism. Codeine is a prodrug, with 10% transformed to morphine by 2D6 activity. Drug inhibition of this enzyme (e.g., paroxetine or fluoxetine) or its absence due to a recessively inherited deficiency (10% of Whites) decreases analgesia without abrogating the side effects.[33] Similarly, care should be exercised with another weak opioid, hydrocodone, since it is also metabolized by the 2D6 gene to the active metabolite, hydromorphone.

Genetic polymorphisms and drug interactions may be important in a significant subset of patients taking "weak" opioids who may have attenuated levels of analgesia but still experience side effects. Care should be taken when considering a dose increase, since fewer side effects may be experienced by changing to a "stronger" opioid like morphine.

ADDICTION

Substance abuse and addiction may be underestimated in cancer patients. Patients with a history of addiction are susceptible to dose escalation and, therefore, are at increased risk for opioid toxicity. As many as 25% of patients admitted to a palliative care unit have a positive screening test for alcoholism.[34] This number may rise to almost 50% for patients with head and neck cancers.

Abuse and addiction in patients with cancer who have no prior history of substance abuse are rare. Large surveys of patients who were administered opioids while in hospital appear to confirm this low risk.[35] Younger patients may not have had time to reveal a propensity for substance abuse, but there is no evidence that exposure to opioids will substantially increase their risk Patients need to be reassured that there is a very small risk of addiction if they have no prior history of alcohol or drug abuse. The difference between physical dependence, which occurs in all patients (characterized by withdrawal when an opioid is abruptly discontinued), and addiction (compulsive use of and overwhelming involvement in acquiring a substance despite adverse social, physical, or psychological consequences) should also be clarified.

Aberrant behavior such as multiple unsanctioned dose escalations or prescription losses may be indicative of abuse, although a couple of episodes of unsanctioned dose escalation or aggressive complaints about the need for higher doses may, in fact, be pseudoaddiction due to unrelieved pain. Treatment of this syndrome requires eliminating aberrant behavior with pain relief.[36]

OTHER SIDE EFFECTS

▶ Allodynia/hyperalgesia

Rare complications of opioids such as allodynia (pain in response to innocuous stimuli) and hyperalgesia (an exaggerated pain in response to noxious stimuli) should also be considered in the patient who continues to complain of pain or cutaneous hypersensitivity. These events may present as a result of intrathecal or systemic opioids; with morphine, the mechanism is thought to be accumulation of the metabolites M3G, normorphine, and hydromorphone. Despite their rarity, allodynia and hyperalgesia are particularly important because escalation of the dose in response to complaints of pain will worsen symptoms of sedation and the pain itself. This counterintuitive situation is similarly present in disinhibited, delirious patients who complain of increased pain. Treatment should include opioid rotation, educating medical staff members who are unfamiliar with these sequelae, and information given to the patient and family.

▶ Pruritus

Opioid-induced pruritus is most likely to be caused by spinal administration of opioids,[26] and is attributed to a peripheral or central release of histamines. While seldom a significant clinical problem, treatment with antihistamines may exacerbate sedation and anticholinergic side effects. Rotation of opioids may be an effective strategy. Fentanyl is a reasonable choice if pruritus is an ongoing problem, since it does not appear to cause the release of histamine. A future alternative is the antagonist methylnaltrexone, which could reverse or prevent side effects such as pruritus without reversing central analgesia.[18]

▶ Urinary retention

Urinary retention is more common with intraspinal opioids, and opioid-naïve patients; however, tolerance usually develops within a few days. Urinary catheterization is seldom required.

▶ Pulmonary edema

Massive increases in doses[37] seem to be associated with this life-threatening condition, whose etiology is unknown, but is noncardiogenic.

Some rare side effects such as biliary spasm are of questionable clinical significance.

REFERENCES

1. Gilson AM, Joranson DE. Controlled substances and pain management: changes in knowledge and attitudes of state medical regulators. *J Pain Symptom Manage.* 2001;21:227–237.
2. Daeninck PJ, Bruera E. Opioid use in cancer pain. Is a more liberal approach enhancing toxicity? *Acta Anaesthesiol Scand.* 1999;43: 924–938.
3. Nestler EJ, Malenka RC. The addicted brain. *Sci Amer.* 2004;290:78–85.
4. Lawlor PG. The panorama of opioid-related cognitive dysfunction in patients with cancer: a critical literature appraisal. *Cancer.* 2002;94: 1836–1853.
5. Strasser F, Willey J, Bertolino M, et al. Methadone versus morphine as a first-line strong opioid for cancer pain: a randomized, double-blind study. *J Clin Oncol.* 2004;22:185–192.
6. Manfredi PL, Ribeiro S, Chandler SW, Payne R. Inappropriate use of naloxone in cancer patients with pain. *J Pain Symptom Manage.* 1996;11:131–134.
7. Kaye AD, Gevirtz C, Bosscher HA, et al. Ultrarapid opiate detoxification: a review. *Can J Anaesth.* 2003;50:663–671, 2003.
8. Bruera E, Miller MJ, Macmillan K, Kuehn N. Neuropsychological effects of methylphenidate in patients receiving a continuous infusion of narcotics for cancer pain. *Pain.* 1992;48:163–166.
9. Wilwerding MB, Lop F, Athmann LM. A randomized, crossover evaluation of methylphenidate in cancer patients receiving strong narcotics. *Support Care Cancer.* 1995;3:135–138.
10. Bruera E, Chadwick S, Brenneis C, et al. Methylphenidate associated with narcotics for the treatment of cancer pain. *Cancer Treat Rep.* 1987;71:67–70.
11. Bruera E, Driver L, Barnes EA, et al. Patient-controlled methylphenidate for the management of fatigue in patients with advanced cancer: a preliminary report. *J Clin Oncol.* 2003;21:4439–4443.
12. Bruera E, Strasser F, Shen L, et al. The effect of donepezil on sedation and other symptoms in patients receiving opioids for cancer pain: a pilot study. *J Pain Symptom Manage.* 2003;26:1049–1054.
13. Slatkin NE, Rhiner M. Treatment of opiate-related sedation: utility of the cholinesterase inhibitors. *J Support Oncol.* 2003;1:53–63.
14. Mercadante S. Pathophysiology and treatment of opioid-related myoclonus in cancer patients. *Pain.* 1998;74:5–9.
15. Lawlor PG, Gagnon B, Mancini IL, et al. Occurrence, causes, and outcome of delirium in patients with advanced cancer: a prospective study. *Arch Intern Med.* 2000;160:786–794.
16. Vella-Brincat J, Macleod AD. Haloperidol in palliative care. *Palliat Med.* 2004;18:195–201.
17. Ponec RJ, Saunders MD, Kimmey MB. Neostigmine for the treatment of acute colonic pseudo-obstruction. *New Engl J Med.* 1999;341:137–141.
18. Yuan CS. Clinical status of methylnaltrexone, a new agent to prevent and manage opioid-induced side effects. *J Supp Oncol.* 2004;2:111–117.
19. Wolff BG, Michelassi F, Gerkin TM, et al. Avimopam Postoperative Ileus Study Group. Alvimopam, a novel, peripherally acting mu opioid antagonist: results of a multicenter, randomized, double-blind, placebo-controlled phase III trial of major abdominal surgery and postoperative ileus. *Ann Surg.* 2004;240:728–734.
20. Bruera E, Moyano JR, Sala R, et al. Dexamethasone in addition to metoclopramide for chronic nausea in patients with advanced cancer: a randomized controlled trial. *J Pain Symptom Manage.* 2004;28:381–388.
21. Davis MP, Khawam E, Pozuelo L, Lagman R. Management of symptoms associated with advanced cancer: olanzapine and mirtazapine. A World Health Organization project. *Expert Rev Anticancer Ther.* 2002;2:365–376.
22. Roy S, Charboneau RG, Barke RA. Morphine synergizes with lipopolysaccharide in a chronic endotoxemia model. *J Neuroimmunol.* 1999;95:107–114.
23. Wang J, Barke R, Charbonoeau RG, Roy S. Morphine impairs host innate immune response and increases susceptibility to Streptococcus pneumoniae lung infection. *J Immunol.* 2005;174(1):426–434.
24. McCarthy L, Wetzel M, Sliker JK, et al. Opioids, opioid receptors, and the immune response. *Drug Alcohol Depend.* 2001;62:111–123.
25. Wei G, Moss J, Yuan C. Opioid–induced immunosuppression: is it centrally mediated or peripherally mediated? *Biochem Pharmacol.* 2003;65:1761–1766.
26. Abs R, Verhelst J, Maeyaert J, et al. Endocrine consequences of long-term intrathecal administration of opioids. *J Clin Endocrinol Metab.* 2000;85:2215–2222.
27. Finch PM, Roberts LJ, Price L, et al. Hypogonadism in patients treated with intrathecal morphine. *Clin J Pain.* 2000;16:251–254.
28. Daniell HW. Hypogonadism in men consuming sustained-action oral opioids. *J Pain.* 2002;3:377–384.
29. Rajagopal A, Vassilopoulou-Sellin R, Palmer JL, et al. Symptomatic hypogonadism in male survivors of cancer with chronic exposure to opioids. *Cancer.* 2004;100:851–858.
30. Walker PW, Klein D, Kasza L. High dose methadone and ventricular arrhythmias: a report of three cases. *Pain.* 2003;103:321–324.
31. Krantz MJ, Lewkowiez L, Hays H, et al. Torsades de pointes associated with very-high-dose methadone. *Ann Intern Med.* 2002;137:501–504.
32. Reddy S, Fisch M, Bruera E. Oral methadone for cancer pain: o indication of Q-T interval prolongation or torsades de pointes. *J Pain Symptom Manage.* 2004;28:301–303.
33. Eckhardt K, Li S, Ammon S, et al. Same incidence of adverse drug events after codeine administration irrespective of the genetically determined differences in morphine formation. *Pain.* 1998;76:27–33.
34. Bruera E, Moyano J, Seifert L, et al. The frequency of alcoholism among patients with pain due to terminal cancer. *J Pain Symptom Manage.* 1995;10:599–603.
35. Porter J, Jick H. Addiction rare in patients treated with narcotics. *New Engl J Med.* 1980;302:123.
36. Passik SD, Portenoy RK, Ricketts PL. Substance abuse issues in cancer patients: Part 1: prevalence and diagnosis. *Oncology (Huntingt).* 1998;12:517–521.
37. Bruera E, Miller MJ. Non-cardiogenic pulmonary edema after narcotic treatment for cancer pain. *Pain.* 1989;39:297–300.

Application of Pain Management Principles in Specific Cancer Care Settings

Michael J. Fisch

INTRODUCTION

The principle goals of pain management are to prolong survival, maximize comfort, and to restore function. These goals do not change even when the settings in which patients are evaluated and managed differ. However, patients and clinicians realize that the setting in which care is applied has a significant impact on the approach to cancer pain management. The most important factors influencing cancer pain management are the relationship between the treating physician and the patient, and the skill and experience of the treating physician in cancer pain management. Patients become apprehensive when facing pain management by clinicians who do not already know them and who are not experts in cancer or cancer pain. At our cancer center, patients frequently drive for several hours and pass numerous local emergency rooms to seek care by physicians who are familiar with them or at least with cancer pain in general.

Within a given cancer center's system of care, various diverse settings influence the personnel involved in cancer pain management as well as the nature and range of approaches used to treat pain (see Table 4-1). This chapter addresses distinct issues that arise in the various settings in which cancer pain care is delivered.

EMERGENCY ROOM

When cancer patients develop significant new health problems, it is often not clear whether the problem is related to the underlying neoplasm, the cancer treatment, or to one or more comorbid medical conditions. Cancer care tends to dominate the medical landscape for individual patients who are under active evaluation or treatment for malignancy. And new problems, regardless of the cause, often have impact on the established plan for managing the malignancy. Cancer patients who experience significant pain often present to an emergency room (ER) associated with the cancer center that has been treating them, or may be referred to the ER from their physician's office with or without an initial attempt to manage the pain in the office setting. Recent data indicate that no less than 9% of patients who died with advanced cancer paid more than one visit to an emergency center in the last month of life.[1]

At the University of Texas M. D. Anderson Cancer Center, pain is the chief complaint at triage for 17% of patients who arrive at the emergency center.[2] Severe cancer pain (8 or greater on a 0–10 visual analog numerical rating scale) is considered an emergent problem for triage purposes. Mild to moderate cancer pain is considered

urgent. For reference, other urgent problems include conditions such as neutropenic fever, hemoptysis, and recent seizure. A problem such as exacerbation of chronic nonmalignant low back pain would be considered nonurgent (along with problems such as cough, dysuria, fatigue).[3]

The assessment of patients in the emergency center includes the assessment and treatment of the pain, and also the crucial evaluation of the underlying problem. Pain is a symptom, not a diagnosis. Oncologic emergencies are explicitly considered and ruled out when appropriate. Common oncologic emergencies presenting as pain problems include spinal cord compression, pathological fracture or impending fracture, brain metastases, and obstruction of a hollow viscus. Other urgent conditions that commonly arise in cancer patients and that may contribute to pain are infection, hemorrhage, and hypercalcemia.

The management of moderate to severe abdominal pain in cancer patients is distinct from the typical evaluation of the "acute abdomen" patient in a general hospital. Whereas fewer than 10% of general surgeons and only about 20% of ER physicians administer analgesics to a patient with significant abdominal pain in a general hospital ER,[4] the use of opioid analgesics for patients with chronic cancer pain localizing to the abdomen is generally indicated and usually given. Another distinguishing feature in the evaluation of moderate to severe abdominal pain in the cancer patient is that severe constipation is frequent enough as either the cause of or a significant contributor to the pain syndrome, and that it is considered in the differential diagnosis so that the amount of stool visualized on abdominal radiographs is noted carefully by ER physicians in cancer centers.

The assessment of cancer pain is described in detail in Chap. 1, and the principles of assessment apply well to the emergency center setting as well. However, it is worth highlighting common causes of pain exacerbation in the patient with stable, chronic cancer pain (see Table 4-2). Regarding the category of factors that shift the dose-response curve for analgesia, it is important to note that codeine, hydrocodone, tramadol, and oxycodone require the cytochrome P-450 liver enzyme 2D6 (CYP2D6) to form the active metabolite for analgesia.[5] As such, these drugs may become less effective when concomitant drugs are prescribed that inhibit CYP2D6.[6,7] Drugs that may inhibit CYP2D6 are summarized in Table 4-3. Another drug interaction to be aware of is inducement of CYP3A4, because opioids such as methadone and fentanyl are metabolized by this enzyme and other drugs that activate this metabolic process may decrease analgesia by these drugs. A common example is rifampin. Rifampin is used to treat infections such as tuberculosis and

Table 4-1

Settings for Cancer Pain Management

Episodic care settings
  Emergency center
  Periprocedural
    Venipuncture
    Tissue biopsy
    Lumbar puncture
    Bone marrow aspirate/biopsy
  Postoperative

Hospital
  Intensive care unit
  Hospital floor
  Palliative care inpatient unit

Outpatient clinic
  Primary care
  Oncology/hematology
  Palliative care
  Pain clinic
    Anesthesiology
    Neurology
    Physical medicine and rehabilitation

Nonhospital chronic care facility
  Nursing home
  Inpatient hospice

Home

Table 4-2

Common Causes of Unstable Pain in Chronic Cancer Pain Patients

Tumor progression
  New site of involvement
  Growth of an existing lesion

Shift in dose-response curve for analgesics
  Concomitant prescribing of a CYP2D6 inhibitor
  Concomitant prescribing of a CYP3A4 inducer
  Change in renal function

Change in medication absorption or compliance
  Mental status changes
  Nausea/vomiting
  Bowel obstruction
  Financial distress
  Opiophobia (patient or family)

Complication of cancer therapy
  Mucositis
  Vertebral compression fracture
  Herpes zoster
  Chemotherapy-related neuropathy

Hypercalcemia

Constipation

Table 4-3

CYP2D6 Inhibitors and CYP3A4 Inducers

Generic Name	Trade Name
CYP2D6 Inhibitors	
Antidepressants: e.g.:	
Clomipramine	Anafranil
Paroxetine	Paxil
Sertraline	Zoloft
Antipsychotic agents: e.g.:	
Chlorpromazine	Thorazine
Haloperidol	Haldol
Antimalarials: e.g.:	
Chloroquine	Aralen
Quinine	Legatrin
Antifungals: e.g.:	
Ketoconazole	Nizoral
Miconazole	Lotrimin
Antihistamines: e.g.:	
Diphenhydramine	Benadryl
Tripelennamine	Di-Delamine
Antivirals: e.g.:	
Delavirdine	Rescriptor
Ritonavir	Norvir
Lidocaine	Xylocaine
Isoniazid	Nydrazid
Amiodarone	Cordarone
Methimazole	Tapazole
Cimetidine	Tagamet
Cocaine	
Methadone	
CYP3A4 Inducers	
Aminoglutethimide	Cytadren
Antibiotics: e.g.:	
Rifabutin	Rifadin
Rifampin	Mycobutin
Anticonvulsants: e.g.:	
Carbamazepine	Tegretol
Phenytoin	Dilantin
Pentobarbital	Nembutal
Phenobarbital	Luminal
Hypericum perforatum[2]	St. John's Wort

methicillin-resistant *Staphylococcus aureus*. Rifampin causes significant CYP3A4 inducement and can make pain control worsen quickly. Finally, for patients with renal dysfunction, opioid metabolites may accumulate and cause opioid toxicities such as opioid-induced hyperalgesia. As such, a change in renal function can be associated with unstable pain, irrespective of the cause of the renal problem.

In the ER setting (or a similar urgent care environment), intravenous (IV) opioids are the most commonly used strategy for managing cancer pain. Because the preponderance of urgent cancer pain problems are A-delta and C fiber related (somatic and visceral pain), the use of opioids is a rational approach to treatment. Morphine,

Table 4-4

Rapid Titration of IV Opioids for Cancer Pain Emergencies (Pain ≥7/10)

Author, year of publication	Soares, 2003[11]	Hagen, 1997[9]	Mercadante, 2002[10]
Number of patients	20	10	45
Prior opioid dose as factor in the protocol? (yes/no)	Yes	No	No
IV bolus dose of opioid	Fentanyl at 10% of the IV morphine/ 24 h equivalent dose*	10–20 mg morphine or equianalgesic dose of another IV opioid	2 mg morphine
Pain threshold for repeat dosing	≥4/10	≥6/10	Not specified
Time interval for repeat dosing	5 min	30 min	2 min
Maximum number of doses per protocol	3	1 (doubled from the initial dose)	Not specified

*Convert oral morphine to intravenous morphine using a 3:1 ratio, and then to fentanyl using a ratio of 1:100

hydromorphone, and fentanyl are the most commonly used opioids and are most frequently administered via the IV route. A systematic review of research trials of rapid analgesia for severe cancer pain identified fewer than 10 studies, and each of these had major methodological limitations.[8] It is, however, clear that respiratory depression is not an issue in treating these patients for severe pain. Three rapid analgesia protocols[9–11] are summarized in Table 4-4. It is noteworthy that for successful achievement of rapid analgesia, the initial dose and dose frequency are clearly more important than the choice of opioid or the prior opioid dose. Given the paucity of published data to guide the care of these patients, expert pain assessment and clinician experience are likely to be key factors in achieving successful outcomes in the ER setting.

Other IV opioids that are sometimes used for managing acute cancer pain in the ER setting include meperidine and methadone. Meperidine is acceptable as a very brief treatment of acute pain,[5] but its central nervous system (CNS) toxicity is greater relative to the other available opioids so that it is not of particular practical value, since the other available opioids are easier to convert into oral or transdermal doses for continuing chronic pain control. Methadone can be given in low doses (1–5 mg IV) for acute cancer pain, but it is intrinsically long-acting and is not ideal for repeat dosing in the urgent care setting. Moreover, the proper initial dosing depends heavily on prior opioid dose, thus requiring the clinician to be skilled in being able to determine the morphine-equivalent opioid dose at baseline as well as the proper initial dosing of methadone. Other opioids are more robust regarding the range of clinicians who can prescribe them skillfully in this setting.

What about non-IV opioid analgesic approaches? First, it should be noted that morphine, hydromorphone, and fentanyl may each be given via subcutaneous injection or infusion. Moreover, oral transmucosal fentanyl citrate (OTFC) has been utilized for acute pain management in opioid-tolerant cancer pain patients. Because fentanyl is about 7000 times more lipophilic than morphine and 75–200 times more potent,[11] it can be formulated for transmucosal administration with the aim of rapid analgesia with time to onset of analgesia in the 5–15 minute range. In a retrospective series, Burton and colleagues described the use of OTFC in an outpatient clinic and its utility in averting the need for an emergency center visit.[12] In the initial multicenter trial that evaluated OTFC for the treatment of breakthrough cancer pain in patients receiving an oral morphine-equivalent dose of at least 60 mg/day, Portenoy and colleagues found that OTFC was safe and effective in nearly three-quarters of patients.[13] Although the most effective OTFC dose did not

correlate well with the prior opioid dose in this study, as a rough guide, 200 mcg dosing appears to be similar to 2 mg of IV morphine, and 800 mcg appears to produce results similar to 10 mg of IV morphine.[14]

Nonopioid adjuvants most likely to be used in the ER setting to treat cancer pain are corticosteroids and nonsteroidal anti-inflammatory agents (NSAIDs). Corticosteroids are most useful for managing widespread osseous pain due to metastases, patients with chronic, malignant bowel obstruction, hepatic pain due to capsular swelling, and for patients with headaches due to brain metastases or skull lesions. It should be noted that corticosteroids are preferred over opioids for managing headache pain from cerebral edema. The risk of respiratory depression and resulting increase in cerebral pressure makes opioids a poor choice for a patient with severe cerebral edema. A typical steroid dose for managing cancer pain is dexamethasone 4–6 mg given every 6–8 hours (or the appropriate dose of an alternate steroid). Higher doses are often used when the indication is cerebral edema. For patients with an intolerance or contraindication to this kind of steroid dosing, ketorolac may be used as an IV NSAID for managing severe cancer pain. Ketorolac should be used for very brief treatment of pain and dose adjustment is needed when it is applied to elderly patients or those with renal dysfunction. In this regard, ketorolac is similar to meperidine in that both drugs need to be used with caution.

PERIPROCEDURAL PAIN

The need for invasive procedures is common in cancer care, and as a result patients are at risk for experiencing acute pain (and sometimes chronic pain). Common procedures that may cause pain in cancer patients include venipuncture, tissue biopsy (such as prostate, breast, lung), lumbar punctures, and bone marrow aspirate/ biopsy. Depending on the procedure, factors that have been associated with the level of pain experienced by patients include the experience of the personnel performing the procedure, the size of the needle, the presence or absence of local anesthesia, the use of systemic analgesics or conscious sedation, and the age and sex of the patient. Just as appropriate prevention of nausea and vomiting with emetogenic chemotherapy can reduce the risk of nausea and vomiting with subsequent cycles of treatment, the same principle applies to pain with invasive procedures. Outcomes can be improved with appropriate patient and family education about the purpose of the procedure and its risks and benefits. The patient's experience with prior procedures should be explored, followed by an explicit discussion of the risk of pain and what measures can be utilized to prevent and control pain and anxiety. Moreover, it is critical to devise a specific plan for monitoring the patient for pain and anxiety during and after the procedure.

Venipuncture is so common in cancer care that its associated discomforts are sometimes overlooked. One way to minimize discomfort is to coordinate blood drawing to limit the frequency of venipuncture whenever possible. The eutectic mixture of local anesthetics (EMLA) can be applied to the skin over the venipuncture site to reduce the pain of the needlestick or insertion of an IV line. EMLA is effective in reducing pain in about 85% of patients,[15] and is particularly helpful for pediatric patients.[16] For adult oncology patients, a common approach is placement of a permanent vascular access device (VAD) to mitigate venipuncture-related pain. Discomforts associated with VADs are cited by almost 30% of patients and include site soreness, sleep disturbance, and the inconvenience of anticoagulation to maintain patency of the catheter. Nevertheless, more than 90% of patients report improved quality of life with VAD placement for this purpose.[17]

Tumor biopsies are another source of acute pain in cancer patients. This topic has not been the subject of extensive research, but there are data related to common procedures such as prostate biopsy or breast biopsy. For example, for fine needle aspirates of the breast, Daltrey and colleagues reported a randomized trial demonstrating that the use of a 23-gauge needle without local anesthetic was less painful than the use of a 21-gauge needle with local anesthetic.[18] For patients receiving transrectal ultrasound-guided biopsy of the prostate, various approaches have been investigated, including use of 2% rectal lidocaine gel, 40% dimethyl sulfonamide mixed with lidocaine and placed in the rectal vault for 10 minutes prior to the procedure, or injections of lidocaine into the prostate or the periprostatic area.[19–22] These methods all have efficacy in pain relief, although the comparison data are fairly limited.

Bone marrow aspirate and biopsy are commonly needed for patients with hematologic malignancy, bone marrow transplant patients, and occasionally for patients with solid tumors. More than 80% of patients experience pain with this procedure, with about one-third experiencing moderate to severe pain.[23] For children, the appropriate approach to managing pain associated with this procedure varies with the age of the patient. For example, in the 6–24-month age group, either general anesthesia or conscious sedation using IV sedatives (such as diazepam or midazolam) plus or minus opioids (such as fentanyl or morphine) is recommended.[24,25] For some adults, this approach may also be necessary. However, the vast majority of adults (more than 95% in one series) get satisfactory results with a topical anesthetic such as lidocaine injected into the periosteum prior to the procedure.[26] Sometimes, systemic oral analgesics are used in addition to topical treatment,[23,27] but this approach can cause bothersome side effects such as nausea, pruritus, and/or sedation.[27]

Finally, lumbar puncture is a frequent procedure in cancer care because of the need to treat or prevent the spread of malignancy to the leptomeningeal space. This procedure is particularly common in leukemia and lymphoma, and can also be necessary for solid tumors (particularly breast cancer). Postdural puncture headache often results from the procedure, occurring in 25%–40% of patients. The headache occurs within 3 days in more than 90% of patients, is worse with standing, and more than 75% of patients experience resolution of the symptom within 7 days.[28] To reduce the frequency and severity of this headache, patients are generally asked to remain supine for 1 or 2 hours after the procedure. More prolonged bed rest has not demonstrated benefit.[29] Other interventions that have been explored but have not shown efficacy include the use of desmopressin acetate, adrenocorticotrophic hormone, caffeine, and sumatriptan. The epidural blood patch is the most effective and most commonly used intervention for preventing or relieving a postdural puncture headache. This procedure involves injecting 20–30 mL of autologous blood into the epidural space at the level of the dural puncture or one intervertebral space below. It is effective in 70%–98% of patients if applied within 24 hours of the initial procedure, and repeat procedures can be helpful if the headache does not resolve.[28]

POSTOPERATIVE PAIN MANAGEMENT

In 2000, it was estimated by the president of the American Pain Society that only about 25% of the 23 million patients who undergo surgery annually in the United States obtain adequate relief of acute pain.[30] Fortunately, postoperative pain has been more effectively managed in cancer care in recent years due to increased attention to pain management at the policy level, advances in surgical techniques, systemic chemotherapy, opioid delivery and dosing, and improved psychosocial assessment and care. At the policy level, the Joint Commission on the Accreditation of Healthcare Organizations (JCAHO) added pain severity and quality assessment to its standard for postprocedure management. In the surgical realm, the most significant advance has been the use of laparoscopic surgical techniques rather than open surgery for various procedures such as colectomy, adrenalectomy, and prostatectomy. Over time, the scope of such procedures has expanded and the outcomes have improved due to advances in surgical training, instrumentation, and understanding of the pathophysiology associated with the procedures.[31] The evidence favors improved pain control for laparoscopic colectomy[32] and adrenalectomy,[33] but thus far the evidence in favor of improved pain control with laparoscopic prostatectomy is lacking.[34,35] Other advances in cancer surgery that have reduced postprocedure pain include the use of sentinel lymph node dissections for breast cancer and melanoma staging procedures, and downsizing of primary tumors before surgery with the advent of neoadjuvant chemotherapy approaches in diseases such as breast cancer, head and neck cancers, and other solid tumors.

In the past 10 years, the use of IV opioids on an "as-needed" basis delivered by the provider postoperatively has given way to patient-controlled analgesia and also to the use of neuraxial opioid delivery (epidural or intrathecal) in the early perioperative period (usually about 3 days). In general, pain control is excellent with a variety of modern methods, and thus comparative studies tend to show no significant differences in overall pain control among methods. There can, however, be differences in costs or side effects. For example, patient-controlled epidural analgesia may produce fewer motor side effects than continuous infusion epidural analgesia.[36] Also, comparing patient-controlled IV analgesia alone to epidural or intrathecal analgesia or in combination with IV opioids reveals improved early postoperative pain control in the intrathecal analgesia group with a small to imperceptible increased risk of complications such as infection or catheter leakage.[37–39] Elements of an institutional guideline for epidural analgesia in the postoperative setting are summarized in Table 4-5.

In addition to opioids and local anesthetics, other adjuvants that have been found to be potentially useful in the postoperative period include NSAIDs,[40] gabapentin and pregabalin,[41] and dextromethorphan[42]

Table 4-5

Key Elements of a Policy for Epidural Use in Postoperative Pain Management

Qualifications of personnel
Pain anesthesiologist and designated nurses

Patient education
Preoperative and postoperative teaching

Necessary equipment
Need for IV access
Designated (approved) pumps

Monitoring
Pulse oximetry (continuously for 24 hours, then every 4 hours until removal)
Nursing assessment (global) every 8 hours
Pain anesthesiologist assessment once daily

Medical prescribing guidelines
Final concentration of each drug should be specified when ordering narcotic/local anesthetic combinations
Anticoagulant, antiplatelet, and CNS depressant medications should be approved by the pain anesthesiologist before administration

Table 4-6

Summary of the 2001 JCAHO Six Standards in Pain Management

Recognize the right of individuals to appropriate pain management
If pain exists, determine this and also assess the nature and intensity
Establish policies and procedures to support ordering safe, effective pain medication
Educate patients and families about effective pain management
Consider pain management needs in the discharge planning process
Incorporate pain management in the organization's performance improvement process

among others. No adjuvant approach has emerged as a standard for consistent use in postoperative cancer care, although adjuvants may be considered in individual cases. Preemptive approaches (preprocedure dosing of medication) have not been helpful when agents such as morphine, ketamine, or clonidine have been used.[43]

Finally, it has been established that poor postoperative pain outcomes are highly associated with preprocedure levels of psychological distress.[44–46] This has led to increased attention to the need for preoperative teaching, counseling, and distress screening to achieve the best possible postoperative pain and symptom control.

PAIN CARE IN HOSPITALIZED CANCER PATIENTS

Uncontrolled cancer pain is an enormous problem in both developing and industrialized countries. Data from the World Health Organization indicated, in 1990, that about 4.5 million patients worldwide die each year in uncontrolled pain.[47] Cancer patients, particularly those with advanced disease, often spend time in the hospital. In the last month of life, about 9% of older adults on Medicare have more than one hospital admission, and almost 12% spend more than 14 days in the hospital. The care of cancer patients and other hospitalized patients with pain in the United States received new attention in 2001 when pain management standards were adopted by the JCAHO, an independent, not-for-profit organization that serves as the primary organization setting health care standards in the United States. The new standards (summarized in Table 4-6) brought about a shift in hospital-based pain management by making it a patients' rights issue and an education and training issue, by emphasizing quantitative aspects of pain assessment, and by emphasizing systematic assessment and safe management.[30] Of note, the JCAHO standards did not assert a right to actual pain relief, as pain is a complex phenomenon. Unfortunately, a guarantee of pain relief is not a realistic goal for all patients because the cognitive, affective, and behavioral meanings of pain vary for each individual and influence response to therapy.[48] Another misconception

is that these JCAHO standards elevated pain as a "fifth vital sign" like the Department of Veterans Affairs had done. It turns out that the fifth vital sign mentality may help improve pain awareness, but it is impractical and inappropriate in some settings and for some patients. For example, patients who do not have pain or painful conditions can become irritated if they are asked to rate their pain on a 0–10 scale every 8 hours when their vital signs are taken. Also, it may not be appropriate for the staff who are responsible for vital signs to be designated to ask patients about their pain instead of staff members who may be more familiar to and trusted by the patient.

A good starting point in understanding hospital-based pain management is the rules of 80% (see Table 4-7). We know that pain is prevalent in cancer patients and that it is readily manageable in 80% of patients,[49] and these patients are generally cared for by their oncologists or hospitalists. It is the approximately 20% of patients whose pain management is more difficult that leads to inpatient consultations from one of several kinds of primary disciplines with expertise in pain management: palliative care, anesthesiology pain management, neurology, physical medicine and rehabilitation, and psychology. This subgroup of more difficult patients with pain may manifest one or more problems such as refractory pain, significant opioid side effects, psychological and perhaps spiritual/existential distress, and complex clinical comorbidities. Careful multidimensional assessment is needed for these patients, ideally in the context of a multidisciplinary team. Whereas pain assessment has been, in principle, mandated in United States hospitals, pain treatment remains the subject of considerable variation. This is because there is a pervasive lack of comparative trials of analgesic drug therapy, and thus there is controversy and practice variation ranging from the choice of first-line and subsequent analgesics to the route of administration, assessment of pain outcomes, and side effects of analgesics.[50,51] It is safe to assert that IV opioids are commonly administered for hospitalized cancer patients with pain crisis, and this may be given

Table 4-7

The Cancer Pain Rules of 80%

More than 80% of patients with cancer develop pain before death
Cancer pain can be controlled with simple treatments in more than 80% of cases
About 80% of patients with cancer will not be able to take oral opioids for some period before their death
About 80% of inpatient pain documentation is recorded by nurses and nurse assistants

by patient-controlled analgesia (except for patients with delirium, aberrant drug taking behaviors, or other contraindications).[52]

INTENSIVE CARE UNIT PAIN ISSUES

A significant proportion of patients with cancer will experience an admission to the intensive care unit (ICU) at some point in their care. For example, based on Medicare claims data from 1996, almost 12% of older adults on Medicare were admitted to the ICU in their last month of life.[53] For cancer patients in the ICU, pain and other physical symptoms are prevalent, with more than half of patients reporting a significant symptom burden and additional issues such as sleep disturbance and difficulty communicating that often accentuate their discomfort.[54] Data from the landmark SUPPORT study (Study to Understand Prognoses and Preferences for Outcomes and Risks of Treatments) indicate that adverse outcomes such as attempted resuscitation, readmission to the hospital, or death while receiving ventilatory assistance were 60% more likely for cancer patients in the ICU who preferred life-extending therapy as opposed to therapy directed at pain relief.[53] In other research, the level of patient comfort and use of nursing resources was not found to be influenced by the presence or absence of "do-not-resuscitate" orders.[55] However, there may be differences in the level of knowledge about pain and symptom management between ICU nurses and other hospital nurses. For instance, in a large survey assessing pain management knowledge among nurses, ICU nurses in Taiwan were found to have significantly lower scores than other nurses.[56]

One way to avoid pain and discomfort associated with aggressive care in the ICU is to improve the selection of patients who enter such a unit. The most appropriate patients for ICU admission are those with newly diagnosed cancer and life-threatening cancer-related events such as bulky mediastinal disease, tumor lysis syndrome, or leukostasis in the setting of acute leukemia.[57] Hospitalized cancer patients who experience unanticipated cardiac arrest due to rhythm disturbances, acute airway obstruction, or pulmonary embolization have a 20%–25% of survival to hospital discharge,[58] and they may be appropriate candidates for ICU care depending on their end-of-life preferences. However, in a series published using M. D. Anderson Cancer Center data, 0 of 171 patients survived to discharge

when they experienced an unanticipated cardiac arrest in the setting of gradual deterioration and subsequent sepsis, acidosis, cardiogenic shock, or multiorgan dysfunction.[58] Given these data, it is clear that effective communication with patients and families provides an avenue for prevention of pain and unnecessary suffering. Back and Arnold have described useful communication tools for addressing conflict related to aggressiveness of care, including active listening, self-disclosure, explaining, empathizing, reframing, and brainstorming.[59] Expanding training and skills in counseling and communication can improve the care of cancer patients with pain or for those who are at risk for pain.

PALLIATIVE CARE PROGRAMS

Some hospitalized cancer patients have access to secondary palliative care, which refers to consultation and specialty care provided by palliative care physicians working in a multidisciplinary team.[60] As defined by Morrison and Meier, the aim of palliative care is to relieve suffering and improve quality of life for patients with advanced illness and their families.[61] It is based on an interdisciplinary approach offered simultaneously with other appropriate medical treatments, which may include chemotherapy or radiation therapy. A conceptual model for the trajectory of cancer patients toward the end of life is summarized in Fig. 4-1. Most patients who receive aggressive anticancer therapy are those with acceptable quality of life and function. Once patients become frail, they are more likely to receive supportive care alone or therapy that is modified significantly to account for their poor health status. Patients then develop dynamic multiorgan dysfunction due to infection, bleeding, thrombosis, metabolic disarray, frank tumor progression, or other factors. There is considerable variability in this final trajectory toward death. As such, the interdisciplinary palliative care team is particularly valuable as it is configured to help manage physical symptoms, provide psychological support and care, communicate with the patient and family about prognosis and options for treatment, assist with the choice of appropriate settings for care, and mobilize other necessary resources.

The scope of services from a typical palliative care team is summarized in Table 4-8. Based on data from the 1998 American

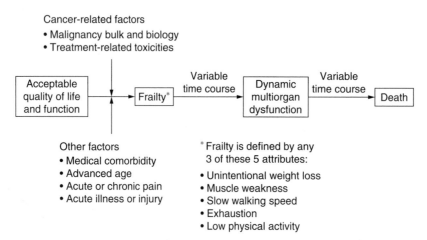

FIGURE 4-1 End-of-life trajectory in cancer patients.

Table 4-8

The Scope of a Typical Palliative Care Multidisciplinary Team

Medical care
Nursing
Psychosocial care
Spiritual care
Pharmacy
Adjunctive therapies (physical, occupational, massage, others)
Volunteers
Administration

Hospital Association survey, 337 (30%) hospitals reported having a hospital-based palliative care unit, and another 228 (20.4%) had plans to establish one.[62] These units are an example of secondary palliative care and are most commonly structured as an inpatient consultation service and hospital-based hospice. They tend to be housed in oncology, general medicine, and geriatrics.[62] The increase in hospital-based palliative care access has also been reported in other countries. For example, Centeno and colleagues reported that since 1990 in Spain there has been an average increase of 18 new programs per year so that about 10% of patients dying from cancer have accessed hospital-based palliative care.[63]

Tertiary palliative care units have also become increasingly common. *Tertiary palliative care* refers to palliative care that is practiced, researched, and taught at academic medical centers.[60] Tertiary palliative care teams are often led by oncologists, and pain (along with fatigue) is a prevalent and treatment-responsive symptom that is among the chief problems addressed in tertiary inpatient units. Elsayem and colleagues reported the early experience in tertiary palliative care at M. D. Anderson Cancer Center and reported that the 61% of patients assessed had pain of 5 or greater on a 0–10 numerical rating scale, with a baseline mean pain score of 6.2, which fell to a follow-up mean of 2.7 with comprehensive treatment.[64] Of note, in the M. D. Anderson Center palliative care unit, 52% of patients were discharged to hospice, 23% died in the unit, and 14% were discharged home without hospice care.[64] The patient disposition distributions vary widely in hospital-based palliative care programs, reflecting differences in referral patterns, patient preferences, and local resources.

Whereas traditional palliative care teams have practiced mostly in hospital, hospice, or nursing home settings, there is a growing trend toward outpatient palliative care. Meyers and Linder described the concept of "simultaneous care" in 2003 to address the fact that too many patients with advanced malignancy were provided with the unsatisfying option of choosing palliative care or systemic cancer therapy, but not both options. Since most systemic cancer therapy is now being given on an outpatient basis, the provision of simultaneous palliative care would require outpatient access to this care as well.[65] Outpatient palliative care programs have been described in the United States,[66–69] Spain,[70] and England.[71] As expected, there is considerable heterogeneity in these programs due to diverse referral patterns. With the growth of these programs and the resulting trend toward earlier referral, the median survival time of the patient population referred to some of these programs is years rather than months.[68] It is clear that cancer patients predominate in these programs and that patients referred to outpatient palliative care programs

have significant symptom burden. For example, Porta-Sales and colleagues described 534 patients with outpatient palliative care appointments during the course of 1 year, 38% of whom had at least three visits.[70] In this sample, one-third of patients had a numerical rating pain score of >4, but only one-fourth of patients were receiving strong opioids at the time of referral. Pain scores improved significantly in this sample of patients. In contrast, a model of outpatient palliative care in the United States that involved only consulting advice reported improved outcomes for dyspnea, anxiety, and spiritual well-being, but not pain control.[72] The absence of improved pain control in that series was attributed to lack of adherence to the recommendations provided by the palliative care consultants.

NURSING HOME CARE

Nursing homes are a common site for patient care toward the end of life. By 2030, more than 20% of Americans and Europeans will be older than age 65. Greater than 50% of those Americans over age 65 are expected to enter a nursing home at some time before they die.[73] Dying nursing home residents are known to experience high rates of untreated pain and other symptoms. A classic study by Bernabei and colleagues reviewed the nursing home experience of cancer patients aged 65 or older and found that at least one-quarter of the patients experienced daily pain, and more than one-quarter of those patients did not receive any pain medication.[74] This finding has persisted in other recent surveys.[75] There are various barriers to pain management in the nursing home setting (see Table 4-9). Lack of pain management knowledge and fear of addiction are common barriers. Nursing home clinicians are sensitive to the need to reduce medication exposures to reduce falls and medication side effects. High-risk medications in older adults include benzodiazepines and other sleep medications, neuroleptics, antidepressants, and anticonvulsants.[76] Pain medications are appropriate for older adults in nursing homes, with the exception of meperidine. Meperidine should not be used because of its association with an increased risk of delirium or seizures in this population due to the metabolite normeperidine.[77] Assessment problems unique to the elderly include differences in pain expression in older adults[78] and dealing with cognitive impairment.

Interventions that have been effective in improving pain management in nursing homes include educational interventions and the provision of interdisciplinary care and comprehensive geriatric assessment.[79–81] Hospice care, which is a specific program for interdisciplinary, comprehensive care of dying patients, is available in nursing homes in some instances. Unfortunately, hospice use varies by region and only 10%–15% of dying nursing home residents are served by hospice.[82,83]

Table 4-9

Barriers to Pain Management in Nursing Homes

Lack of pain management knowledge in nursing home staff and physicians
Lack of standardized approaches and institutional commitment
Fear of addiction and analgesic overdose
Difficulty in assessing cognitively impaired patients

Table 4-10

Major Aspects of Discussing Hospice

Establishing the proper context
  Clarifying the patient and caregiver's understanding
  Elucidating the patient and caregiver's preference for detail
  Negotiating who should be present for hospice discussion
  Negotiating who should deliver the information
Key steps in the discussion
  Discussion of overall goals of care
  Responding to emotions
  Exploring hospice compared to other options to achieve the stated
    goals
  Establishing a concrete plan

HOSPICE

The modern definition of *hospice* refers to the concept of providing comprehensive, interdisciplinary care to dying patients and their families. Hospice care originated in England and has become increasingly prevalent in the United States since the 1970s. In the United States, the word hospice is often used to refer specifically to care provided by the Medicare Hospice Benefit that was established in 1982. This benefit applies to terminally ill patients with an expected survival of 6 months or less. Such patients may elect to surrender all other Medicare benefits (except for the attending physician's services) in favor of care under a hospice program that provides a package of core services. These include physician services, skilled nursing services, social services, spiritual care, drugs and biologics related to the care of the terminal illness, and counseling (including bereavement care). There is considerable variability in services provided by hospice programs depending on whether the hospice program is for profit or not-for-profit,[84] how much philanthropy is attracted, and its relationship to the community and other healthcare organizations.[85]

Provision of care in the context of a hospice program is one effective way to provide comprehensive, interdisciplinary, and skillful care of terminally ill patients with cancer pain and other problems. One of the major challenges in providing hospice care to eligible patients is for healthcare providers to introduce the topic and discuss it effectively with patients and their family caregivers. Numerous, excellent reviews provide guidance on this sort of discussion.[59,86–90] Major points in approaching the topic of hospice with patients are summarized in Table 4-10.

REFERENCES

1. Earle CC, Neville BA, Landrum MB, et al. Trends in the aggressiveness of cancer care near the end of life. *J Clin Oncol.* 2004;22:315–321.
2. Escalante CP, Meltzer BA. Emergency care at comprehensive cancer centers. In: Yeung SJ, Escalante CP, eds. *Oncologic Emergencies.* Hamilton, BC Decker; 2002:1–5.
3. Liu W, Ho T, Lee EL, et al. Triage. In: Yeung SJ, Escalante CP, eds. *Oncologic Emergencies.* Hamilton, BC Decker; 2002:6–12.
4. Graber MA, Ely JW, Clarke S, et al. Informed consent and general surgeons' attitudes toward the use of pain medication in the acute abdomen. *Am J Emerg Med.* 1999;17:113–116.
5. Institute for Clinical Systems Improvement (ICSI). *Assessment and Management of Acute Pain.* Bloomington, ICSI; 2004:66.
6. Heiskanen T, Olkkola KT, Kalso E. Effects of blocking CYP2D6 on the pharmacokinetics and pharmacodynamics of oxycodone. *Clin Pharmacol Ther.* 1998;64:603–611.
7. Otton SV, Wu D, Joffe RT, et al. Inhibition by fluoxetine of cytochrome P450 2D6 activity. *Clin Pharmacol Ther.* 1993;53:401–409.
8. Davis MP, Weissman DE, Arnold RM. Opioid dose titration for severe cancer pain: a systematic evidence-based review. *J Palliat Med.* 2004;7:462–468.
9. Hagen NA, Elwood T, Ernst S. Cancer pain emergencies: a protocol for management. *J Pain Symptom Manage.* 1997;14:45–50.
10. Mercadante S, Villari P, Ferrera P, et al. Rapid titration with intravenous morphine for severe cancer pain and immediate oral conversion. *Cancer.* 2002;95:203–208.
11. Soares LG, Martins M, Uchoa R. Intravenous fentanyl for cancer pain: a "fast titration" protocol for the emergency room. *J Pain Symptom Manage.* 2003;26:876–881.
12. Burton AW, Driver LC, Mendoza TR, et al. Oral transmucosal fentanyl citrate in the outpatient management of severe cancer pain crises: a retrospective case series. *Clin J Pain.* 2004;20:195–197.
13. Portenoy RK, Payne R, Coluzzi P, et al. Oral transmucosal fentanyl citrate (OTFC) for the treatment of breakthrough pain in cancer patients: a controlled dose titration study. *Pain.* 1999;79:303–312.
14. Lichtor JL, Sevarino FB, Joshi GP, et al. The relative potency of oral transmucosal fentanyl citrate compared with intravenous morphine in the treatment of moderate to severe postoperative pain. *Anesth Analg.* 1999;89:732–738.
15. Fetzer SJ. Reducing venipuncture and intravenous insertion pain with eutectic mixture of local anesthetic: a meta-analysis. *Nurs Res.* 2002;51:119–124.
16. Rogers TL, Ostrow CL. The use of EMLA cream to decrease venipuncture pain in children. *J Pediatr Nurs.* 2004;19:33–39.
17. Chernecky C. Satisfaction versus dissatisfaction with venous access devices in outpatient oncology: a pilot study. *Oncol Nurs Forum.* 2001;28:1613–1616.
18. Daltrey IR, Kissin MW. Randomized clinical trial of the effect of needle gauge and local anaesthetic on the pain of breast fine-needle aspiration cytology. *Br J Surg.* 2000;87:777–779.
19. Mutaguchi K, Shinohara K, Matsubara A, et al. Local anesthesia during 10 core biopsy of the prostate: comparison of 2 methods. *J Urol.* 2005;173:742–745.
20. Kravchick S, Peled R, Ben-Dor D, et al. Comparison of different local anesthesia techniques during TRUS-guided biopsies: a prospective pilot study. *Urology.* 2005;65:109–113.
21. Inal G, Yazici S, Adsan O, et al. Effect of periprostatic nerve blockade before transrectal ultrasound-guided prostate biopsy on patient comfort: a randomized placebo controlled study. *Int J Urol.* 2004;11:148–151.
22. Ozden E, Yaman O, Gogus C, et al. The optimum doses of and injection locations for periprostatic nerve blockade for transrectal ultrasound guided biopsy of the prostate: a prospective, randomized, placebo controlled study. *J Urol.* 2003;170:2319–2322.
23. Vanhelleputte P, Nijs K, Delforge M, et al. Pain during bone marrow aspiration: prevalence and prevention. *J Pain Symptom Manage.* 2003;26:860–866.
24. Litman RS. Conscious sedation with remifentanil and midazolam during brief painful procedures in children. *Arch Pediatr Adolesc Med.* 1999;153:1085–1088.
25. Zeltzer LK, Altman A, Cohen D, et al. American Academy of Pediatrics Report of the Subcommittee on the Management of Pain Associated with Procedures in Children with Cancer. *Pediatrics.* 1990;86:826–831.
26. Giannoutsos I, Grech H, Maboreke T, et al. Performing bone marrow biopsies with or without sedation: a comparison. *Clin Lab Haematol.* 2004;26:201–204.
27. Schechter NL, Weisman SJ, Rosenblum M, et al. The use of oral transmucosal fentanyl citrate for painful procedures in children. *Pediatrics.* 1995;95:335–339.
28. Turnbull DK, Shepherd DB. Post-dural puncture headache: pathogenesis, prevention, and treatment. *Br J Anaesth.* 2003;91:718–729.
29. Thoennissen J, Herkner H, Lang W, et al. Does bed rest after cervical or lumbar puncture prevent headache? A systematic review and meta-analysis. *CMAJ.* 2001;165:1311–1316.
30. Phillips DM. JCAHO pain management standards are unveiled. Joint Commission of Accreditation and Healthcare Organizations. *JAMA.* 2000;284:428–429.
31. Are C, Talamini MA. Laparoscopy and malignancy. *J Laparoendosc Adv Surg Tech A.* 2005;15:38–47.

32. Veldkamp R, Kuhry E, Hop WC, et al. Laparoscopic surgery versus open surgery for colon cancer: short-term outcomes of a randomized trial. *Lancet Oncol.* 2005;6:477–484.

33. Rubinstein M, Gill IS, Aron M, et al. Prospective, randomized comparison of transperitoneal versus retroperitoneal laparoscopic adrenalectomy. *J Urol.* 2005;174:442–445.

34. Webster TM, Herrell SD, Chang SS, et al. Robotic assisted laparoscopic radical prostatectomy versus retropubic radical prostatectomy: a prospective assessment of postoperative pain. *J Urol.* 2005;174:912–914; discussion 914.

35. Remzi M, Klingler HC, Tinzl MV, et al. Morbidity of laparoscopic extraperitoneal versus transperitoneal radical prostatectomy verus open retropubic radical prostatectomy. *Eur Urol.* 2005;48:83–89.

36. Standl T, Burmeister MA, Ohnesorge H, et al. Patient-controlled epidural analgesia reduces analgesic requirements compared to continuous epidural infusion after major abdominal surgery. *Can J Anaesth.* 2003;50:258–264.

37. de Leon-Casasola OA, Parker BM, Lema MJ, et al. Epidural analgesia versus intravenous patient-controlled analgesia. Differences in the postoperative course of cancer patients. *Reg Anesth.* 1994;19:307–315.

38. Elit LM, Thomas H, Trim K, et al. Evaluation of postoperative pain control for women undergoing surgery for gynaecologic malignancies. *J Obstet Gynaecol Can.* 2004;26:1051–1058.

39. Devys JM, Mora A, Plaud B, et al. Intrathecal + PCA morphine improves analgesia during the first 24 hr after major abdominal surgery compared to PCA alone. *Can J Anaesth.* 2003;50:355–361.

40. Diblasio CJ, Snyder ME, Kattan MW, et al. Ketorolac: safe and effective analgesia for the management of renal cortical tumors with partial nephrectomy. *J Urol.* 2004;171:1062–1065.

41. Dahl JB, Mathiesen O, Moiniche S. 'Protective premedication': an option with gabapentin and related drugs? A review of gabapentin and pregabalin in the treatment of post-operative pain. *Acta Anaesthesiol Scand.* 2004;48:1130–1136.

42. Weinbroum AA, Bender B, Nirkin A, et al. Dextromethorphan-associated epidural patient-controlled analgesia provides better pain- and analgesics-sparing effects than dextromethorphan-associated intravenous patient-controlled analgesia after bone-malignancy resection: a randomized, placebo-controlled, double-blinded study. *Anesth Analg.* 2004;98:714–722.

43. Holthusen H, Backhaus P, Boeminghaus F, et al. Preemptive analgesia: no relevant advantage of preoperative compared with postoperative intravenous administration of morphine, ketamine, and clonidine in patients undergoing transperitoneal tumor nephrectomy. *Reg Anesth Pain Med.* 2002;27:249–253.

44. Montgomery GH, Bovbjerg DH. Presurgery distress and specific response expectancies predict postsurgery outcomes in surgery patients confronting breast cancer. *Health Psychol.* 2004;23:381–387.

45. Ozalp G, Sarioglu R, Tuncel G, et al. Preoperative emotional states in patients with breast cancer and postoperative pain. *Acta Anaesthesiol Scand.* 2003;47:26–29.

46. Yang JC, Clark WC, Tsui SL, et al. Preoperative Multidimensional Affect and Pain Survey (MAPS) scores predict postcolectomy analgesia requirement. *Clin J Pain.* 2000;16:314–320.

47. Foley KM. Dismantling the barriers: providing palliative and pain care. *J Am Med Assoc.* 2000;283:115.

48. Meldrum ML. A capsule history of pain management. *JAMA.* 2003;290:2470–2475.

49. Bruera E, Kim HN. Cancer pain. *JAMA.* 2003;290:2476–2479.

50. Foley KM. Treatment of cancer-related pain. *J Natl Cancer Inst Monogr.* 2004;32:103–104.

51. Carr DB, Goudas LC, Balk EM, et al. Evidence report on the treatment of pain in cancer patients. *J Natl Cancer Inst Monogr.* 2004;32: 23–31.

52. Hill HF, Chapman CR, Kornell JA, et al. Self-administration of morphine in bone marrow transplant patients reduces drug requirement. *Pain.* 1990;40:121–129.

53. Weeks JC, Cook EF, O'Day SJ, et al. Relationship between cancer patients' predictions of prognosis and their treatment preferences. *JAMA.* 1998;279:1709–1714.

54. Nelson JE, Meier DE, Oei EJ, et al. Self-reported symptom experience of critically ill cancer patients receiving intensive care.[see comment]. *Crit Care Med.* 2001;29:277–282.

55. Kaplow R. Use of nursing resources and comfort of cancer patients with and without do-not-resuscitate orders in the intensive care unit. *Am J Crit Care.* 2000;9:87–95.

56. Lai YH, Chen ML, Tsai LY, et al. Are nurses prepared to manage cancer pain? A national survey of nurses' knowledge about pain control in Taiwan. *J Pain Symptom Manage.* 2003;26:1016–1025.

57. Thiery G, Azoulay E, Darmon M, et al. Outcome of cancer patients considered for intensive care unit admission: a hospital-wide prospective study. *J Clin Oncol.* 2005;23:4406–4413.

58. Ewer MS, Kish SK, Martin CG, et al. Characteristics of cardiac arrest in cancer patients as a predictor of survival after cardiopulmonary resuscitation. *Cancer.* 2001;92:1905–1912.

59. Back AL, Arnold RM. Dealing with conflict in caring for the seriously ill: "it was just out of the question." *JAMA.* 2005;293:1374–1381.

60. von Gunten CF. Secondary and tertiary palliative care in U.S. hospitals. *JAMA.* 2002;287:875–881.

61. Morrison RS, Meier DE. Clinical practice. Palliative care. *N Engl J Med.* 2004;350:2582–2590.

62. Pan CX, Morrison RS, Meier DE, et al. How prevalent are hospital-based palliative care programs? Status report and future directions. *J Palliat Med.* 2001;4:315–324.

63. Centeno C, Hernansanz S, Flores LA, et al. Spain: palliative care programs in Spain, 2000: a national survey. *J Pain Symptom Manage.* 2002;24:245–251.

64. Elsayem A, Swint K, Fisch MJ, et al. Palliative care inpatient service in a comprehensive cancer center: clinical and financial outcomes. *J Clin Oncol.* 2004;22:2008–2014.

65. Meyers FJ, Linder J, Beckett L, et al. Simultaneous care: a model approach to the perceived conflict between investigational therapy and palliative care. *J Pain Symptom Manage.* 2004;28:548–556.

66. Meyers FJ, Linder J. Simultaneous care: disease treatment and palliative care throughout illness. *J Clin Oncol.* 2003;21:1412–1415.

67. Nelson KA, Walsh D. The business of palliative medicine—Part 3: The development of a palliative medicine program in an academic medical center. *Am J Hosp Palliat Care.* 2003;20:345–352.

68. Palmer JL, Fisch MJ. Association between symptom distress and survival in outpatients seen in a palliative care cancer center. *J Pain Symptom Manage.* 2005;29:565–571.

69. Casarett DJ, Hirschman KB, Coffey JF, et al. Does a palliative care clinic have a role in improving end-of-life care? Results of a pilot program. *J Palliat Med.* 2002;5:387–396.

70. Porta-Sales J, Codorniu N, Gomez-Batiste X, et al. Patient appointment process, symptom control and prediction of follow-up compliance in a palliative care outpatient clinic. *J Pain Symptom Manage.* 2005;30: 145–153.

71. Oliver D. The development of an interdisciplinary outpatient clinic in specialist palliative care. *Int J Palliat Nurs.* 2004;10:446–448.

72. Rabow MW, Dibble SL, Pantilat SZ, et al. The comprehensive care team: a controlled trial of outpatient palliative medicine consultation. *Arch Intern Med.* 2004;164:83–91.

73. Kemper P, Murtaugh CM. Lifetime use of nursing home care. *N Engl J Med.* 1991;324:595–600.

74. Bernabei R, Gambassi G, Lapane K, et al. Management of pain in elderly patients with cancer. SAGE Study Group. Systematic Assessment of Geriatric Drug Use via Epidemiology. *JAMA.* 1998;279:1877–1882.

75. Buchanan RJ, Barkley J, Wang S, et al. Analyses of nursing home residents with cancer at admission. *Cancer Nurs.* 2005;28:406–414.

76. Tinetti ME. Clinical practice. Preventing falls in elderly persons. *N Engl J Med.* 2003;348:42–49.

77. Knight EL, Avorn J. Quality indicators for appropriate medication use in vulnerable elders. *Ann Intern Med.* 2001;135:703–710.

78. Kemp CA, Ersek M, Turner JA. A descriptive study of older adults with persistent pain: use and perceived effectiveness of pain management strategies [ISRCTN11899548]. *BMC Geriatr.* 2005;5:12.

79. Hanson LC, Reynolds KS, Henderson M, et al. A quality improvement intervention to increase palliative care in nursing homes. *J Palliat Med.* 2005;8:576–584.

80. Extermann M, Aapro M, Bernabei R, et al. Use of comprehensive geriatric assessment in older cancer patients: recommendations from the task force on CGA of the International Society of Geriatric Oncology (SIOG). *Crit Rev Oncol Hematol.* 2005;55:241–252.

81. Vandenberg EV, Tvrdik A, Keller BK. Use of the quality improvement process in assessing end-of-life care in the nursing home. *J Am Med Dir Assoc.* 2005;6:334–339.

82. Hanson LC, Sengupta S, Slubicki M. Access to nursing home hospice: perspectives of nursing home and hospice administrators. *J Palliat Med.* 2005;8:1207–1213.

83. Zerzan J, Stearns S, Hanson L. Access to palliative care and hospice in nursing homes. *JAMA.* 2000;284:2489–2494.

84. Carlson MD, Gallo WT, Bradley EH. Ownership status and patterns of care in hospice: results from the National Home and Hospice Care Survey. *Med Care.* 2004;42:432–438.

85. von Gunten CF, Ryndes T. The academic hospice. *Ann Intern Med.* 2005;143:655–658.

86. Clayton JM, Butow PN, Tattersall MH. When and how to initiate discussion about prognosis and end-of-life issues with terminally ill patients. *J Pain Symptom Manage.* 2005;30:132–144.

87. Lynn J. Perspectives on care at the close of life. Serving patients who may die soon and their families: the role of hospice and other services. *JAMA.* 2001;285:925–932.

88. Von Gunten CF. Discussing hospice care. *J Clin Oncol.* 2003; 21: 31–36.

89. Back AL, Arnold RM, Baile WF, et al. Approaching difficult communication tasks in oncology. *CA Cancer J Clin.* 2005;55:164–177.

90. Hanson LC, Ersek M. Meeting palliative care needs in post acute-care settings: "To help them live until they die." *JAMA.* 2006;295: 681–686.

Basic Neurobiology of Cancer Pain

CHAPTER

5

Juan P. Cata
Han-Rong Weng
Patrick M. Dougherty

INTRODUCTION

The sensation of pain is normally a response associated with the application of noxious or injurious stimuli. In cancer patients, pain stimuli occur as a result of trauma secondary to surgical/medical procedures, invasion and compression of tumor cells into peripheral nerves and spinal cord, and chemotherapy and radiation therapy. Pain in cancer patients thus involves multiple components and mechanisms, including those mediating acute somatic pain, primary and secondary hyperalgesia, and those mediating neuropathic pain.[1] This chapter reviews the basic physiology of the neural apparatus that responds to noxious stimuli. This is followed by a synopsis of the neural mechanisms and neurochemical mediators of acute primary and secondary hyperalgesia, and finally by a review of the mechanisms of neuropathic pain. Our goal is to provide an informed basis for selecting intervention strategies for each of these sources of pain.

PAIN FROM UNINJURED TISSUE

▶ Peripheral neural mechanisms

The initial neural encoding of pain depends upon the properties of nociceptors, a distinct class of primary afferent fibers that respond selectively to noxious stimuli. The responses of these fibers to natural stimuli correlate with the pain reported by subjects to the same stimuli. Primary afferent nociceptors are generally subdivided according to whether the parent nerve fiber is unmyelinated (C fiber) or myelinated (A fiber).

C-fiber nociceptors

Cutaneous C-fiber nociceptors studied in anesthetized nonhuman primates typically are responsive to stimuli over a receptive field area of about 20 mm². Most C-fiber nociceptors respond to numerous diverse stimulus modalities applied throughout the receptive field, including heat, chemical, and mechanical stimuli, and are often termed *polymodal nociceptors*. Several lines of evidence indicate that C-fiber nociceptors are essential for the normal perception of pain. C-fiber nociceptors recorded from monkey and from humans exhibit a monotonically increasing discharge frequency with heat applied to skin that correlates with changes in human judgments of pain. The latency for heat pain sensation to thermal stimuli applied to skin matches the conduction time of C-fiber nociceptors. Intraneural electrical stimulation of identified C-fiber nociceptors

in humans elicits the sensation of pain, and C-fiber blocks prevent thermal pain perception at the normal heat pain threshold. Finally, microscopic examination of the peripheral nerves of patients with congenital insensitivity to pain is marked by the absence of C fibers.

A-fiber nociceptors

A-fiber nociceptors respond to mechanical, heat, and chemical stimuli and are also termed *polymodal*. Two types of A-fiber nociceptors have been identified based on their profile of response to heat stimuli. Type I A-fiber nociceptors have very high thresholds for activation by mechanical stimuli applied to skin under normal circumstances, and, because of this, are often referred to as high threshold mechanoreceptors. However, many of these fibers also respond well to intense heat stimuli. Type I A-fiber nociceptors are particularly prevalent on the glabrous skin of the hands in monkeys and have been described in cats, rabbits, and man. The mean conduction velocity for type I A-fiber nociceptors in monkeys is 30 m/s and extends as high as 55 m/s. Thus, by conduction velocity criteria, these nociceptors fall into a category between that of A-d and A-b fibers.

Type II A-fiber nociceptors are found exclusively on hairy skin and exhibit the major distinguishing feature of a substantially lower heat activation threshold than that of Type I A-fiber nociceptors. In addition, the mean conduction velocity of Type II A-fiber nociceptors is 15 m/s, which is lower than that of the Type I A fibers. Rapid heat stimuli applied to hairy skin evoke a fast onset sharp pricking sensation, followed by a slower onset burning sensation. Type II A-fiber nociceptors appear to mediate the first sharp pricking heat pain sensation. The thermal threshold of Type II fibers is near the threshold temperature for first pain, and the conduction velocity of myelinated afferent fibers corresponds to the latency of response to first pain. Type II A-fiber nociceptors yield a burst of activity at the onset of a heat stimulus that is consistent with the perception of a momentary pricking sensation. Finally, the absence of the first pain sensation to heat stimuli applied to the palm of the human hand correlates with the failure to find Type II A-fiber nociceptors in glabrous skin.

Mechanically insensitive afferents

Recent evidence suggests that about one-half of A-fiber nociceptors and one-third of C-fiber nociceptors either have very high mechanical thresholds or are unresponsive to mechanical stimuli and so are referred to as mechanically insensitive afferents. Similar afferent fibers have been reported in knee joint, viscera, and cornea. Some cutaneous mechanically insensitive afferents may be chemo-specific receptors. Others respond to intense cold or heat stimuli.

▶ Central mechanisms

Following transduction by peripheral afferents, nociceptive information flows to the central nervous system (CNS) where it is processed, registered, and a reaction formulated. Figures 5-1 and 5-2 are schematic diagrams of the flow of somatosensory information through the anterolateral and dorsal spinal pathways. The spinal dorsal horn, and to a much lesser extent the dorsal column nuclei, provide the first link in the central nociceptive pathways. From here, nociceptive information is distributed to sites in the brainstem, midbrain, hypothalamus, thalamus, and finally to sensory and so-called limbic cortices.

The spinal dorsal horn

The cells of the dorsal horn are arranged in layers that are defined by anatomic and physiologic methods first described by Rolando, and later schematized by Rexed.

Primary afferent fibers make well-defined connections with spinal neurons. A-δ and C afferents primarily terminate in layer I and the outer part of layer II. The targets include cells intrinsic to the dorsal horn (interneurons) as well as cells whose axons leave the spinal cord and ascend (projection neurons) to more rostral targets in the brainstem and diencephalon. The larger myelinated afferents end upon cells deeper in the spinal cord, especially layers III to V and perhaps the inner aspect of layer II.

The functional properties of dorsal horn cells reflect their innervation. Many of the neurons in laminae I and II respond exclusively to noxious inputs. These cells are often called *nociceptive-specific (NS)* or *high-threshold (HT)* neurons. NS neurons studied in anesthetized preparations usually have ongoing background activity, although this is not always the case in awake preparations. Nevertheless, NS cells in anesthetized animals have a lower level of spontaneous activity than other sensory cells, averaging around 2 Hz. NS cells also tend to have relatively small excitatory polymodal receptive fields. These are confined to a single digit or small patch of skin and are responsive to cutaneous mechanical, heat, chemical, and, in some cases, cooling stimuli.

A second group of spinal cord cells responds only to nonnoxious stimuli. This group is composed of low-threshold (LT) neurons. LT cells have a higher mean level of spontaneous activity (in the anesthetized preparation) than NS neurons, averaging around 10 Hz. The excitatory receptive fields are usually larger than for HT cells, often covering two or more digits, and often covering both glabrous and hairy skin. LT cells are especially prevalent in lamina II, and many of these may be inhibitory interneurons. LT neurons that project from the spinal cord primarily ascend to the dorsal column nuclei, with relatively few of these cells projecting to the brainstem, midbrain, or diencephalon.

The final classes of sensory spinal neurons are the wide dynamic range (WDR) and multireceptive (MR) cells. Both of these respond to noxious and nonnoxious stimuli with the difference being that WDR cells show a discharge rate that is graded with stimulus intensity, whereas the MR stimulus-intensity function is flat. WDR and MR cells in laminae I to VI include interneurons and projection neurons. The inputs from nociceptors to these cells may be passed via contacts from more superficial intrinsic cells or may be passed via contacts of afferent fibers on dorsal dendrites that penetrate into the superficial laminae. WDR neurons found in lamina I may be the key neural substrates for the transmission of cooling and warm

(nonnoxious thermal) stimuli. WDR and MR cells in laminae III to V respond to both cutaneous mechanical and heat stimuli, but rarely show responses from deep tissues. WDR and MR projection neurons in these laminae are found to innervate all rostral targets of the spinal cord. Cells in laminae VI and VII especially tend to show responses from deep tissue and visceral receptors.

The responses of typical NS, WDR, and LT neurons to different intensities of mechanical stimuli are shown in Fig. 5-3. As mentioned above, WDR neurons demonstrate responses to noxious and nonnoxious stimuli, whereas NS neurons respond only to stimuli well above the intensity needed to provoke the sensation of pain, which are often sufficient to cause tissue damage. Based on these observations it has been suggested that WDR neurons provide the neural substrate for the detection and discrimination between noxious and nonnoxious stimuli. This property allows the organism to detect cutaneous stimuli as they approach an intensity that would be tissue damaging, which permits a reaction that prevents actual damage. NS cells under this scheme only inform the organism that actual tissue damage has occurred. Another possibility is that WDR cells provide a "nonspecific alerting or conditioning input," which primes more rostral neurons for the more specific inputs of the NS neurons.

The dorsal column nuclei

The dorsal column nuclear complex is composed of two subdivisions, the nucleus gracilis that processes sensory information for the body surface approximately below T6, and the nucleus cuneatus that processes information for the upper half of the trunk, arms, and neck. The dorsal column nuclei receive direct primary afferent innervation that has ascended in the dorsal (posterior) spinal funiculi as well as input from at least two groups of dorsal horn projection neurons, the postsynaptic dorsal column pathway and the spinocervical tract. The cells of the dorsal column nuclei largely respond to innocuous stimuli alone, and the lemniscal system in primates does not appear to encode painful stimuli. The primary information carried in this path to the nucleus is from hair follicle receptors, Pacinian corpuscles, and types I and II slowly adapting receptors. In addition, the nucleus cuneatus responds to muscle afferents such as muscle spindles and Golgi tendon organs (this information for the lower half of the body is processed in Clark's nucleus in the thoracic spinal cord and ascends to the cerebellum in the dorsal spinocerebellar tract in the dorsal lateral spinal funiculus). However, several lines of evidence suggest that dorsal column nuclei participate in nociceptive transmission in special circumstances. For example, the recurrence of pain following a lesion of the anterolateral spinal quadrant and the reference of pain to other regions of the body immediately after anterolateral chordotomy are often cited. Although most afferent input to dorsal column nuclei is from large myelinated afferents, neuropathic pains are, in fact, largely conveyed by myelinated fiber inputs. In addition, an input from nonmyelinated afferents to the dorsal column nuclei has also been shown and a small number of nociceptive dorsal column neurons have been reported. Although not yet demonstrated in man, the two spinal tracts which ascend to the dorsal column nuclei mentioned above are often nociceptive. Finally, research over the past several years suggests the presence of a novel pain pathway running in the dorsal columns that mediates the perception of visceral pain.

Rostral CNS areas involved in pain perception

Other rostral targets innervated by dorsal horn projection neurons include the medullary reticular formation (spinoreticular tract),

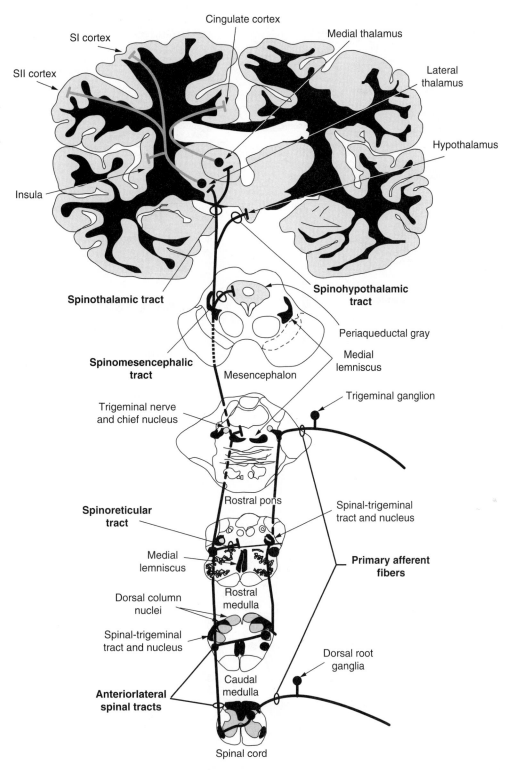

FIGURE 5-1 Schematic diagram of the anterior-lateral spinal nociceptive pathways. Primary afferent fibers are illustrated as entering the neuraxis from the right of the figure via spinal nerves with cell bodies in the dorsal root ganglia (lower right), and via the trigeminal nerve with cell bodies in the trigeminal ganglion (center right). Primary afferents from the body are shown as synapsing in the spinal dorsal horn, and then second-order axons cross the midline in the anterior white commissure and gather into the anterior-lateral spinal columns (tracts). The primary afferent nociceptive fibers for the head are shown to descend in the spinal trigeminal tract to the spinal trigeminal nucleus where these fibers synapse and collect with those from the body. The combined second-order axons ascend with collaterals exiting to the reticular formation, midbrain, and hypothalamus prior to the remainder of the fibers, terminating in either the lateral or medial thalamus. Third-order thalamic neurons project to various cortical areas.

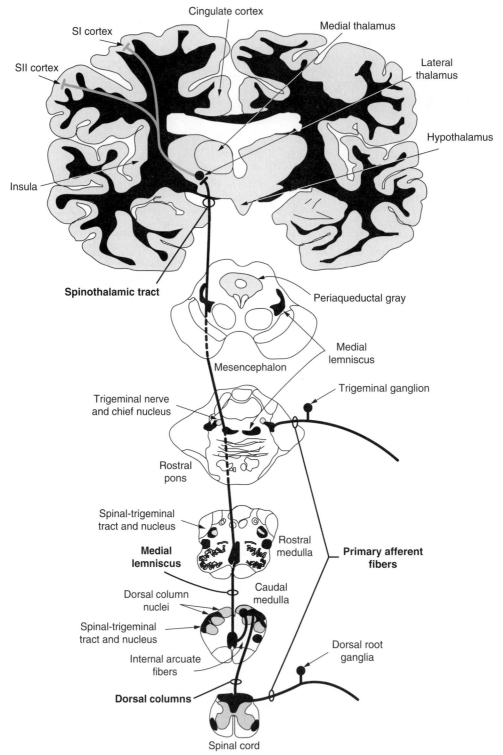

FIGURE 5-2 Schematic diagram of the dorsal column-medial lemniscal sensory pathways. Primary afferent fibers are illustrated as entering the neuraxis from the right of the figure via spinal nerves with cell bodies in the dorsal root ganglia (lower right), and via the trigeminal nerve with cell bodies in the trigeminal ganglion (center right). Primary afferents from the body are shown to ascend in the dorsal (posterior) spinal columns to synapse in the dorsal column nuclei, and then second-order axons cross the midline in the internal arcuate fibers and gather to form the medial lemniscus. The primary afferent sensory fibers for the head are shown as entering and synapsing in the chief (main) sensory trigeminal nucleus, and the second-order fibers cross the midline and collect with those from the body. The combined second-order axons ascend and terminate in the lateral thalamus. Third-order thalamic neurons project to SI and SII cortical areas.

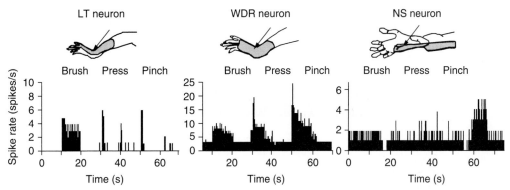

FIGURE 5-3 The rate histograms show responses of primate spinothalamic tract neurons representative of low-threshold (LT), wide dynamic range (WDR), and nociceptive-specific (NS) classes. The responses of these cells were evoked by application of a series of mechanical stimuli of graded intensity to multiple sites across the receptive field for each cell. The times and sites of each stimulus application are indicated by the lines and labels at the top of each histogram. The brush stimulus was provided by a soft camel hair brush while the large, medium, and small clip stimuli were provided by applications of increasingly intense compressive arterial clips to the skin. The WDR cell in the center of the figure shows responses that are graded with the intensity of the stimuli. The NS neuron shows no significant responses to any stimuli but the most intense, whereas the LT neuron responds to innocuous brushing of the skin alone (the transient responses with the application and removal or the arterial clips are due to the touch stimuli provided at contact). Finally, the diagrams of the hind limbs show the receptive field locations of each neuron (shaded region) and the sites on skin where each of the mechanical stimuli were applied (spots and numerals).

the mesencephalic periaqueductal gray and neighboring area (spinomesencephalic), the hypothalamus (spinohypothalamic tract), and finally, the sensory regions of thalamus (spinothalamic tract), including the ventral posterior lateral (VPL) nucleus, the posterior-inferior thalamic region, and to a more limited extent the central-lateral nucleus of the thalamus.

Among the higher nociceptive centers, the thalamus and the spinothalamic tract are the most studied. The spinothalamic tract has received special attention because these neurons encode stimuli that correlate well with the perceptions of humans to noxious stimuli. This characteristic is well illustrated by comparing the psychophysical ratings of humans and the physiological responses of spinothalamic neurons in primates with graded intensities of cutaneous stimuli. Figure 5-4 shows that the responses of spinothalamic neurons to

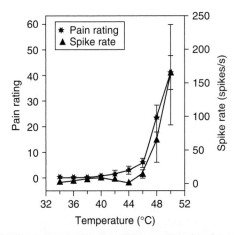

FIGURE 5-4 Comparison of pain ratings of human subjects (stars) to graded heat stimuli with the discharges of monkey spinothalamic neurons (triangles) to the identical stimuli. The y-axis is labeled in units for the pain ratings on the left and for the neuron discharge rates on the right. *(Adapted from Simone DA, Sorkin LS, Oh U, et al. Neurogenic hyperalgesia: central neural correlates in responses of spinothalamic tract neurons. J Neurophysiol. 1991;66:228–246.)*

graded heat stimuli applied to the skin correlate well with the rating of pain intensity given by human subjects to the same stimuli. Each of the other spinal pathways (e.g., the spinoreticular, spinomesencephalic, and spinohypothalamic tracts) has some neurons with response profiles that resemble those for the spinothalamic cells. Indeed, many spinothalamic neurons send collaterals into many of these other targets. But such additional pathways also include subsets of cells that solely innervate their respective targets and do not correlate with human ratings of pain intensity. For example, it is not uncommon to find cells projecting to the reticular formation or mesencephalon that have receptive fields spread over large body areas and that are composed of zones where sensory stimuli evoke increases in discharge, and other zones where sensory stimuli evoked decreases in discharge. The relationship between these complex responses and human ratings of stimulus intensity are not readily apparent, and so the specific functions of these pathways remain poorly defined. It is possible that brainstem, midbrain, and hypothalamic pathways are engaged in the affective/motivational and vegetative (autonomic and neuroendocrine) aspects of nociception.

Each of the primary targets of spinal projection neurons project in turn to more rostral targets. The dorsal column nuclei project via the medial lemniscus to an area of the ventral posterior thalamus just anterior to the termination of the spinothalamic tract. Readers may also find this region termed the "core" of the ventral posterior nucleus, whereas the area of spinothalamic termination may be called the matrix region, the posterior-inferior nuclear region, or ventromedial preoptic nucleus (VMpo). Neurons in the somatosensory thalamus project to the SI, SII, and retroinsular cortexes, with those thalamic cells receiving lemniscal inputs, especially projecting to the more rostral SI and SII areas and the cells receiving spinothalamic input especially projecting to the posterior-inferior retroinsular area. The rostral targets of the brainstem reticular formation, the mesencephalic gray, and the hypothalamus are very diffuse, and outputs from these structures can also include pathways that descend back to the spinal cord.

The same types of neurons present in the spinal dorsal horn have also been described for each of these higher sites in the central

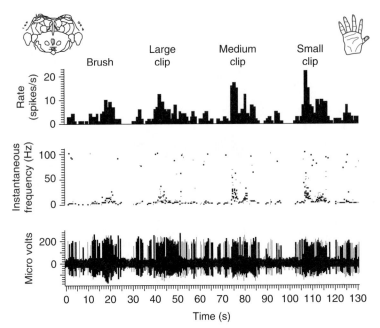

FIGURE 5-5 Responses of a WDR neuron in the nonhuman somatosensory thalamus (VPL) to noxious and nonnoxious mechanical stimuli. The bottom line shows an oscilloscope sweep of analog recordings of the cell to the mechanical stimuli, whereas compiled rate histograms and instantaneous frequency plots for each of the stimuli are shown in the top and middle lines. The outline at top left shows the estimated recording site in thalamus and the drawing of the forepaw at top right shows the location of the neuron's receptive field. *(Adapted from Dougherty, 2005.)*

nociceptive pathways. Figure 5-5, for example, shows the responses of a WDR neuron in the chief sensory nucleus of the nonhuman primate thalamus to graded thermal, mechanical, and cooling stimuli. Also present in the thalamus, but not illustrated, are LT and HT neurons as described previously for the dorsal horn. The LT neurons are especially prevalent in the "core" or "rod zone" of the ventral posterior nucleus that receives inputs largely from the medial lemniscus via the dorsal column nuclei. The NS neurons in thalamus are concentrated especially in the posterior-inferior area of the thalamus, which some term the matrix area of the thalamus.

▶ Neurochemistry of somatosensory transmission

Excitatory neurotransmitters

As illustrated in Fig. 5-6, multiple neurotransmitters and neuropeptides are involved in somatosensory neurotransmission. The main excitatory neurotransmitters are the amino acids glutamate and aspartate. Glutamate (referred to as aspartate from here on) mediates excitatory transmission at each of the afferent connections in the somatosensory system, including the synaptic connection between primary afferent fibers and spinal neurons, from spinal neurons to thalamic neurons, and others. There are four excitatory amino acid receptor subtypes in the somatosensory system. Each receptor subtype was originally named for the synthetic agonist by which it is best activated, but they are now known to be encoded by distinct gene families.

One very important subtype in pain signaling is termed the *N*-methyl-*D*-aspartate (NMDA) receptor. NMDA receptors comprise several subunits: NR1, NR2A–D, and NR3A and NR3B. The NR1 subunit is essential to the structure of the receptor, and the NR2 subunit confers many of the conductance channel's molecular and functional features. NR2A and NR2B are high-conductance channels, whereas

NR2C and NR2D receptors are low-conductance channels. The NMDA receptor has two key pharmacologic features that have important physiologic effects. First, for the receptor to be activated, glutamate binding must occur during sustained membrane depolarization so that a resting Mg^{2+}-dependent blockade of the receptor can be released. This results in the NMDA receptor functioning as a coincidence and intensity detector and as such it is normally only activated by nociceptive stimuli. Second, once the NMDA receptor is activated, a marked influx of monovalent and especially divalent calcium ions occurs; this increases cellular excitability and also leads to the activation of various intracellular signaling pathways. These events result in increased expression of immediate early genes and neurotrophic factors, release of arachidonic acid and nitric oxide synthase, each of which contributes to sustained increases in cellular excitability. More is discussed in this regard later during the consideration of mechanisms of hyperalgesia.

The second broad class of receptors not activated by NMDA (non-NMDA receptors) includes three subtypes, a kainate receptor (KAR), an AMPA [(R,S)-a-amino-3-hydroxy-5-methylisoxazole-4-proprionic acid] receptor, and the metabotropic glutamate receptors. The kainate and AMPA receptors are linked to sodium channels and are considered to mediate the majority of the fast synaptic afferent signaling in this system for all modalities and intensities of stimuli. Five members of the KAR family have been cloned: GluR5, GluR6, GluR7, KA-1, and KA-2, whereas four subunits GluR1–4 form AMPA receptors. The GluR1 subunit was the first to be discovered and cloned with the other subunits subsequently identified. GluR1–4 are permeable to Ca^{2+} ions and their activation evokes inward rectifying currents. The intracellular domain of the GluR2/3/4 subunits interacts with different intracellular proteins and thereby serve in multiple cellular functions: as clustering receptors in the plasma membrane, in receptor trafficking, and as coupling receptors between signaling and cytoskeletal molecules.[2] The

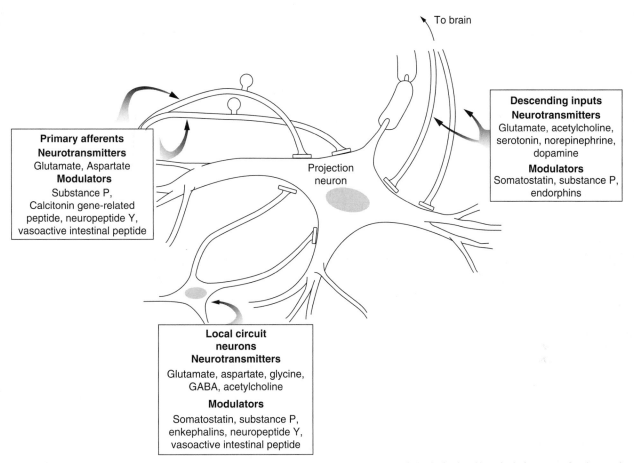

FIGURE 5-6 The schematic summarizes the neurochemical pathways involved in somatosensory neurotransmission in the dorsal horn. Intrinsic sources of each transmitter are indicated by each of the labeled boxes.

AMPA/kainate and NMDA receptors are also frequently considered to mediate mono- and polysynaptic contacts of primary afferent fibers to dorsal horn neurons.

Finally, the metabotropic receptors, first known as the ACPD (trans-($\pm$)-1-amino-cyclopentane-1,3-dicarboxylate) receptor, is in fact a large family of G protein-linked sites that in turn include three functional subdivisions. Group I metabotropic receptors are coupled via G_q to phospholipase C and includes mGlu1 and mGlu5. The group II receptors, mGlu2 and mGlu3, are coupled to G_i and inhibit the formation of cyclic adenosine monophosphate (cAMP). Finally, the group III metabotropic receptors, mGlu4, 6, 7, and 8 are also coupled to G_i. Group I receptors (mGlu1 and mGlu5) modulate nociceptive transmission by controlling the presynaptic release of neurotransmitter[3] and by modulating postsynaptic NMDA-mediated currents.[4] Group II and III metabotropic receptors generally reduce neuronal excitability and synaptic transmission in many areas of the brain and spinal cord and inhibit voltage-gated Ca^{2+} channels.

A second type of excitatory substance that appears to have a transmitter role in the somatosensory system is adenosine triphosphate (ATP). There are two families of purinoreceptors, the P2X and P2Y subtypes. P2X receptors are ligand-gated ion channels that evoke inward currents.[5] P2Y subtypes are G protein-coupled metabotropic receptors that trigger activation of phospholipase C and the breakdown of PIP_2 to IP_3 and diacylglycerol.[6] P2X receptors are located on small non-peptide-containing sensory afferents by which high concentrations of ATP evoke depolarization and lower concentrations evoke inhibition. $P2Y_1$ and $P2Y_2$ are localized in small, medium, and large sensory afferent fibers, where their activation induces thermal hyperalgesia and sensitizes C fibers to thermal inputs.[7] The expression of purinergic receptors is upregulated in sensory afferents and spinal cord neurons of rats with neuropathic pain suggesting that these receptors have a particularly important role in chronic pain conditions.[8]

Inhibitory neurotransmitters

The primary inhibitory neurotransmitters of the somatosensory system include the amino acids glycine and g-aminobutyric acid (GABA). Glycine is particularly important at spinal levels while GABA is the predominate inhibitory transmitter at higher levels. Glycine has two receptor sites, a chloride-linked strychnine-sensitive inhibitory receptor as well as a strychnine-insensitive modulatory site on the NMDA glutamate receptor complex. GABA binds to three receptors that are found in pre- and postsynaptic terminals, referred to as $GABA_A$, $GABA_B$, and $GABA_C$ receptors. The $GABA_A$ receptor has affinity to bicuculline, insensitivity to baclofen, and a pentameric transmembrane structure that after activation generates a fast inhibitory response (inotropic) linked to chloride channels. Conversely, high affinity to baclofen, insensitivity to bicuculline, and slow generating response (metabotropic) are characteristics of the $GABA_B$ receptor. This receptor belongs to the family of guanosine triphosphate (GTP)-binding proteins and is linked to membrane Ca^{2+} and K^+ channels. $GABA_B$ receptors can be further subclassified as $GABA_{B1}$ and $GABA_{B2}$. The $GABA_C$ receptor has a pentameric structure that is coupled to chloride channels and is insensitive to both bicuculline and baclofen.

Alterations in the functions of the inhibitory neurotransmitters may be particularly important with the induction of hyperalgesia and following the development of neuropathic pain. For example, a $GABA_A$-mediated link between large myelinated fibers and C-fiber nociceptors has been proposed as a mechanism for the development of allodynia following intradermal injection of the irritant capsaicin. Additionally, a selective loss of inhibitory interneurons at both spinal and thalamic levels has been suggested as contributing to some neuropathic pain conditions.

Norepinephrine is an important inhibitory neurotransmitter in descending brainstem projections to the dorsal horn. The adrenergic receptors include two broad classes termed the alpha and beta receptors, each of which in turn have several subtypes. The alpha-2 adrenergic receptor is the primary form found in the spinal dorsal horn that provides an inhibitory function of neurotransmission of sensory information. However, it should be noted that the function of norepinephrine following injury to the nervous systems might become reversed from an inhibitory, analgesic role to one of promoting and/or sustaining an ongoing chronic pain state.

Another important inhibitory neurotransmitter at spinal levels is the purine adenosine. There are at least four types of adenosine receptors, A1, $A2_A$, $A2_B$, and A3, which are coupled to pertussis toxin-sensitive G proteins. A1 receptors inhibit NMDA-induced release of excitatory amino acids, whereas $A2_A$ receptors have excitatory effects. $A2_B$ receptors modulate the activity of glial cells during the inflammatory process. Finally, A3 receptors have paradoxical effects depending on the experimental model of pain being studied. Adenosine receptors are localized pre- and postsynaptically in many brain regions with a particular concentration in superficial spinal lamina. Activation of these receptors has a major effect on the inhibitory control of synaptic transmissions; these effects appear to be related to the modulation of K^+ and Ca^{2+} channels, and due to a strong interaction with $GABA_B$ receptors. Morphine induces the release of adenosine by activating m receptors, and this effect is also Ca^{2+}-dependent. The spinal administration of adenosine has analgesic effects that are mediated by A1 receptors,[9] and the level of adenosine in the cerebrospinal fluid appears to be lower than normal in patients with neuropathic pain. The spinal administration of adenosine kinase inhibitors also produces analgesia in several experimental models of pain; however, the administration of methylxanthines inhibits spinal analgesia by morphine. The peripheral effects of adenosine remain controversial; and it seems that whether analgesic or hyperalgesic effects occur depends upon whether adenosine binds to A1 or $A2_A$ receptors. Moreover, studies in mice have demonstrated that the activation of A3 receptors is involved in carrageenan-induced hyperalgesia.

Acetylcholine is yet another neurotransmitter that appears to mediate antinociception at the level of the spinal dorsal horn. The antinociceptive effects appear to be mediated by the muscarinic and not by the nicotinic acetylcholine receptor subtypes.

Finally, serotonin has been proposed as an inhibitory transmitter in pathways descending to the spinal dorsal horn from the midbrain raphe nuclei. There are multiple serotonin receptor subtypes, including 5HT-1, 2, and 3 receptors. Each of these major types also has several subtypes. Controversy remains concerning which of these subtypes mediate the analgesic properties of serotonin. In part, this controversy may be due to the fact that some serotonin receptor subtypes in fact promote nociception while others are inhibitory.

Neuropeptides

Multiple neuropeptides contribute to signaling somatosensory information. The excitatory neuropeptides in the somatosensory system include substance P and neurokinin A. These peptides are especially concentrated in primary afferent fibers that express tyrosine kinase A (TrkA) receptors and that terminate in spinal lamina I and II outer but also may be present in intrinsic neurons of the spinal dorsal horn and thalamus. The receptors for these peptides include the neurokinin 1 and 2 sites, each of which has been associated with elevation of intracellular calcium levels, perhaps through liberation of inositol phosphate. At the spinal level these peptides are released only following application of noxious stimuli that are sufficient to produce sustained discharges in C nociceptors, although some small myelinated (A-d) fibers may also contain substance P. These peptides do not appear to signal as synaptic transmitters but rather as transsynaptic transmitters. Thus, once released the peptides are not confined to a site of action on the immediate postsynaptic membrane but instead tend to spread throughout the dorsal horn, potentially acting on multiple synapses at some distance from their point of release. It has been suggested that stimuli of particular modalities (e.g., mechanical vs. thermal) are associated with selective release of one peptide versus another; however, this suggestion has not been corroborated. Activation of neurokinin 1 and/or 2 receptors by substance P and/or neurokinin A are agreed as being key steps needed for the induction of sensitization and hence the expression of hyperalgesia following cutaneous injury. It has been further proposed that the mechanism of neurokinin receptor involvement in the expression of sensitization is through facilitation of the synaptic actions of the excitatory amino acid neurotransmitters.

The inhibitory neuropeptides at spinal levels include somatostatin, the enkephalins, and possibly dynorphin. These peptides are contained both in intrinsic neurons of the dorsal horn and in the fibers descending to the dorsal horn from various brainstem nuclei. At thalamic levels, the inhibitory neuropeptides also include the endorphins, which are contained in ascending antinociceptive pathways. The receptor types for the opioid peptides include the m, d, and k receptor subtypes at all levels of the somatosensory system. These receptors are associated with modulation of both intracellular cAMP and potassium levels. There is also an important cooperative functional link between m opioid and alpha-2 adrenergic receptors that has yet to be fully exploited in clinical applications.

Finally, numerous neuropeptides are present in the somatosensory system whose functions have not been fully clarified and so they are considered as a third category. These peptides include calcitonin gene-related peptide (CGRP), vasoactive intestinal peptide (VIP), neuropeptide Y (NPY), and cholecystokinin (CCK), among others. CGRP is found in primary afferents of the dorsal horn. CGRP binds to CGRP1 receptors, which are formed by a complex of seven transmembrane domains that modulate the production of cAMP and PKA and PKC. When CGRP is injected intrathecally, mechanical and thermal hyperalgesia result. This effect is reversed by the administration of $CGRP_{8-37}$ (a CGRP receptor antagonist) and PKA and PKC inhibitors.[10] CGRP enhances the release of excitatory amino acids in the spinal cord, increases the background and evoked activity of nociceptive-specific neurons and wide dynamic neurons to AMPA and NMDA, and facilitates substance P-induced pain behavior by enhancing the release and inhibiting the degradation of substance P.[11] CGRP is involved in capsaicin-induced hyperalgesia and sensitization of spinal WDR neurons.[10]

Galanin is a 29-amino acid peptide that is widely distributed in the brain, spinal cord, and gut. Fewer than 5% of neurons in the dorsal root ganglia (DRG) express galanin; however, the levels of expression increase dramatically after nerve injury. Galanin is expressed in approximately half of the unmyelinated sensory neurons that contain CGRP; the levels of this peptide in large myelinated fibers are low. In lamina II of the dorsal horn, galanin is found in local neurons that coexpress enkephalins and neuropeptide Y. Galanin binds to three receptors: GAL1, GAL2, and GAL3.[12] GAL1 and GAL2 are localized in large myelinated and small myelinated fibers, respectively, and all three receptors are expressed in spinal cord neurons.[13] The GAL1 receptor is coupled to G proteins that open inwardly rectifying K$^+$ channels, reducing the concentration of cAMP and increasing MAP kinase activity. GAL2 receptor modulates the activity of phospholipase C and inhibits cAMP accumulation. GAL3 is linked to G protein-coupled, inwardly rectifying K$^+$ channels.[12] Behavioral and electrophysiologic studies suggest that galanin has a paradoxical dose-dependent response in pain processing: The administration of galanin at low doses shows a hyperalgesic effect, but hand pain-related behaviors are reduced when this peptide is injected at high doses or is infused over a long period of time.[14] This paradoxical effect may be associated with the activation of different receptors since agonists of GAL1 and GAL2 show antihyperalgesic and hyperalgesic properties, respectively.[15]

NPY is an abundant 36-amino acid peptide that binds to three receptors known as NPY$_1$, NPY$_2$, and NPY$_3$. NPY is highly expressed in the spinal cord but poorly expressed in primary afferents; however, after nerve injury, NPY levels increase, predominantly in large myelinated fibers. NPY$_1$ and NPY$_2$ receptors are found in small to medium primary afferents and one-third of the NPY$_1$ receptor-expressing peripheral afferents also coexpress substance P and double stain for IB4. Coupling of NPY$_1$ receptor to G protein leads to changes in the intracellular concentration of Ca^{2+}. NPY levels are increased in laminae III and IV of animals with the chronic constriction injury (CCI) model of neuropathic pain, and the degree of hyperalgesia is correlated with increased NPY. Short-term spinal injections of NPY reverse thermal hyperalgesia in inflammatory models of pain; however, when NPY is administered over long periods to animals with neuropathic pain, hyperalgesia is exacerbated.

CCK is another enigmatic peptide present in the brain and spinal cord. Two types of receptors exist, CCK-A (also known as CCK$_1$) and CCK-B (CCK$_2$), and are highly expressed in the CNS. The amount of spinally released CCK is normally very low; however, CCK levels like the other peptides just reviewed increase markedly following nerve injury. The exogenous administration of CCK attenuates morphine-induced antinociception, and intrathecal injections of a selective CCK-B receptor antagonist reverse mechanical hyperalgesia and potentiate the analgesic effect of opioids in animals with neuropathic pain.[16] CCK$_B$$^{-/-}$ mutant mice are resistant to neuropathic pain. Moreover, these animals show hyperalgesia after spinal injection of naloxone, which suggests that in pathologic conditions increased spinal CCK levels modulate the antinociceptive efficacy of endogenous and exogenous opioids, probably by regulating the expression of proopiomelanocortin.[16–18]

VIP is a 28-amino acid peptide originally isolated from porcine small intestine but that is also found at especially high levels in the lumbosacral spinal cord in fine fibers reaching laminae I and II from the gut. VIP binds with high affinity to two receptors: VIP$_1$ (or VACP1) and VIP$_2$ (or VACP2), and also binds to membrane-bound calmodulin. Both receptors are G protein-coupled receptors that stimulate the cAMP pathway, which ultimately leads to PKA activation.

Intrathecal administration of VIP modulates somatosensory processing in a bimodal, concentration-dependent response characterized by an early antinociceptive effect and subsequent hyperalgesic behaviors.[19] The expressions of VIP and VIP receptors change in neuropathic conditions. VIP levels are significantly increased after nerve damage, whereas VIP$_1$ and VIP$_2$ receptor mRNA expressions are markedly decreased and increased, respectively. The electrical activity of multireceptive neurons of the spinal dorsal horn is also modulated by VIP$_1$ and VIP$_2$ receptors, which appear to be involved in exaggerated responses to noxious stimuli in mustard oil-induced activity of neuropathic animals. Selective blockade of the VIP$_2$ receptors results in significant antihyperalgesia in rats injected with mustard oil.[20]

HYPERALGESIA FOLLOWING TISSUE INJURY AND INFLAMMATION

Hyperalgesia develops after injury or inflammation of cutaneous and deep tissue such as that occurring with surgery in the cancer patient. Hyperalgesia is characterized by a decreased pain threshold, increased pain in response to suprathreshold stimuli, and ongoing pain. Hyperalgesia occurs at the site of injury and also in the surrounding uninjured area. Hyperalgesia at the site of injury is termed *primary hyperalgesia*, whereas hyperalgesia in the uninjured skin surrounding the injury is termed *secondary hyperalgesia*.

The characteristics of primary and secondary hyperalgesia differ. A burn to the glabrous skin of the hand leads to a marked hyperalgesia to heat and to mechanical stimuli applied at the injury site. The pain threshold for both modalities is dramatically reduced, and pain to suprathreshold stimuli is greatly increased in this primary zone of hyperalgesia. In contrast, when stimuli are applied away from the site of injury, hypersensitivity to mechanical stimuli but not to thermal stimuli is present in the zone of secondary hyperalgesia. Indeed, at least two forms of mechanical hyperalgesia have been reported in the secondary zone. Hyperalgesia to light touch or stroking stimuli, often referred to as allodynia, and hyperalgesia to sharp stimuli such as VonFrey probes, referred to as punctate hyperalgesia, are each present and appear to have different neural mechanisms.

▶ Primary afferent sensitization and primary hyperalgesia

Primary hyperalgesia is mediated by sensitization of nociceptors. *Sensitization* is defined as a leftward shift of the stimulus-response function that relates magnitude of the neural response to stimulus intensity. Sensitization is characterized by a decreased threshold, an augmented response to suprathreshold stimuli, and ongoing spontaneous activity. The changes in responses of primary afferent fibers recorded in anesthetized monkeys after injury correlates with the changes in subjective ratings of pain in humans following the same injury. When test heat stimuli were applied to the glabrous skin of the hand before and after a burn, prominent hyperalgesia resulted in human subjects. C-fiber nociceptors showed a decreased response following the burn, whereas the type I A-fiber nociceptors were markedly sensitized. Thus, A-fiber nociceptors play an important role in primary hyperalgesia in glabrous skin. In contrast, C-fiber nociceptors in hairy skin are sensitized following injury, and so C-fiber and A-fiber nociceptors mediate primary hyperalgesia that occurs in hairy skin. In the knee joint, mechanically insensitive afferents become responsive to mechanical stimuli after inflammation.

Similar sensitization to mechanical stimuli after administration of inflammatory agents or after cutaneous injury has also been observed in cutaneous mechanically insensitive afferents. Thus, mechanically insensitive afferents also have an important role in the mechanical hyperalgesia resulting from both cutaneous and deep tissue injury.

▶ Spinal neuron sensitization and secondary hyperalgesia

The idea that sensitization of spinal neurons accounts for secondary hyperalgesia remained controversial for a prolonged period. Lewis first proposed that the spreading sensitization of primary afferents, wherein activation and sensitization of an initial nociceptor leads to sensitization of neighboring nociceptors due to the effects of a sensitizing substance released from the initial nociceptor, accounted for secondary hyperalgesia. However, injury adjacent to a nociceptor-receptive field or indeed even to one-half of a receptive field does not produce sensitization of the nociceptor fibers outside the area of injury. Similarly, antidromic stimulation of nociceptive fibers does not cause sensitization of primary afferent endings.

Psychophysical studies provided the earliest evidence that spinal neurons mediate secondary hyperalgesia. Intradermal injection of capsaicin, the active ingredient in hot peppers, produces intense pain at the injection site and a large zone of secondary hyperalgesia surrounding the injection site. When capsaicin is administered under conditions of a proximal anesthetic nerve block to spare the spinal cord from the nociceptive barrage generated at the time of injection but leaving the peripheral nervous system effects of the capsaicin unaffected, no secondary hyperalgesia is present even after the block has worn off. An alteration in central processing therefore plays a major role in secondary hyperalgesia. When the capsaicin injection site is cooled or anesthetized after the injection, signs of secondary hyperalgesia to light touch are eliminated or substantially reduced while hyperalgesia to punctate stimuli remains largely unaffected. Thus, ongoing input from primary afferent neurons at the site of injury is required to maintain some types of secondary hyperalgesia, while other types become independent of nociceptor input after the provoking nociceptor barrage. These two forms of secondary mechanical hyperalgesia are transmitted by different primary afferent types. Selectively blocking large myelinated fibers using pressure causes pain to light touch to disappear when touch sensation is lost, but heat and cold sensations are still present. Similarly, intraneural microstimulation of large diameter (A-b) fibers in awake human subjects evoked tactile paresthesias in normal skin but hyperalgesic pain in skin with capsaicin. Meanwhile, other lines of psychophysical evidence indicate that punctuate secondary mechanical hyperalgesia is mediated by small diameter (A-d) fibers.

Neurophysiologic investigations have shown that the characteristics of secondary hyperalgesia are well explained by properties of dorsal horn neurons after injury. As mentioned earlier, the responses of spinothalamic cells to noxious stimuli correlate well with the pain ratings of humans to the same stimuli. Similarly, spinothalamic cell responses after injury also correlate with the development of secondary hyperalgesia. As shown in Fig. 5-7, the responses of dorsal horn neurons to mechanical stimuli are increased in magnitude to a given stimulus following an injury. In addition, the receptive field areas of single neurons become expanded. This expansion of receptive field area results in a greater number of cells responding to a stimulus delivered to any given area of skin. Thus, both more pain

signaling cells are responding to a given mechanical stimulus, and these responses are increased in magnitude. Meanwhile, the response of dorsal horn neurons to heat is enhanced only for stimuli applied in the area of primary hyperalgesia at the site of injury but is either unchanged or reduced for heat stimuli applied in the adjacent secondary hyperalgesia areas of undamaged skin.

Controversy remains regarding the specific roles that functional subsets of dorsal horn neurons play in generating secondary hyperalgesia. Most WDR dorsal horn neurons are sensitized by a variety of peripheral injuries suggesting that this subtype of neurons is important for the detection and discrimination of tissue-damaging stimuli and in the generation of secondary hyperalgesia. NS cells sensitize less frequently after peripheral injury than do WDR neurons, and so NS cells have often been assigned a less prominent role in the generation of secondary hyperalgesia. However, since even the signaling of nonsensitized NS cells would be superimposed on that of sensitized WDR cells, a role for NS cells in secondary hyperalgesia should not be minimized. LT cells have not been reported to acquire nociceptive inputs following injury, but rather often show a loss of all excitatory responses.[21] At first blush, these data suggest that this group of neurons have little or no role in the generation of secondary hyperalgesia. Yet, some characteristics of secondary hyperalgesia, such as the uniform intensity of pain throughout the zone and the sharp borders to the zone of hyperalgesia, could involve a subtraction-type of signal like that shown by LT neurons.

▶ Hyperalgesia and plasticity in rostral CNS structures

Finally, neurons in higher CNS areas also show enhanced responses after injury. For example, the responses of neurons in the thalamus and cortex of rats to cutaneous mechanical stimuli have been shown to increase with the induction of both experimental arthritis and experimental neuropathy. Similarly, neuronal activity in the thalamus of humans with chronic pain also demonstrates alterations. Although these changes in responses of thalamic and cortical neurons may only reflect changes that have taken place in the primary afferents and spinal cord neurons under each of these conditions, it should be noted that anatomic and neurochemical changes also take place in the thalamus and cortex under each of these conditions. Thus, neuronal substrates exist to support a third or even fourth component to hyperalgesia.

▶ Neurochemistry of primary afferent and central sensitization

Primary afferent sensitization

Mechanistically, primary afferent fibers are sensitized by the release of the inflammatory soup arising from damaged tissues and from activated immune and inflammatory cells. These mediators, many of which directly cause pain, include bradykinin, serotonin, histamine, prostaglandins, leukotrienes, excitatory amino acids, adenosine triphosphate, substance P, cytokines, nerve growth factor, nitric oxide, and various physiochemical stimuli. Specific primary afferent fibers are often sensitive to only one or a few of these substances and specific substances often produce hyperalgesia to only a specific modality of sensation. For example, bradykinin only produces thermal hyperalgesia when injected into human skin. Other components of the soup, most notably the prostaglandins, do not directly cause pain or hyperalgesia, but sensitize the fibers to other mediators of the

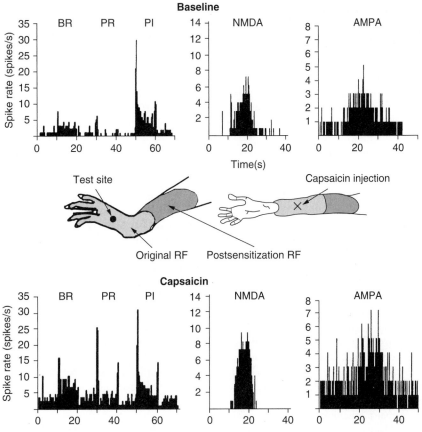

FIGURE 5-7 The rate histograms at the left in each row show the background activity and responses of a representative wide dynamic range spinothalamic tract neuron to mechanical stimulation of the hind limb before and after an intradermal injection of capsaicin. The baseline responses to the mechanical stimuli are shown in the upper row, while the matching records after capsaicin are shown in the lower row. The mechanical stimuli were applied to the sites shown on the drawing of the leg in the middle of the figure. The "X" shows the site at which capsaicin was delivered. The lightly stippled area shows the receptive field during the baseline recordings, whereas the heavily stippled area shows the expansion in receptive field induced by capsaicin. The rate histograms in the center and at right in each row show the responses of this cell to excitatory amino acids applied by microiontophoresis before (upper row), and then following sensitization by capsaicin (lower row). The times of each drug application are shown by the lines over each set of histograms. NMDA = N-methyl-D-aspartate, AMPA = a-amino-3-hydroxy-5-methyl-isoxazolepropionic acid.

soup. Nevertheless, a final common biochemical pathway shared by almost all of these mediators in their effects on primary afferent fibers is through activation of adenyl cyclase.

The role of the transient receptor potential (TRP) family of receptors in the signaling and sensitization of primary afferent fibers has generated particular interest in current research circles. TRPV1 receptors are expressed in small nociceptive neurons in the DRG and trigeminal ganglia, and are activated by capsaicin and by sudden increases in temperature.[22] Activated TRPV1 receptors are highly permeable to Ca^{2+}, which in turn regulates the activity of various intracellular messengers and membrane-bound lipids. These include phorbol esters, diacylglycerol, and phosphoinositol,[23,24] which then regulate additional downstream molecular cascades, including the p38 mitogen-activated protein (MAP) and extracellular signal-regulated kinases (ERK) in small sensory neurons and in a small population of medium-caliber A fibers. Thus, TRPV1 receptors have gained recognition as key regulators of excitability and sensitization in primary afferent fibers. TRPV2 and TRPV3 receptors respond to hot (50°C–60°C) and warm (35°C–45°C) temperatures, respectively; with TRPV3 receptors primarily found in keratinocytes and TRPV2 receptors in DRG neurons.[25–27] The role of these receptors in primary afferent signaling and sensitization is still being defined.

Central neural sensitization

The wide variety of chemical mediators involved in regular sensory neurotransmission as reviewed above can all influence the sensitization process in the spinal dorsal horn. However, as illustrated in Fig. 5-7, the key event in spinal sensitization is facilitation of excitatory amino acid neurotransmission between primary afferent fibers and dorsal horn neurons by coreleased neuropeptides. Tachykinin neuropeptides, substance P and neurokinin A, released from C fibers with noxious stimulation produce an immediate increase in the postsynaptic effects of the excitatory amino acids, glutamate, and aspartate that are released from either nociceptive or nonnociceptive primary afferents. Facilitation of responses by tachykinins at AMPA-type glutamate receptors requires continuous activation at tachykinin receptors, and thus provides a neurochemical mechanism for the signs of secondary hyperalgesia that are readily reversible with anesthesia of the site of injury. In contrast, facilitation of responses by tachykinins at NMDA-type glutamate receptors is often very long-lasting after a single coordinated coactivation of these receptors by both types of ligands. Thus, neurokinin-induced facilitation of glutamate NMDA receptors provides a neurochemical mechanism for the characteristics of secondary hyperalgesia such as punctuate hyperalgesia that outlast anesthesia of the injury site.

HYPERALGESIA FOLLOWING NERVE INJURY

▶ Symptomatology and psychophysics of neuropathic pain

Traumatic injury to soft tissue, bone, and/or nerve leads, in certain cases, to a chronic pain state that is characterized by ongoing pain and hyperalgesia. Intriguingly, in some patients pain and hyperalgesia depend upon sympathetic innervation of the affected area (sympathetically maintained pain, SMP), whereas in others pain is independent of the sympathetics (SIP). Clinically, both SMP and SIP patients often present with similar signs and symptoms.

Several lines of evidence indicate that activity in LT mechanoreceptors evokes pain in neuropathic pain patients. Thus, touch-evoked pain disappears during a selective A-fiber block and the latency for touch-evoked pain is short. Similarly, weak electrical stimulation of involved peripheral nerves such that only A-b fibers are activated evokes pain in patients with SMP before, but only tingling after, a sympathetic block.

Although primary afferent nociceptor sensitization accounts for certain aspects of hyperalgesia in tissue injury (described earlier in the chapter), the touch-evoked pain commonly seen in neuropathic pain states appears to be due to a central sensitization. Central neurons, activity which leads to the sensation of pain, develop an enhanced response to input from nonnociceptive afferents such as LT mechanoreceptors. Such a central sensitization of dorsal horn neurons following cutaneous injury has been demonstrated by several investigators (described earlier in the chapter). This central sensitization may be selective in that mechanical hyperalgesia can be present in the absence of hyperalgesia to heat. Thus, the mechanical hyperalgesia observed in neuropathic pain is similar to the secondary hyperalgesia observed after cutaneous injury.

▶ Animal models for the study of neuropathic pain

Plasticity in the nervous system after nerve injury has been studied following axotomy, rhizotomy following various types of partial injuries to nerves innervating the hind limbs, and most recently following the chronic infusion of various cancer chemotherapy drugs.[28–30]

Justification of these injuries as models for the study of human neuropathic pain is based on the behaviors shown by animals with these injuries. For example, a few days to a week after rhizotomy or axotomy, animals show an increased sensitivity to mechanical stimuli and may self-mutilate the deafferented limb (autotomy). In contrast, animals with partial nerve injury or treated with chemotherapy drugs rarely autotomize yet do exhibit other behavioral changes consistent with a neuropathic pain state. These symptoms are observed within hours or several days after the partial nerve injury or drug treatment.[28–30] The posture of the rats is altered so that the hind limb appears to be maintained in a "guarded" position. In addition, the rats exhibit enhanced behavioral responses to noxious thermal, mechanical, and sometimes cooling stimuli.[28–30]

▶ Physiologic changes in peripheral nerves after nerve injury

Peripheral nerves show an initial afferent barrage when traumatically injured that may be briefly quite intense, but which usually resolves within no more than several minutes. This injury barrage appears to be a very important event in provoking many of the sequelae of nerve injury. Although injury barrage following partial nerve injury models has not been directly measured, indirect evidence suggests that such an injury barrage does in fact take place with these models. For example, anesthesia of the sciatic nerve prior to injury reduces both the severity and duration of the thermal hyperalgesia which later develops. Similarly, administration of MK-801, an antagonist for the NMDA-type glutamate receptor activated by intense afferent barrages, reduces the severity of partial nerve injury-induced hyperalgesia as do antagonists for the nitric oxide cascade.

Once the injury discharges subside, the injured axons enter a period of quiescence. The transected axons are clearly no longer connected to the peripheral transducers. Similarly, many axons in partially injured nerves fail to conduct through the nerve injury site, and the dorsal root potentials and afferent volleys are reduced.

Three to five days following axotomy, rhizotomy, or partial nerve injury, spontaneous discharges develop in the severed nerves. This activity following overt nerve section reaches a peak frequency at about day 14 after injury and then slowly tapers to a low level, which is sustained for many weeks. Most of the spontaneously active fibers have conduction velocity of small myelinated fibers, although some unmyelinated fibers also show spontaneous discharges. Ectopic discharges arise from sites both at the cut ends of fibers in the neuroma as well as near the cell bodies in the DRG. Many fibers in a neuroma are sensitive to mechanical or chemical stimuli, some alter their discharge rates upon heating or cooling, and some may form direct electrical (ephaptic) connections with neighboring fibers within the neuroma. However, it is not clear whether the ectopic activity in neuroma or injured axons parallels the behaviors shown by animals with nerve injuries.

▶ Physiologic changes in central neurons after nerve injury

CNS neurons, like primary afferents, also show a large discharge at the time of nerve transection. The time course of the injury discharges observed in the CNS parallels that found in primary afferents. Once the injury discharges subside, spinal neurons also enter a period of quiescence, which is characterized by a decrease in excitatory inputs. Indeed for many spinal neurons, the decrease in excitatory input is global so that receptive fields become more difficult to identify in the dorsal horn, especially for cells immediately contiguous to the entry zone of the severed nerve.

A few days following nerve injury, many CNS neurons develop changes in spontaneous activity. These changes lag behind the development of spontaneous discharges in afferent fibers by 1–3 days. Cells either show a continuous, regular discharge of high frequency, or are relatively silent except for sudden high frequency bursts. Most of the cells showing these changes after nerve section are in the center of a deafferented zone and have no defined peripheral receptive field. However, some cells at the margins of the deafferented zones exhibit responses to cutaneous stimuli as well as changes in spontaneous activity. Higher percentages than normal of these cells respond only to noxious stimuli. Similar changes in the spontaneous activity of dorsal horn cells was also shown after partial nerve injury, although most dorsal horn cells retained receptive fields. Altered spontaneous discharges develop in the dorsal horn and dorsal column nuclei as soon as a week following peripheral nerve injury, while similar changes in the thalamus and cortex are not reported until later time points. Moreover, alterations in spontaneous activity are not limited to experimental animals but have also been shown in the human spinal cord and thalamus after nerve injury.

Reappearance of receptive fields for dorsal horn neurons that were originally deafferented occurs about 1–2 weeks after injury.

Many of these new receptive fields are somatotopically inappropriate, usually located in body areas corresponding to dermatomes neighboring the deafferented areas. The receptive fields often have unusual sizes varying from very large to very small, and are often split. Many of these neurons respond only to low-intensity mechanical stimuli. The development of inappropriate somatotopy has also been reported to take place in the human thalamus following nerve injury and in the cortex of experimental animals.

Dorsal horn neurons studied in animals with partial nerve injuries do not usually show altered receptive fields. Instead these neurons have elevated baseline firing rates and a propensity for very prolonged afterdischarges. Cells in monkeys with a partial nerve injuries show elevated responses to all cutaneous stimuli at the margins of the

nerve injured zone. As illustrated in Fig. 5-8, these types of changes in physiology are also commonly seen in spinal neurons of animals with hyperalgesia due to chronic exposure to chemotherapy drugs.

▶ Neurochemistry of neuropathic pain

The neurochemistry underlying neuropathic pain shares much in common with that underlying acute primary and secondary hyperalgesia reviewed above. Thus, inflammatory mediators near primary afferent nerve endings produce sensitization of these fibers, and excitatory amino acids and neurokinin peptides contribute to sensitization of spinal neurons. However, given that neuropathic pain by definition involves damage to the nervous system, it should not be

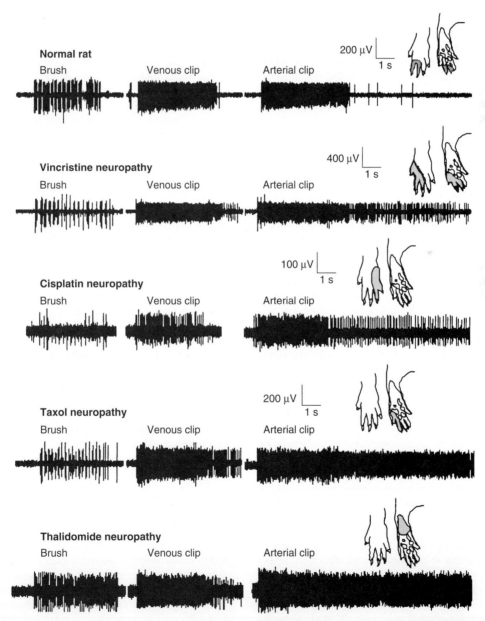

FIGURE 5-8 The analog recordings of neuron activity from spinal cord show excess afterdischarges to cutaneous stimuli in rats with hyperalgesia after being treated for 3–5 days with various chemotherapy drugs. The times of each stimulus application are indicted by the lines over each trace and the receptive fields locations are shown in the drawings at the right.

surprising that this neurochemistry is further complicated due to both degenerative as well as regenerative processes in both primary afferent and central neurons. Not only does cell loss and attempted regrowth complicate the neurochemical milieu in the somatosensory system, but the morphologic responses to injury and attempted tissue repair are also likely culprits that underlie the refractory and long-term nature of neuropathic pain.

The most obvious of the degenerative changes occurring with peripheral nerve damage is the loss of primary afferent drive to the spinal dorsal horn. The gate theory of pain control posits that inputs in large diameter fibers inhibit spinal processing of signals from small diameter nociceptors. A disinhibition of pain signaling in cells that normally have convergent input could easily be envisaged as a consequence of nerve damage that preferentially affects large fiber inputs to this cell or group of cells. A less-obvious degenerative change thought to contribute to neuropathic pain after peripheral nerve injury is the transsynaptic loss of inhibitory neurons in the spinal cord following peripheral nerve injury. A similar loss of inhibitory neurons in the thalamus may contribute to central pain following spinal cord injury.[31] Wallerian degeneration of peripheral axons and digestion of lost central neurons provoke the activation of both central and peripheral glial elements as well as inflammatory cells. Activation of these cells increases the levels of perineural inflammatory cytokines that can further activate nociceptive neurons and generate pain.[32,33]

Following the phase of axonal/neuronal degeneration due to injury is the stimulation of regrowth of surviving injured axons and proliferation of neurons that adjoin deafferented neural and peripheral targets. Neurons that are injured will attempt to restore connectivity that is lost to an original innervation target, and uninjured neurons will attempt to establish innervation to targets that have become deprived of neural input. Competition between these two sets of growing neurons almost ensures that inappropriate connectivity, both within the CNS and in the periphery, will result. In addition, as neurons grow they discharge spontaneously, thus increasing signal traffic throughout the somatosensory axis. Gene expression is also changed in neurons,[34] resulting in changes in cell phenotype that may include alteration of cell surface ion channels,[35] neurotransmitter and neuropeptide receptors, surface growth-associated proteins, and changes in neurotransmitter and neuropeptide content and synaptic release. Invasion of DRG by sympathetic nerves and the de novo expression of adrenergic receptors on peripheral nerves are examples of phenotypic changes resulting in pain. Finally, the expression of nerve growth factors is upregulated with neuronal proliferation, which directly produces pain when administered to experimental animals.[36]

Cytokines have key roles in the pathogenesis of several preclinical models of neuropathic and inflammatory pain. Glial fibrillary acidic protein (GFAP)-positive activated astrocytes, a source for the cytokines tumor necrosis factor (TNF), interleukin-1b (IL-1b), IL-15, and IL-6,[37] are increased in the spinal cord segments to which the nerves affected by neuropathic and inflammatory pain project. Neuropathic pain can be induced by surrounding a peripheral nerve with chromic gut suture or producing structural damage to peripheral axons, which leads to an inflammatory reaction at the site of injury, or by simply surrounding peripheral nerves with an immune stimulant such as zymosan.[38] Inflammatory cells infiltrate the site, levels of cytokines increase (IL-1, and particularly TNF), and endoneural swelling and neuropathic pain ensue.[38] Mechanisms by which cytokines might produce pain are by directly producing discharges of nociceptors,[33,39] altering the trafficking of growth factors

along nerve fibers resulting in phenotypic changes in sensory endings, inducing an alteration of glial cell-mediated support of neural activities such as synaptic glutamate reuptake,[40] or inducing the degeneration of neurons and the retraction of cell processes.[41] The inflammatory cascade leading to nerve constriction pain can be blocked by thalidomide, a TNF antagonist,[42] whereas inflammatory neuritis is blocked by either thalidomide or the immunosuppressant cyclosporin A.[38] The reduction in constriction neuropathy-induced pain by thalidomide is paralleled by reductions in endoneural levels of TNF-a.[42]

Chemotherapy-induced neuropathy can similarly result due to the induction of proinflammatory cytokines around nerve endings. Cytokines are released from both animal and human tissues following exposure to chemotherapy drugs in vitro, and coadministration of chemotherapeutic drugs with cytokines, for example, vincristine in combination with granulocyte-macrophage colony-stimulating factor (GM-CSF), markedly increases the severity and magnitude of treatment-induced pain and other neurologic impairments. The cytokines interferon (IFN)-a/g, TNF-a, IL-1, and IL-6 are increased in vitro by cisplatin, Taxol,[43] and by both ionizing and ultraviolet irradiation.[44] The pattern of cytokine gene induction, synthesis, and release induced by Taxol is identical to that induced by lipopolysaccharide (LPS).[45] Cell sources for the cytokines induced by cisplatin and Taxol include macrophages, monocytes, tumor, and endothelial cells. Neurons and glial cells are another potential source of proinflammatory cytokines[37,46] that have not yet been tested. Vincristine increases GM-CSF[47] and IL-15 and downregulates TNF-a receptors.[47] All three chemotherapy drugs directly activate the NF-kB signaling pathway that is shared with LPS, IL-1, IL-6, IFN, and TNF.

The effects of cytokines on Schwann cells could explain the clinical presentation of chemoneuropathy and account for the known risk and protective factors. Both myelinating and nonmyelinating Schwann cells express receptors for TNF, IFN, IL-1, and IL-6 and activation of these receptors leads to activation of NF-kB and c-jun pathways that in turn result in downregulation of myelin synthesis, increased expression of the p75 nerve growth factor (NGF) receptor, dedifferentiation, and proliferation.[48,49] Exposure of peripheral nerves to inflammatory cytokines thus results in extirpation of myelin and perineural swelling like that observed in the early stages of Wallerian degeneration and in neural biopsies from chemotherapy-treated animals and humans, as described above. These phenotypic changes would consequently have a pronounced impact on A-b fiber function that is heavily dependent on extensive myelination, but less so on C fibers, thus generating a clinical picture like that observed in the patient studies. Moreover, because of the plethora of proinflammatory cytokines that are found in cells resident in the skin, such as tissue macrophages, Langerhans cells, and most especially keratinocytes that are in close proximity to myelinated nerve endings outside the blood-brain barrier, the dieback pattern is only to be expected. As individual Schwann cells become activated and exposed to proinflammatory cytokines, these Schwann cells themselves begin to synthesize and release proinflammatory cytokines,[49,50] affecting neighboring Schwann cells and thus closing a positive feedback loop that can sustain the neuropathy. Prolonged or high-dose exposure of Schwann cells leads to apoptosis, which could further explain the persistence of pain in some chemotherapy patients.[51] Finally, NGF, insulin-like growth factor (IGF), and neurotrophin-3 (NT-3), all of which offer protection to chemotherapy-induced pain in animals, inhibit NF-kB signaling[52] and prevent or reverse the effects of inflammatory cytokines on Schwann cells.[53,54]

SUMMARY

The physiologic basis of pain sensation from skin can be summarized as a series of neuronal linkages that run from the skin to the spinal cord and then on to a number of more rostral centers located in the brainstem, midbrain, diencephalon, and finally the cortex. Cancer pain occurs as a result of alterations in the usual manner by which both noxious and nonnoxious stimuli are processed by these networks of neurons. It involves the routine processing of acute nociceptive stimuli, processes of short-term sensitization of peripheral and central neurons, and long-term processes associated with neuropathic pain. Each of these pain processes share signaling pathways and also have shared as well as unique neurochemical and physiological components. Thus, treatment of pain in cancer patients requires identification of the specific pain mechanisms that have been activated and subsequently a tailoring of treatment to best remedy each specific pain component.

REFERENCES

1. Wilkie D, Huang H-Y, Reilly N, Cain K. Nociceptive and neuropathic pain in patients with lung cancer: a comparison of pain quality descriptors. *J Pain Symptom Manage.* 2002;22:899–910.
2. Garry EM, Fleetwood-Walker SM. A new view on how AMPA receptors and their interacting proteins mediate neuropathic pain. *Pain.* 2004;109:210–213.
3. Bordi F, Ugolini A. Group I metabotropic glutamate receptors: implications for brain diseases. *Prog Neurobiol.* 1999;59:55–79.
4. Spooren W, Ballard T, Gasparini F, et al. Insight into the function of Group I and Group II metabotropic glutamate (mGlu) receptors: behavioural characterization and implications for the treatment of CNS disorders. *Behav Pharmacol.* 2003;14:257–277.
5. Ueno S, Tsuda M, Iwanaga T, Inoue K. Cell type-specific ATP-activated responses in rat dorsal root ganglion neurons. *Br J Pharmacol.* 1999;126:429–436.
6. Abbracchio MP, Boeynaems JM, Barnard EA, et al. Characterization of the UDP-glucose receptor (re-named here the P2Y14 receptor) adds diversity to the P2Y receptor family. *Trends Pharmacol Sci.* 2003;24:52–55.
7. Moriyama T, Iida T, Kobayashi K, et al. Possible involvement of P2Y2 metabotropic receptors in ATP-induced transient receptor potential vanilloid receptor 1-mediated thermal hypersensitivity. *J Neurosci.* 2003;23:6058–6062.
8. Xiao HS, Huang QH, Zhang FX, et al. Identification of gene expression profile of dorsal root ganglion in the rat peripheral axotomy model of neuropathic pain. *Proc Natl Acad Sci USA.* 2002;99:8360–8365.
9. Eisenach JC, Curry R, Hood DD. Dose response of intrathecal adenosine in experimental pain and allodynia. *Anesthesiology.* 2002;97: 938–942.
10. Sun RQ, Tu YJ, Lawand NB, et al. Calcitonin gene-related peptide receptor activation produces PKA- and PKC-dependent mechanical hyperalgesia and central sensitization. *J Neurophysiol.* 2004;92:2859–2866.
11. Ebersberger A, Charbel Issa P, Vanegas H, Schaible H-G. Differential effects of calcitonin gene-related peptide and calcitonin gene-related peptide 8-37 upon responses to N-methyl—aspartate or (R,S)-alpha-amino-3-hydroxy-5-methylisoxazole-4-propionate in spinal nociceptive neurons with knee joint input in the rat. *Neuroscience.* 2000;99:171–178.
12. Branchek TA, Smith KE, Gerald C, Walker MW. Galanin receptor subtypes. *Trends Pharmacol Sci.* 2000;21:109–117.
13. O'Donnell D, Ahmad S, Wahlestedt C, Walker P. Expression of the novel galanin receptor subtype GALR2 in the adult rat CNS: distinct distribution from GALR1. *J Comp Neurol.* 1999;409:469–481.
14. Kerr BJ, Cafferty WB, Gupta YK, et al. Galanin knockout mice reveal nociceptive deficits following peripheral nerve injury. *Eur J Neurosci.* 2000;12:793–802.
15. Liu HX, Brumovsky P, Schmidt R, et al. Receptor subtype-specific pronociceptive and analgesic actions of galanin in the spinal cord: selective actions via GalR1 and GalR2 receptors. *Proc Natl Acad Sci USA.* 2001;98:9960–9964.
16. Coudore-Civiale MA, Courteix C, Fialip J, et al. Spinal effect of the cholecystokinin-B receptor antagonist CI-988 on hyperalgesia, allodynia and morphine-induced analgesia in diabetic and mononeuropathic rats. *Pain.* 2000;88:15–22.
17. Kurrikoff K, Koks S, Matsui T, et al. Deletion of the CCK2 receptor gene reduces mechanical sensitivity and abolishes the development of hyperalgesia in mononeuropathic mice. *Eur J Neurosci.* 2004;20: 1577–1586.
18. Pommier B, Beslot F, Simon A, et al. Deletion of CCK2 receptor in mice results in an upregulation of the endogenous opioid system. *J Neurosci.* 2002;22:2005–2011.
19. Yeomans DC, Onyuksel H, Dagar S, et al. Conformation-dependent effects of VIP on nociception in rats. *Peptides.* 2003;24:617–622.
20. Dickinson T, Mitchell R, Robberecht P, Fleetwood-Walker SM. The role of VIP/PACAP receptor subtypes in spinal somatosensory processing in rats with an experimental peripheral mononeuropathy. *Neuropharmacology.* 1999;38:167–180.
21. Dougherty PM, Schwartz A, Lenz FA. Responses of primate spinomesencephalic tract cells to intradermal capsaicin. *Neuroscience.* 1999;90: 1377–1392.
22. Caterina MJ, Julius D. The vanilloid receptor: a molecular gateway to the pain pathway. *Annu Rev Neurosci.* 2001;24:487–517.
23. Hwang SW, Cho H, Kwak J, et al. Direct activation of capsaicin receptors by products of lipoxygenases: endogenous capsaicin-like substances. *Proc Natl Acad Sci USA.* 2000;97:6155–6160.
24. Zygmunt PM, Petersson J, Andersson DA, et al. Vanilloid receptors on sensory nerves mediate the vasodilator action of anandamide. *Nature.* 1999;400:452–457.
25. Caterina MJ, Rosen TA, Tominaga M, et al. A capsaicin-receptor homologue with a high threshold for noxious heat. *Nature.* 1999;398:436–441.
26. Peier AM, Reeve AJ, Andersson DA, et al. A heat-sensitive TRP channel expressed in keratinocytes. *Science.* 2002;296:2046–2049.
27. Xu H, Ramsey IS, Kotecha SA, et al. TRPV3 is a calcium-permeable temperature-sensitive cation channel. *Nature.* 2002;418:181–186.
28. Cata JP, Weng H-R, Dougherty PM. Clinical and experimental findings in humans and animals with chemotherapy-induced peripheral neuropathy. *Minerva Anes.* 2005. (In Press).
29. Polomano RC, Mannes AJ, Clark US, Bennett GJ. A painful peripheral neuropathy in the rat produced by the chemotherapeutic drug, paclitaxel. *Pain.* 2001;94:293–304.
30. Weng H-R, Cordella JV, Dougherty PM. Changes in sensory processing in the spinal dorsal horn accompany vincristine-induced hyperalgesia and allodynia. *Pain.* 2003;103:131–138.
31. Ralston DD, Dougherty PM, Lenz FA, et al. Plasticity of the inhibitory circuits of the primate ventrobasal thalamus following lesions of the somatosensory pathways. In: Devor M, Rowbotham MC, Wiesenfeld-Hallin Z, eds. *Proceedings of the 9th World Congress on Pain.* Vol. 16. Seattle: IASP Press; 2000:427–434.
32. Milligan ED, Twining C, Chacur M, et al. Spinal glia and proinflammatory cytokines mediate mirror-image neuropathic pain in rats. *J Neurosci.* 2003;23:1026–1040.
33. Sorkin LS, Doom CM. Epineurial application of TNF elicits an acute mechanical hyperalgesia in the awake rat. *J Peripher Nerv Syst.* 2000;5:96–100.
34. Okamoto K, Martin DP, Schmelzer JD, et al. Pro- and anti-inflammatory cytokine gene expression in rat sciatic nerve chronic constriction injury model of neuropathic pain. *Exp Neurol.* 2001;169:386–391.
35. Dib-Hajj SD, Fjell J, Cummins TR, et al. Plasticity of sodium channel expression in DRG neurons in the chronic constriction injury model of neuropathic pain. *Pain.* 1999;83:591–600.
36. Kanaan SA, Saade NE, Karam M, et al. Hyperalgesia and upregulation of cytokines and nerve growth factor by cutaneous leishmaniasis in mice. *Pain.* 2000;85:477–482.
37. Wieseler-Frank J, Maier SF, Watkins LR. Glial activation and pathological pain. *Neurochem Int.* 2004;45:389–395.
38. Bennett GJ. A neuroimmune interaction in painful peripheral neuropathy. *Clin J Pain.* 2000;16:S139–S143.
39. Leem JG, Bove GM. Mid-axonal tumor necrosis factor-alpha induces ectopic activity in a subset of slowly conducting cutaneous and deep afferent neurons. *J Pain.* 2002;3:45–49.
40. Honore P, Menning PM, Rogers SD, et al. Neurochemical plasticity in persistent inflammatory pain. *Prog Brain Res.* 200;129:357–363.

41. Allan SM. The role of pro- and antiinflammatory cytokines in neurodegeneration. *Ann N Y Acad Sci.* 2000;917:84–93.

42. George A, Marziniak M, Schafers M, et al. Thalidomide treatment in chronic constrictive neuropathy decreases endoneurial tumor necrosis factor-alpha, increases interleukin-10 and has long-term effects on spinal cord dorsal horn met-enkephalin. *Pain.* 2000;88:267–275.

43. Zaks-Zilberman M, Zaks TZ, Vogel SN. Induction of proinflammatory and chemokine genes by lipopolysaccharide and paclitaxel (Taxol) in murine and human breast cancer cell lines. *Cytokine.* 2001;15:156–165.

44. Ibuki Y, Goto R. Contribution of inflammatory cytokine release to activation of resident peritoneal macrophages after in vivo low-dose gamma-irradiation. *J Radiat Res (Tokyo).* 1999;40:253–262.

45. Ding AH, Porteu F, Sanchez E, Nathan CF. Shared actions of endotoxin and taxol on TNF receptors and TNF release. *Science.* 2002;248:370–372.

46. Hanisch U-K. Microglia as a source and target of cytokines. *Glia.* 2002;40:140–155.

47. Ogura K, Ohta S, Ohmori T, et al. Vinca alkaloids induce granulocyte-macrophage colony stimulating factor in human peripheral blood mononuclear cells. *Anticancer Res.* 2000;20:2383–2388.

48. Conti G, De Pol A, Scarpini E, et al. Interleukin-1 beta and interferon-gamma induce proliferation and apoptosis in cultured Schwann cells. *J Neuroimmunol.* 2002;124:29–35.

49. Shubayev VI, Myers RR. Endoneurial remodeling by TNFa- and TNFa-releasing proteases. A spatial and temporal co-localization study in painful neuropathy. *J Peripher Nerv Syst.* 2002;7:28–36.

50. Ohtori S, Takahashi K, Moriya H, Myers RR. TNF-alpha and TNF-alpha receptor type 1 upregulation in glia and neurons after peripheral nerve injury: studies in murine DRG and spinal cord. *Spine.* 2004;29:1082–1088.

51. Benn T, Halfpenny C, Scolding N. Glial cells as targets for cytotoxic immune mediators. *Glia.* 2001;36:200–211.

52. Otten U, März P, Heese K, et al. Cytokines and neurotrophins interact in normal and diseased states. *Ann N Y Acad Sci* 2000;917: 322–330.

53. Cheng HL, Steinway ML, Xin X, Feldman EL. Insulin-like growth factor-I and Bcl-X(L) inhibit c-jun N-terminal kinase activation and rescue Schwann cells from apoptosis. *J Neurochem.* 2001;76: 935–943.

54. Teare KA, Pearson RG, Shakesheff KM, Haycock JW. A-MSH inhibits inflammatory signaling in Schwann cells. *Neuroreport.* 2004;15: 493–498.

PART 2

MANAGEMENT OF SPECIFIC CANCER PAIN SYNDROMES

Bone Pain

CHAPTER 6

Kyle G. Halvorson
Lucy J. Sullivan
Patrick W. Mantyh

INTRODUCTION

More than 1.3 million cases of cancer will be diagnosed in 2006 in the United States alone and 90% of patients with advanced cancer will experience significant, life-altering cancer-induced pain. Bone cancer pain is the most common pain in patients with advanced cancer as most common tumors, including breast, prostate, and lung, have a remarkable affinity to metastasize to bone. Currently, the factors that drive cancer pain are poorly understood; however, several recently introduced models of cancer pain are not only providing insight into the mechanisms that drive bone cancer pain but are guiding the development of novel mechanism-based therapies to treat the pain and skeletal remodeling that accompanies metastatic bone cancer. As analgesics can also influence disease progression, findings from these studies may lead to therapies that have the potential to improve the quality of life and survival of patients with skeletal malignancies.

THE CHALLENGE OF BONE CANCER PAIN

Although bone is not a vital organ, most common tumors have a strong predilection for bone metastasis. Tumor metastases to the skeleton are major contributors to morbidity and mortality in metastatic cancer. Tumor growth in bone results in anemia, increased susceptibility to infection, pain, skeletal fractures, and decreased mobility with resulting cardiovascular dysfunction, all of which compromise the patient's survival and quality of life.[1] Once tumor cells have metastasized to the skeleton, tumor-induced bone pain is usually described as dull in character, constant in presentation, and gradually increasing in intensity with time.[2] As bone remodeling progresses, severe spontaneous pain frequently occurs[2] and given that the onset of this pain is both acute and unpredictable, this component of bone cancer pain can be particularly debilitating to the patient's functional status and quality of life.[1,2] Breakthrough pain, which is an intermittent episode of extreme pain, can occur spontaneously, or more commonly, is induced by movement of or weight-bearing on the tumor-bearing bone(s).[3]

Currently, the treatment of pain from bone metastases involves the use of multiple complementary approaches, including radiotherapy, chemotherapy, bisphosphonates, and analgesics.[2] However, bone cancer pain is one of the most difficult of all persistent pains to fully control[2] as the metastases are generally not limited to a single site and the analgesics that are most commonly used to treat bone cancer pain—the nonsteroidal anti-inflammatory drugs (NSAIDs)[2] and opioids[2,4–6]— are limited by significant adverse side effects.[7,8] For example, nonselective NSAIDs can cause intestinal bleeding, whereas some selective cyclooxygenase-2 (COX-2) inhibitors, while causing less bleeding, have significant cardiovascular and renal safety issues.[9,10] Opioids are effective in attenuating bone cancer pain but are frequently accompanied by side effects such as constipation, sedation, nausea, vomiting, and respiratory depression.[11] Individuals with primary bone tumors such as sarcomas or those with prostate tumors, which metastasize primarily to bone and not other vital organs such as lung, liver, or brain, tend to live for a significant period of time (on average, 55 months for prostate cancer patients) beyond their initial diagnosis.[12] Although the length of survival continues to increase for cancer patients,[12] to maintain the patient's quality of life and functional status, it is essential that new therapies be developed that can be administered over several years to control bone pain without the side effects commonly encountered with the currently available analgesics.

In the past 6–7 years, the first animal models of bone cancer pain were developed and in terms of tumor growth, bone remodeling, and bone pain, these models appear to mirror several aspects of human bone cancer pain.[13–17] While information engendered from these models has begun to provide insight into the mechanisms that generate and maintain bone cancer pain, a major unanswered question is how the primarily osteolytic animal models (which are the models that have been the most utilized to date) compare with common osteoblastic tumors that avidly metastasize to bone in regard to bone remodeling (Fig. 6-1) and tumor-induced bone pain. Here, the similarities and differences between a primarily osteolytic sarcoma tumor versus a primarily osteoblastic prostate tumor are examined in terms of bone destruction, bone formation, tumor growth, macrophage infiltration, osteoclast and osteoblast number, and type and severity of bone cancer-related pain. Additionally, the remodeling of the sensory innervation of bone in osteolytic and osteoblastic bone cancer models is discussed as are recent advances in our understanding and development of mechanism-based therapies to treat bone cancer pain.

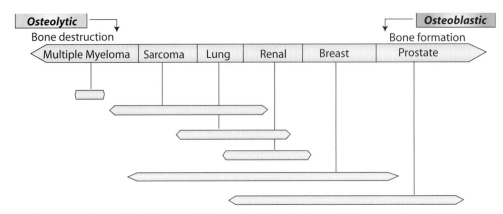

FIGURE 6-1 Representative spectrum of tumor-induced bone remodeling extending from primarily osteolytic tumors, such as multiple myeloma, to primarily osteoblastic tumors, such as prostate, which have metastasized to bone. Arrows represent the approximate degree of osteolytic or osteoblastic nature of each tumor type. Importantly, the figure illustrates how tumors that metastasize to bone often are highly variable within individual patients as well as between patients suffering from the same type of metastatic tumor burden. *(Adapted from Mundy G. Metastasis to bone: causes, consequences, and therapeutic opportunities. Nat Rev Cancer. 2002;2:584–593.)*

TUMOR GROWTH, SKELETAL REMODELING, AND PAIN INDUCED BY PRIMARILY OSTEOLYTIC OR OSTEOBLASTIC TUMORS

Previous studies examining tumor-induced bone pain have primarily utilized tumor lines that generate marked bone destruction with only modest bone formation. When primarily osteolytic 2472 murine osteosarcoma tumor cells are injected and confined to the intramedullary space of the femur, these tumor cells grow in a highly reproducible fashion as they proliferate, replacing the hemopoietic cells that are normally present in the intramedullary canal.[15,17] Thus, at 14 days following tumor cell injection and confinement of these primarily osteolytic cells to the femur, the entire marrow space is homogeneously filled with tumor cells and tumor-associated inflammatory/immune cells. In contrast, following injection and confinement of the primarily osteoblastic angiotensin-converting enzyme-1 (ACE-1) prostate cells into the mouse femur, the tumor cells are present in small clonal colonies throughout the marrow space of the femur and these small colonies of osteoblastic tumor cells are separated from each other by extensive matrices of newly formed woven bone at the day 19 end point.

The marked differences in tumor growth when comparing a primarily osteolytic tumor such as the 2472 osteosarcoma versus the primarily osteoblastic ACE-1 prostate cells are even more dramatic in comparing the bone remodeling induced by these two types of tumor cells. Fourteen days following injection and confinement of the 2472 osteosarcoma cells to the femur, there is significant bone destruction, with no significant bone formation. Interestingly, the bone destruction occurs almost exclusively in the proximal and distal head of the femur with little evidence of significant bone destruction in the intervening diaphysis of the bone.

In sharp contrast to the tumor-induced bone remodeling observed in the 2472 osteosarcoma model, the ACE-1 prostate tumor cells induce significant formation of new woven bone at day 19 in the proximal and distal head of the femur as well as the diaphysis of the bone. The marked bone formation induced by the ACE-1 prostate cells is also accompanied by bone destruction, giving the tumor-bearing femur a unique scalloped appearance when viewed radiographically (Fig. 6-2) or with traditional histological

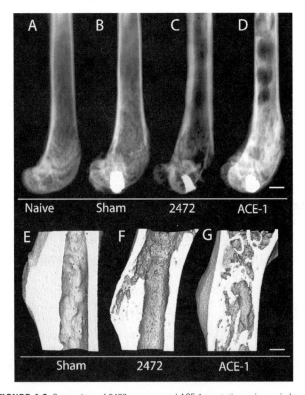

FIGURE 6-2 Comparison of 2472 sarcoma and ACE-1 prostatic carcinoma-induced bone remodeling. Sham-injected mice femurs (B) present neither bone formation nor bone destruction and are highly similar to naïve mouse femurs (A). 2472 sarcoma-injected femurs primarily display osteolytic appearances and are visible as regions of radiolucency at the distal head (C). ACE-1 prostatic carcinoma-injected femora present a mixed osteolytic and osteoblastic appearance visible radiographically at the day 19 endpoint, which is characterized by bone formation surrounding pockets of radiolucencies as diaphyseal bridging and mineral densities similar to those found in the trabecular regions at both the proximal and distal heads (D). Sham-injected mice femurs (E) present neither bone formation nor bone destruction, whereas 2472 sarcoma-injected femurs display primarily osteolytic appearances and are visible as regions of apparent bone mineral resorption throughout the diaphysis of the femur and, in this example, near the gluteal tuberosity (F) when analyzed with micro-CT imaging. Micro-CT analysis of ACE-1 prostatic carcinoma-induced bone remodeling presents extensive bone formation visible as bridging structures (white bone mass between the cortical walls) in the proximal diaphysis surrounding pockets of either normal hematopoietic or tumor cells (G). Scale bar = 4 mm.

methodology (Fig. 6-3), which is similar in appearance to that observed in human patients with prostate tumor metastases.[18] The concurrent bone destruction and formation in the ACE-1 model is quite distinct from that observed in tumors such as sarcoma[16,19] or breast,[20] where the tumor was primarily osteolytic as bone destruction predominates.[16,19] This mixed bone remodeling in the ACE-1 tumor-bearing femurs is marked by an increase in the number of osteoclasts throughout the intramedullary space. These serve to drive osteolytic bone remodeling in addition to the increased number of macrophages scattered throughout the tumor and remaining hematopoietic spaces in the bone. These macrophages may be involved in the inflammatory and neuropathic component of this tumor-induced bone pain (Fig. 6-4). Though the 2472 sarcoma cell line used in most of our previous studies does indeed induce an upregulation in the number of osteoclasts and macrophages (to an approximately twofold greater increase in macrophages than the ACE-1 line), it is the simultaneous upregulation in osteoblastic bone formation and the increase in the number of osteoblasts found throughout the tumor-bearing intramedullary space that ultimately separates the ACE-1 tumor from the primarily osteolytic bone tumors in which a minimal increase in osteoblasts is observed and little or no bone formation occurs (Table 6-1).

Patients with bone cancer pain often guard their tumor-bearing limb or affected body region, and movement of the limb or region often exacerbates the pain. Mice with bone cancer pain also guard their tumor-bearing bone and show significantly increased guarding and flinching behaviors as the tumor cells proliferate throughout the femur. Additionally, nonnoxious palpation of the tumor-bearing limb is used normally as a measure of palpation-evoked pain and mimics allodynia, the condition in which a normally innocuous sensation is perceived as noxious, commonly experienced in patients with advanced cancer. Mice bearing 2472 and ACE-1 spent more time guarding and had a greater number of flinches compared to corresponding sham mice following palpation. Interestingly, while the osteolytic 2472 cells induced greater ongoing and palpation-evoked pain behaviors than ACE-1-injected mice, both mice displayed significant tumor-induced pain-related behaviors. One reason that the primarily osteolytic tumor appears to generate greater palpation-induced pain behaviors than the osteoblastic tumors is that the woven bone formed by the osteoblastic tumor may convey some mechanical stability to the bone so that the palpation-evoked mechanical distortion of the sensory fibers in the periosteum is less in the osteoblastic ACE-1 tumor versus the osteolytic 2472-bearing femur (Fig. 6-5).

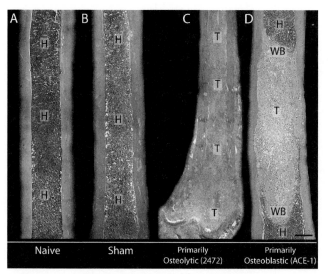

FIGURE 6-3 Hematoxylin and eosin-stained histological comparison of 2472 sarcoma and ACE-1 prostatic carcinoma-induced bone remodeling. Sham-injected mice femurs (B) present neither bone formation or bone destruction and are highly similar to naïve mouse femurs (A) when viewed with hematoxylin and eosin staining (H&E). 2472 sarcoma-injected femurs primarily display osteolytic characteristics and are visible as regions of bone resorption at the distal head (C) where tumor-induced acidosis has occurred. ACE-1 prostatic carcinoma-injected femurs present a mixed osteolytic and osteoblastic appearance visible histologically at the day 19 endpoint (D) as woven bone formation surrounding pockets of tumor cells which generates diaphyseal bridging structures with mineral densities similar to those found in the trabecular regions at both the proximal and distal heads (D). Scale bar = 4 mm. T = tumor; H = hematopoietic cells; WB = ACE-1-induced woven bone formation.

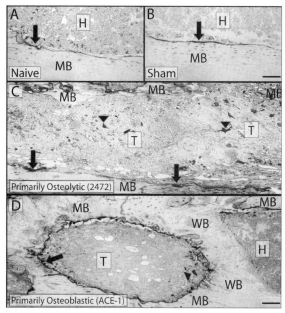

FIGURE 6-4 ACE-1 prostatic carcinoma and 2472 sarcoma tumor-induced osteoclastogenesis and macrophage infiltration. TRAP-stained images of naïve (A), sham-injected (B), 2472 tumor-injected (C), and ACE-1 tumor-injected (D) femurs illustrate that osteoclast proliferation occurs in both models along regions of tumor-induced bone remodeling (arrows). ACE-1 macrophage infiltration is less intense than 2472-associated macrophage infiltration (arrowheads), although both models present macrophages with similar morphology. Sham (B) mice present osteoclast numbers and morphology, and macrophages, which are not significantly different from naïve mice (A). Scale bar = 50 mm. Arrows = osteoclasts; arrowheads = macrophages; MB = mineralized bone; H = hematopoietic cells; T = tumor.

Table 6-1

Histological and Radiological Quantification of Bone Remodeling and Tumor Progression in ACE-1 and 2472-Injected Animals

	Sham (C3H/HeJ)	Sham (nude)	Primarily osteolytic (2472)	Primarily osteoblastic (ACE-1)
1. Bone histomorphometry				
Osteoclasts (OC) (OC #/mm^2 diaphyseal intramedullary space)	16±10	16±1	55±5*	47±3†
Osteoblasts (OB) (OB #/mm^2 diaphyseal intramedullary space)	72±5	81±4	70±15	127±7†
Macrophages (Ms) (Ms/mm^2 diaphyseal intramedullary space)	2±1	2±1	50±3*	27±2†
Tumor-induced new bone formation (% Diaphyseal intramedullary space occupied)	0±0	0±0	0±0	14±2†
Tumor cells (% intramedullary space occupied)	0±0	0±0	95±5*	60±7†
Hematopoietic cells (% Intramedullary space occupied)	100±0	100±0	5±5*	26±8†
2. Radiological bone density score				
% Normalized transmission $\frac{(1/[\text{antilog optical density}])}{(\text{naive transmission})} \times 100\%$	115±2	105±2	76±9*	109±5‡

*$P < 0.05$ versus sham (C3H/HeJ) (one way ANOVA, Fisher's PLSD).
†$P < 0.05$ versus sham (nude).
‡Total bone density similar to sham, however less dense woven bone has replaced a great portion of the intramedullary space.

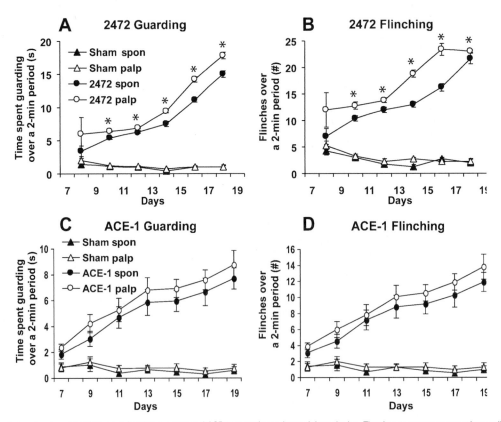

FIGURE 6-5 Tumor-induced, pain-related behaviors in 2472 sarcoma and ACE-1 prostatic carcinoma-injected mice. The time spent spontaneously guarding, the time spent guarding after palpation, the number of spontaneous flinches, and the number of flinches after palpation of the afflicted limb over a 2-minute observation period were used as measures of ongoing pain. Spontaneous pain behaviors in 2472 tumor-injected mice (2472 spontaneous; filled circles) (A) as compared to palpation-induced, pain-related behaviors (2472 palpation; open circles) (B), were significantly different at most time points. Spontaneous pain behaviors in ACE-1 tumor-injected mice (ACE-1 spontaneous; filled circles) (C) as compared to palpation-induced, pain-related behaviors (ACE-1 palpation; open circles) (D), were very similar in magnitude. Both guarding and flinching in the sham-injected mice of both strains were significantly different from either ACE-1 or 2472-injected mice respectively, across disease progression. Error bars represent SEM. *$P < 0.05$ vs. spontaneous response.

TUMOR-INDUCED REMODELING OF THE SENSORY INNERVATION OF BONE: NEUROPATHIC COMPONENT OF BONE CANCER PAIN

Primary afferent sensory neurons are the gateway by which sensory information from peripheral tissues is transmitted to the spinal cord and brain.[21] The cell bodies of sensory fibers that innervate the head and body are housed in ganglia that maintain distinct dermatomes from head to toe.[21] There are two major types of sensory fibers: myelinated A fibers and smaller diameter unmyelinated C fibers. Nearly all large diameter myelinated A-beta fibers normally conduct nonpainful stimuli applied to the skin, joints, and muscles, and thus in a normal situation, do not conduct noxious stimuli.[22] In contrast, most small diameter sensory fibers—unmyelinated C fibers and finely myelinated A-delta fibers—are specialized sensory neurons known as *nociceptors*.[21] Their major function is to detect and convert environmental stimuli that are perceived as harmful into electrochemical signals that are transmitted to the central nervous system. Unlike primary sensory neurons involved in vision or olfaction, which are required to detect only one type of sensory stimulus (light or chemical odorants, respectively), individual primary sensory neurons of the pain pathway have the remarkable ability to detect a wide range of stimulus modalities, including those of a physical and chemical nature.[23,24] To accomplish this, nociceptors express a diverse repertoire of receptors and transduction molecules that can sense forms of noxious stimulation (thermal, mechanical, and chemical) albeit with varying degrees of sensitivity (Fig. 6-6).

Numerous studies have demonstrated that the periosteum is densely innervated by both sensory and sympathetic fibers,[25–27] and that it receives the greatest density of nerve fibers per area. Using a combination of minimal decalcification techniques (using regular radiographic assessment of the extent of decalcification) and antigen amplification techniques, it has also been demonstrated that the bone marrow, mineralized bone, and periosteum all receive a significant innervation by both sensory and sympathetic nerve fibers that are associated with blood vessels.[28–30] Since sensory and sympathetic neurons are present within the bone marrow, mineralized bone, and periosteum, and all aspects of the bone are ultimately impacted by fractures, ischemia, or the presence of tumor cells, sensory fibers in any of these compartments may play a role in the generation of bone cancer pain.

In examining the changes in the sensory innervation of bone induced by the primarily osteolytic 2472 cells at the 14-day endpoint, it was noted that tumor cells were found to grow within the bone, come into contact with, injure, and then destroy the very distal processes of sensory fibers that innervate the bone marrow and mineralized bone. Thus, while sensory fibers were observed at and within the leading edge of the tumor in the deep stromal regions of the tumor, sensory nerve fibers displayed a discontinuous and fragmented appearance, suggesting that following initial activation by the osteolytic tumor cells, the distal processes of the sensory fibers were ultimately injured by the invading tumor cells (Fig. 6-7). In contrast, in examining the sensory innervation of bone following injection of the primarily osteoblastic ACE-1 prostate cells at the 19-day endpoint, it was noted that there is simultaneous injury and sprouting of sensory fibers in the bone (Fig. 6-7). Thus, within the body of the ACE-1 tumor cells present in the intramedullary space of the bone, the density of sensory fibers is significantly higher than that observed in the normal marrow space (Fig. 6-8).

In 2472 sarcoma-injected animals, there was expression of activating transcription factor-3 (ATF-3) in the nucleus of sensory neurons that innervate the femur. ATF-3 is a member of the ATF/CREB

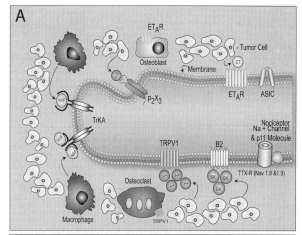

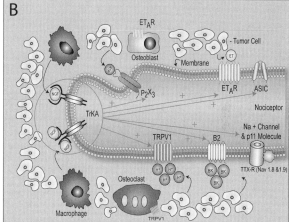

FIGURE 6-6 Detection by sensory neurons of noxious stimuli produced by tumors. Nociceptors (pink) use several different types of receptor to detect and transmit signals about noxious stimuli that are produced by cancer cells (yellow) or other aspects of the tumor microenvironment. The vanilloid receptor-1 (TRPV1) detects extracellular protons (H+) that are produced by cancer cells, whereas endothelin-A receptors (ET$_A$R) detect endothelins (ET) that are released by cancer cells. The dorsal-root acid-sensing ion channel (ASIC) detects mechanical stimuli as tumor growth mechanically distends sensory fibers. Nerve growth factor (NGF) released by macrophages binds to the tyrosine kinase receptor TrkA, whereas extracellular ATP binds to the purinergic P$_2$X$_3$ receptor (A). Activation of these receptors as illustrated in panel B increases the excitability of the nociceptor, inducing the phosphorylation of the 1.8 and/or 1.9 sodium channel (Na+ channel) and decreasing the overall threshold required for nociceptor excitation.

family of transcription factors, which is not expressed at detectable levels in normal sensory neurons or in sensory neurons following peripheral inflammation, but is strongly expressed in sensory neurons following injury to peripheral nerves in neuropathic pain models.[31] It is likely that the expression of ATF-3 in sensory neurons of tumor-bearing animals is a result of peripheral nerve destruction within the tumor-bearing femur.[32]

This tumor-induced injury of sensory nerve fibers in the 2472 sarcoma model is accompanied by an increase in ongoing and movement-evoked pain behaviors, an upregulation of ATF-3 and galanin by sensory neurons that innervate the tumor-bearing femur, upregulation of glial fibrillary acidic protein (GFAP) and hypertrophy of satellite cells surrounding sensory neuron cell bodies within the ipsilateral dorsal root ganglia (DRG), and macrophage infiltration of the DRG ipsilateral to the tumor-bearing femur.[19,33,34] Similar neurochemical changes have been described following peripheral nerve injury and in other noncancerous neuropathic pain states.[35] Chronic

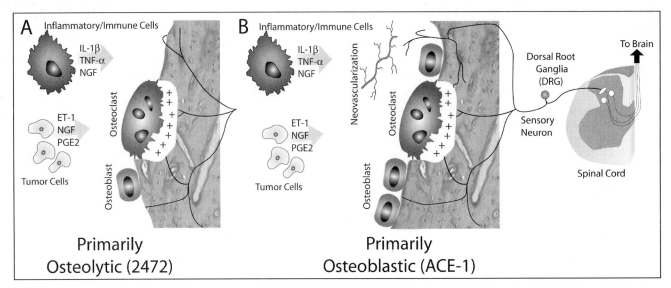

FIGURE 6-7 Schematic of the sensory innervation of the intramedullary canal and mineralized bone and the bone remodeling that occurs in the 2472 sarcoma and prostatic carcinoma (ACE-1) tumors. In this schematic, the normal mineralized bone is pink in color as it is stained with hematoxylin and eosin and woven bone appears orange/tan. The 2472 sarcoma is primarily a bone-destroying tumor as illustrated by the large osteoclast and accompanying resorption bay (purple cells with large black nuclei near + symbols) and few osteoblasts (orange/yellow cells) (A), whereas the ACE-1 prostatic carcinoma is a "mixed" tumor that induces significant bone formation and some bone destruction (B). Bone formation is accomplished by an increase in activated osteoblasts (orange/yellow cells); however, this newly formed bone (woven bone), which is created by the mixed tumor, does not have the mechanical strength of normal mineralized bone. Also present in the ACE-1 model is an extensive degree of sensory neuron sprouting and neovascularization. In both models, tumor or inflammatory cell-released factors may play a role in the generation and maintenance of cancer-induced bone pain and may mediate neurochemical reorganization in the dorsal root ganglia or the spinal cord with advanced disease.

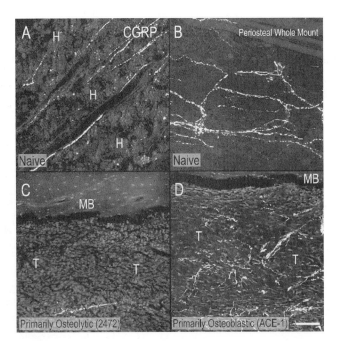

FIGURE 6-8 Naive femurs show a characteristic distribution and appearance of calcitonin gene-related peptide immunoreactive (CGRP-IR) sensory fibers in the femur and there was no observable difference in the levels of immunofluorescence or density of CGRP-IR fibers between naive mice (A). 2472-injected femurs present minimal maintenance of CGRP-IR fibers and those that are preserved are often truncated and sparsely distributed (C). ACE-1 injected femurs present heavily increased density of CGRP-IR sensory fibers (D) comparable to the number and intensity of those found in a periosteal whole mount (B). Scale bar = 50 mm. T = tumor; H = hematopoietic cells; MB = mineralized bone.

treatment with gabapentin in the 2472 model also did not influence tumor growth, tumor-induced bone destruction, or the tumor-induced neurochemical reorganization that occurs in sensory neurons or the spinal cord, but it did attenuate both ongoing and movement-evoked bone cancer-related pain behaviors.[19] These results suggest that even when the tumor is confined within the bone, a component of bone cancer pain is due to tumor-induced injury to primary afferent nerve fibers that normally innervate the tumor-bearing bone.

SKELETAL REMODELING AND ACIDOSIS IN BONE CANCER PAIN

Recent experiments in a murine model of bone cancer pain have reported that osteoclasts play an essential role in cancer-induced bone loss, and that osteoclasts contribute to the etiology of bone cancer pain.[16,36] Osteoclasts are terminally differentiated, multi-nucleated, monocyte lineage cells that resorb bone by maintaining an extracellular microenvironment of acidic pH (4.0–5.0) at the osteoclast-mineralized bone interface.[37] Tumor-induced release of protons and acidosis may be particularly important in the generation of bone cancer pain. Both osteolytic (bone destroying) and osteoblastic (bone forming) cancers are characterized by osteoclast proliferation and hypertrophy.[38]

Bisphosphonates, a class of antiresorptive compounds which induce osteoclast apoptosis, have also been reported to reduce pain in patients with osteoclast-induced skeletal metastases.[39–41] Bisphosphonates are pyrophosphate analogues that display high affinity for calcium ions, causing them to rapidly target the mineralized matrix of bone.[42] These drugs have been reported to act directly on osteoclasts, inducing their apoptosis by impairing either the synthesis of ATP or cholesterol—both of which are necessary for cell survival.[43,44] Osteoclasts treated with bisphosphonates undergo morphologic changes, including cell shrinkage, chromatin condensation, nuclear fragmentation, and loss of the ruffled border that are indicative of apoptosis.[42] Studies in both clinical[39–41] and animal[45–47] models of bone cancer have reported antiresorptive effects of bisphosphonate therapy, although the effect on long-term survival rates and tumor growth remain controversial.

In a recent study of the bisphosphonate alendronate in the 2472 sarcoma model, a reduction in the number of osteoclasts and osteoclast activity was noted, as evidenced by the reduction in tumor-induced bone resorption and a reduction in the number of osteoclasts displaying the clear zone at the basal bone-resorbing surface that is characteristic of highly active osteoclasts.[48] In this model, alendronate also attenuates ongoing and movement-evoked bone cancer pain, and the neurochemical reorganization of the peripheral and central nervous system while at the same time promoting both tumor growth and tumor necrosis. The present results suggest that in bone cancer, alendronate can simultaneously modulate pain, bone destruction, tumor growth, and tumor necrosis, and that administration of alendronate along with a tumoricidal agent may synergistically improve the survival and quality of life of patients with bone cancer pain. In other studies with nonmalignant bone loss in humans, ibandronate, a nitrogen-containing bisphosphonate has been shown to be effective with intermittent dosing and illustrates that the total cumulative dose of bisphosphonate administered determines the response, independent of the dosing regimen.[43] The mechanism by which ibandronate alleviates bone loss in nonmalignant disease and its effectiveness at low concentrations with multiple bioeffective routes of administration as compared to alendronate or other bisphosphonates may also be involved in ibandronate's potential pain-relieving efficacy in patients who suffer from bone cancer pain. These data emphasize that it is essential to utilize a model in which pain, skeletal remodeling and tumor growth can be simultaneously assessed, as each of these can significantly impact patient quality of life and survival (Table 6-2).[49]

Table 6-2

Mechanism-Based Therapies Currently Available or under Investigation in Animal Models such as the 2472 Sarcoma or ACE-1 Prostatic Carcinoma for the Treatment of Specific Components of Bone Cancer Pain

Drug Class	Site of Action	Osteolytic		Osteoblastic	
		Pain	Disease Progression	Pain	Disease Progression
Tumor/Inflammatory Products					
Selective COX-2 inhibitors	Prostaglandin synthesis in the CNS and PNS	↓	↓	↔	↔
Endothelin receptor antagonsits	Nerve fibers (CNS, PNS) & smooth muscle cells (PNS)	↓	↔	↓	↔
Anti-NGF antibody	trkA receptor in the PNS	↓	↔	↓	↔
Acid sensitive ion channels (TRPV1; ASIC)	Blockade of H+ ion channels in the CNS and PNS	↓	↔	↔	↔
Purinergic receptor antagonists	Blockade of P2X receptors in the CNS and PNS	↓	↔	↔	↔
Opioids	Opioid receptors in the CNS and PNS	↓	?/↑	↓	?/↑
Bone Remodeling					
Osteoprotegerin (AMG-162)	Inhibitor of osteoclast mediated osteolysis in bone	↓	?/↓	↔	?/↓
Bisphosphonates	Pro-osteoclast apoptotic action in bone	↓	?/↓	↓	?/↓
TRPV1 antagonists	TRPV1 receptor blockade in the CNS and PNS	↓	↔	↔	?
Nerve Injury					
Anticonvulsants (gabapentin, pregabalin)	Regulators of calcium channel activity and GABAergic neuronal discharge in the CNS and PNS	↓	↔	?	?
Antidepressants (cymbalta)	Selective serotonin and Dopaminergic reuptake inhibitors in the CNS	?	?	?	?
Sodium channel blockers (NAV 1.8, 1.9)	Blockade of sodium channels in the CNS and PNS	?	?	?	?
GDNF therapy (artemin)	Stimulation of GDNF receptor in the CNS and PNS	?	?	?	?

COX = cyclooxygenase; NGF = nerve growth factor; TRPV1 = transient receptor potential V1; ASIC = acid-sensing ion channel; GDNF = glial-derived neurotrophic factor. ↔ = no significant change observed; ? = potential therapeutic target for which data has not yet been generated; CNS = central nervous system; PNS = peripheral nervous system

While bisphosphonates are currently being used to reduce tumor-induced bone destruction and have been shown to reduce bone cancer pain induced by both primarily osteolytic and osteoblastic tumors, the use of osteoprotegerin (OPG) or antibodies that have OPG-like activities holds significant promise for alleviating bone cancer pain (Table 6-2). OPG is a secreted soluble receptor that is a member of the tumor necrosis factor receptor (TNFR) family.[50] This decoy receptor prevents the activation and proliferation of osteoclasts by binding to and sequestering OPG ligand (OPGL; also known as receptor for activator of NFκB ligand, RANKL).[44,50–52] While OPG has been shown to decrease pain behaviors in the 2472 sarcoma model of bone cancer,[36] a monoclonal antibody (AMG-162) that also blocks the interaction of OPGL and RANK is being developed for treating skeletal pain. These results suggest that a substantial part of the actions of OPG seem to result from inhibition of tumor-induced bone destruction via a reduction in osteoclast function. The reduction of osteoclast function, in turn, inhibits the neurochemical changes in the spinal cord that are thought to be involved in the generation and maintenance of cancer pain. These results demonstrate that excessive tumor-induced bone destruction is involved in the generation of bone cancer pain, and that bisphosphonates or molecules with OPG-like effects may provide an effective palliative treatment.

The finding that sensory neurons can be directly excited by protons or acid originating from cells like osteoclasts in bone has generated intense clinical interest in pain research.[53,54] Studies have shown that subsets of sensory neurons express different acid-sensing ion channels.[24,55] The two major classes of acid-sensing ion channels expressed by nociceptors are TRPV1[56,57] and the acid-sensing ion channel-3 (ASIC-3).[53,55,58] Both of these channels are sensitized and excited by a decrease in pH. Tumor stroma[59] and areas of ischemic necrosis[60] such as that observed in the 2472 or ACE-1 prostate bone cancer model typically exhibit lower extracellular pH than surrounding normal tissues. As inflammatory cells invade tumor stroma, they release protons that generate local acidosis. The large amount of apoptosis that occurs in the tumor environment may also contribute to the acidotic environment.

It has been shown that TRPV1 is present on a subset of sensory neuron fibers and on those that innervate the mouse femur, and that in an in vivo model of bone cancer pain, acute or chronic administration of a TRPV1 antagonist or disruption of the TRPV1 gene results in a significant attenuation of both ongoing and movement-evoked nocifensive behaviors.[34] In addition, previous studies have also shown in the 2472 model that administration of a TRPV1 antagonist retains its efficacy at early, middle, and late stages of tumor growth.[34] The ability of a TRPV1 antagonist to maintain its analgesic potency with disease progression is probably influenced by the fact that sensory nerve fibers innervating the tumor-bearing mouse femur maintain their expression of TRPV1 even as tumor growth and tumor-induced bone destruction progresses. These results suggest that the TRPV1 channel plays a role in the integration of nociceptive signaling in a severe pain state, and that antagonists of TRPV1 may be effective in attenuating difficult to treat mixed chronic pain states, such as that encountered in patients with bone cancer pain (Table 6-2).

TUMOR-DERIVED PRODUCTS IN GENERATION OF BONE CANCER PAIN

The tumor stroma is made up of many different cell types apart from cancer cells, including immune cells such as macrophages, neutrophils, and T lymphocytes. They secrete various factors that have been shown to sensitize or directly excite primary afferent neurons, such as prostaglandins,[61,62] tumor necrosis factor-alpha (TNF-α),[63–66] endothelins,[67,68] interleukins-1 and -6,[63,69,70] epidermal growth factor,[71] transforming growth factor-beta,[72,73] and platelet-derived growth factor.[74–76] Receptors for many of these factors are expressed by primary afferent neurons. While each of these factors may play an important role in the generation of pain in particular forms of cancer, drugs that target prostaglandins and endothelins are the only drugs currently used to control pain in cancer patients.[77,78]

Cancer cells and tumor-associated macrophages have both been shown to express high levels of COX isoenzymes, leading to high levels of prostaglandins.[79–83] Prostaglandins are lipid-derived eicosanoids that are synthesized from arachidonic acid by COX isoenzymes COX-1 and COX-2. Prostaglandins have been shown to be involved in the sensitization and/or direct excitation of nociceptors by binding to several prostanoid receptors expressed by nociceptors that sensitize or directly excite nociceptors.[84] Prostaglandins have also been implicated in a number of biologic and pathologic processes, including mediating pain and inflammation,[24] bone homeostasis,[85] and tumorigenesis.[86] NSAIDs inhibit both COX-1 and COX-2 and while clinically effective in attenuating acute non-malignant skeletal pain, NSAIDs are generally not indicated for extended use in cancer patients as they have significant side effects such as gastrointestinal ulceration, neutropenia, enhanced bleeding, and disruptions in renal function.[87] However, the advent of selective COX-2 inhibitors has significantly improved the side-effect profile of anti-inflammatory drugs while maintaining analgesic efficacy.

Studies have shown in the 2472 sarcoma model of bone cancer pain that chronic inhibition of COX-2 activity with selective COX-2 inhibitors significantly attenuated bone cancer pain behaviors as well as many of the neurochemical changes suggestive of both peripheral and central sensitization.[16] In addition, prostaglandins have been shown to be involved in tumor growth, survival, and angiogenesis.[88–94] Therefore, as well as having the ability to block cancer pain, COX-2 inhibitors are also capable of retarding tumor growth within bone.[16] Chronic administration of a selective COX-2 inhibitor significantly reduced tumor burden in sarcoma-bearing bones, which may, in turn, reduce factors released by tumor cells capable of exciting primary afferent fibers.[67] Acute or chronic administration of a selective COX-2 inhibitor significantly attenuated both ongoing and movement-evoked pain. Whereas acute administration of a COX-2 inhibitor presumably reduces prostaglandins capable of activating sensory or spinal cord neurons, chronic inhibition of COX-2 also appears to simultaneously reduce osteoclastogenesis, bone resorption, and tumor burden. Together, suppression of prostaglandin synthesis and release at multiple sites by selective inhibition of COX-2 may synergistically improve the survival and quality of life of patients with bone cancer pain (Table 6-2).

Endothelin antagonists are another group of pharmacological agents that offer promise in the management of cancer pain.[95] Endothelins (endothelin-1, -2, and -3) are a family of vasoactive peptides that are expressed at high levels by several types of tumors, including those that arise from the prostate.[68] Clinical studies have shown a correlation between the severity of the pain and plasma levels of endothelins in prostate cancer patients.[96] Endothelins could contribute to cancer pain by directly sensitizing or exciting nociceptors, as a subset of small unmyelinated primary afferent neurons express endothelin A receptors.[97] Furthermore, direct application of endothelin to peripheral nerves induces activation of primary afferent fibers and an induction of pain-related behaviors.[98] Like prostaglandins, endothelins that are produced by cancer cells are also thought to be involved in regulating angiogenesis[99] and tumor growth.[100] These findings indicate that endothelin antagonists may be useful in inhibiting cancer pain and in reducing tumor growth and metastases.

In our 2472 sarcoma model, acute or chronic administration of the endothelin A receptor (ET_AR)-selective antagonist ABT-627 significantly attenuated ongoing and movement-evoked bone cancer pain and chronic administration of ABT-627 reduced several neurochemical indices of peripheral and central sensitization without influencing tumor growth or bone destruction.[78] As tumor expression and release of ET-1 has been shown to be regulated by the local environment, location-specific expression and release of ET-1 by tumor cells may provide insight into the mechanisms that underlie the heterogeneity of bone cancer pain that is frequently observed in humans with multiple skeletal metastases (Table 6-2).

Bradykinin is another potential target for the development of selective analgesics to treat cancer pain. Previous studies have shown that bradykinin and related kinins are released in response to tissue injury and these kinins play a significant role in driving acute and chronic inflammatory pain.[101] The action of bradykinin is mediated by two receptors termed B_1 and B_2. Although the B_2 receptor is constitutively expressed at high levels by sensory neurons, the B_1 receptor is normally expressed at low but detectable levels by sensory neurons and these B_1 receptors are significantly upregulated following peripheral inflammation and/or tissue injury.[102] Tumor metastases to the skeleton induce significant bone remodeling with accompanying tissue injury, which presumably induces the release of bradykinin. It has been demonstrated that both bone cancer-induced ongoing and movement-evoked nocifensive behaviors were reduced following the pharmacologic blockade of the B_1 receptor.[103] We have also shown that administration of B_1 antagonists not only reduces bone cancer-induced, pain-related behaviors but that this efficacy is retained in advanced bone cancer pain (Table 6-2).[103]

One important concept that has emerged over the past decade is that in addition to nerve growth factor (NGF) being able to directly activate sensory neurons that express the TrkA receptor, NGF modulates expression and function of a wide variety of molecules and proteins expressed by sensory neurons that express the TrkA or p75 receptor. Some of these molecules and proteins include neurotransmitters (substance P and CGRP), receptors (bradykinin R), channels (P_2X_3, TRPV1, ASIC-3, and sodium channels), transcription factors (ATF-3), and structural molecules (neurofilaments and the sodium channel anchoring molecule p11).[104–111] Additionally, NGF has been shown to modulate the trafficking and insertion of sodium channels such as Nav 1.8[108] and TRPV1[109] in the sensory neurons as well as modulating the expression profile of supporting cells in the DRG and peripheral nerve, such as nonmyelinating Schwann cells and macrophages.[112] Therefore, anti-NGF antibody therapy may be particularly effective in blocking bone cancer pain as NGF appears to be integrally involved in the upregulation, sensitization, and disinhibition of multiple neurotransmitters, ion channels, and receptors in the primary afferent nerve and DRG fibers that synergistically increase nociceptive signals originating from the tumor-bearing bone.

In two recent studies, where the same analgesic therapy was used in the primarily osteolytic 2472 sarcoma and the primarily osteoblastic ACE-1 prostate bone cancer model, it was demonstrated that administration of an anti-NGF antibody was not only highly efficacious in reducing both early and late stage bone cancer pain-related behaviors (Table 6-2) but that this reduction in pain-related behaviors was greater than that achieved with acute administration of

10 or 30 mg/kg of morphine sulfate.[14,33] In light of these findings, a critical question that requires further investigation is what are the mechanisms that contribute to the efficacy of anti-NGF in blocking sarcoma or prostate tumor-induced bone pain? In summary, however, all of these findings together suggest that products derived from the tumor microenvironment may be excellent potential therapeutic targets for the attenuation of bone cancer-related pain.

CONCLUSIONS

For the first time, animal models of cancer pain are now available that effectively mirror the clinical picture observed in humans with bone cancer pain. Information generated from these models has begun to provide insight into the mechanisms that generate and maintain bone cancer pain and helped target potential mechanism-based therapies to treat this chronic pain state. It is noteworthy that in these models analgesics such as a bisphosphonate, osteoprotegerin, and a COX-2 inhibitor appear to influence disease progression in the tumor-bearing bone. Together these and other studies using models of bone cancer suggest that it may be possible to develop novel mechanism-based therapies that not only reduce tumor-induced bone pain but may provide added benefit in synergistically abrogating disease progression. Successful development and clinical use of these therapies has the potential to positively impact survival, and also to improve the cancer patient's quality of life.

REFERENCES

1. Coleman RE. Skeletal complications of malignancy. *Cancer.* 1997;80:1588–1594.
2. Mercadante S. Malignant bone pain: pathophysiology and treatment. *Pain.* 1997;69:1–18.
3. Mercadante S, Arcuri E. Breakthrough pain in cancer patients: pathophysiology and treatment. *Cancer Treat Rev.* 1998;24:425–432.
4. Cherny N. New strategies in opioid therapy for cancer pain. *J Oncol Manag.* 2000;9:8–15.
5. Hanks GW, Conno F, Cherny N, et al. Morphine and alternative opioids in cancer pain: the EAPC recommendations. *Br J Cancer.* 2001;84:587–593.
6. Portenoy RK, Lesage P. Management of cancer pain. *Lancet.* 1999;353:1695–1700.
7. Foley KM. Misconceptions and controversies regarding the use of opioids in cancer pain. *Anticancer Drugs.* 1995;6:4–13.
8. Weber M, Huber C. Documentation of severe pain, opioid doses, and opioid-related side effects in outpatients with cancer: a retrospective study. *J Pain Symptom Manage.* 1999;17:49–54.
9. Mukherjee D, Nissen SE, and Topol EJ. Risk of cardiovascular events associated with selective COX-2 inhibitors. *JAMA.* 2001;286:954–959.
10. Davies NM, Jamali F. COX-2 selective inhibitors cardiac toxicity: getting to the heart of the matter. *J Pharm Pharm Sci.* 2004;7:332–336.
11. Mercadante S. Problems of long-term spinal opioid treatment in advanced cancer patients. *Pain.* 1999;79:1–13.
12. Jemal A, Murray T, Ward E, et al. Cancer statistics, 2005. *CA Cancer J Clin.* 2005;55:10–30.
13. Guise TA. Parathyroid hormone-related protein and bone metastases. *Cancer.* 1997;80:1572–1580.
14. Halvorson KG, Kubota K, Sevcik MA, et al. A blocking antibody to nerve growth factor attenuates skeletal pain induced by prostate tumor cells growing in bone. *Cancer Res.* 2005;65:9426–9435.
15. Honore P, Rogers SD, Schwei MJ, et al. Murine models of inflammatory, neuropathic and cancer pain each generates a unique set of neurochemical changes in the spinal cord and sensory neurons. *Neuroscience.* 2000;98:585–598.
16. Sabino MA, Ghilardi JR, Jongen JL, et al. Simultaneous reduction in cancer pain, bone destruction, and tumor growth by selective inhibition of cyclooxygenase-2. *Cancer Res.* 2002;62:7343–7349.

17. Schwei MJ, Honore P, Rogers SD, et al. Neurochemical and cellular reorganization of the spinal cord in a murine model of bone cancer pain. *J Neurosci.* 1999;19:10886–10897.

18. Body JJ. Metastatic bone disease: clinical and therapeutic aspects. *Bone.* 1992;13:S57–S62.

19. Peters CM, Ghilardi JR, Keyser CP, et al. Tumor-induced injury of primary afferent sensory nerve fibers in bone cancer pain. *Exp Neurol.* 2005;193:85–100.

20. Boyce BF, Yoneda T, Guise TA. Factors regulating the growth of metastatic cancer in bone. *Endocr Relat Cancer.* 1999;6:333–347.

21. Nolte J. *The Human Brain: An Introduction to Its Functional Anatomy.* St. Louis, Missouri: Mosby, Inc.; 2002.

22. Djouhri L, Bleazard L, Lawson SN. Association of somatic action potential shape with sensory receptive properties in guinea-pig dorsal root ganglion neurones. *J Physiol.* 1998;513:857–872.

23. Basbaum AI, Jessel TM. The perception of pain. In: Kandel ER, JH Schwartz, TM Jessell, eds. *Principles of Neural Science.* New York: McGraw-Hill; 2000:472–490.

24. Julius D, Basbaum AI. Molecular mechanisms of nociception. *Nature.* 2001;413:203–210.

25. Asmus SE, Parsons S, Landis SC. Developmental changes in the transmitter properties of sympathetic neurons that innervate the periosteum. *J Neurosci.* 2000;20:1495–1504.

26. Bjurholm A. Neuroendocrine peptides in bone. *Int Orthop.* 1991;15:325–329.

27. Hukkanen M, Konttinen YT, Rees RG, et al. Innervation of bone from healthy and arthritic rats by substance P and calcitonin gene related peptide containing sensory fibers. *J Rheumatol.* 1992;19:1252–1259.

28. Bjurholm A, Kreicbergs A, Brodin E, et al. Substance P- and CGRP-immunoreactive nerves in bone. *Peptides.* 1988;9:165–171.

29. Bjurholm A, Kreicbergs A, Terenius L, et al. Neuropeptide Y-, tyrosine hydroxylase- and vasoactive intestinal polypeptide-immunoreactive nerves in bone and surrounding tissues. *J Auton Nerv Syst.* 1988;25:119–125.

30. Tabarowski Z, Gibson-Berry K, Felten SY. Noradrenergic and peptidergic innervation of the mouse femur bone marrow. *Acta Histochem.* 1996;98:453–457.

31. Tsujino H, Kondo E, Fukuoka T, et al. Activating transcription factor 3 (ATF3) induction by axotomy in sensory and motoneurons: a novel neuronal marker of nerve injury. *Mol Cell Neurosci.* 2000;15:170–182.

32. Honore P, Luger N, Sabino M, et al. Osteoprotegerin blocks bone cancer-induced skeletal destruction, skeletal pain and pain-related neurochemcial reorganization of the spinal cord. *Nat Med.* 2000;6:521–528.

33. Sevcik MA, Ghilardi JR, Peters CM, et al. Anti-NGF therapy profoundly reduces bone cancer pain and the accompanying increase in markers of peripheral and central sensitization. *Pain.* 2005;115:128–141.

34. Ghilardi JR, Rohrich H, Lindsay TH, et al. Selective blockade of the capsaicin receptor TRPV1 attenuates bone cancer pain. *J Neurosci.* 2005;25:3126–3131.

35. Obata K, Yamanaka H, Fukuoka T, et al. Contribution of injured and uninjured dorsal root ganglion neurons to pain behavior and the changes in gene expression following chronic constriction injury of the sciatic nerve in rats. *Pain.* 2003;101:65–77.

36. Luger NM, Honore P, Sabino MA, et al. Osteoprotegerin diminishes advanced bone cancer pain. *Cancer Res.* 2001;61:4038–4047.

37. Delaisse JM, Vaes G. Mechanism of mineral solubilization and matrix degradation in osteoclastic bone resorption. In: Rifkin BR, CV Gay, eds. *Biology and Physiology of the Osteoclast.* Ann Arbor: CRC; 1992:289–314.

38. Clohisy DR, Perkins SL, Ramnaraine ML. Review of cellular mechanisms of tumor osteolysis. *Clin Orthop Rel Res.* 2000;373:104–114.

39. Berenson JR, Rosen LS, Howell A, et al. Zoledronic acid reduces skeletal-related events in patients with osteolytic metastases. *Cancer.* 2001;91:1191–1200.

40. Fulfaro F, Casuccio A, Ticozzi C, et al. The role of bisphosphonates in the treatment of painful metastatic bone disease: a review of phase III trials. *Pain.* 1998;78:157–169.

41. Major PP, Lipton A, Berenson J, et al. Oral bisphosphonates: a review of clinical use in patients with bone metastases. *Cancer.* 2000;88:6–14.

42. Rogers MJ, Gordon S, Benford HL, et al. Cellular and molecular mechanisms of action of bisphosphonates. *Cancer.* 2000;88:2961–2978.

43. Gatti D, Adami S. New bisphosphonates in the treatment of bone diseases. *Drugs Aging.* 1999;15:285–296.

44. Rodan GA, Martin TJ. Therapeutic approaches to bone diseases. *Science.* 2000;289:1508–1514.

45. Hiraga T, Williams PJ, Mundy GR, et al. The bisphosphonate ibandronate promotes apoptosis in MDA-MB-231 human breast cancer cells in bone metastases. *Cancer Res.* 2001;61:4418–4424.

46. Yoneda T, Michigami T, Yi B, et al. Actions of bisphosphonate on bone metastasis in animal models of breast carcinoma. *Cancer.* 2000;88:2979–2988.

47. Sasaki A, Boyce B, Story B, et al. Bisphosphonate risedronate reduces metastatic human breast cancer burden in bone in nude mice. *Cancer Res.* 1995;55:3551–3557.

48. Horton A, Nesbitt S, Bennett J, et al. Integrins and other cell surface attachment molecules of bone cells. In: Bilezikian JP, Raisz LG, Rodan GA, eds. *Principles of Bone Biology.* San Diego: Academic Press; 2002:265–286.

49. Sevcik MA, Luger NM, Mach DB, et al. Bone cancer pain: the effects of the bisphosphonate alendronate on pain, skeletal remodeling, tumor growth and tumor necrosis. *Pain.* 2004;111:169–180.

50. Simonet WS, Lacey DL, Dunstan CR, et al. Osteoprotegerin—a novel secreted protein involved in the regulation of bone density. *Cell.* 1997;89:309–319.

51. Anderson DM, Maraskovsky E, Billingsley WL, et al. A homologue of the TNF receptor and its ligand enhance T-cell growth and dendritic-cell function. *Nature.* 1997;390:175–179.

52. Yasuda H, Shima N, Nakagawa N, et al. Osteoclast differentiation factor is a ligand for osteoprotegerin/osteoclastogenesis-inhibitory factor and is identical to TRANCE/RANKL. *Proc Natl Acad Sci USA.* 1998;95:3597–3602.

53. Sutherland S, Cook S, McCleskey EW. Chemical mediators of pain due to tissue damage and ischemia. *Prog Brain Res.* 2000;129:21–38.

54. Woolf CJ, American College of Physicians, American Physiological Society. Pain: moving from symptom control toward mechanism-specific pharmacologic management. *Ann Intern Med.* 2004;140:441–451.

55. Olson TH, Riedl MS, Vulchanova L, et al. An acid sensing ion channel (ASIC) localizes to small primary afferent neurons in rats. *Neuroreport.* 1998;9:1109–1113.

56. Caterina MJ, Schumacher MA, Tominaga M, et al. The capsaicin receptor: a heat-activated ion channel in the pain pathway. *Nature.* 1997;389:816–824.

57. Tominaga M, Caterina MJ, Malmberg AB, et al. The cloned capsaicin receptor integrates multiple pain-producing stimuli. *Neuron.* 1998;21:531–543.

58. Bassilana F, Champigny G, Waldmann R, et al. The acid-sensitive ionic channel subunit ASIC and the mammalian degenerin MDEG form a heteromultimeric H+-gated Na+ channel with novel properties. *J Biol Chem.* 1997;272:28819–28822.

59. Griffiths JR. Are cancer cells acidic? *Br J Cancer.* 1991;64:425–427.

60. Deigner HP, Kinscherf R. Modulating apoptosis: current applications and prospects for future drug development. *Curr Med Chem.* 1999;6:399–414.

61. Galasko CS. Diagnosis of skeletal metastases and assessment of response to treatment. *Clin Orthop Relat Res.* 1995;312:64–75.

62. Nielsen OS, Munro AJ, Tannock IF. Bone metastases: pathophysiology and management policy. *J Clin Oncol.* 1991;9:509–524.

63. DeLeo JA, Yezierski RP. The role of neuroinflammation and neuroimmune activation in persistent pain. *Pain.* 2001;90:1–6.

64. Watkins LR, Maier SF, Goehler LE. Immune activation: the role of pro-inflammatory cytokines in inflammation, illness responses and pathological pain states. *Pain.* 1995;63:289–302.

65. Watkins LR, Maier SF. Implications of immune-to-brain communication for sickness and pain. *Proc Natl Acad Sci USA.* 1999;96:7710–7713.

66. Nadler RB, Koch AE, Calhoun EA, et al. IL-1beta and TNF-alpha in prostatic secretions are indicators in the evaluation of men with chronic prostatitis. *J Urol.* 2000;164:214–218.

67. Davar G. Endothelin-1 and metastatic cancer pain. *Pain Med.* 2001;2:24–27.

68. Nelson JB, Carducci MA. The role of endothelin-1 and endothelin receptor antagonists in prostate cancer. *BJU Int.* 2000;85:45–48.

69. Opree A, Kress M. Involvement of the proinflammatory cytokines tumor necrosis factor-alpha, IL-1 beta, and IL-6 but not IL-8 in the development of heat hyperalgesia: effects on heat-evoked calcitonin gene-related peptide release from rat skin. *J Neurosci.* 2000;20:6289–6293.

70. Watkins LR, Goehler LE, Relton J, et al. Mechanisms of tumor necrosis factor-alpha (TNF-alpha) Hyperalgesia. *Brain Res.* 1995;692:244–250.

71. Stoscheck CM, King LE, Jr. Role of epidermal growth factor in carcinogenesis. *Cancer Res.* 1986;46:1030–1037.

72. Poon RT, Fan ST, Wong J. Clinical implications of circulating angiogenic factors in cancer patients. *J Clin Oncol.* 2001;19:1207–1225.

73. Roman C, Saha D, Beauchamp R. TGF-beta and colorectal carcinogenesis. *Microsc Res Tech.* 2001;52:450–457.

74. Silver BJ. Platelet-derived growth factor in human malignancy. *Biofactors.* 1992;3:217–227.

75. Daughaday WH, Deuel TF. Tumor secretion of growth factors. *Endocrinol Metab Clini North Am.* 1991;20:539–563.

76. Radinsky R. Growth factors and their receptors in metastasis. *Semin Cancer Biol.* 1991;2:169–177.

77. Lassiter LK, Carducci MA. Endothelin receptor antagonists in the treatment of prostate cancer. *Semin Oncol.* 2003;30:678–688.

78. Peters CM, Lindsay TH, Pomonis JD, et al. Endothelin and the tumorigenic component of bone cancer pain. *Neuroscience.* 2004;126:1043–1052.

79. Shappell SB, Manning S, Boeglin WE, et al. Alterations in lipoxygenase and cyclooxygenase-2 catalytic activity and mRNA expression in prostate carcinoma. *Neoplasia.* 2001;3:287–303.

80. Kundu N, Yang QY, Dorsey R, et al. Increased cyclooxygenase-2 (cox-2) expression and activity in a murine model of metastatic breast cancer. *Int J Cancer.* 2001;93:681–686.

81. Ohno R, Yoshinaga K, Fujita T, et al. Depth of invasion parallels increased cyclooxygenase-2 levels in patients with gastric carcinoma. *Cancer.* 2001;91:1876–1881.

82. Molina MA, Sitja-Arnau M, Lemoine MG, et al. Increased cyclooxygenase-2 expression in human pancreatic carcinomas and cell lines: growth inhibition by nonsteroidal anti-inflammatory drugs. *Cancer Res.* 1999;59:4356–4362.

83. Dubois RN, Radhika A, Reddy BS, et al. Increased cyclooxygenase-2 levels in carcinogen-induced rat colonic tumors. *Gastroenterology.* 1996; 110:1259–1262.

84. Vasko MR. Prostaglandin-induced neuropeptide release from spinal cord. *Prog Brain Res.* 1995;104:367–380.

85. Pilbeam CC, Harrison JR, Raisz LG. Prostaglandins and bone metabolism. In: Bilezikian JP, Raisz LG, Rodan GA, eds. *Principles of Bone Biology.* San Diego: Academic Press; 2002.

86. Gupta RA, Dubois RN. Colorectal cancer prevention and treatment by inhibition of cyclooxygenase-2. *Nat Rev Cancer.* 2001;1:11–21.

87. Thun MJ, Henley SJ, Patrono C. Nonsteroidal anti-inflammatory drugs as anticancer agents: mechanistic, pharmacologic, and clinical issues [Review]. *J Natl Cancer Inst.* 2002;94:252–266.

88. Sonoshita M, Takaku K, Sasaki N, et al. Acceleration of intestinal polyposis through prostaglandin receptor EP2 in Apc(Delta 716) knockout mice. *Nature Med.* 2001;7:1048–1051.

89. Sheng H, Shao J, Kirkland SC, et al. Inhibition of human colon cancer cell growth by selective inhibition of cyclooxygenase-2. *J Clin Invest.* 1997;99:2254–2259.

90. Williams CS, Tsujii M, Reese J, et al. Host cyclooxygenase-2 modulates carcinoma growth. *J Clin Invest.* 2000;105:1589–1594.

91. Masferrer JL, Leahy KM, Koki AT, et al. Antiangiogenic and antitumor activities of cyclooxygenase-2 inhibitors. *Cancer Res.* 2000;60:1306–1311.

92. Harris RE, Alshafie GA, Abou-Issa H, et al. Chemoprevention of breast cancer in rats by celecoxib, a cyclooxygenase 2 inhibitor. *Cancer Res.* 2000;60:2101–2103.

93. Reddy BS, Hirose Y, Lubet R, et al. Chemoprevention of colon cancer by specific cyclooxygenase-2 inhibitor, celecoxib, administered during different stages of carcinogenesis. *Cancer Res.* 2000;60:293–297.

94. Lal G, Ash C, Hay K, et al. Suppression of intestinal polyps in Msh2-deficient and non-Msh2-deficient multiple intestinal neoplasia mice by a specific cyclooxygenase-2 inhibitor and by a dual cyclooxygenase-1/2 inhibitor. *Cancer Res.* 2001;61:6131–6136.

95. Carducci MA, Nelson JB, Bowling MK, et al. Atrasentan, an endothelin-receptor antagonist for refractory adenocarcinomas: safety and pharmacokinetics.[erratum appears in *J Clin Oncol* 2003 Jun 15;21(12):2449]. *J Clin Oncol.* 2002;20:2171–2180.

96. Nelson JB, Hedican SP, George DJ, et al. Identification of endothelin-1 in the pathophysiology of metastatic adenocarcinoma of the prostate. *Nature Med.* 1995;1:944–949.

97. Pomonis JD, Rogers SD, Peters CM, et al. Expression and localization of endothelin receptors: implication for the involvement of peripheral glia in nociception. *J Neurosci.* 2001;21:999–1006.

98. Davar G, Hans G, Fareed MU, et al. Behavioral signs of acute pain produced by application of endothelin-1 to rat sciatic nerve. *Neuroreport.* 1998;9:2279–2283.

99. Dawas K, Laizidou M, Shankar A, et al. Angiogenesis in cancer: the role of endothelin-1. *Ann R Coll Surg Engl.* 1999;81:306–310.

100. Asham EH, Loizidou M, Taylor I. Endothelin-1 and tumor development. *Eur J Surg Oncol.* 1998;24:57–60.

101. Couture R, Harrisson M, Vianna RM, et al. Kinin receptors in pain and inflammation. *Eur J Pharmacol.* 2001;429:161–176.

102. Fox A, Wotherspoon G, McNair K, et al. Regulation and function of spinal and peripheral neuronal B1 bradykinin receptors in inflammatory mechanical hyperalgesia. *Pain.* 2003;104:683–691.

103. Sevcik MA, Ghilardi JR, Halvorson KG, et al. Analgesic efficacy of bradykinin B1 antagonists in a murine bone cancer pain model. *J Pain.* 2005;6:771–775.

104. Rueff A, Dawson AJ, Mendell LM. Characteristics of nerve growth factor induced hyperalgesia in adult rats: dependence on enhanced bradykinin-1 receptor activity but not neurokinin-1 receptor activation. *Pain.* 1996;66:359–372.

105. Verge VM, Tetzlaff W, Bisby MA, et al. Influence of nerve growth factor on neurofilament gene expression in mature primary sensory neurons. *J Neurosci.* 1990;10:2018–2025.

106. Averill S, Michael GJ, Shortland PJ, et al. NGF and GDNF ameliorate the increase in ATF3 expression which occurs in dorsal root ganglion cells in response to peripheral nerve injury. *Eur J Neurosci.* 2004;19:1437–1445.

107. Donnerer J, Schuligoi R, Stein C. Increased content and transport of substance P and calcitonin gene-related peptide in sensory nerves innervating inflamed tissue: evidence for a regulatory function of nerve growth factor in vivo. *Neuroscience.* 1992;49:693–698.

108. Gould HJ, 3rd, Gould TN, England JD, et al. A possible role for nerve growth factor in the augmentation of sodium channels in models of chronic pain. *Brain Res.* 2000;854:19–29.

109. Ji RR, Samad TA, Jin SX, et al. p38 MAPK activation by NGF in primary sensory neurons after inflammation increases TRPV1 levels and maintains heat hyperalgesia. *Neuron.* 2002;36:57–68.

110. Ramer MS, Bradbury EJ, McMahon SB. Nerve growth factor induces P2X(3) expression in sensory neurons. *J Neurochem.* 2001;77:864–875.

111. Mamet J, Lazdunski M, Voilley N. How nerve growth factor drives physiological and inflammatory expressions of acid-sensing ion channel 3 in sensory neurons. *J Biol Chem.* 2003;278:48907–48913.

112. Heumann R, Korsching S, Bandtlow C, et al. Changes of nerve growth factor synthesis in nonneuronal cells in response to sciatic nerve transection. *J Cell Biol.* 1987;104:1623–1631.

Neuropathic Pain

Ricardo A. Cruciani
Helena Knotkova

INTRODUCTION

The prevalence of chronic pain in patients with cancer ranges from 40% to 60%.[1] Several prospective studies suggest that adequate pain relief could be achieved in 90% of cancer patients with chronic pain if the recommendations by the World Health Organization (WHO) are followed.[2,3]

However, the prevalence is still 20%–40% in the outpatient setting, climbing to more than 80% at the end of life.[4] These disappointing outcomes could be improved by understanding the different types of pain, and recognizing the more common pain syndromes and the current strategies for cancer pain management. Indeed, the ability to recognize the different etiologies and physiopathologic mechanisms of pain syndromes will result in a better selection of therapeutic strategies, increase the success rate, and circumvent unnecessary suffering.

Nociceptive pain (see later) is the most common type of pain but in as many as 40% of cases it is accompanied by a neuropathic component. The underlying mechanism(s) in both types of pain is very different and has important implications for the selection of the treatment. Indeed, the treatment of neuropathic pain, contrary to nociceptive pain, relies on a combination of adjuvant analgesia and opioid therapy. Research into neuropathic pain in cancer patients has been very challenging and most of the strategies currently utilized are the result of extrapolation from the noncancer population. Although there are differences between the two patient populations, there are enough common grounds to justify this reasoning. Currently, many ongoing studies are designed to elucidate the mechanism of cancer-related neuropathic pain and to improve treatment outcomes.[5,6] This chapter discusses the diagnosis, physiopathology, and treatment strategies of cancer-related neuropathic pain.

TYPES OF PAIN

Two major types of pain have been described: nociceptive (visceral or somatic) and neuropathic. Nociceptive pain is the result of the activation of nociceptors at the level of the affected structures. Nociceptors are free nerve endings that can be activated by elements released by the injured tissue (potassium, decreased pH) or by substances secreted by mast cells as a response to injury (substance P, bradykinin). Essentially, the activation of any one of them results in the generation of action potentials that travel centripetally through the axon of the pseudobipolar dorsal root ganglia (DRG) neurons to the posterior horn of the spinal cord. There, this so-called primary afferent neuron synapses with a projection neuron that conveys the pain information through the spinothalamic tract to a third-order neuron localized in the postero-ventricular-lateral (PVL) and the postero-ventricular-medial (PVM) nucleus of the thalamus where pain can be identified. At that level, the pain sensations can be felt but not localized. An example frequently seen in clinical practice comes from patients with stroke that involves some area of the somatosensory cortex. These patients can feel painful stimulation because the pathways to thalamus are intact but, in response to painful stimuli, they withdraw the limb or move it randomly, failing to identify the area from where the pain originated. From the thalamus a third-order neuron transmits the action potentials to the sensory cortex where, with the participation of association areas, the pain sensation can be localized to a specific body region (the patient can localize the pain). This normal physiologic response alerts the individual to the presence of a noxious stimulus, allowing protective measures to be taken (e.g., immobilization of the injured body part). The other type of pain, called neuropathic, is the result of injury to the nerve tissue itself, and it can occur at any level of the nervous system. The presentation of the symptoms varies with the site of the lesion and can be the result of an acute or chronic insult. In cancer patients, certain types of neuropathic lesions present most frequently and are caused by direct invasion or compression of nerve structures by tumor. Depending on the level of involvement they can be mononeuropathies, polyneuropathies, plexopathies, or radiculopathies. Radiculopathies are most common and are caused by compression of the nerve root by metastatic disease to the vertebral body. The pain can be constant or intermittent and lancinating or dysesthetic. Approximately two-thirds of the underlying causes of neuropathic pain syndromes in cancer patients are the result of direct action of the tumor, whereas one-third are due to side effects from the therapies used to treat cancer.

WHAT IS NEUROPATHIC PAIN?

The definition of neuropathic pain has evolved over time. The International Association for the Study of Pain (IASP) defines neuropathic pain as "pain initiated or caused by a primary lesion or dysfunction in the nervous system." However, for many investigators *neuropathic pain* implies abnormal processing of information, which is not clearly accounted for in this definition. The symptoms that result from compression (e.g., metastatic disease to vertebral bodies in prostate cancer) of a nerve root or trunk (e.g., electric current or burning sensation in a radicular distribution) may well be the product of the activation of normal nociceptors that innervate the nerve itself (nervi nervorum). This pertains to the mechanism in regard to nociceptive pain as discussed above. However, if abnormal sensory processing also develops (e.g., allodynia and hyperalgesia), then the pain progresses and becomes a classic neuropathic pain syndrome. Hence, from a practical clinical perspective, defining neuropathic pain as "abnormal persistent pain that results from a direct injury to the nervous system" would be a more helpful characterization.

▶ Types of neuropathic pain

There are many classifications but the one based on the location of the generator of the pain into central and peripheral pain seems to be the most useful. Indeed, neuropathic pain is very complex and encompasses various mechanisms that involve the central or the peripheral nervous system.

Central pain: This is the result of a lesion in the central nervous system (CNS) and it has been associated with CNS tumors, postradiation, myelopathy, and stroke. It is not frequently seen in cancer patients and is more resistant to treatment than the peripheral counterpart. Mechanisms of central pain have not yet been determined. However, several hypotheses have been considered. Most theories were based initially on human studies, but the recent development of several animal models has allowed further investigation of the molecular and neurohumoral basis of neuronal pathology related to central pain. Central disinhibition and central sensitization leading to neuronal hyperexcitability have been considered as possible mechanisms of central pain.[7] Also, numerous functional imaging studies suggest that functional plasticity and reorganization within somatosensory centers and the motor cortex play an important role in the development of central pain.[8,9]

Peripheral pain: It may involve the plexus (brachial, lumbar, sacral) or individual nerves (mononeuropathy, polineuropathy, peripheral neuropathy). Interestingly, although the lesion occurs in the peripheral nervous system, the generator can be localized in the periphery, the CNS, or both, a distinction that has implications for treatment strategies and prognosis. Peripheral neuropathic pain associated with oncologic diseases was observed in patients with lymphomas; head and neck malignancies can cause painful cranial neuropathies, pelvic cancer can invade the lumbosacral plexus, and metastasis or lymphomas can cause meningeal carcinomatosis and affect multiple spinal roots.[10,11] Peripheral neuropathic pain is more commonly seen, is easier to treat, responds better to pharmacologic approaches, in certain cases can be treated with interventional techniques (nerve block, radiation, direct injection of local anesthetics), and has a better overall prognosis.

A pathophysiologic classification is also widely utilized: (1) peripheral mononeuropathies or polyneuropathies (possibly due to abnormal processing of the peripheral nervous system); (2) deafferentation pain (result of injury to the peripheral or CNS), believed to be caused by abnormal central processing of the sensory input; (3) sympathetically mediated pain (caused by an abnormal sympathetic response).

This broad definition includes a large number of symptoms that should be recognized and identified independently to assure rapid and effective intervention.

The pathophysiology of neuropathic pain is highly complex and may present with multiple types of sensory abnormalities, suggesting the presence of multiple underlying mechanisms. After an injury to the peripheral nervous system or CNS, the following pathophysiologic changes may occur: nociceptors acquire new characteristics; regenerating nerve sprouts may discharge spontaneously (which may be associated with spontaneous dysesthesia); activation thresholds may be decreased (resulting in pain after non-noxious stimuli or allodynia); the stimulus-response function may shift to the left (such that a noxious stimulus causes more pain than normal or hyperalgesia). Although all of these events are usually considered to drive any type of neuropathic pain, newer research suggests that specific types of sensory abnormalities, such as allodynic responses or cold hyperesthesia, may be associated with specific abnormalities in neural processing.[12] It is hoped that in the future, an increased understanding of the pathophysiology of specific types of neuropathic pain will lead to mechanism-based treatment decision-making.

Numerous membrane components that are putatively relevant in the development and maintenance of pathologic pain have recently been identified. These neural structures represent potential targets for analgesic drugs and therapeutic interventions designed to relieve pathologic pain:

Purine receptors. Purinergic receptors (P2X3, P2X2/3) are localized on peripheral sensory afferents. They are involved in the development of hyperalgesia and mechanical allodynia in neuropathic pain.[8]

Proton-gated ion channels (ASIC1, 3; ASIC/DRASIC). These structures are amiloride-sensitive channels activated by low pH, and play a role in the development of bone pain. ASICs are activated by the acidic microenvironment produced by osteoclasts during bone resorption.[13, 14]

Transient receptor potential vanilloid channels (TRPV-1–4). TRPV-1 plays a crucial role in inflammatory pain and thermal hyperalgesia. Activation of TRPV-1 leads to the release of neuropeptides, including substance P, which can also activate osteoclasts and mast cells.[15]

Proteinase-activated receptor-2 (PAR-2). This receptor is a member of the G protein-coupled, seven transmembrane domain receptor family, and it is activated by mast cell-derived tryptase and other proteinases. PAR-2 appears in primary sensory neurons and it is involved in hyperalgesia.[16] This receptor is a recently discovered potential treatment target.[17]

Voltage-gated sodium channels (TTX-R Na (v) 1.8; TTX-S Na (v) 1.7). The TTX-R Na (v) 1.8 channel is expressed exclusively in primary nociceptive sensory neurons, and it plays a crucial role in inflammatory pain. TTX-S Na (v) 1.7 also may contribute to pain associated with inflammation,[18] and both TTX-S and TTX-R sodium channels are upregulated during chronic inflammation. Mutations in the gene encoding the TTX-S Na (v) 1.7 sodium channel contribute to neuropathic pain related to a disorder known as *primary erythermalgia*, an autosomal dominant genetic disorder characterized by episodic attacks of reddening of the skin, due to vasodilation of the dermis.[19]

Cannabinoid receptors (CB1, CB2). An increasing body of evidence supports the hypothesis of the role of CB1 and CB2 in central and peripheral mechanisms of nociception, particularly during inflammation and neuropathic pain.[20,21] Recent research results suggest a potential role for CB1 and CB2 as anti-inflammatory and antihyperalgesic agents, and in the potentiation of opioid analgesia.[22]

Voltage-gated calcium channels. The role of calcium channels in the control of transmitter release from nociceptive terminals is well known. However, there is evidence that some anticonvulsant drugs (gabapentin, pregabalin) that have been used to treat neuropathic pain act via voltage-gated calcium channels. Both gabapentin and pregabalin bind with high affinity to the alpha-2-delta subunit of the N- and P/Q-type voltage-gated calcium channels and decrease intracellular calcium influx.[23,24]

Bradykinin receptors. Expression of B1 receptors is induced by tissue injury, and B1 contributes significantly to inflammatory hyperalgesia. The B2 receptor, which acts via a pertussis toxin-sensitive G protein that stimulates phospholipase CB1, is a key player in inflammatory hyperalgesia.[25,26]

Adenosine receptors (A1, A2A, A2B, and A3). Spinally injected adenosine induces antinociception in animal models of neuropathic pain, and intrathecal adenosine appears to induce some degree of analgesia and relieve neuropathic pain in humans.[27,28]

Most conditions of neuropathic pain develop after partial injury of the peripheral nervous system. Research on animal models reveals that both injured and neighboring uninjured nerve fibers contribute to the generation of neuropathic pain.[29,30]

NEUROHUMORAL CHANGES RELATED TO NEURAL INJURY

The microenvironment of nerve fibers changes substantially after injury as a result of Wallerian degeneration of lesioned fibers and responses in Schwann cells, satellite cells around the cell bodies of primary sensory neurons in the DRGs, and various components of the immune system. Cellular changes, including dedifferentiation and proliferation of Schwann cells, promote regrowth of surviving neurons in the proximal stump of a lesioned nerve. In the distal part of a damaged nerve, macrophages are recruited to clear axonal and myelin tissue. Neurotrophic factors, cytokines, and their receptors are upregulated during this process. As a result, primary sensory neurons become hyperexcitable and may exhibit spontaneous activity.

▶ Neurotrophic factors

Transection of a peripheral nerve leads to an increased expression of nerve growth factor (NGF) in skin keratinocytes within the area of the damaged nerve. In Schwann cells, an increased transcription of brain-derived neurotrophic factor (BDNF) occurs, together with enhanced production of NGF and neurotrophin-4 (NT-4). In DRGs, neurotrophic factors contribute to pain hypersensitivity that develops after injury. It was shown that inactivation of NGF, BDNF, and NT-4 reduces the development of mechanical allodynia.

▶ Signaling between sensory neurons and the sympathetic nervous system

Following injury, efferent sympathetic fibers sprout into DRGs and form compact structures around the cell bodies of large diameter A-beta neural fibers. The release of neurotrophins critically contributes to the creation of this abnormal connection. A blockade of the action of BDNF, NGF, and neurotrophic factor decreases the sprouting of sympathetic efferents.[31]

▶ Cytokines

The cytokine tumor necrosis factor-alpha (TNF-alpha) has been shown to play a role in pain hypersensitivity that occurs following a neural injury.[32] There is also an upregulation of interleukin 1-beta,

interleukin-6, and interleukin-10, with a different temporal pattern. TNF-alpha accumulates at the site of injury after release from Schwann cells, and this increase coincides with the invasion of macrophages and T-lymphocytes. Proliferating satellite cells represent another potential source of the increase of TNF-alpha in DRGs.

▶ Upregulation of ion channels

After a neural injury, the proportion of sensory neurons expressing the purinoreceptor (P2X3) transiently increases, and intense immunoreactivity occurs at the injury site. Knockdown of the P2X3 receptor reduces mechanical hyperalgesia and allodynia related to neuropathic pain.[33]

▶ Pathologic changes in cell bodies of injured neurons

The ectopic discharge from injured fibers exhibits a rhythmic pattern that is caused by the emergence of sinusoidal subthreshold membrane potential oscillation and is maintained by depolarizing afterpotentials. Hyperpolarization-activated "pacemaker" channels in the membranes of cell bodies of injured neurons are responsible for the spontaneous activity of A-beta neural fibers. These channels, which are permeable to sodium and potassium ions, are also responsible for part of the spontaneous activity in A-delta fibers. Blockade of these pacemaker channels reduces mechanical allodynia.

DIAGNOSIS OF NEUROPATHIC PAIN

The diagnosis is derived from taking a careful history and a detailed physical examination. Patients frequently describe their pain as tingling, burning, stabbing, or electrical. On occasion, patients mention that they cannot tolerate contact with clothing or sheets at night, and women may stop using a bra to avoid the pressure and contact to their skin.[2,34] This is typically seen in postherpetic neuralgia (PHN; a type of neuropathic pain) that affects a thoracic dermatome. Special attention should be devoted to the location of the pain. When the thoracic spine is affected, radicular pain caused by a nerve root being compressed by a collapsed vertebral body secondary to metastatic disease to the bone can present with pain in a band distribution in the chest. If the lesion is in the lumbar spine, it may radiate to the internal aspect of the thigh (L2-3), the posterior aspect of the leg down to the dorsum of the foot involving the big toe (L4-5), or the bottom of the foot (L5-S1). When the cervical spine is involved, the pain radiates in the internal aspect of the arm to the small finger (C8) or the thumb (C6).

The pain in patients with a lesion to the CNS (e.g., stroke, myelopathy) does not follow a dermatomal or a radicular distribution but tends to involve the entire limb. This type of pain is called central and patients may complain of pain in the entire hemibody contralateral to the site of the lesion.

A glove-and-stocking distribution can be seen in patients undergoing chemotherapy with *cis*-platinum, carboplatin, or vincristine. *Cis*-platinum characteristically involves the long fibers so that although light touch and proprioception are affected, temperature and pinprick sensation are spared. These patients may have a clear worsening of the gait with frequent falls. Paraneoplastic syndromes can also present with a glove-and-stocking distribution but tend to affect both long and short fibers. A variation in the intensity of the pain over the course of the day may be an indicator as well. The pain is usually worse at night, which should be a factor when administering medications over a 24-hour period of time. Activity usually exacerbates the pain. When there is sympathetic involvement, patients may complain of "freezing" of the limb while objective changes in temperature may be only minimal. The opposite, increased temperature in the limb, is also sometimes reported.

CHARACTERISTICS OF THE PHYSICAL EXAMINATION

The need for a thorough neurologic examination cannot be emphasized enough. The physical examination is often significant for abnormal sensations that include hypesthesia (a numbness or lessening of feeling), paresthesias (spontaneous abnormal nonpainful sensations such as tingling, cold, or itching), dysesthesias (spontaneous abnormal painful sensations such as burning, stinging, shooting, lancinating, shock-like), hyperalgesia (increased perception of painful stimuli), hyperpathia (exaggerated pain response), and allodynia (pain induced by nonpainful stimuli such as light touch, cool air),[18] as described in Table 7-1 that lists somatosensory abnormalities found on physical examination.

Reduced vibration sense or decreased proprioception may reveal involvement of long fibers, as seen with cisplatin chemotherapy. The presence of mechanical allodynia can be determined by a gentle stroke with a cotton ball. Thermal allodynia can be tested with a cool reflex hammer or a tuning fork gently applied to the putatively affected area for a few seconds. Mechanical hyperalgesia can be tested with a disposable safety pin used to gently prick the area in question.

With a careful examination of the affected region, two distinct areas can be delineated in some patients. The area of primary hyperalgesia is characterized by the presence of heat and mechanical allodynia, but not cold allodynia, which delineate the area of the lesion. When cold allodynia is present in addition to mechanical and heat hyperalgesia/allodynia in the periphery of the area of primary hyperalgesia, the presence of central sensitization is suggested, which is called secondary hyperalgesia.

Deep tendon reflexes may be decreased or absent. The motor examination may be significant for distal weakness that is more common in peripheral neuropathies as opposed to proximal weakness that is more characteristic of myopathies (e.g., corticosteroids). A foot drop is another common finding in peripheral neuropathies.

Table 7-1

Somatosensory Abnormalities Found on Physical Examination

Dysesthesias	Spontaneous abnormal painful sensations (burning, stinging, shooting, lancinating); shock-like abnormal sensations
Hyperalgesia	Increased perception of painful stimuli
Hypesthesia	Numbness or decreased feeling; increased pain threshold
Allodynia	Pain induced by nonpainful stimuli (light touch, cool air, contact with clothing)
Numbness	Can occur with normal threshold to touch
Prolonged after sensations	More common in central pain

PATHOPHYSIOLOGY OF NEUROPATHIC PAIN

After trauma or compression of a neural structure, some fibers may be injured or sectioned but a variable number remains intact. This concept is very important because neuropathic pain is a complex phenomenon caused by the changes that occur not only in the distal part of the sectioned or injured axons but also in the proximal segment, the DRG neurons where these axons originate, and the remaining intact fibers. Soon after the injury, the distal part of the injured fibers undergoes Wallerian degeneration while the proximal part of the axon starts the regenerating process within hours. When the newly generated axons (smaller, thinner fibers) find their way into the myelin sheath, successful regeneration occurs. The resultant nerve will be thinner, wrapped by a characteristically abnormal myelin sheath, and will show abnormal conduction velocities. On the other hand, the axons that don't find the myelin sheath produce a chaotic number of fibers at the end of the proximal sectioned axon that is known as *Medusa head*. These structures, called neuromas, can be a source of abnormal impulses, which are initially mediated by A-delta and later by C fibers. Such abnormal electrical activity, also known as injured nerve currents, can be increased by mechanical and chemical stimulation, including a decrement in pH that occurs during the inflammatory response. The mechanism underlying this electrical activity has not been elucidated. Changes in sympathetic fibers, including sprouting of sympathetic fibers into DRG neurons, has been observed. However, alpha-2 receptor blockers have been shown to be ineffective, indicating that the changes observed in neuroma formation may occur independently from the sympathetic system.

The observation that excitability increases in the remaining intact fibers has been a topic of great interest. The most important modifications seem to be at the level of the sodium channels. The sodium channels are important structures in the generation of action potentials. Those localized in the neuronal body remain the same, whereas the sodium channels that are in the axons are redistributed and accumulate. These changes seem to be responsible for some, but not all, of the symptoms observed in neuropathic pain. Indeed, intrathecal application of antisense oligodeoxynucleotides reverses thermal hyperalgesia and hypersensitivity but does not alter thermal or mechanical nociception. As a result, neural activity may occur independently from peripheral noxious stimuli and fire spontaneously. P2X are the receptors for adenosine triphosphate (ATP), which is released after injury along with potassium and other intracellular elements. P2X is also upregulated and has been correlated with the development of allodynia. In addition, vallinoid receptors (now known as TRP V1), which are structures activated by heat and localized in C and A fibers, are also upregulated but their role in neuropathic pain has not been clearly established. It has been observed that glial cells and immune cells experience activation and produce cytokines. In contrast, Schwann cells and keratinocytes release BDNF and NGF, increasing the excitability of the remaining normal fibers. In normal conditions, these neurons are activated by their physiologic neurotransmitter (substance P, glutamate) or by the application of voltage (~10 mV). However, changes in the surrounding tissue make them very excitable so that they can spontaneously fire action potentials. Schwann cells seem to play an important role in the development of these changes, as manifested by the increased expression of NGF and NT-4. The changes that result from injury to a neural structure are not limited to the vicinity of the lesion and can extend to the cell bodies of the DRG. These neurons increase the expression of NGF, which has a pivotal role in the development of the postinjury sequelae. After NGF binds the TrkA receptors, they are internalized as a complex and transported to the cell body where they initiate gene transcription of sodium channels, receptors, and the neuropeptides that participate in pain transmission. Indeed, it has been shown that NGF has a tonic effect on the expression of substance P in nociceptors. The changes in sodium channels are very complex. Sodium channels transport positively charged sodium atoms across the cell membrane. These ions subsequently produce the upstroke velocity of action potentials. Thus, the generation of action potentials depends upon sodium channels. After an injury occurs, the properties of sodium channels change as well as the expression of different types of sodium channels, among other changes. Two main types of sodium channels have been described: TTX sensitive and TTX resistant. Although the sodium channels remain unchanged in the DRG cell body, they are redistributed on the cell membrane, which results in the generation of "nerve injury discharges." Ultimately, the sympathetic efferent fibers sprout into the A-delta fiber cell bodies, forming basket-like structures that are responsible for sympathetically-mediated pain. Preclinical studies in mice have shown that when the effect mediated by NGF, BDNF, and NT-3 is blocked, sympathetic sprouting is decreased. This finding suggests that early intervention following injury could have an important impact on the outcome of neuropathic pain. However, the role of the sympathetic fibers in the development of neuropathic pain remains unclear. Transgenic mice lacking functional alpha-2 adrenoceptors respond similarly to the wild-type phenotype. Although it has been suggested that sympathetic changes (sprouting, increased expression of the presynaptic alpha-2 receptors) are transient phenomena producing no long-term impact on neuropathic pain, it is currently accepted that such changes are responsible, at least in part, for the development of sympathetically mediated neuropathic chronic pain.

NEUROPATHIC PAIN SYNDROMES

The patients with cancer pain may present a variety of pain syndromes as described in Table 7-2.

▶ Radiculopathy or cauda equina syndrome

Involvement of vertebral bodies with extradural compression of the spinal cord or its nerve roots is an important complication of multiple myeloma. Paraspinal or retroperitoneal lymph node involvement may lead to spinal cord compression in lymphoma patients. Approximately 4% of lymphoma and 11% of myeloma patients develop spinal cord or cauda equina compression during the course of their illness.[35,36] Radicular pain, (often aggravated by coughing, sneezing, or straining), night pain, as well as an exacerbation of known back pain, are early signs. These occur in approximately 50% of patients prior to the development of muscle weakness. This condition is a medical emergency, which requires immediate investigation via magnetic resonance imaging (MRI). Once motor weakness is established it may be irreversible.

▶ Plexopathy

Disease-related plexopathy

Cervical, axillary, paraaortic, or retroperitoneal lymph nodes may infiltrate their respective plexus, resulting in cervical, brachial, or lumbosacral plexopathy. Due to the close proximity of lymph nodes

Table 7-2
Common Cancer-Related Neuropathic Pain Syndromes

Chemotherapy-induced neuropathy
   Cisplatin
   Oxiliplatin
   Paclitaxel
   Thalidomide
   Vincristine
   Vinblastine

Cranial neuropathies
   Jugular foramen syndrome

CRPS
   Type I
   Type II

Direct nerve lesion (tumor infiltration, compression) mononeuropathies
   Plexopathies
      Brachial
      Lumbosacral
      Radiculopathy

Leptomeningeal metastasis

Postherpetic neuralgia

Postradiation plexopathy

Neuropathies due to surgical procedures
   Phantom pain
   Postmastectomy syndrome
   Postthoracotomy syndrome
   Radical neck dissection
   Neuroma formation

CISPS = complex regional pain syndrome

and the nerve plexus, plexopathy is a common feature of patients with advanced lymphoma. Pain is the most common symptom, followed by muscle weakness and sensory abnormalities.[37] Rapidly developing excruciating pain and neurologic deficit usually points to a neoplastic etiology, whereas a more insidious onset of mild symptoms may indicate radiation-induced plexopathy.

Radiation-induced plexopathy

In patients who have been treated with radiotherapy, the appearance of plexopathy may be due to irradiation and not due to the underlying disease. Symptoms do not usually occur until after a latent period of 6 months although the interval may be much longer, sometimes many years. Slowly progressing symptoms, electromyographic recording of myokymic discharges, and absence of a space-occupying mass in MRI-imaging studies suggest radiation-induced plexopathy. Pain is usually milder than in disease-related plexopathy.

▶ Peripheral neuropathy

Disease-related peripheral neuropathy

Peripheral neuropathy is a classic complication in the course of IgM paraproteinemia such as Waldenström's macroglobulinemia, occurring in 5%–10% of patients.[38] The paraprotein reacts with neural antigens resulting in demyelination. The resultant neuropathy manifests as a sensory syndrome with distal numbness, paresthesias, reduced proprioception, and Romberg's sign, and progresses gradually. Tremor, generalized areflexia, and gait ataxia are also common findings. Limb weakness develops in most cases but rarely overshadows the sensory findings.[39,40]

Between 3% and 5% of patients with multiple myeloma develop a diffuse, progressive sensorimotor polyneuropathy; 50% of these cases are associated with amyloid production.

Chemotherapy-induced peripheral neuropathy

Given that most hematology patients are treated with chemotherapy protocols until shortly before they die, chemotherapy-induced peripheral neuropathy can be a significant problem. Even though part of the nerve damage might be reversible over time, most of these patients will not live to see the effects of nerve regeneration. Preexisting nerve damage[41] such as diabetic or alcoholic neuropathy or disease-related peripheral neuropathy (discussed earlier in the chapter) can add to the risk of chemotherapy-induced neuropathy. Assessment relies mainly on patient report and clinical examination since there is no technical method available for detecting and evaluating neuropathy at an early stage. Extrapolating from studies in noncancer patients with peripheral neuropathy is a common approach to treating patients with chemotherapy-induced peripheral neuropathy. However, caution should be exercised. A double-blind, placebo-controlled study in cancer patients with chemotherapy-induced peripheral neuropathy produced no improvement in pain in cancer patients treated with up to 100 mg/day of nortriptyline, whereas this is an effective treatment for patients without cancer suffering from peripheral neuropathy. These results suggest that there may be substantial differences in the underlying physiopathology of the two entities.[42] Several chemotherapeutic agents have been identified as neurotoxic either at the level of the CNS, peripheral level, or a combination of the two.[43]

Oxiliplatin This is a relatively new agent recently approved by the U.S. Food and Drug Administration for the treatment of colon cancer. It has been observed that this agent can produce dose-dependent peripheral neuropathy that is characterized by paresthesias and dysesthesias.[44] A unique, frequent, acute sensory neuropathy that is triggered or aggravated by exposure to cold that resolves rapidly occurs in 80%–85% of patients, whereas chronic symptoms are reported by 16%.[45] The acute neurologic symptoms reflect a state of peripheral nerve hyperexcitability that is suggestive of a transient channelopathy.[46] With cumulative doses of 1020 mg/m^2, peripheral neuropathies of grades 1, 2, and 3 have been observed in 48%, 31%, and 12% of patients, respectively.[47] A long-term follow-up study reported persistent nerve conduction abnormalities a year after the last treatment while the results from motor studies remained normal.[54,48] This is an important finding, because the addition of bevacizumab to oxiliplatin in combination with infusional 5-fluorouracil/leucovorin (FOLFOX, FUFOX) for advanced colorectal cancer could conceivably prolong progression-free survival. However, neurotoxicity rather than tumor progression could become the dominating treatment-limiting issue in first-line therapy for these patients.

Cisplatin This drug is often substituted for by other less-toxic derivatives but is still very useful, particularly in head and neck cancer. Peripheral neuropathy occasionally results from cumulative doses of as little as 200 mg/m^2 and is usual after 400 mg/m^2. The degree of neuropathy correlates directly with the cumulative dose of

platinum and with each individual dose.[49] The peripheral neuropathy starts with tingling, that is occasionally painful, in the toes and later in the fingers.[54] It then spreads proximally to affect both legs and arms. The deep tendon reflexes disappear (ankle jerk first), and proprioceptive loss can be so severe that patients become unable to feed themselves and walk. Nerve conduction study findings are consistent with sensory axonopathy (decreased conduction velocities and diminished amplitude of sensory nerve potentials). The first neuropathic symptoms may not appear until cisplatin treatment is completed and may progress for several months before stabilizing. DRG neurons are probably the primary site of pathology. Pathologic examination of nerve roots reveals axonal loss with secondary demyelination. Axonal loss is observed in dorsal (sensory) but not ventral (motor) roots, with secondary degeneration of posterior columns. It has been suggested that a careful clinical evaluation combined with a detailed electrophysiological evaluation of the patient prior to the chemotherapy could predict the final neurologic outcome of the cisplatin- or/and paclitaxel-based chemotherapy.[60]

Vincristine This is the most neurotoxic of the *vinca* alkaloids. Although it primarily affects the peripheral nervous system, it can also cause CNS toxicity. Almost all patients show a dose-limiting sensorimotor neuropathy that starts with tingling and paresthesias of the fingertips followed by the toes and loss of ankle reflexes. Fine movements are often impaired. Motor weakness is typical at the dorsiflexion of the feet (unilateral or bilateral foot droop) and wrist extension. On occasion, motor weakness may develop months after the treatment has been completed. Infrequently, the neuropathy may involve the cranial nerves and the patient may develop ophthalmoplegia, vocal cord paralysis, and ptosis. Nerve conduction studies and biopsy findings, although rarely needed, are consistent with axonal neuropathy. It has been observed that the nutritional status, abnormal liver enzymes, and other chemotherapeutic agents (etoposide, teniposide, cyclosporine) may enhance toxicity. The sensory symptoms, weakness, and loss of reflexes are reversible, although recovery may take as long as several months after stopping chemotherapy.[53]

Paclitaxel Approximately 60% of patients receiving paclitaxel at doses of 250 mg/m^2 develop hand and foot paresthesias. Cumulative dosages greater than 1000 mg/m^2 are invariably associated with gradual development of sensorimotor peripheral neuropathy that involves all sensory modalities. In most patients, the symptoms do not progress and may even resolve despite continued therapy, but in some patients it can be dose-limiting. Interestingly, itching can be a manifestation of neuropathy. It can sometimes produce proximal weakness of neuropathic rather than myopathic origin that can resolve or reappear with repeated treatments.[53]

Thalidomide The neuropathy produced by this drug is treatment-duration dependent and most frequently seen with doses ranging from 25 to 1600 mg/day. The neuropathy is sensory axonal and has been reported in some cases to be nonreversible. In a more recent study, improvement was reported after treatment, suggesting that the site of the lesion is the axon rather than the DRG neuron itself.[61]

▶ Phantom pain

Phantom pain refers to the pain experienced where an amputated body part used to be. In the case of an amputated lower extremity, the patient may complain of excruciating pain in a missing foot that can be exacerbated by the imaginary movement of the missing leg. That the pain exists at all may be very disturbing to patients, who may think that it is impossible to have such sensations and as a result may begin to question their own sanity. The entity, first described after the Civil War in the United States by wounded soldiers, is frequently encountered in cancer patients. Classically, it has been described after a limb amputation (e.g., Edwin sarcoma) but can occur after other surgical treatments as well (mastectomy, eye removal secondary to an astrocytoma, anus). The incidence of phantom pain correlates with the intensity of pain present prior to the amputation and for that reason preemptive therapy has been proposed. The pain improves spontaneously, with only 2% of patients suffering from this condition 1 year after surgery. A sign of improvement is the feeling that the limb is becoming shorter. The patient has the sensation that the distal part of the extremity is immediately adjacent to the stump. This symptom, called *telescoping*, is an excellent prognostic sign. In addition to phantom pain, patients may have other pain syndromes. The stump itself may be painful to touch, suggesting a neuropathic component. The pain may be accompanied by redness, change in temperature, and muscle trophism, indicating the presence of sympathetically mediated pain. After amputation, the surgeon buries the free end of a transected nerve into neighboring soft tissue structures to avoid pressure and irritation. Nonetheless, neuromas can form and cause extreme pain. A neuroma is the normal evolution of a sectioned nerve and it is characterized by anarchic regeneration of the end of the nerve, in a phenomenon that has been compared to a Medusa head. Removal of the neuroma can be helpful in certain cases, but it may regenerate with the same or worse symptoms. The literature indicates that when there are more than three interventions, pain almost never improves and may worsen. The pain tends to be localized in a specific area that corresponds to the underlying neuroma and it can be reproduced or aggravated by pressing on it. Phantom pain can also be accompanied by neuropathic pain in the area of the surgical incision.

Pain resulting from an amputated limb is a good model that can be used to review the various strategies available for the treatment of neuropathic pain because of the simultaneous occurrence of several types of pain that may require specific individual attention. The phantom pain itself may be helped by a combination of adjuvant analgesics (e.g., anticonvulsants, antidepressants), opioids, and rehabilitation. The patient is encouraged to exercise the missing limb, resulting in better pain control, presumably due to normalization of the changes in plasticity at the level of the sensorimotor cortex that resulted from the amputation.[62–67]

Physical therapy of the amputated limb can be difficult for the patient because he/she cannot visualize the missing body part. To facilitate the therapy, the patient can utilize a box with mirrors inside that are placed so that the patient can visualize an image where the missing limb would be. The visualization of the limb allows the patient to do motor exercises.[68–72]

The pain caused by the neuroma may improve with injections of local anesthetics to the site of the pain. Surgical exploration of the stump to release the free nerve ending from pressure or to bury it in the surrounding muscles to protect it from microtraumas may be helpful as well. Local application of topical lidocaine to the stump can improve local pain. A block with local anesthetics of the sympathetic structure that innervates the affected area (e.g., satellite ganglia for the upper extremity) may alleviate, if present, the component of sympathetically mediated pain. In addition, if the pain is refractory to medications a plexus infusion may allow temporary release. Spinal cord stimulation is a treatment option for phantom pain that is localized in a limb. Patients who achieve a degree of relief with opioids but experience severe side effects may benefit from a trial of intrathecal opioids and adjuvants (e.g., clonidine, baclofen).

▶ Postcerebral infarct pain

In addition to the common causes of stroke in the general population (long-standing hypertension, poorly controlled diabetes), cancer patients have unique risk factors. Interestingly, hypercholesterolemia is less frequently seen in these patients than in the general population. It has been speculated that poor nutrition and cachexia may result in the reversal of previously formed cholesterol plaques. Whatever the mechanism might be, various studies have shown that patients with malignant melanoma, and breast and lung cancer presented with fewer atherosclerotic lesions in the circle of Willis than patients with nonmalignant diseases.

Cerebral infarct can involve arterial or venous territories (more commonly, the venous sinuses). Infarct in the arterial territory is more commonly embolic in nature, including bacterial or fungal endocarditis, nonbacterial thrombotic endocarditis, tumor, mucin, fat, bone marrow, and calcified valves.

Disseminated intravascular coagulation (DIC) occurs in as many as 75% of patients with disseminated disease, particularly leukemias, although it can also be seen in patients with breast or lung cancer. In autopsies, 1%–2% reveal brain involvement. Although many structures can be affected, the superior sagital sinus is most frequently involved. Once the coagulation factors are dissipated, the infarct may become hemorrhagic. Hypercoagulability can be secondary to chemotherapy with L-asparaginase, with the mechanism apparently being depletion of antithrombin III by L-asparaginase.

Although the classical description of poststroke pain occurs in a stroke that involves the thalamus, virtually any stroke can produce chronic central pain. Of the patients that survive the event, 20% may experience pain in the area affected by the stroke. The pain does not follow a radicular or nerve distribution and can be extremely severe and refractory to treatment. The affected patients complain of classical symptoms of neuropathic pain such as allodynia and hyperalgesia.

▶ Herpes zoster and postherpetic neuralgia

This condition results from reactivation of the varicella zoster virus that remains dormant in DRG neurons after *chicken pox* infection in childhood. For unclear reasons, reactivation occurs in about 1% of immunocompetent individuals and in 10% of immunocompromised patients, with an increased incidence with age. In 90% of cases, it resolves in days to weeks, but 10% of patients progress into a debilitating chronic painful condition known as PHN. The virus replicates in the DRG causing an inflammatory response with swelling, hemorrhage, areas of necrosis, and neuronal loss. Subsequently, the virus travels centrifugally along the nerve (producing in its wake nerve inflammation and damage) to the skin where it forms a self-limiting rash known as *shingles*. In 50% of immunocompromised patients, this cascade produces a generalized life-threatening viral dissemination involving the CNS. The most commonly affected areas are the thoracic dermatomes, preferentially T10. The ophthalmic branch of the trigeminal nerve is the most commonly affected cranial nerve, which on occasion invades the eye, producing keratitis and/or uveitis. Aggressive treatment is crucial to avoid subsequent scarring and compromised vision. In addition, involvement of cranial nerves III,

IV, and VI with palsies occurs frequently. When shingles affect the ear, Ramsay Hunt syndrome, facial paralysis, hearing loss, and vertigo can occur. Inspection of the external auditory canal can reveal blisters in the tympanic membrane.

Herpes zoster usually starts with a prodromal phase characterized by pain, paresthesias (numbness/tingling) and dysesthesias (unpleasant sensations) in the affected dermatomes in a "belt-like fashion" that does not cross the midline. A few days later a maculopapular rash develops, which evolves into vesicles that usually scab within 10 days and heal in a month. Sometimes, the prodrome has no cutaneous involvement (zoster sine herpete). When lesions do form, they are not contagious after the scab forms. Once resolved, the scarred areas are less sensitive than normal skin and are often anesthetic. During active infection, the skin may exhibit marked superficial pain with light touch (allodynia) or an increased sensitivity to noxious stimulation (hyperesthesia). The normal progression is res-. olution of the vesicles accompanied by decreased pain.

PHN is the most common complication of herpes zoster. This self-limiting condition is defined as pain persisting beyond 3 months after the resolution of the skin lesions. The symptoms may be very intense and disabling. Antiviral therapy in combination with amitriptyline early in the initial viral infection may reduce the incidence of progression into PHN.[73] Symptoms tend to abate over time. Fewer than 25% of patients still experience pain 6 months after the herpes zoster eruption, and fewer than one in twenty has pain at 1 year. Patients may complain of a steady burning or aching pain with or without paroxysmal lancinating pain. Both can occur spontaneously and can be aggravated by even the lightest contact. It is not unusual for patients to complain that they cannot tolerate contact with clothing or the bedsheets at night. Some have to stay away from fans or air conditioning; even the light breeze provoked by fast walking can cause significant discomfort. Lack of allodynia in the early stages of herpes zoster infection is a predictor of good recovery by 3 months.[74]

Physical activity, temperature change, and emotional upsets may exacerbate the pain. The patient's quality of life can become severely affected and depression may develop. The pain is caused by changes in the posterior horn of the spinal cord that lead to deafferentation and hypersensitivity. There is no role for antiviral therapy in treating PHN. For patients with a poor response to a pharmacologic approach, laminectomy and electrocoagulation of the dorsal root entry zone have been advocated. However, since this is an invasive procedure and the pain can worsen as a result of additional deafferentation, the procedure is not frequently utilized. There is evidence that spinal cord stimulation may give some relief.

▶ Complex regional pain syndrome

Complex regional pain syndrome (CRPS) is a condition characterized by spontaneous pain, allodynia, hyperalgesia, edema, trophic changes of the skin, and nails with or without sympathetic involvement. This syndrome was initially named reflex sympathetic dystrophy (RSD) in reference to the sympathetically mediated responses that were observed in the affected body part. Later, a second syndrome with similar symptoms to RSD but caused by nerve injury was described and named causalgia. In an effort to clarify the syndrome, a change in taxonomy was adopted in 1992 and named complex regional pain syndrome type I and II. CRPS type I (formerly known as RSD) is caused by injury to nonnerve tissue, whereas in CRPS II (causalgia) a clear history of nerve injury could be documented. This classification is not mechanistic and does not take into consideration the presence or absence of sympathetic features.

Hence, CRPS type I and II can present with or without sympathetic involvement. This is in contrast to the old classification where sympathetic compromise was part of RSD.

Although there are several reports of CRPS in cancer patients, this condition is frequently undiagnosed. Due to mixed presentations in this patient population, specific signs of CRPS may be unrecognized. As an example, patients with Pancoast syndrome who present with a red, swollen arm may be diagnosed with venous stasis and plexopathy without considering CRPS as a differential diagnosis. The mechanical pressure of the tumor on the plexus can cause CRPS to develop in this subgroup of patients. Since CRPS can be triggered by trauma, surgery, or immobilization of a body part, cancer patients are at risk. Due to the lack of correlation between the intensity of the pain and the triggering trauma (that on occasion cannot be found at all), it is usually misdiagnosed or undertreated. Surgery or trauma is the most common culprit. However, why some patients develop this condition while others undergoing similar procedures do not is unclear. The clinical presentation is characterized by acute onset of pain that does not follow the distribution of a root or nerve. It is more common in the upper extremities than the lower ones and can involve the entire arm or only the hand. The affected area initially may not show visible changes but a careful neurologic examination may reveal hyperalgesia and allodynia. If these changes are not present, the diagnosis should be revised.

Autonomic abnormalities: These findings are not constant and do not define the syndrome. When abnormalities of the sympathetic nervous system are detected, the syndrome is said to have "sympathetically-mediated pain." The skin of the area involved may show changes in coloration that can alternate between redness or being pale. The temperature of the affected area is also unstable. The same area may present with a decrease in temperature at one visit while on other occasions may demonstrate an increase in temperature. In cases for which the diagnosis is difficult to determine, a temperature probe is applied and small differences in temperature can be detected. The syndrome, for prognostic purposes, has been divided into four phases. During the neurologic examination, in the early stages only pain and mild changes in temperature are observed. In advanced disease, atrophy of the skin and nails, muscle atrophy due to disuse, and changes visualized on a three-phase bone scan became apparent. A three-phase bone scan has been advocated as a diagnostic tool. However, the third phase is positive in only 20%.

▶ Paraneoplastic syndromes

A paraneoplastic syndrome can be defined as neurologic abnormalities not caused by the spread of cancer, but it is commonly described as the remote effects of cancer on the nervous system. It can affect any portion of the nervous system, with both central and/or peripheral components. This section focuses on paraneoplastic syndromes that can cause neuropathies. Although the incidence of paraneoplastic syndromes is low, it is important for clinicians to recognize its occurrence because the neurologic symptoms may precede and signal the diagnosis of systemic cancer. It also should be differentiated from metastatic disease, metabolic or nutritional disorders, and cancer treatment-related side effects. It has been reported that most peripheral neuropathies in patients with lung cancer are likely related to weight loss and nutritional disturbances rather than being truly paraneoplastic. Sensory neuronopathy can be present when the spinal cord and DRG are involved. Encephalomyelitis may present as the result of multiple levels of central and peripheral nervous system involvement. When peripheral nerves are involved, it can be manifested as a subacute or chronic sensorimotor peripheral neuropathy, mononeuritis multiplex, brachial neuritis, peripheral neuropathy with islet-cell tumors, and peripheral neuropathy associated with paraproteinemia.

Subacute sensory neuropathy is a rare syndrome that is not limited to patients with cancer and can also affect patients with autoimmune diseases. Symptoms typically begin in midlife without a gender preference. When the neurologic symptoms precede the diagnosis of cancer, the diagnosis usually turns out to be small-cell lung cancer. Most of these patients that test positive for anti-HU antibodies are women. The initial symptoms include dysesthesias and pain in the lower extremities. The symptoms can progress over days or weeks, eventually affecting all four limbs, the trunk, and on occasion the face. Subacute sensory neuropathy compromises all sensory modalities in contrast to *cis*-platinum, which spares pinprick and temperature sensations. The pathology is significant for inflammatory infiltration of the DRG with neuronal loss that can progress into the peripheral nerves and posterior horns and columns of the spinal cord.

Subacute sensory-motor neuropathy can cause a predominantly distal symmetric polyneuropathy, which is more pronounced in the lower extremities and can precede a diagnosis of cancer by 3–5 years. Characteristically, patients demonstrate weakness and sensory deficits in a glove-and-stocking distribution. The course of the disorder tends to progress more rapidly in patients with cancer than in patients with other diseases such as diabetes. Pathology is significant for axonal degeneration with lymphocytic infiltration of peripheral nerves and spinal root demyelination.

In general, treatment of paraneoplastic syndromes is disappointing and patients may be left with severe neurologic deficits.

STRATEGIES FOR THE TREATMENT OF NEUROPATHIC PAIN

In patients whose neuropathic pain had responded to opioid treatment in the past but who later experience increased pain intensity, changed pain characteristics must be comprehensively reassessed as the initial step in management. The goal is to determine whether specific contributing factors can be identified that could be amenable to primary therapeutic strategies such as chemotherapy and/or radiotherapy to address disease progression associated with loss of analgesic effectiveness. Other potential factors underlying the exacerbation of preexisting pain such as cord compression, systemic or local infection, and psychological distress (e.g., depression) should be ruled out prior to nonspecific modification of the treatment strategy.

▶ Therapeutic strategies that target the cause of the pain

Primary therapy directed at the etiology of the pain should be considered whenever assessment of the patient with poorly opioid responsive neuropathic pain suggests that such an approach is viable. Patients who suffer from pain during the course of refractory or relapsed lymphoma or myeloma can benefit dramatically from palliative chemotherapy or radiotherapy. Figure 7-1 shows an algorithm for the treatment of neuropathic pain.

▶ Pharmacologic interventions

The pharmacologic options available for neuropathic pain have advanced rapidly in the past years and clinical experience suggests that most patients with neuropathic cancer pain that is poorly responsive to opioids can be managed with the addition of an adjuvant analgesic.[2]

However, very few adjuvant analgesics have been studied in the palliative care setting and the information used to develop dosing guidelines has generally been extrapolated from other patient populations. Caution is usually appropriate as adjuvant analgesics are used in a medically ill population. Low initial doses and gradual dose escalation may avoid early side effects and identify dose-dependent analgesic effects. These can be explored to improve the balance between pain relief and adverse effects. The use of low initial doses and dose titration may delay the onset of analgesia, however, and patients must be informed about this possibility to improve compliance.

Anticonvulsants

Originally, anticonvulsants were thought to be most effective in syndromes characterized by lancinating or paroxysmal neuropathic pain such as trigeminal neuralgia. Recent data, however, support their usefulness in a broad variety of neuropathic pain syndromes including PHN, and peripheral diabetic neuropathy (PDN). Controlled studies show that as many as two-thirds of patients obtain good pain relief.[75] The anticonvulsants more commonly utilized for the treatment of neuropathic pain are listed in Table 7-3.

Gabapentin In two large controlled studies of patients with PDN and PHN, gabapentin was shown to be efficacious for the treatment of pain and its interference with sleep, mood, and quality of life.[76,77] In an uncontrolled study of 22 cancer patients whose neuropathic pain was not completely controlled with opioids, the addition of gabapentin resulted in decreased pain in 20 patients.[78] Gabapentin significantly reduced pain in 48% of patients with chemotherapy-induced peripheral neuropathy.[79] Gabapentin is a chemical analogue of γ-aminobutyric acid (GABA) but does not act as a GABA-receptor agonist. It binds to a receptor site in the CNS, gabapentin-binding protein, and interacts with calcium channels in the CNS. It increases GABA synthesis and release but its exact mechanism of action is still not fully understood. Gabapentin has an acceptable adverse effect profile, is not metabolized in the liver, and has no known drug-drug interactions. The most common side effects include somnolence, dizziness, ataxia, and peripheral edema. Treatment usually starts with 100–300 mg/day, and dose titration continues until benefit occurs, side effects supervene, or the total daily dose is at least 2700–3600 mg/day (see Table 7-4). A slow titration of the dose is recommended in patients who are elderly, have renal impairment, or are receiving other CNS-depressant drugs. Some do not reach a maximal response until the dose is increased to 6000 mg/day or even higher. Dose adjustment is recommended in patients with renal impairment or those undergoing hemodialysis. The daily dose is usually administered in three equal parts, but if daytime sedation remains a problem, a single nighttime dose can be used for analgesia and sleep-related benefits. In patients taking antacids containing aluminium or magnesium, the administration of gabapentin should be separated by at least 2 hours. If required, the capsules can be opened and the contents mixed with water, fruit juice, and other beverages.[80] Recent data suggest that gabapentin in combination with morphine produces more pain relief than each agent individually.[81] Although this combination is very commonly used in clinical practice, the double blind, placebo-controlled, three-arm study reported here provides the first evidence that supports this strategy.

Other Anticonvulsants Pregabalin is a new anticonvulsant available in Canada and Europe that has been recently approved in the United States. Its mechanism of action is similar to gabapentin, but with

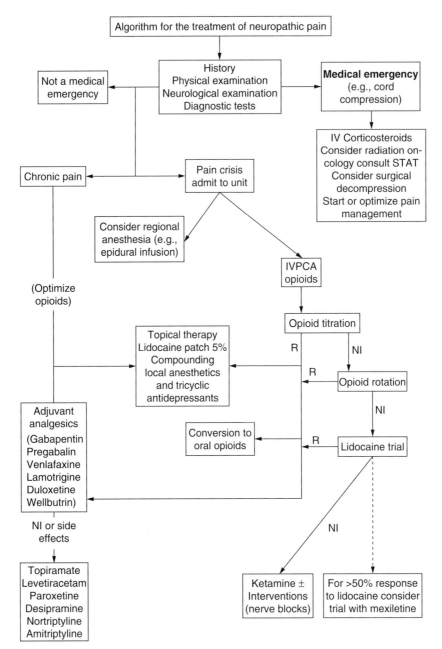

FIGURE 7-1 Proposed algorithm to treat patients with pain in various possible scenarios. R = pain relief, NI = no improvement, IV = intravenous.

more predictable pharmacokinetics. The dose ranges between 200 and 600 mg/day. A double-blind, placebo-controlled study in patients with neuropathic PDN showed significant pain improvement.[82,83] Similar results were observed in the treatment of PHN although the improvement was not significantly better than with traditional therapy. Withdrawal due to adverse events was also more frequent with pregabalin than with placebo.[84] The most common adverse events were dizziness, peripheral edema, weight gain (not affecting diabetes control), and somnolence. Data of its use for cancer neuropathic pain are not yet available.

Lamotrigine is another new anticonvulsant, which is effective for treating neuropathic pain and putatively acts by decreasing glutamate release through blocking presynaptic sodium channels.[85,86] Several randomized studies suggest a role for lamotrigine in the treatment of nonmalignant neuropathic pain and trigeminal neuralgia.[87,88] In a double-blind, placebo-controlled study in 30 adult patients with central pain, it was shown that 200 mg/day of lamotrigine decreased pain by 50%.[89] In addition, various case studies have been described.[90]

Oxcarbazepine, a metabolite of carbamazepine, has a similar spectrum of indications and better tolerability than the parent drug. Levetiracetam, topiramate, zonisamide, and tiagabine also demonstrate efficacy. Levetiracetam, gabapentin, and pregabalin have few drug-drug interactions.

Carbamazepine, phenytoin, valproate, and clonazepam have been used for many years. Despite its high effectiveness, the utility of carbamazepine in the cancer population is limited by its potential to suppress bone marrow production in as many as 7% of cases,[91] and to alter the liver metabolism of other drugs.

Table 7-3

Anticonvulsants Used as Adjuvant Analgesics

Drug	Daily Dose (mg)	Dosing Interval	Side Effects	Mechanism of Action	Evidence
Gabapentin	300–3600 (6000)	At bedtime to four times daily	Sedation	Ca++ channel	CT
Carbamazepine	100–1600	Twice a day to four times a day	Hyponatremia, neutropenia	Na+ channel	CT
Valproate	400–1200	Twice a day	Nausea, tremor, weight gain, hair loss, hepatic toxicity	Na+ channel	OLT
Phenytoin	100–300	Daily	Ataxia, rush, sedation, neuropathy, gingival hyperplasia, hirsutism	Na+ channel	CT
Clonazepam	1–10	Twice a day	Sedation, addiction, tolerance	Cl- conductance	OLT
Lamotrigine	150–500	Twice a day	Rush, Steven-Johnson's	Na+ channel	CT
Topiramate	25–400	Twice a day	Weight loss, renal calculi, sedation, attention, and memory difficulties	Na+ channel	CT
Pregabalin	200–600	Daily		Ca++ channel	CT
Oxcarbazepine	300–2400	Twice a day		Na+ channel	OLT

Abbreviations: CT = controlled trials, OLT = open-label trials.
Source: Modified from Farrar JT, Portenoy RK. Neuropathic cancer pain: the role of adjuvant analgesics. *Oncology (Williston Park).* 2001;15:1435–1442.

During the past few years, gabapentin has become the most commonly used first-line adjuvant analgesic to treat neuropathic pain. The onset of action varies, but a trial usually requires several weeks to allow for dose adjustment and determination of efficacy. Sequential trials of different agents may be needed to identify the most useful one. Clonazepam may be particularly useful if pain is associated with anxiety.

Antidepressants

Although widely accepted as adjuvant drugs, there have been no randomized trials of antidepressants for cancer-related neuropathic pain. Most indications and recommendations for treatment have been extrapolated from neuropathic pain in noncancer patients, such as those suffering from diabetes and PHN. Realistic goals should be discussed with patients and they should be told that although their pain could improve, complete pain relief is unusual. Table 7-5 lists the antidepressants that are more commonly used as adjuvant analgesics.

Table 7-4

Dose Escalation for Gabapentin

	Fast	Slow
Day 1	300 mg at bedtime	100 mg at bedtime
Day 2	300 mg BID	
Day 3	300 mg TID	
Day 4	400 mg TID	100 mg TID
Day 7	(Then increase by 300 mg/day until benefit occurs, side effects supervene, or the total daily is at least 2700–3600 mg/day)	300 mg TID
Day 14		600 mg TID
Day 21		900 mg TID
Day 28		1200 mg TID

Source: Modified from Twycross R, Wilcock A, Charlesworth S, Dickman A, eds. *Palliative Care Formulary.* 2nd ed. Abingdon: Radcliffe Medical Press; 2002.

Table 7-5

Antidepressants Used as Adjuvant Analgesics

Drug	Daily Dose	Dosing Interval	Evidence
Tricyclic Antidepressants			
Tertiary Amines			
Amitriptyline	10–200 mg/d	Every day	CT
Imipramine	10–200 mg/d	Daily to twice a day	CT
Secondary Amines			
Nortriptyline	20–80 mg/d	Daily to twice a day	CT
Desipramine	10–300mg/d	Daily to twice a day	CT
Second- and Third-Generation Agents			
Trazodone	50–200 mg/d	Three times daily	CR
Maprotiline	25–225 mg/d	Daily	CT
Selective Serotonin-Reuptake Inhibitors			
Citalopram	20–80 mg/d	Daily	CT
Fluoxetine	20–80 mg/d	Daily	CT
Paroxetine	20–80 mg/d	Daily	CT
Sertraline	50–250 mg/d	Daily	OLT

Abbreviations: CT = controlled trials, OLT = open-label trials, CR = case report.

Tricyclic Antidepressants Tricyclic antidepressants have been found to be effective in the treatment of PHN and PDN independently from their antidepressant effects.[92] Nortriptyline has been shown to be as effective as, and better tolerated than, amitriptyline in patients with PHN.[93] In the treatment of PDN, desipramine seems comparable to amitriptyline. A recent crossover design, randomized, controlled study of 25 patients with PDN compared amitriptyline with gabapentin, finding no difference in pain relief or adverse effects.[94] However, clinical experience suggests a better tolerability of gabapentin, particularly in the elderly in whom the anticholinergic side effects of the tricyclics are more pronounced.

The most commonly utilized antidepressants are the selective serotonin reuptake inhibitors (SSRIs) because they are better tolerated by cancer patients than other antidepressants. Patients with metastatic disease may experience even more severe side effects from these agents than patients undergoing cancer treatment. Nonetheless, most of the data on chronic pain treatment are from studies with tricyclics used in patients with noncancer neuropathic pain, so if possible, they should be tried first. This group of medications may have severe side effects due to their anticholinergic properties. In a study of 15 patients with postmastectomy syndrome treated with amitriptyline, 5 of the 8 women who had a good response did not want to continue due to adverse events (the order of importance being tiredness, dry mouth, and constipation).[95] Urinary retention, confusion, and orthostatic hypotension are less common. Cardiotoxicity (e.g., conduction defects, arrhythmias) is very uncommon. Patients who have significant heart disease, including conduction disorders, arrhythmia, or heart failure, should not be treated with tricyclic antidepressants. Amitriptyline is the best studied and, on this basis, may be the optimal choice after a failed trial with gabapentin. Patients who are not able to tolerate the common side effects might be considered for a trial with a secondary amine tricyclic, such as nortriptyline or desipramine. The secondary amine tricyclic drugs are less anticholinergic and, therefore, better tolerated than the tertiary amines. They also are less likely to cause orthostatic hypotension, somnolence, and confusion. A trial with paroxetine or bupropion is appropriate for patients who cannot tolerate a secondary amine tricyclic drug or have contraindications to a tricyclic trial.[96] To decrease the likelihood of side effects, tricyclics should be started with low initial doses. In the elderly and those predisposed to side effects such as hypotension, one might begin with 10 mg at night; in others one might start with 25 mg at night. The dose should be increased every 2–3 days by the size of the starting dose. The optimal dose usually ranges from 50 to 150 mg. Dry mouth may be a good indicator that the drug is achieving a significant blood level. For higher doses, blood levels of the drug should be determined to avoid toxicity.

Selective Serotonin Reuptake Inhibitors Adverse effects are even less likely with the SSRIs (Table 7-5), but evidence of analgesic efficacy for these drugs is very limited. Several controlled studies, however, do suggest efficacy for drugs with a mixed mechanism of action (combined serotonin and norepinephrine [NE] uptake inhibitors) such as venlafaxine, paroxetine, duloxetine, or bupropion (dopaminergic agonist).[96] A double-blind, placebo-controlled trial in diabetic patients with painful PDN had a 50% improvement on extended release bupropion at 150 mg administered twice daily.[97] A recent double-blind, placebo-controlled, randomized study in patients with PDN showed an improvement of about 50% in pain scores in patients taking duloxetine 30–60 mg twice daily for 4 weeks.[98] Another double-blind, placebo-controlled study showed that paroxetine 30–70 mg/day induces pain improvement in patients with PDN.[99] The analgesic effect shown in both studies was independent of the antidepressive action. On the other hand, SSRIs such us fluoxetine seem to be ineffective. To avoid side effects, the SSRI should be started at a low therapeutic dose, with the dose being increased after 1–2 weeks, based on the effect.

Failure to respond to one type of antidepressant does not predict a failure to respond to another. In the case of poor response to a particular agent, a rotation to another antidepressant of the same or different class should be attempted. If the reason for the rotation is intolerable side effects, particularly if observed at low doses, a rotation to a different class of antidepressant may be preferable. If there is no major benefit (e.g., pain reduction >50%) despite reasonable doses and length of trial (4–6 weeks), or if the side effects are substantial despite gradual dose escalation, the antidepressant should be discontinued. Withdrawal symptoms and insomnia following discontinuation of antidepressants can occur so the drug should be tapered over the course of at least 1 week. However, the antidepressant should be continued if the patient shows signs of depression. There is a high comorbidity of depression in patients with chronic pain and cancer.

There has been considerable speculation regarding the mechanism involved in the analgesic effect of antidepressants. An overview of the pathways involved in pain mechanisms and the interaction with serotonin and noradrenergic pathways may help to clarify the issue. For a more in-depth understanding, see Chap. 5 "Basic Neurobiology of Cancer Pain." Primary afferent fibers (A-delta and C) synapse in the posterior horn of the spinal cord with the projection neurons that eventually convey pain information to the thalamus and from there to the sensory cortex. The neurotransmitters involved in this pathway are glutamate and substance P. As a response to noxious stimuli these neurotransmitters are released and excite selective postsynaptic receptors, facilitating the transmission of pain signals. The synapse is modulated negatively by enkephalins that are released from interneurons localized at the same level. The enkephalins bind both to pre- and postsynaptic opioid receptors. This binding abrogates the release of glutamate and substance P by the primary afferent neuron and decreases the responsiveness of the postsynaptic neurons, respectively, hence decreasing pain information. It is noteworthy that interneurons are modulated by descending pathways with cell bodies localized in the periaqueductal grey area (brainstem). Normally this pathway is inhibited by GABA (an inhibitory neurotransmitter), so enkephalins are not released and pain transmission occurs. However, as a response to pain, the descending pathway is disinhibited and enkephalins are released to the interphase. This release decreases the response to glutamate and substance P, which ultimately results in the transmission of less pain information. The descending pathway utilizes NE and serotonin as neurotransmitters. Since the antidepressants increase serotonin and/or NE levels, it has been postulated that the release of descending pathways by the antidepressant is the underlying mechanism, which functions by inducing an analgesic effect independently from the antidepressant properties. Moreover, amitriptyline has been shown to increase the plasma concentration of morphine in cancer patients.

Local anesthetics

The use of local anesthetics for nerve blocks is a common practice, however, the use of intravenous (IV) infusion for the treatment of neuropathic pain is less frequently utilized. IV lidocaine has been found to be useful for patients with neuropathic pain due to phantom limb pain, diabetic neuropathy, and herpes zoster, which are all conditions that can be found in cancer patients.[100] In patients with pain crisis, it can be utilized to "break the cycle." In some centers, IV trials with local anesthetics are used to identify responders who are then placed on long-term therapy with equivalent PO formulations. The mechanism of action is unclear but seems to be related to stabilization of membranes through blockade of sodium channels with the subsequent interference of initiation and propagation of nerve fiber depolarization. Lidocaine is used most commonly for systemic infusion via subcutaneous (SC) or IV routes. The rapid onset of effect makes it useful in the treatment of patients with severe, rapidly progressing neuropathic pain. Baseline laboratory work that includes basic electrolytes, liver function tests, and an electrocardiogram (ECG) should be done. With monitoring, 1–2 mg/kg of lidocaine is infused over 30 minutes in an IV line. Because a dose response can ensue, a prudent approach involves an initial low-dose infusion, which is followed, if unsuccessful, by infusions at incrementally higher doses. The dose is repeated every 10 minutes up to a dose of 100 mg for the adult patient. The effect of a lidocaine infusion can last 3–21 days. For patients needing frequent IV lidocaine infusions, a continuous SC infusion of 1–2 mg/kg/h lidocaine can be considered. A plasma concentration of 2–5 µg/mL should be achieved to determine whether lidocaine is effective. Common side effects of lidocaine are either neurologic (paresthesias, tremor, nausea of central origin, lightheadedness, hearing disturbances, slurred speech, and convulsions) or cardiovascular (bradycardia, hypotension, and cardiac arrhythmias). Patients with a history of myocardial dysfunction or arrhythmia may be at increased risk of serious cardiac events and should undergo an appropriate cardiac evaluation before local anesthetic therapy is initiated. Given the increased risk of arrhythmias, tricyclic antidepressants should be stopped at least 48 hours before starting lidocaine or mexiletine. Verbal analog scores are recorded before and after the trial is completed. Some clinicians advocate that a decrease of 50% or more in pain scores warrants a trial with an oral local anesthetic (mexiletine). The data are inconsistent but a select group of patients can experience a significant improvement using this strategy. In a prospective study, pain relief following an IV lidocaine test correlated with the subsequent response to mexiletine.[101] On the other hand, in a pilot study evaluating oral anesthetics for the treatment of cancer-related neuropathic pain, 90% of the patients didn't benefit from the treatment and 5 of 8 patients experienced intolerable nausea/gastrointestinal distress.[102] The trial medication delivered by the oral route is started with a dose of 150 mg at bedtime and, if tolerated, the dose is increased to a three-times-a-day schedule. Titration of the dose should be at 150 mg increments every 3–7 days, with a maximum dose of 1200 mg/day. Mexiletine can have significant side effects, such as gastrointestinal distress/nausea, dry mouth, and CNS symptoms, including sleep disturbance, headaches, and drowsiness. Treatment usually involves the infusion over 30 minutes of a dose that ranges between 2 and 5 mg/kg. A trial with an oral local anesthetic usually is considered after antidepressant and anticonvulsant drugs have been tried. IV or SC lidocaine may be useful in the treatment of severe, rapidly increasing neuropathic pain.

N-methyl-D-aspartate (NMDA) receptor antagonists

Excitatory amino acids play a fundamental role in pain transmission at the level of the spinal cord. Noxious stimuli activate A-delta and C fibers of pseudobipolar DRG neurons that project their axons to the posterior horn of the spinal cord. There they synapse with projection neurons that are localized in the laminae I and II. The neurotransmitters involved in this pathway are glutamate and substance P. Substance P is a peptide, which is inactivated rapidly. There

are no stable antagonists at this point that can be successfully utilized in clinical practice. On the other hand, glutamate is an excitatory amino acid that can be blocked with several stable drugs that are currently in use in clinical practice for other indications, including ketamine (anesthesia), dextromethorphan (antitussive), and mamentine (advanced Alzheimer's disease). For this reason, glutamate-mediated responses have received more attention than those mediated by substance P. Once in the biophase the two neurotransmitters, glutamate and substance P, activate projection neurons by binding selectively to postsynaptic receptors. The receptor activated by glutamate has been named after the NMDA ligand that also binds to it with high affinity. Under physiologic conditions, the response to painful stimuli is mediated by the normal release of glutamate at the level of primary afferent neurons in the posterior horn of the spinal cord.

Excitatory amino acids have been implicated in the development of abnormal responses that occur in neuropathic pain syndromes and also in the development of tolerance to opioids. Preclinical studies have established that NMDA receptors are involved in the sensitization of central neurons following injury and in the development of the "windup" phenomenon, a change in the response of central neurons. Trujillo and Akil,[103] in preclinical studies, suggested that hyperalgesia (one of the abnormal sensory findings in neuropathic pain) and the development of tolerance to opioids can be ameliorated by blocking the NMDA receptors. Shortly after clinical trials were conducted to determine a possible role for dextromethorphan and ketamine, these two NMDA receptor antagonists were widely utilized in the clinical setting. Although the affinity of dextromethorphan for the NMDA receptors is weak, it was found to be safe and well tolerated when utilized as an antitussive. Pierce and coworkers[104] studied the analgesic efficacy of dextromethorphan in PDN and PHN, two widely utilized models for neuropathic pain. The design was a double-blind placebo-controlled crossover study. A decrease in pain was observed in patients with PDN, whereas patients with PDN/PHN did not experience improvement. Patients were allowed to titrate the dose to obtain pain relief or relief from side effects. The doses required to produce pain relief were too high and most patients experienced side effects, indicating a very limited clinical tool. Clinical studies with ketamine were also performed and showed moderate benefit as well (see below). Preclinical studies by Pierce and coworkers[104] suggested that pretreatment with dextromethorphan could prevent the development of tolerance to morphine in mice. They assayed several combinations of the two compounds with an optimal ratio of about 1:1. Based on their data several clinical trials were conducted in patients with neuropathic pain using the same ratio of dextromethorphan to morphine (1:1), suggesting a role for this treatment modality.

Ketamine is an NMDA receptor antagonist utilized extensively in anesthesia due to its dissociative properties. Because of its toxicity and side effects, it is considered to be a third-line drug for the treatment of neuropathic pain. When combined with opioids it can be very effective. Indeed, the addition of oral ketamine significantly reduced pain scores in 7 of 9 cancer patients with severe neuropathic pain that were treated with opioids, sodium valproate, amitriptyline, or a combination of the above.[105] Ketamine can be utilized as an oral formulation or by IV or SC infusion. Oral ketamine can be added to the existing drug regime in a dose of 0.5 mg/kg three times a day. Continuous IV or SC infusion should be started at a dose of 2.5–5 mg/kg/24h and can be gradually increased by 50–100 mg/24h up to 500 mg/24h. Concomitant administration of antipsychotics or diazepam may reduce the risk of psychomimetic effects, such as derealization, visual or auditory hallucinations, nightmares, and delirium, that are limiting. Ketamine is contraindicated in patients with intracranial hypertension or seizures. There is some evidence that oral ketamine has a more favorable side-effect profile than parenteral ketamine, with drowsiness being the most common side effect to which the patient may develop tolerance over a 3-week period of time.

Opioids

The notion that neuropathic pain would not respond to opioid therapy was widely accepted and resulted in unnecessary suffering. About a decade ago, Portenoy and others[106] reported that as many as 50% of patient with this condition can respond to this form of therapy. Since then, many studies have been published showing similar results. More recently, the importance of aggressive treatment for neuropathic pain with opioids has been addressed. Studies in amputees with phantom pain showed changes in the cortical representation of the missing limb. Indeed, the cortical representation of the amputated arm decreased while neighboring areas (mouth) took over that region. Flor and coworkers showed that the sensory cortical representation of the lips will extend into the missing limb cortical area and that this takeover correlates with increased pain.[63] Of these patients, 50% responded to opioids and the reduction in pain correlated with reexpansion of the cortical representation of the missing limb. This study illustrates that aggressive opioid treatment of phantom pain, and perhaps other forms of neuropathic pain, can reverse plastic changes at the level of the sensory cortex. More studies are required to determine if long-lasting phantom pain changes in plasticity are reversible. In the study by Flor, morphine was the opioid of choice; however, any opioid can be utilized for the treatment of neuropathic pain.[63] The current recommendation by the WHO—the so-called "ladder approach"—is an excellent strategy for the treatment of pain in this patient population, including patients with neuropathic pain. The recommendation is to start treatment with the least potent agent and switch to a more potent opioid if maximal dosing has been achieved and pain control is inadequate. All full opioid agonists (codeine, morphine, oxycodone, fentanyl, methadone) have the potential of achieving a maximal therapeutic effect if there are no side effects and a gradual dose escalation can be accomplished. Methadone is an opioid that may produce an additional benefit compared to the classical mu agonists. In the United States, this agent is commercially available as a combination of the L- and D-enantiomers. The L-enantiomer produces analgesia through the activation of mu opioid receptors, whereas the D-enantiomer is a weak blocker of NMDA receptors. These receptors are activated by the naturally occurring excitatory amino acid glutamate and may be responsible for the development of allodynia and hyperalgesia, two cornerstone symptoms of neuropathic pain. In addition, Trujillo and Akil suggested a role for this excitatory neurotransmitter in the development of tolerance to opioids.[103] Hence, methadone could be accomplishing two important functions at once: analgesia plus blocking hyperalgesia and prevention of tolerance. Because of its long-lasting effect and low cost, many pain specialists are beginning to utilize methadone as a first-line agent for the treatment of neuropathic pain. This recent reemergence of methadone as an analgesic justifies a more detailed discussion of its unusual properties. Although it was originally developed as an analgesic during the World War II by the Germans, in the 1960s it was introduced for the treatment of opioid addiction. Based on the work by Dole[107] and Nyswander,[108] which proposed that drug addicts had an endogenous deficiency of opioids and that opioid utilization was a way to supplement this deficiency, clinics were created to provide methadone to this patient population. In time, methadone became stigmatized and identified by patients and the general public as a drug for drug addicts and was largely eliminated from the pain armamentarium. When using methadone to treat pain, a note of caution is the patient-to-patient half-life variability that can result in accumulation of the drug and toxicity. In addition, methadone has been identified as a drug with potential to prolong the QTc interval. This cardiac side effect was reported by Krantz and coworkers who reported several cases of fatal "torsades de pointes" in intensive care unit patients receiving methadone.[109] Some of the patients, however, had electrolyte abnormalities that could account for the tragic events. Most recently, Cruciani and coworkers[110] studied more than 100 patients who had received a wide range of methadone dosages for pain treatment or maintenance (up to 1.5 g/day) and did not find a single case of "torsades de pointes." Another study of IV methadone showed that the vehicle for this drug was responsible for the cardioelectrical abnormalities rather than the methadone itself.[111]

For patients with cancer-related neuropathic pain and comorbidity of drug abuse, who are currently enrolled in a methadone maintenance treatment program (MMTP), methadone can be prescribed for the treatment of pain in addition to using the maintenance dose. This strategy requires coordination with the patient's counselor in the program. The patient continues going to the program and receives his dose on a daily or weekly basis, depending on the patient, so that the pain practitioner then prescribes methadone solely for the treatment of pain. The schedule includes additional prescribed methadone divided into three or four doses, which are separate from the patient's daily morning maintenance dose. This additional amount of methadone can be titrated to pain and side effects, independently of the maintenance dose that may remain constant. The adjustment of the maintenance program would be done by the MMTP clinic, utilizing the usual criteria for the treatment of drug abuse.

Several approaches have been described to facilitate the switch from morphine to methadone.[112] In a recent publication, morphine was stopped and immediately substituted for with methadone, using different methadone:morphine ratios based on the patients' daily morphine doses: 1:4 (1 mg of oral methadone = 4 mg of oral morphine) for patients receiving less than 90 mg morphine per day, 1:8 for patients receiving 90–300 mg/day, and 1:12 for patients receiving more than 300 mg/day of morphine.[113] This changing equianalgesic ratio is based on the observation that the potency of methadone increases in patients with substantial prior opioid exposure. This observation may be explained by reversal of tolerance produced by the *d*-isomer. Practical aspects of prescribing methadone are outlined by another contributor in App. D.

Other drug classes

Several other drug classes may be useful for managing neuropathic pain (Table 7-6).

Corticosteroids Patients with cancer can present with diverse pain syndromes that may be ameliorated by the use of corticosteroids.[114,115]

Patients with metastatic disease to the spine can present with symptoms that are suggestive of spinal cord compression. In this situation IV dexamethasone 20–100 mg, followed by 60–90 mg daily in three divided doses is the drug of choice. This presentation is a medical emergency and steroids should be initiated before confirmatory ancillary studies are done. In addition, immediate consultation with radiation oncology should be requested. Steroids can be continued at this dose level until radiation is instituted (when applicable), after which the dose of corticosteroids is tapered gradually. Compression

Table 7-6

Other Oral Adjuvant Analgesics

Drug	Daily Dose	Dosing Interval	Evidence
Local Anesthetics			
Mexiletine	150–900 mg/d	Three times a day	CT
NMDA Antagonists			
Ketamine	1.5 mg/kg	Three times a day	OLT
Corticosteroids			
Prednisone	10–20 mg/d	Daily to twice a day	CR
Dexamethasone	2–4 mg/d	Daily to twice a day	CR
GABA Agonists			
Baclofen	30–200 mg/d	Three times a day	CT
Benzodiazepines			
Clonidine	1–10 mg/d	Twice a day	OLT
Alprazolam	0.75–1.5 mg/d	Three times a day	OLT
Diazepam	5–20 mg/d	Twice a day	CR

Abbreviations: CT = controlled trials, OLT = open-label trials, CR = case report.

of nerve roots by metastatic breast or prostate cancer to the vertebral bodies can also result in neuropathic pain. This syndrome can also benefit from radiation therapy or nerve blocks. Lymphoma-related neuropathy has a significant inflammatory and mass effect component and may benefit from corticosteroids as well. Doses can range from 5 to 10 mg prednisone or 1–2 mg dexamethasone once or twice daily. Initiation of treatment with adjuvant analgesics like gabapentin is recommended. Once therapeutic gabapentin levels are reached, corticosteroids can be tapered off.

Baclofen Baclofen is a muscle relaxant that binds to $GABA_B$ postsynaptic receptors, inducing increased K^+ conductance and reduced neuronal excitability. It has been shown to be effective in the treatment of trigeminal neuralgia and may be a useful drug for neuropathic pain in the medically ill.[116] In addition to its direct effectiveness for neuropathic pain, baclofen decreases muscle spasms and the pain associated with it. The benzodiazepines may have a similar effect through a different mechanism of action. When started at low doses (2.5–5 mg TID), the most common side effects of drowsiness, dizziness, and gastrointestinal distress are usually well tolerated. The dose should then be increased, if tolerated and necessary, by 5–10 mg every other day. Baclofen cannot be discontinued abruptly after prolonged use, as hallucinations, manic psychotic episodes, or seizures may occur.[116] Baclofen may be especially useful for patients with paroxysmal neuropathic pain.

Benzodiazepines A survey of cancer patients with mixed types of neuropathic pain suggested that alprazolam might have analgesic effects.[117] Pain can result in the development of muscle spasms, which in turn can cause more pain. The centrally mediated muscle relaxant effect of the benzodiazepines may contribute to a decrease in pain. Whether or not this group of pharmacologic agents has a direct analgesic effect is not entirely clear. However, patients with cancer pain commonly experience anxiety and muscle spasms, phenomena that may exacerbate the intensity of pain and respond well to other benzodiazepines, such as diazepam. Changes in mental status can occur during dose titration and must be monitored closely. Dosing should be started at the lowest possible dose.

Alpha-2 Adrenergic Agonists This group of agents activates the autoreceptors localized in the presynapses of noradrenergic neurons, decreasing the release of endogenous NE. Clonidine, the prototype of this family, has been utilized to treat hypertension for many years and has been successfully used to treat nonmalignant neuropathic pain. The severity of side effects and its limited benefit makes clonidine a second-line agent, which is utilized for refractory neuropathic pain only after other agents have failed. It can be administered orally, transdermally, or intraspinally. This route of administration is particularly useful in patients who are only partially responsive to opioids.

Tizanidine is a more selective alpha-2-adrenergic receptor agonist than clonidine and causes less hypotension. Current data support its use in myofascial pain syndrome as an antispasmodic and also in the prophylaxis of chronic daily headache. However, some positive reports for its use in treating neuropathic pain justify a trial after other adjuvants have failed.

Neuroleptics Olanzapine, a new generation neuroleptic, has been shown to improve pain and decrease the use of opioids in cancer patients. In a case series olanzapine improved cognitive function and decreased anxiety.[118] However, due to its potential severe side effects that include tardive dyskinesia and neuroleptic, malignant syndrome, and diabetes the recommendation is to use neuroleptics only in the presence of delirium or psychosis.

Bisphosphonates Bisphosphonates reduce bone reabsorption by inhibiting osteoclastic activity.[119] They have been shown to have analgesic properties in various disorders but the mechanism of action remains unclear. Pamidronate, the most extensively studied of the bisphosphonates, has been shown to have an analgesic effect in bone metastasis of patients with breast cancer and multiple myeloma. In addition, it has been shown to decrease the number of pathological fractures, to decrease the incidence of cord compression, and to decrease the need for radiation, as well as decreasing the occurrence of hypercalcemia. Although in general, pamidronate is well tolerated, it can cause a flu-like syndrome and hypocalcemia. The selection of patients for the prescription of pamidronate and other drugs of the same family has to be done on an individual basis due to the recent report of osteonecrosis of the jaw. The dose and frequency of treatment that can cause this side effect is still not clear and more data are necessary to draw definite guidelines. It should be avoided in patients with poor dental care.

Recently, more potent analogs have been introduced. Zoledronic acid, an analog, which is threefold more potent than pamidronate, has been shown to reduce pain in lung cancer, multiple myeloma,[120] and breast and prostate cancer. In a long-term follow-up study of 122 patients with prostate cancer skeletal-related events, the side effects were similar to those experienced with pamidronate. Zoledronic acid can be infused safely at a dose of 4 mg every 3 weeks. In contrast to pamidronate, the dose does not need to be adjusted for renal failure. Fatigue, nausea, and arthralgia are the most frequently observed side effects.

Clodronate is another agent of the same family that can be administered by mouth at a dose of 1600 mg/day.[121] The drug is not available in the United States and the analgesic effect in prostate cancer and multiple myeloma is not conclusive. However, clodronate was effective in the treatment of skeletal complications from prostate cancer. There was an objective response in 91.4% of treated patients, with a marked improvement in the subjective visual pain scale evaluation as well as on Karnofsky's index, with low side effects.

Etidronate, like clodronate, triggers apoptosis by generating a toxic analog of adenosine triphosphate, which then targets the mitochondria. Its inhibition suppresses protein geranylgeranylation, which is essential for the basic cellular processes required for osteoclastic bone resorption.

Calcitonin Data on the analgesic effect of calcitonin are inconclusive. A double-blind, placebo-controlled study in patients with CRPS type I found no positive effect.[122] However, positive results in patients with neuropathic pain in diverse diseases, including cancer, justify a trial with the intranasal formulation. The initial dose should be 200 IU, alternating nostrils to avoid epistaxis. The dose can be increased if no effects are observed but the maximal dose has not been well established. Although calcitonin has also been utilized SC and IV, the intranasal route of administration is more convenient.

Cannabinoids Animal studies suggest that cannabinoids may be useful analgesics for neuropathic pain.[123,124] CB1 acts on pathways that partly overlap with those affected by opioids such as morphine, but also acts through pharmacologically distinct mechanisms. There is evidence that oral delta-9-tetrahydrocannabinol (THC) and other cannabinoids can improve appetite, reduce nausea and vomiting, and alleviate moderate neuropathic pain in patients with cancer. CB1 is widely distributed throughout the CNS and peripheral nervous system, reaching high concentrations in periaqueductal grey matter.[125] Due to the similarities in the physical distribution of their receptors, cannabinoids and opioids may have additive or synergistic analgesic effects. Studies of analgesia in humans with experimentally induced pain have shown mixed results;[123] however, similar to the analgesic effects of opioids,[103] better analgesic results have been observed in clinical studies of cannabinoids in patients with severe, persistent cancer pain that was resistant to traditional analgesics.[123–125] These double-blind, placebo-controlled trials showed that cannabinoids had analgesic effects equal to those of codeine, and also improved mood, well-being, and appetite. In the setting of chronic pain, a series of well-designed studies[124,125] using THC, cannabidiol, both, or placebo are good evidence of the efficacy of cannabinoids and suggest that they may have a role in managing neuropathic pain, but have lesser efficacy for treating nociceptive pain.[124] A study of a cannabinoid analog in a few patients demonstrated a substantial analgesic effect for chronic pain, with fewer psychotropic effects.[126] In this 7-day, placebo-controlled trial, the cannabinoid analog significantly reduced pain 3 hours after use and the benefit lasted 6 hours. Water-soluble cannabinoids such as delta-8-THC-11-oic acid have a wider range of medication formulations and drug-delivery methods than THC but need to be studied in adequately powered clinical studies to assess their analgesic and other therapeutic effects.[127]

Topical analgesic therapies

Topical Lidocaine Lidocaine can be applied as a gel, cream, or patch. The lidocaine patch has become very popular because it is easy to apply and has a low profile of side effects. Lidocaine systemic absorption is minimal with no systemic side effects for up to three patches at a time (although monitoring for toxicity at initiation of treatment is recommended). Application of more than three patches may be useful for some patients, but this approach should be accompanied by initial monitoring for local anesthetic toxicity. An adequate trial may require several weeks of observation. The most frequently reported adverse event is mild to moderate skin redness, rash, or irritation at the site of the patch. Since lidocaine has a local mode of action it should be applied directly to the area where the pain is felt. Although the patch shouldn't be kept on for more than 12 hours at a time to avoid tachyphylaxis (acute tolerance), limited data suggest that it is safe to use lidocaine around the clock.[128] The 12-hour period of time should be customized to the patient's specific problem. If the pain is localized to the foot, it would probably be better to use it during the night so the patch stays in place.[128] The patch may be utilized in combination with other drugs that may be helpful in the treatment of neuropathic pain. In one study,[129] the simultaneous use of lidocaine patches with oral gabapentin, for example, showed that the total effect was greater that the sum of the effect of each individual agent.

Capsaicin Capsaicin is a peptide that depletes substance P, which along with glutamate, is the most important neurotransmitter for pain transmission in small primary afferent neurons in the posterior horn of the spinal cord. Capsaicin is applied locally in a 0.05% formula (starting dose) to the affected area. The application has to be done carefully and the mucosa should be avoided. The patient or patient's caretaker has to be warned to utilize disposable gloves because capsaicin can inadvertently cause painful irritation of the conjunctiva. Immediately after the first application, it may cause a severe burning sensation limited to the area of application that may result in abandonment of the treatment. Simultaneous application of 5% lidocaine may decrease the intensity of the initial burning. Despite this side effect, in a recent study on cancer patients with surgical neuropathic pain (e.g., postmastectomy syndrome), capsaicin was found to significantly decrease pain and was preferred by 60% of the patients.[130] If results are not seen in a week, it is unlikely that further treatment will result in pain relief.

▶ Nonpharmacologic interventions

There is good evidence that in patients with neuropathic pain that is poorly responsive to conservative management, invasive techniques such as peripheral nerve blocks and sympathetic neurolytic blocks can reduce analgesic requirements.[131] However, in neurolysis, exacerbation of pain through central sensitization may occur so that the use of these blocks has to be considered carefully and only after the pain syndrome is shown to be refractory to several trials of adjuvant drugs. Different techniques, including psychological interventions (e.g., guided imagery, hypnosis, and other approaches), physical therapy, and neurostimulation (e.g., transcutaneous electrical nerve stimulation), have shown benefit in some clinical trials and from clinical experience.

Intraspinal therapy

Opioids in combination with adjuvant therapy benefit most patients. However, for a small percentage of patients with severe, intractable neuropathic pain, intrathecal or epidural application of analgesic drugs can help. This strategy may also reduce the need for systemic opioids in patients who experience unacceptable side effects. Most patients undergoing these procedures still require a certain amount of systemic therapy as well.[132] Neuropathic pain is poorly responsive to spinal opioids alone but in combination with local anesthetics or alpha-2-adrenergic agonists (e.g., clonidine), they may be efficacious.[132] In one study, the epidural infusion of bupivacaine 0.1%–0.5% in addition to morphine was very helpful. Sensory loss was observed only at bupivacaine concentrations above 0.25%, and motor weakness at concentrations over 0.35%.[133] In an uncontrolled study in patients with severe refractory cancer pain, a constant intrathecal infusion of 0.5 mg/mL morphine plus 4.75 mg/mL bupivacaine resulted in good pain relief.[133] Side effects that included urinary retention, paresthesias, paresis, and gait impairment were observed in approximately one-third of the patients but these did not interfere with the trial. In addition, a controlled study in 85 cancer patients with refractory pain syndromes demonstrated adequate neuropathic relief in more than 50% of the patients treated with 30 μg/h epidural clonidine together with rescue epidural morphine.[134] Most common side effects are hypotension and bradycardia, and patients should be monitored thoroughly during the first treatment days. Baclofen has demonstrated powerful antinociceptive effects in experimental animal models at doses that produce little or no motor-blocking effects but has rarely been used as a spinal analgesic agent in patients without spasticity. So far, three studies have shown it to be effective in patients with peripheral nociceptive or neuropathic pain mechanisms. In clinical and animal studies, combinations of baclofen and morphine or clonidine have demonstrated greater efficacy than each drug alone.[135]

PHN may be very resistant to treatment. In a double-blind, placebo-controlled study of 277 patients, Kotani et al.[136] showed significant improvement in pain symptoms in intractable PHN with the administration of intrathecal methylprednisolone.[136]

Current strategies to prevent the development of peripheral neuropathy induced by chemotherapy

With longer disease-free intervals due to advances in cancer therapy, quality of life has become increasingly important in selecting the right chemotherapeutic regimen for individual patients. At present, there is no specific treatment for toxic neuropathy, and in most cases the effects of neuropathic pain on quality of life are not reversible. Therefore, prevention or attenuation of toxic neuropathy remains a major goal. In addition, recent data suggest that a subset of patients, including those with a history of diabetes and those in whom neuropathy is present at the time of chemotherapy, and patients receiving high-dose regimens, are at higher risk for developing neuropathy. Since the development of neuropathy is often the dose-limiting factor, the prevention of this toxicity might allow the use of higher doses of chemotherapeutic agents and potentially improve their efficacy.[137]

Oxiliplatin in addition to FOLFOX has become a first-line treatment for colon cancer. Oxiliplatin can induce acute cold-triggered painful neuropathy (self-limiting) and cumulative chronic neuropathy, which is seen most frequently in patients who received ≥ 540 mg/m². It has been suggested that the neuropathy is induced by the liberation of the metabolite oxalate, which alters the normal functioning of neuronal voltage-gated Na channels. The effect of calcium and magnesium, which are oxalate chelators, was studied in a double-blind, placebo-controlled study in 161 patients. Ninety six patients were infused with Ca gluconate (1 g) and Mg sulfate (1 g) before and after oxiliplatin infusion. Only 4% of patients withdrew for neurotoxicity

in the Ca/Mg group versus 31% in the control group. In this study, calcium and magnesium solutions reduced the severity of symptoms without affecting tumor response to chemotherapy.[138,139] Although *cis*-platinum has been replaced by carboplatin in most chemotherapy regimens due to its toxicity, it is still utilized for the treatment of neck and head cancer. Peripheral neuropathy secondary to *cis*-platinum is well documented. Once the neuropathy has developed it cannot be reversed. Some degree of protection against the development of peripheral neuropathy induced by *cis*-platinum has been reported with an adrenocorticotropic 4-9 hormone analog (ORG 2766) and the radioprotective agent WR2721 and nimodipine, and delayed development of neuropathy and tolerability of higher doses of vincristine or a combination of *cis*-platin and paclitaxel in the rat model. There are phase II and III clinical trials that evaluated the effect of recombinant human nerve growth factor (rhNGF) on human immunodeficiency virus (HIV) and diabetic peripheral neuropathy. In addition, gangliosides, glutamic acid, isaxonine, prednisone, pyridoxine, folic acid, and ORG 2766, induced some improvement in vincristine-associated toxic peripheral neuropathy. However, none of these strategies are routinely utilized in clinical practice.[57] Low levels of vitamin E were reported after 2–4 cycles of cisplatin and a correlation with neuropathy was suggested.[140] The neuroprotective effect of vitamin E on neuropathy induced by cisplatin, paclitaxel, or their combination has been tested in a pilot, randomized, open label with blind assessment, controlled trial. The mean peripheral neuropathy scores were 3.4 ± 6.3 for the treatment group and 11.5 ± 10.6 for the control ($p = 0.026$). These data suggest that vitamin E supplementation in cancer patients may have a neuroprotective effect.[141] A recent report suggests a possible role for topiramate and venlafaxine in oxiliplatin-induced disabling permanent neuropathy.[142] Nonpharmacologic strategies, including light weightlifting and stretching exercises, can result in mild improvement of symptoms.

New strategies for the treatment of hyperalgesia

In the early 1990s, Trujillo and Akil recognized the role of excitatory amino acids in hyperalgesia and development of tolerance to opioids.[103] In addition, Mao et al. explored the benefits of simultaneous administration of opioids and dextromethorphan in the animal model.[100] Based on this observation, several clinical trials utilizing various NMDA antagonists alone or in combination with opioids were designed. In view of the disappointing results other strategies were explored. About a decade ago Crain and Shen[143] observed that ultra-low doses of naltrexone, an opioid antagonist used to reverse opioid overdose, can potentiate the effect of most opioids tested. This so-called bimodal effect is the result of the simultaneous activation of opioid-mediated excitation (caused by ultra-low doses of opioids) and inhibition (elicited by a "pharmacologic" dose of identical opioids). The way the system works is that excitation (hyperalgesia) can be blocked with ultra-low doses of the antagonist, potentiating inhibition. Cruciani and Pasternak suggested that the mechanism is mediated by G_s alpha protein by intrathecal administration of antisense oligonucleotides directed against G_s alpha mRNA.[144] These results were in agreement with in vitro experiments by Crain and Shen.[143] The notion of two systems mediating hyperalgesia in neuropathic pain suggests that successful intervention can occur only if the two systems are simultaneously shut down. The design of clinical studies focusing on concomitant blockade of NMDA receptors and ultra-low dose opioid antagonists may prove to be the successful model.

CONCLUSION

The treatment of neuropathic pain in cancer patients can be very challenging and may require several trials with different types of drugs before equilibrium between side effects and pain relief can be achieved. We are proposing an algorithm to help navigate a decision tree that is not always clear to the nonpain practitioners (Fig. 7-1). The armamentarium for the treatment of neuropathic pain has increased rapidly in the last few years, presenting the practitioner with many different options. Adequate knowledge of the pain syndromes in cancer patients and available treatment options will assist the practitioner in selecting a successful treatment regimen. In general, opioids combined with adjuvant analgesics may be the best combination for most patients.

REFERENCES

1. Caraceni A, Portenoy RK. An international survey of cancer pain characteristics and syndromes. IASP Task Force on Cancer Pain. International Association for the Study of Pain. *Pain.* 1999;82:263–274.
2. Grond S, Radbruch L, Meuser T, et al. Assessment and treatment of neuropathic cancer pain following WHO guidelines. *Pain.* 1999;79: 15–20.
3. Anderson KO, Syrjala KL, Cleeland CS. How to assess cancer pain. In: Turk DC, Melzack R, eds. *Handbook of Pain Assessment.* New York, London: The Guilford Press; 2001:579–600.
4. Cleeland CS, Gonin R, Hatfield R, et al. Pain and its treatment in outpatients with metastatic cancer. *N Engl J Med.* 1994;330:592–596.
5. Katz N. Neuropathic pain in cancer and AIDS. *Clin J Pain.* 2000;16:S41–S48.
6. Boucher TJ, Okuse K, Bennett DL, et al. Potent analgesic effects of GDNF in neuropathic pain states. *Science.* 2000;290:124.
7. Empl M, Renaud S, Erne B, et al. TNF-alpha expression in painful and nonpainful neuropathies. *Neurology.* 2001;56:1371–1377.
8. McGaraughty S, Wismer CT, Zhu CZ, et al. Effects of A-317491, a novel and selective P2X3/P2X2/3 receptor antagonist, on neuropathic, inflammatory and chemogenic nociception following intrathecal and intraplantar administration. *Br J Pharmacol.* 2003;140:1381–1388.
9. Jin SX, Zhuang ZY, Woolf CJ, et al. p38 mitogen-activated protein kinase is activated after a spinal nerve ligation in spinal cord microglia and dorsal root ganglion neurons and contributes to the generation of neuropathic pain. *J Neurosci.* 2003;23:4017–4022.
10. Dworkin RH, Backonja M, Rowbotham MC et al. Advances in neuropathic pain: diagnosis, mechanisms, and treatment recommendations. *Arch Neurol.* 2003;60:1524–1434.
11. Chen R, Cohen LG, Hallett M. Nervous system reorganization following injury. *Neuroscience.* 2002;111:761–773.
12. Elbert T, Flor H, Birbaumer N, et al. Extensive reorganization of the somatosensory cortex in adult humans after nervous system injury. *Neuroreport.* 1994;5:2593–2597.
13. Harris AJ. Cortical origin of pathological pain. *Lancet.* 1999;354: 1464–1466.
14. Maihofner C, Handwerker HO, Neundorfer B, et al. Patterns of cortical reorganization in complex regional pain syndrome. *Neurology.* 2003;61:1707–1715.
15. Peyron R, Schneider F, Faillenot I, et al. An fMRI study of cortical representation of mechanical allodynia in patients with neuropathic pain. *Neurology.* 2004;63:1838–1846.
16. Martin LA, Hagen NA. Neuropathic pain in cancer patients: mechanisms, syndromes, and clinical controversies. *J Pain Symptom Manage.* 1997;14:99–117.
17. Amato AA, Collins MP. Neuropathies associated with malignancy. *Semin Neurol.* 1998;18:125–144.
18. Farrar JT, Portenoy RK. Neuropathic cancer pain: the role of adjuvant analgesics. *Oncology (Williston Park).* 2001;15:1435–1442.
19. Luger NM, Mach DB, Sevcik MA, et al. Bone cancer pain: from model to mechanism to therapy. *J Pain Symptom Manage.* 2005;29:S32–S46.
20. Lerner UH. Neuropeptidergic regulation of bone resorption and bone formation. *J Musculoskelet Neuronal Interact.* 2002;2:440–447.
21. Davis JB, Gray J, Gunthorpe MJ, et al. Vanilloid receptor-1 is essential for inflammatory thermal hyperalgesia. *Nature.* 2000;405:183–187.
22. Vergnolle N, Bunnett NW, Sharkey KA, et al. Proteinase-activated receptor-2 and hyperalgesia: a novel pain pathway. *Nat Med.* 2001;7:821–826.
23. Knotkova H, Pappagallo M. Pharmacology of pain transmission and modulation. II. Peripheral mechanisms. In: Pappagallo M, ed. *The Neurological Basis of Pain.* New York: McGraw-Hill; 2005:53–60.
24. Black JA, Liu S, Tanaka M, et al. Changes in the expression of tetrodotoxin-sensitive sodium channels within dorsal root ganglia neurons in inflammatory pain. *Pain.* 2004;108:237–247.
25. Waxman SG, Dib-Hajj SD. Erythromelalgia: a hereditary pain syndrome enters the molecular era. *Ann Neurol.* 2005;57:785–788.
26. Ross RA, Coutts AA, McFarlane SM, et al. Actions of cannabinoid receptor ligands on rat cultured sensory neurones: implications for antinociception. *Neuropharmacology.* 2001;40:221–232.
27. Piomelli D, Beltramo M, Giuffrida A, Stella N, et al. Endogenous cannabinoid signaling. *Neurobiol Dis.* 1998;5:462–473.
28. Calignano A, La Rana G, Giuffrida A, et al. Control of pain initiation by endogenous cannabinoids. *Nature.* 1998;394:277–281.
29. Marais E, Klugbauer N, Hofmann F. Calcium channel alpha(2) delta subunits—structure and Gabapentin binding. *Mol Pharmacol.* 2001;59:1243–1248.
30. Sutton KG, Martin DJ, Pinnock RD. Gabapentin inhibits high-threshold calcium channel currents in cultured rat dorsal horn ganglion neurones. *Br J Pharmacol.* 2002;135:257–265.
31. Lai J, Hunter JC, Porreca F. The role of voltage-gated sodium channels in neuropathic pain. *Curr Opin Neurobiol.* 2003;13:291–297.
32. Davis AJ, Perkins MN. Induction of B1 receptors in vivo in a model of persistent inflammatory mechanical hyperalgesia in the rat. *Neuropharmacology.* 1994;33:127–133.
33. Seabrook GR, Bowery BJ, Heavens R, et al. Expression of B1 and B2 bradykinin receptor mRNA and their functional roles in sympathetic ganglia and sensory dorsal root ganglia neurones from wild-type and B2 receptor knockout mice. *Neuropharmacology.* 1997;36:1009–1017.
34. Gomes JA, Li X, Pan HL, et al. Intrathecal adenosine interacts with a spinal noradrenergic system to produce antinociception in nerve-injured rats. *Anesthesiology.* 1999;91:1072–1079.
35. Khandwala H, Zhang Z, Loomis CW. Inhibition of strychnine-allodynia is mediated by spinal adenosine A1- but not A2-receptors in the rat. *Brain Res.* 1998;808:106–109.
36. Pappagallo M, Gaspardone A, Tomai F, et al. Analgesic effect of bamiphylline on pain induced by intradermal injection of adenosine. *Pain.* 1993;53:199–204.
37. Sawynok J. Adenosine receptor activation and nociception. *Eur J Pharmacol.* 1998;347:1–11.
38. Zhu CZ, Mikusa J, Chu KL, et al. A-134974: a novel adenosine kinase inhibitor, relieves tactile allodynia via spinal sites of action in a peripheral nerve injured rats. *Brain Res.* 2001;905:104–110.
39. Suzuki R, Chapman V, Dickenson AH. The effectiveness of spinal and systemic morphine on rat dorsal horn neuronal responses in the spinal nerve ligation model of neuropathic pain. *Pain.* 1999;80:215–228.
40. Matthews EA, Dickenson AH. Effects of spinally delivered N- and P-type voltage-dependent calcium channel antagonists on dorsal horn neuronal responses in a rat model of neuropathy. *Pain.* 2001;92:235–246.
41. Zhou XF, Deng YS, Xian CJ, et al. Neurotrophins from dorsal root ganglia trigger allodynia after spinal nerve injury in rats. *Eur J Neurosci.* 2000;12:100–105.
42. Schafers M, Svensson CI, Sommer C, et al. Tumor necrosis factor-alpha induces mechanical allodynia after spinal nerve ligation by activation of p38 MAPK in primary sensory neurons. *J Neurosci.* 2003;23: 2517–2525.
43. Jarvis MF, Burgard EC, McGaraughty S, et al. A-317491, a novel potent and selective non-nucleotide antagonist of P2X3, and P2X2/3 receptors, reduces chronic inflammatory and neuropathic pain in the rat. *Proc Natl Acad Sci USA.* 2002;99:17179–17185.
44. Boureau F, Doubrere JF, Luu M. Study of verbal description in neuropathic pain. *Pain.* 1990;42:145–152.
45. Wallington M, Mendis S, Premawardhana U, et al. Local control and survival in spinal cord compression from lymphoma and myeloma. *Radiother Oncol.* 1997;42:43–47.

46. Correale J, Monteverde JA, Bueri JA, et al. Peripheral nervous system and spinal cord involvement in lymphoma. *Acta Neurol Scand.* 1991;83:45–51.

47. Vecht CJ. Cancer pain: a neurological perspective. *Curr Opin Neurol.* 2000;13:649–653.

48. Dimopoulos MA, Alexanian R. Waldenström's macroglobulinemia. *Blood.* 1994;83:1452–1459.

49. Kissel JT, Mendell JR. Neuropathies associated with monoclonal gammopathies. *Neuromuscul Disord.* 1996;6:3–18.

50. Wicklund MP, Kissel JT. Paraproteinemic neuropathy. *Curr Treat Options Neurol.* 2001;3:147–156.

51. Chaudhry V, Chaudhry M, Crawford TO, et al. Toxic neuropathy in patients with pre-existing neuropathy. *Neurology.* 2003;60:337–340.

52. Hammack JE, Michalak JC, Loprinzi CL, et al. Phase III evaluation of nortriptyline for alleviation of symptoms of cis-platinum-induced peripheral neuropathy. *Pain.* 2002;98:195–203.

53. Postma TJ, Hoekman K, van Riel JM, et al. Peripheral neuropathy due to biweekly paclitaxel, epirubicin and cisplatin in patients with advanced ovarian cancer. *J Neurooncol.* 1999;45:241–246.

54. Quasthoff S, Hartung HP. Chemotherapy-induced peripheral neuropathy. *J Neurol.* 2002;249(1):9–17.

55. Grothey A. Clinical management of oxiliplatin-associated neurotoxicity. *Clin Colorectal Cancer.* 2005;5(Suppl. 1):S38–S46.

56. Lehky TJ, Leonard GD, Wilson RH, et al. Oxiliplatin-induced neurotoxicity: acute hyperexcitability and chronic neuropathy. *Muscle Nerve.* 2004;29:387–392.

57. Posner JB. Side effects of chemotherapy. In: Posner JB, ed. *Neurologic Complications of Cancer.* Philadelphia, PA: E.A. Davis Company; 1995:282–310.

58. Krishnan AV, Goldstein D, Friedlander M, et al. Oxiliplatin-induced neurotoxicity and the development of neuropathy. *Muscle Nerve.* 2005;32:51–60.

59. Verstappen CC, Heimans JJ, Hoekman K, et al. Neurotoxic complications of chemotherapy in patients with cancer: clinical signs and optimal management. *Drugs.* 2003;63:1549–1563.

60. Argyriou AA, Polychronopoulos P, Koutras A, et al. Peripheral neuropathy induced by administration of cisplatin- and paclitaxel-based chemotherapy. Could it be predicted? *Support Care Cancer.* 2005;13:647–651.

61. Chaudhry V, Cornblath DR, Corse A, et al. Thalidomide-induced neuropathy. *Neurology.* 2002;59:1872–1875.

62. Birbaumer N, Lutzenberg W, Montoya P, et al. Effects of regional anesthesia on phantom limb pain are mirrored in changes in cortical reorganization. *J Neurosci.* 1997;17:5503–5508.

63. Flor H, Elbert T, Knecht S, et al. Phantom limb pain as a perceptual correlate of massive cortical reorganization following arm amputation. *Nature.* 1995;375:482–484.

64. Karl A, Birbaumer N, Lutzenberger W, et al. Reorganization of motor and somatosensory cortex in upper extremity amputees with phantom limb pain. *J Neurosci.* 2001;21:3609–3618.

65. Kew JJ, Ridding MC, Rothwell JC, et al. Reorganization of cortical blood flow and transcranial magnetic stimulation maps in human subjects after upper limb amputation. *J Neurophysiol.* 1994;72:2517–2524.

66. Pascual-Leone A, Peris M, Tormos JM, et al. Reorganization of human cortical motor output maps following traumatic forearm amputation. *Neuroreport.* 1996;7:2068–2070.

67. Sherman RA, Arena JG. Phantom limb pain: mechanisms, incidence, and treatment. *Clin Rev Phys Rehabil Med.* 1992;4:1–26.

68. Jeannerod M. The representing brain: neural correlates of motor intention and imagery. *Brain Behav Sci.* 1994;17:187–245.

69. Jeannerod M. Mental imagery in the motor context. *Neuropsychologia.* 1995;33:1419–1432.

70. Lotze M, Grodd W, Birbaumer N, et al. Does the use of a myoelectric prosthesis prevent cortical reorganization and phantom limb pain? *Nat Neurosci.* 1999;2:501–502.

71. Lotze M, Flor H, Grodd W, et al. Phantom movements and pain. An fMRI study in upper limb amputees. *Brain.* 2001;124:2268–2277.

72. Pezzin LE, Dillingham TR, MacKenzie EJ. Rehabilitation and the long-term outcomes of persons with trauma-related amputations. *Arch Phys Med Rehabil.* 2000;81:292–300.

73. Johnson R. Herpes zoster—predicting and minimizing the impact of post-herpetic neuralgia. *J Antimicrob Chemother.* 2001;Suppl T1:1–8.

74. Haanpaa M, Laippala P, Nurmikko T. Allodynia and pinprick hypesthesia in acute herpes zoster, and the development of postherpetic neuralgia. *J Pain Symptom Manage.* 2000;20:50–58.

75. Tremonts-Lukats IW, Megeff C, Backonja MM. Anticonvulsants for neuropathic pain syndromes: mechanisms of action and place in therapy. *Drugs.* 2000;60:1029–1052.

76. Backonja M, Beydoun A, Edwards KR, et al. Gabapentin for the symptomatic treatment of painful neuropathy in patients with diabetes mellitus: a randomized controlled trial. *JAMA.* 1998;280:1831–1836.

77. Rowbotham M, Harden N, Stacey B, et al. Gabapentin for the treatment of postherpetic neuralgia: a randomized controlled trial. *JAMA.* 1998;280:1837–1842.

78. Caraceni A, Zecca E, Martini C, et al. Gabapentin as an adjuvant to opioid analgesia for neuropathic cancer pain. *J Pain Symptom Manage.* 1999;17:441–445.

79. Bosnjak S, Jelic S, Susnjar S, et al. Gabapentin for relief of neuropathic pain related to anticancer treatment: a preliminary study. *J Chemother.* 2002;14:214–219.

80. Twycross R, Wilcock A, Charlesworth S, Dickman A, eds. *Palliative Care Formulary.* 2nd ed. Abingdon: Radcliffe Medical Press; 2002.

81. Gilron I, Bailey JM, Tu D, et al. Morphine, gabapentin, or their combination for neuropathic pain. *N Engl J Med.* 2005;31(352):1324–1334.

82. Richter RW, Portenoy R, Sharma U, et al. Relief of painful diabetic peripheral neuropathy with pregabalin: a randomized, placebo-controlled trial. *J Pain.* 2005;6:253–260.

83. Freynhagen R, Strojek K, Griesing T, et al. Efficacy of pregabalin in neuropathic pain evaluated in a 12-week, randomized, double-blind, multicentre, placebo-controlled trial of flexible- and fixed-dose regimens. *Pain.* 2005;115:254–263.

84. Hadj Tahar A. Pregabalin for peripheral neuropathic pain. *Issues Emerg Health Technol.* 2005;67:1–4.

85. Brodie MJ. Lamotrigine. *Lancet.* 1992;339:1397–1400.

86. Guay DR. Oxcarbazepine, topiramate, zonisamide, and levetiracetam: potential use in neuropathic pain. *Am J Geriatr Pharmacother.* 2003;1:18–37.

87. Nakamura-Craig M, Follenfant RL. Effect of lamotrigine in the effect of acute and chronic hyperalgesia induced by PGE2 and in the chronic hyperalgesia in rats with streptozotocin-induced diabetes. *Pain.* 1995;63:33–37.

88. Canavero S, Bonicalzi V. Lamotrigine control of central pain. *Pain.* 1996;68:179–181.

89. Vestergaard K, Andersen G, Gottrup H, et al. Lamotrigine for central post-stroke pain: a randomized controlled trial. *Neurology.* 2001;56: 184–190.

90. Mockenhaupt M, Messenheimer J, Tennis P, et al. Risk of Stevens-Johnson syndrome and toxic epidermal necrolysis in new users of antiepileptics. *Neurology.* 2005;64:1134–1138.

91. Sobotka JL, Alexander B, Cook BL. A review of carbamazepine's hematologic reactions and monitoring recommendations. *DICP.* 1990;24:1214–1219.

92. Max MB, Lynch SA, Muir J, et al. Effects of desipramine, amitriptyline, and fluoxetine on pain in diabetic neuropathy. *N Engl J Med.* 1992;326:1250–1256.

93. Watson CP, Vernich L, Chipman M, et al. Nortriptyline versus amitriptyline in postherpetic neuralgia: a randomized trial. *Neurology.* 1998;51:1166.

94. Morello CM, Lechband SG, Stoner CP, et al. Randomized double blind study comparing the efficacy of gabapentin with amitriptyline in diabetic peripheral neuropathy pain. *Arch Intern Med.* 1999;59:1931–1937.

95. Kalso E, Tasmuth T, Neuvonen P. Amitriptyline effectively relieves neuropathic pain following treatment of breast cancer. *Pain.* 1996;64: 293–302.

96. Ansari A. The efficacy of newer antidepressants in the treatment of chronic pain: a review of current literature. *Harv Rev Psychiatry.* 2000;7:257–277.

97. Semenchuk MR, Sherman S, Davis B. Double-blind, randomized trial of bupropion SR for the treatment of neuropathic pain. *Neurology.* 2001;57:1583–1588.

98. Goldstein DJ, Lu Y, Detke MJ, et al. Duloxetine vs. placebo in patients with painful diabetic neuropathy. *Pain.* 2005;116:109–118.

99. Sindrup SH, Grodum E, Gram LF, et al. Concentration-response relationship in paroxetine treatment of diabetic neuropathy symptoms: a patient-blinded dose-escalation study. *Ther Drug Monit.* 1991;13: 408–414.

100. Mao J, Chen LL. Systemic lidocaine for neuropathic pain relief. *Pain.* 2000;87:7–17.

101. Galer BS, Harle J, Rowbotham MC. Response to intravenous lidocaine infusion predicts subsequent response to oral mexiletine: a prospective study. *J Pain Symptom Manage.* 1996;12:161–167.

102. Chong SF, Bretscher ME, Mailliard JA, et al. Pilot study evaluating local anesthetics administered systemically for treatment of pain in patients with advanced cancer. *J Pain Symptom Manage.* 1997;13:112–117.

103. Trujillo KA, Akil H. Inhibition of morphine tolerance and dependence by the NMDA receptor antagonist MK-801. *Science.* 1991;251:85–87.

104. Pierce TL, Tiong GK, Olley JE. Morphine and methadone dependence in the rat: withdrawal and brain met-enkephalin levels. *Pharmacol Biochem Behav.* 1992;42:91–96.

105. Kannan TR, Saxena A, Bhatnagar S, et al. Oral ketamine as an adjuvant to oral morphine for neuropathic pain in cancer patients. *J Pain Symptom Manage.* 2002;23:60–65.

106. Portenoy RK, Khan E, Layman M, et al. Chronic morphine therapy for cancer pain: plasma and cerebrospinal fluid morphine and morphine-6-glucuronide concentrations. *Neurology.* 1991;41:1457–1461.

107. Dole VP. Implications of methadone maintenance for theories of narcotic addiction. *JAMA.* 1988;260:3025–3029.

108. Nyswander M, Dole VP. The present status of methadone blockade treatment. *Am J Psychiatry.* 1967;123:1441–1442.

109. Krantz MJ, Kutinsky IB, Robertson AD, et al. Dose-related effects of methadone on QT prolongation in a series of patients with torsade de pointes. *Pharmacotherapy.* 2003;23:802–805.

110. Cruciani RA, Sekine R, Homel P, et al. Measurements of QTc in patients receiving chronic methadone therapy. *J Pain Symptom Manage.* 2005;29:385–391.

111. Kornick CA, Kilborn MJ, Santiago-Palma J, et al. QTc interval prolongation associated with intravenous methadone. *Pain.* 2003;105: 499–506.

112. Mercadante S. Opioid rotation for cancer pain: rationale and clinical aspects. *Cancer.* 1999;86:1856–1866.

113. Mercadante S, Cacuccio A, Fulfaro F, et al. Switching from morphine to methadone to improve analgesia and tolerability in cancer patients: a prospective study. *J Clin Oncol.* 2001;19:2898–2904.

114. Vecht CJ, Haaxma-Reiche H, van Putten WL, et al. Initial bolus of conventional versus high-dose dexamethasone in metastatic spinal cord compression. *Neurology.* 1989;39:1255–1257.

115. Watanabe S, Bruera E. Corticosteroids as adjuvant analgesics. *J Pain Symptom Manage.* 1994;9:442–445.

116. Fromm GH. Baclofen as an adjuvant analgesic. *J Pain Symptom Manage.* 1994;9:500–509.

117. Fernandez F, Adams F, Holmes VF. Analgesic effect of alprazolam in patients with chronic, organic pain of malignant origin. *J Clin Psychopharmacol.* 1987;7:167–169.

118. Khojainova N, Santiago-Palma J, Kornick C, et al. Olanzapine in the management of cancer pain. *J Pain Symptom Manage.* 2002; 23: 346–350.

119. Pavlakis N, Schmidt R, Stockler M. Bisphosphonates for breast cancer. *Cochrane Database Syst Rev.* 2005. CD003474.

120. Terpos E, Dimopoulos MA. Myeloma bone disease: pathophysiology and management. *Ann Oncol.* 2005;16:1223–1231.

121. Reszka AA, Rodan GA. Mechanism of action of bisphosphonates. *Curr Osteoporos Rep.* 2003;1:45–52.

122. Kovcin V, Jelic S, Babovic N, Tomasevic Z. A pilot study to assess the efficacy of salmon calcitonin in the relief of neuropathic pain caused by extraskeletal metastases. *Support Care Cancer.* 1994;2(1):71–73.

123. Hohmann AG. Spinal and peripheral mechanisms of cannabinoid antinociception: behavioral, neurophysiological and neuroanatomical perspectives. *Chem Phys Lipids.* 2002;121:173–190.

124. Goya P, Jagerovic N, Hernandez-Folgado L, et al. Cannabinoids and neuropathic pain. *Mini Rev Med Chem.* 2003;3:765–772.

125. Cravatt BF, Lichtman AH. The endogenous cannabinoid system and its role in nociceptive behavior. *J Neurobiol.* 2004;61:149–160.

126. Karst M, Salim K, Burstein S. Analgesic effect of the synthetic cannabinoid CT-3 on chronic neuropathic pain: a randomized controlled trial. *JAMA.* 20003;290:1757–1762.

127. Pertwee RG. Cannabinoid receptors and pain. *Prog Neurobiol.* 2001;63:569–611.

128. Galer BS, Rowbotham MC, Perander J, et al. Topical lidocaine patch relieves postherpetic neuralgia more effectively than a vehicle topical patch: results of an enriched enrollment study. *Pain.* 1999;80: 533–538.

129. White WT, Patel N, Drass M, Nalamachu S. Lidocaine patch 5% with systemic analgesics such as gabapentin: a rational polypharmacy approach for the treatment of chronic pain. *Pain Med.* 2003;4:321–330.

130. Ellison N, Loprinzi CL, Kugler J, et al. Phase III placebo-controlled trial of capsaicin cream in the management of surgical neuropathic pain in cancer patients. *J Clin Oncol.* 1997;15:2974–2980.

131. Abram SE. Neural blockade for neuropathic pain. *Clin J Pain.* 2000;16:S56–S61.

132. Bennett G, Serafini M, Burchiel K, et al. Evidence-based review of the literature on intrathecal delivery of pain medication. *J Pain Symptom Manage.* 2000;20:S12–S36.

133. Du Pen SL, Kharash ED, Williams A, et al. Chronic epidural bupivacaine-opioid infusion in intractable cancer pain. *Pain.* 1992;49:293–300.

134. Eisenach JC, DuPen S, Dubois M, et al. Epidural clonidine analgesia for intractable cancer pain. The Epidural Clonidine Study Group. *Pain.* 1995;61(3):391–399.

135. Slonimski M, Abram SE, Zuniga RE. Intrathecal baclofen in pain management. *Reg Anesth Pain Med.* 2004;29:269–276.

136. Kotani N, Kushikata T, Hashimoto H, et al. Intrathecal methylprednisolone for intractable postherpetic neuralgia. *N Engl J Med.* 2000;343:1514–1519.

137. Visovsky C. Chemotherapy-induced peripheral neuropathy. *Cancer Invest.* 2003;21:439–451.

138. Gamelin L, Boisdron-Celle M, Delva R, et al. Prevention of oxiliplatin-related neurotoxicity by calcium and magnesium infusions: a retrospective study of 161 patients receiving oxiliplatin combined with 5-Fluorouracil and leucovorin for advanced colorectal cancer. *Clin Cancer Res.* 2004;15;10:4055–4061.

139. Cersosimo RJ. Oxiliplatin-associated neuropathy: a review. *Ann Pharmacother.* 2005;39:128–135.

140. Bove L, Picardo M, Maresca V, et al. A pilot study on the relation between cisplatin neuropathy and vitamin E. *J Exp Clin Cancer Res.* 2001; 20:277–280.

141. Argyriou AA, Chroni E, Koutras A, et al. Vitamin E for prophylaxis against chemotherapy-induced neuropathy: a randomized controlled trial. *Neurology.* 2005;64:26–31.

142. Durand JP, Alexandre J, Guillevin L, et al. Clinical activity of venlafaxine and topiramate against oxiliplatin-induced disabling permanent neuropathy. *Anticancer Drugs.* 2005;16:587–591.

143. Crain SM, Shen KF. Ultra-low concentrations of naloxone selectively antagonize excitatory effects of morphine on sensory neurons, thereby increasing its antinociceptive potency and attenuating tolerance/dependence during chronic cotreatment. *Proc Natl Acad Sci USA.* 1995;92: 10540–10544.

144. Cruciani RA, Pasternak GW. Blockade of hyperalgesia by antisense oligodeoxynucleotide to Gs α (abstract). International Narcotic Research Conference, July 15–20, 2000, Seattle, WA.

Skin Pain and Wound Management

Cecelia C. Monge

INTRODUCTION

Pain or the fear of pain also can influence the healing process; unresolved pain is often associated with delayed wound closure.[1,2]

The skin is the largest organ in the body. The skin weighs 6 lb and receives up to one-third of cardiac output. As the body's first line of defense, its main function is to protect, while regulating temperature, storing water and fat, and absorbing and excreting.

The skin is made up of two layers: the epidermis and the dermis. The epidermis is the layer we see and touch. It has cells (melanocytes), which give skin color. This is the layer that prevents transepidermal water loss (TEWL). This layer does not have a blood supply and is in a constant state of renewal with new cells pushing up from the dermis as old cells are being shed. The epidermis protects us from bodily fluids (incontinence) such as urine and feces and the wound exudate.

The second layer of the skin, just under the epidermis, is the dermis. The dermis has a rich blood supply along with oil glands and hair follicles. Its main function is temperature regulation through sweat production and evaporation. The dermis also produces collagen and elastin, which give the skin its strength.[3]

Detailed history taking utilizing listening and observational skills is important when patients are first approached for dressing changes of acute or chronic wound and skin care. Factors that are important to consider for skin care in wound management include the patient's age, nutritional status, comorbidities, drugs or medications, tissue perfusion, infection and bioburden, stress, specific treatments, and whether the patient had prolonged exposure to the sun. It is important to know if patients used precautions while in the sun. An assessment should be made to determine whether the patient is fair skinned, and has a history of sequelae following sun exposure. In older, mature adults, skin and wound problems take longer to heal than in younger individuals and there is less perception of skin damage. The aging skin thins and is easily damaged due to shearing or friction. The removal of dressings, inappropriate management of the patient's bed position, and transfers from bed to chair contribute to skin damage. Because thinning of the skin produces decreased dermal vascularity and diminished inflammatory response, the cascade of wound healing is impaired. Nutritional status in a patient is an important assessment parameter. Albumin and prealbumin levels should be included in the laboratory work. The diet that ensures rapid, efficient wound healing must be adequate in minerals and vitamins (vitamin C 500–2000 mg/day, zinc, iron) as well as incorporating balanced amounts of proteins (1.5–2.0 gm/kg body weight/day), fats, and carbohydrates that will provide sufficient calories (30–35 cal/kg of body weight/day).

Identifying comorbidities is an important part of a complete assessment. Questions to consider are: Does the patient have diabetes? Does the patient have chronic pulmonary and cardiac conditions that can delay wound healing? Are the treatments for the disease processes impairing or delaying the healing process? Drugs such as steroids and chemotherapeutic agents play an important role in interrupting or promoting a delay in wound healing. Disease treatments can cause wounds such as postradiation sequelae of the skin (dry or moist desquamation) or necrosis. Common medications such as antibiotics and antihistamines affect the skin and the healing response, particularly as the skin ages. Invading organisms produce tissue infection so that the patient's bioburden is the metabolic stress imposed on the wound by bacteria. Infection prolongs the inflammatory response and affects vasoconstriction and hemostasis. Physiological and psychological stress also impair the body's ability to heal by delaying the initiation of the inflammatory response via inhibited cellular migration and infiltration, decreased vasoconstriction, and decreased tissue perfusion.[4–6]

Pain control is a mainstay of wound care.

There are many types of skin pain, whose causes include peristomal complications, perineal dermatitis, urinary or fecal incontinence, thermal injuries, chronic leg ulcers, pressure ulcers, surgical wounds, or skin tears. Trauma increases pain and the periwound surface should be protected throughout the healing process: denudement, erythema, maceration, and dermatitis of intact skin delay epithelial activity and increase pain. All reepithelialization is orchestrated from the edges; therefore, special attention to the periwound skin should be part of all dressing changes.[7]

The time invested preparing the patient for the dressing change prior to removal is time well spent. The wound care practitioner should assess the patient at this time for pain and anxiety. The treating clinician should assume the wounds are painful and there will be pain beginning with the removal of dressings. Pain medication should be given 15–30 minutes prior to a dressing change depending upon the route of the medication, the level and strength of the analgesic, whether the patient has been receiving pain medication for an extended period of time, or if this is the first dressing change requiring pain medication prior to the procedure. Antianxiety medication may be administered at this time to lessen perceived pain or expectation of pain upon dressing changes during wound management. Ativan administered intravenously or per mouth is an excellent choice for the relief of anxiety. The patient must also have choices presented of measures available to them that will help reduce feelings of fear, anxiety, and subsequent pain. Patients who feel more pain than previously expected from a procedure such as a scheduled daily, biweekly, or weekly dressing change can become less confident about the clinicians treating them. The result may also be anticipatory anxiety about future wound care.[1]

Patients are often anxious and fear pain at the time of the dressing change when the wound is in the acute stages. If wounds become chronic, patients should have a psychological assessment. Depression often negatively impacts pain perception.[6,7]

SKIN PAIN

Assessment

Skin pain during wound management requires assessment, intervention, and reassessment. It is common practice to alter the treatment plan as the patient reaches certain milestones in wound healing. Optimal care for patients requires taking a patient-centered approach to pain and wound management.

The wound care practitioner should assume that every wound is painful and every patient who has a wound is in pain.[6]

The patient should feel he or she is in a safe, stress-free environment: in a clinic setting the patient should be placed in a private area where the door can be closed, and away from interruptions or sudden intrusions. Practitioners should introduce themselves and colleagues and minimize the number of colleagues observing dressing changes. The patient should be prepared for the procedure to be done: the *gentle* removal of old dressings and the cleansing of the wound and periwound skin, application of topical agents and medications, and the application of the new dressings.

Pain is sometimes associated with skin and wound cleansing and the application of topical prescriptives and dressings. A thorough ongoing assessment of the client's pain is important throughout the treatment process.[2]

A routine should be established for the patient receiving wound care. The patient must be aware of when pain medication will be administered, what steps will be followed for wound care, when the midpoint of a dressing change evolves, when the dressing change has ended, and if and when breakthrough medications are needed at midpoint during the dressing change.

Patient/family teaching

The patient should be positioned to minimize discomfort during dressing changes. The patient/family should be instructed about which steps to follow for the dressing change procedure. This is an important procedure because when the patient is discharged from the hospital to home, the patient/family will be changing the dressings. It is important to continue to use the same steps during each dressing change, with a set pattern that the practitioner, patient, family/caretaker, and nursing staff can follow. The timing of pain medication administration before dressing changes and breakthrough medication administration for particularly long dressing changes is vitally important. The family members who will be involved in wound care as well as the client should be informed of the beginning, midpoint, and end of the dressing change procedure. It is important for the unit nurse to assist the wound care practitioner in the first dressing change in an inpatient setting. This is particularly important so that every dressing change thereafter remains the same for the patient, which will ensure that the procedures followed adhere to an evidence-based, patient-centered practice.

The unit nurse should be aware of the time needed for dressing changes, preprocedure medication, dosage, and route of administration. The unit nurse should be well versed about the topical medications utilized for dressing removal, cleansing agents, and the procedures and protocols for applying new medications and dressings.

Anxiety reduction

Many methods have been identified to facilitate anxiety reduction during dressing changes: (1) the patient identifies triggers of pain and pain reducers, (2) the patient may be involved as much or as little as she/he wishes in the dressing changes, (3) slow rhythmic breathing may be encouraged, and (4) the pace of the dressing change is dictated by the patient with occasional "time-outs" incorporating hand signals for stopping the process until the patient is able to gain control of the pain. Patients may choose to remove their own dressings at their own pace.[1,9]

Occasionally, particularly large wounds complicated by ostomies and fistulas require two clinicians and 3 or more hours to remove old dressings and apply new dressings accompanied by topical medication. Breakthrough pain may occur during the long dressing change and an established routine would alert the unit/patient nursing staff when to deliver additional medication for breakthrough pain.

Pain identification

It is important for the patient to be the person who identifies the pain she/he is feeling. The patient's age and cultural background and other patient-specific parameters should be considered when utilizing pain assessment strategies. Often family members accompanying the client dictate the amount of medication the patient is to receive. Occasionally family members may feel that the patient is taking "too much" medication and should "tough it out" because pain medications are addictive. The patient must, however, be permitted to request breakthrough pain medication without family or staff raising issues related to addiction. Unfounded concerns about addiction may lead to subtherapeutic dressing changes and poor pain control. Patients whose pain is poorly controlled can exhibit behavioral characteristics suggestive of addiction. The term *pseudoaddiction* refers to the perception by nurses or other observers, such as family members, of drug-seeking behavior by patients who have severe pain. These behaviors include drug-seeking behavior, medication taken in larger amounts than prescribed, running out of medications prematurely, tolerance, and withdrawal symptoms. There is an emerging consensus that these behaviors are not often associated with true addiction but are a result of serious undertreatment for pain.

Conversely, a family member may feel the patient is not obtaining enough medication and pain relief is not possible. The practitioner can utilize pain scales when a client is new or when the client presents for a dressing change.

PAIN SCALES

The patient's self-report is the mainstay of pain assessment. To enhance pain management across all settings, clinicians should teach families to use pain assessment tools. The clinician should help the patient describe the pain, location, intensity, severity, aggravating or relieving factors, cognitive response to pain, and goals for pain control.[2,6,8]

Pediatric clinicians often utilize the Wong-Baker Faces Pain Rating Scale. Children point to the face that best matches the type of pain they are feeling at the time of assessment. The Faces Pain Rating Scale may also be used with adults who cannot read but are able to alert the clinician managing the wound dressing change by pointing to the face that best expresses their pain level. In the Wong-Baker Faces Pain Rating Scale, there are six faces ranging from a smiling face depicting "NO HURT" to a crying face depicting "HURTS WORST." Other pain rating scales may be utilized in assessing skin and wound pain such as the visual analogue scale, the numerical rating scale, and the verbal rating scale. The visual analogue scale asks the patient to pick a point on a 0 through 10 continuum that best reflects how she/he is feeling: 0 = no pain and 10 = worst pain. The numerical rating scale asks the patient on a scale of 0–10, where 0 = no pain and 10 = worst pain to choose a number that best describes his/her current level of pain. The verbal rating scale asks the patient which word best describes his/her current level of pain: no pain, mild pain, moderate pain, and severe pain.[2, 6, 8]

Pain assessment is a critical factor and it must occur prior to every dressing change. Dressing removal is considered by practitioners to be the time of greatest perceived pain by the patient, closely followed by wound cleansing.[1,6]

WOUND DRESSING REMOVAL

Wound dressing removal is perceived by most patients as extremely painful, so it is important to moisten the dressings prior to removal. Dried-out dressings and adherent products are most likely to cause pain and trauma at dressing changes (Figs. 8-1 and 8-2).[2,6,9,11]

Skin can be damaged due to poor choice of dressings, leading to stripping of the epidermis, maceration due to inadequate absorption, poor protection of periwound tissue, or erythema due to unrelieved pressure, shearing, and friction. Pressure on skin surfaces can occur over bony prominences if a patient is not repositioned correctly at least every 2 hours while in bed and afforded pressure relief while in a chair. Shearing and friction can occur when a patient slips downward in bed while the head of the bed is elevated or while being transferred from bed to chair.[9] Nesacaine 3% may be used to

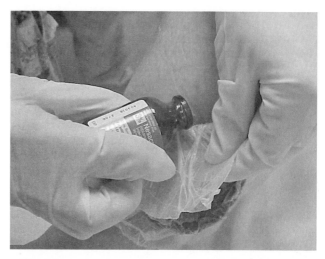

FIGURE 8-2 Use of Nesacaine 3% during removal of NPWT sponge in wound. *(Copyright Woodward L, M. D. Anderson Cancer Center.)*

moisten dressings prior to removal: such as the sponge used in negative pressure wound therapy (NPWT), gauze, or adhesive tapes. Nesacaine 3% may be used with normal saline to premoisten dressings and tape prior to removal. Stockinettes, elastic wraps, gauze wraps, and soft silicone dressings can be used instead of tape when securing dressings over a wound. The periwound skin and peristomal skin should always be protected with a no-sting skin barrier applied at least three times (allowing it to dry between each application) prior to the application of an adhesive dressing or ostomy appliance. Peritube skin (gastric tube, J-tube, or chest tube) can be protected from drainage by applying moisture barrier ointments or petrolatum-impregnated gauze with a silicone foam product to absorb wound drainage.

The skin around wound fistulas or spit fistulas can be protected by applying a skin barrier, thin hydrocolloids, and a pouching appliance.[6]

THE CASCADE OF WOUND HEALING

▶ Inflammatory phase

Healing begins at the time of injury when hemostasis occurs. This phase lasts for 4–6 days. Phagocytic leukocytes (neutrophils) enter the wound to begin the removal of bacteria and debris. Monocytes enter the wound 24–48 hours after the initial injury and transform into macrophages. The macrophages ingest bacteria, necrotic tissue, and dead neutrophils. There is a great deal of wound drainage during this phase of wound healing. If the wound is not cleansed of foreign material and necrotic tissue, it cannot progress to the next phase of wound healing and becomes a chronic wound.

▶ Proliferative phase

Angiogenesis, the formation of new capillaries, occurs and a new vascular bed is formed. Granulation and epithelialization occur in this phase of wound healing. The wound fills with granulation tissue containing fibrin and collagen and it fills as it contracts. The granulation tissue is covered by new epithelium from the wound edges.

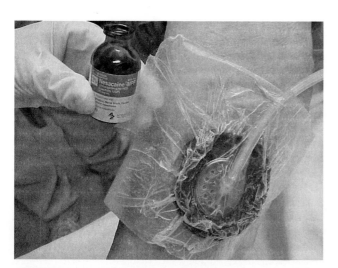

FIGURE 8-1 Use of Nesacaine 3% during removal of NPWT sponge in wound. *(Copyright Woodward L, M. D. Anderson Cancer Center.)*

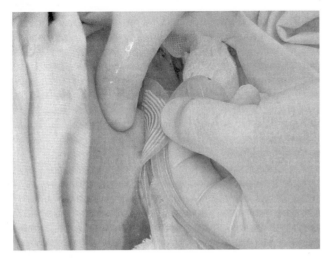

FIGURE 8-3 Push-pull method of ostomy appliance removal to avoid stripping peristomal tissue. *(Copyright Reid A, M. D. Anderson Cancer Center.)*

▶ Maturation phase

Tensile strength begins to increase during this phase and continues for 2 years. Healed wounds will eventually achieve up to 80% of their original tensile strength. The healed tissue is not as elastic as normal dermis, which makes it friable and more easily damaged than uninjured tissue.[4]

WOUND CLEANSING

Wound healing is a multifaceted process, involving the formation of granulation tissue and epithelium, which can be challenged by the presence of debris and bacteria. To minimize pain, warm solutions such as normal saline at room temperature, or warmer if the room is particularly cool, should be used when cleaning wounds. The *best* care requires use of an appropriate cleanser, which should be pH-balanced and specially formulated to gently remove drainage from the periwound tissue.[3,12,13] The periwound skin may be cleansed with normal saline. Some studies show that stool- and urine-contaminated periwound tissue should be cleansed with prepared cleansers to avoid critical contamination of the wound. The ideal skin cleanser should remove only skin debris and dirt while maintaining the skin's two primary functions of protection and water retention.[14] Normal saline-moistened cotton-tipped applicators can be used to gently remove dry or wet drainage from around drainage tube sites and gauze moistened with normal saline or a mixture of normal saline and Nesacaine can be used to remove debris from periwound skin and slough from within the wound bed. Warm moist cloths can assist in the removal of ostomy appliances utilizing a gentle "push and pull" method to avoid skin stripping. Warm moist cloths may also be used to cleanse peristomal skin (Fig. 8-3).

ODOR CONTAINMENT

Wound odor affects the quality of life of the patient experiencing it. The patient and the patient's family are aware of wound odor and are often distressed by it. Wound odor is due to the type and number of bacteria present in the wound. The more bacteria the wound contains, the more obvious the wound odor. Wound odors do not always indicate an infectious process.

Patients tend to isolate themselves and become depressed if wound odor persists. The wound care practitioner can reassure the patient and the family that wound cleansings and dressings will help to decrease and manage odor.[6] Charcoal dressings, metronidazole gel, and SilvaSorb gel are excellent choices for containing odor.

INCONTINENCE

TEWL causes the stratum corneum layer of the skin to lose some of its protective properties and dehydrate. TEWL can be caused by factors that include low humidity, changes in skin pH, normal aging, abraded skin, skin compromised by radiation therapy, shear, thermal injuries, friction, and pressure.

Perineal dermatitis is a common problem in individuals with urine/fecal incontinence. If untreated, denuded skin can rapidly progress to ulceration and secondary infection, including bacterial and yeast infection. A critical immediate defense is a thorough and ongoing assessment of the patient's perineum and prevention. Initially, the mild erythema that occurs in perineal dermatitis and that is associated with urinary or fecal incontinence can progress to a dark red appearance, with blistering, erosion, and serous exudates if left untreated. Prevention of skin problem centers on alleviating urinary or fecal incontinence combined with treatment. Urinary incontinence can be managed by placing the patient on a toileting schedule, prompted voiding schedule, bladder training program, and pelvic muscle rehabilitation combined with pharmacologic treatment (anticholinergic agents and tricyclic antidepressants).[12,15,16]

Fecal incontinence can also be managed with a toileting schedule. If diarrhea is persistent, a bowel management system (Zassi) can be used with stool modification guidelines.

Prevention requires the use of cleansing lotions and body cleansers to remove urine and/or feces. Dry, cracked, and flaky skin can be managed with creams containing skin nutrients and lipid replacements. The skin cream should contain a waterproof ingredient to provide a moisture barrier, protect the skin against further damage, and help block TEWL.

Early intervention for stage I pressure ulcers and to address itchy or abraded skin utilizes cleansing lotions and body cleansers, and an effective, long-lasting dimethicone moisture barrier can be used to protect skin against incontinent episodes. The moisture barrier should also continue to provide relief for dry and abraded or denuded skin, and should offer protection even after multiple washings.

Late intervention for cracked, denuded, macerated, and partial thickness injury to the perineal skin utilizes cleansers containing phospholipids to clean and moisturizers, emollients, humectants, and lipids to provide the highest level of TEWL control. Protectants and barriers provide the most therapeutic and physiologic barrier available against moisture and drainage absorption. All products used should be pH balanced and easy to apply. Fragrance products should be avoided as alcohol is used to insert the fragrance into solution.

Yeast infections or other opportunistic infections caused by change in skin pH from ongoing fecal and urine incontinence are treated with antifungal powders and creams.[9,15,16]

Hospital pharmacies can compound NDX ointment (nystatin, Desitin, and Xylocaine) for the treatment of eroded perineal skin. The following manufacturers often carry a complete product line of skin cleansers, moisture barriers, and therapeutic moisturizers to choose from and the best of these products prevent TEWL: Medline Industries, Inc., Sage Products, Inc., Coloplast, ConvaTec, Smith & Nephew, Swiss-American Products, Inc., Hollister Incorporated, and Calmoseptine, Inc.

MOIST WOUND HEALING

In the past, wounds were dressed with protective bandages to limit blood loss and keep external debris from contaminating newly healing skin. As the germ theory gained acceptance, standard wound care was keeping the wound covered and dry. Advancements soon advocated the use of antimicrobials, warmth, and synthetic materials for enhancing the natural biologic processes of wound healing. After the observation that a blister healed faster when kept intact, researchers sought to discover the benefits of moist wound healing. The rate of wound healing in laboratory animals whose wounds were covered with polyethylene films was double that of wounds covered with a scab. Dressings offering the benefits of moist environments and exudate management were developed. Further study of wounds in humans covered with occlusive dressings demonstrated a greater degree of epithelialization than wounds exposed to air.[4]

Moist wound dressings do not stick to wounds, minimizing trauma to healing tissues. A moist wound environment assists wound healing by accelerating angiogenesis, facilitating cell viability, release of growth factors, and the breakdown of dead tissue. In a moist environment wounds heal faster, produce less scarring, and, most important, are least painful (Table 8-1).[4]

Only epidermis and upper dermis can regenerate. Lower dermis, bone, muscle, and tendon cannot regenerate and such defects are filled with scar tissue. Pressure ulcers cannot be retrostaged once they begin to heal so that a stage III cannot become a stage II, but becomes a "healing stage III" and is charted as such.

WOUND ASSESSMENTS

Wounds should be visually assessed and measured and healing ridges palpated in an incisional wound. In a wound assessment the length, width, depth of wound should be documented in centimeters (7.5 cm L × 3.5 cm W × 2.5 cm D) with the amount of drainage, character, slough, and eschar documented in percentages (40% slough in wound). If patients are unable to reposition themselves, a thorough patient assessment should include the use of a pressure ulcer risk assessment tool. If pressure wounds are covered in eschar, they cannot be staged until necrotic tissue is debrided. Pressure ulcers are charted as stage I, stage II, stage III, and stage IV or as partial thickness and full-thickness wounds.[17]

There must be a thorough understanding of the patient's overall physical and mental status. The healing of pressure ulcers can be impeded by underlying comorbidities such as peripheral vascular disease, diabetes mellitus, immune deficiencies, collagen vascular disease, malignancies, psychosis, and depression. Screening for nutritional deficiencies is an important part of the initial assessment.[18]

▶ Pressure ulcers

Pressure sores develop as a result of a two-step process. First, blood vessels are occluded by external pressure; second, there is endothelial damage of arterioles and microcirculation due to friction and shearing forces. Pressure damage occurs when the skin and other tissues are directly compressed between bone and another hard surface. There is an inverse relationship between time and pressure. A patient can endure a great amount of pressure during a short period of time or a low amount of pressure during a longer period of time without sustaining damage. Pressure multiplied by duration of time results in pressure ulcers.[18]

Ulcer care includes cleansing, debriding, possible application of gels, dressings, and adjunctive therapy. Ulcers should be assessed at least weekly and the efficacy of the ulcer care evaluated. Adjunctive therapy for wounds and ulcers may require water irrigation at pressures of 8–15 psi (pounds per square inch) to enhance the removal of debris from the pressure ulcer. Electrotherapy and hyperbaric oxygen therapy are other adjunctive treatments that enhance the healing rate of pressure ulcers. Support surfaces have been known to provide an environment in which pressure ulcers improve, but are only one component of a comprehensive pressure ulcer treatment plan.[9]

Wounds should be measured by longest length and widest width.[7] Undermining and tunnels in a wound should be documented in centimeters and in a clockwise fashion with the patient's head at 12 o'clock and the patient's lower extremities at 6 o'clock (tunnel at 3 o'clock, approximately 3.25 cm in depth with purulent drainage). It is important to document the condition of the periwound skin. If the periwound tissue is macerated, it may be necessary to apply a protective skin barrier (Fig. 8-4).

Table 8-1

Pressure Ulcer Staging System

Stage I: Nonblanching erythema of intact skin; the heralding sign of skin ulceration. May or may not be reversible. NOTE: In dark-skinned individuals, Stage I presents as area of deepened skin color plus warmth and possibly induration

Stage II: Partial-thickness skin loss involving epidermis and possibly dermis. The ulcer is superficial and presents clinically as an abrasion blister, or shallow crater

Stage III: Full-thickness skin loss involving damage or necrosis of subcutaneous tissue, which may extend down to, but not through, underlying fascia. The ulcer presents clinically as a deep crater with or without undermining of adjacent tissue

Stage IV: Full-thickness skin loss with extensive destruction, tissue necrosis, or damage to muscle, bone, or supporting structures (e.g., tendon, joint capsule, etc.)

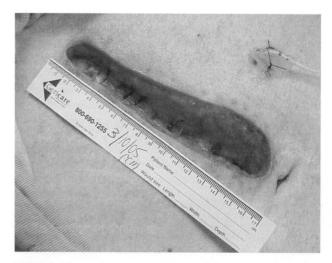

FIGURE 8-4 Thoracic wound measured lengthwise. *(Copyright Monge C, M. D. Anderson Cancer Center.)*

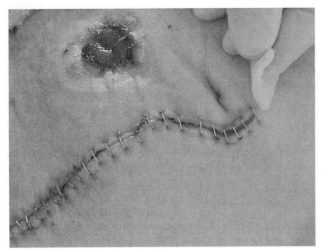

FIGURE 8-5 Using skin prep barrier to seal incision site. *(Copyright Monge C, M. D. Anderson Cancer Center.)*

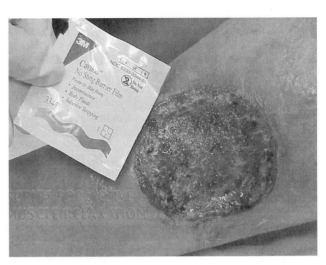

FIGURE 8-7 Using skin prep barrier to protect periwound skin from maceration. *(Copyright Monge C, M. D. Anderson Cancer Center.)*

If the periwound tissue is stripped or erythematous, different dressings may need to be applied and a gentler method of dressing removal and a nonstinging skin barrier spray or wipe used. Photographs can be used when the wound care practitioner cannot coordinate dressing changes with the physician/surgeon's presence. Photographs document the wound at the time of the first dressing. This provides a starting point for the size and scope of the wound and documents improvement of the wound size at subsequent dressing changes.

The photographs can be e-mailed to the physician for input into the dressings and/or other medications/applications to be used, or if the physician is not available during dressing changes (Figs. 8-5, 8-6, and 8-7).

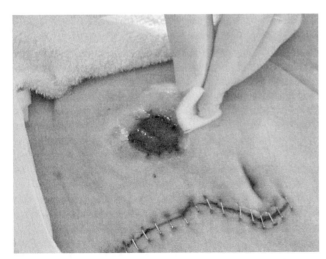

FIGURE 8-6 Using skin prep barrier to protect peristomal tissue. *(Copyright Monge C, M. D. Anderson Cancer Center.)*

WOUND CARE PRODUCTS AND WOUND MANAGEMENT

The following list of wound care products is not all-inclusive. There are hundreds of available wound care products.

The number of manufacturers and distributors of wound care products has increased significantly in the last 10–15 years. Manufacturers compete for placement on national hospital contracts at various levels such as Advanced Wound Care Products. It is important to remember there is parity among most wound care products; for instance, medical/surgical supply companies manufacture silver products for wound care and many companies also produce silver products for wound care. These products include silver foam, which is used to cover a wound, or silver topical in the form of a gel or powder to be used in the wound bed, or a silver transparent sheet. The silver product may be in the form of a polyethylene mesh or an absorbable silver sheet used in combination with other gels or ointments under dressings. While all of the silver products are not identical, there is parity because they are utilized for wound care. In the case of the silver dressings, gels, foams, and meshes, the silver products all protect the wound against bacterial penetration.

The advantages, limitations, applications, absorption, and moisture vapor transference rate (MVTR) of the various wound care products are listed below. The most common of the varied wound care products are listed with the name of the manufacturer in parentheses.

▶ Gauze/nonwoven dressings

Gauze is manufactured and distributed with different names and by different companies.

Fluftex (DeRoyal), Kerlix (Tyco-Kendall), ABD Pads (Medline Industries, Inc.), Packing Strips (Alba Health LLC), Telfa Island Dressing (Tyco-Kendall), CovRSite Wound Cover Dressing (Smith & Nephew), Curity Cover Sponges (Tyco-Kendall), Cover-Roll (BSN-Jobst), Medipak Gauze Bandage Rolls (McKesson Medical Surgical), and Surgical Gauze Packing (Hermitage Hospital Products, Inc.).

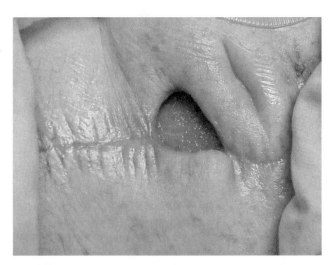

FIGURE 8-8 Dehisced abdominal wound. *(Copyright Reid A, M. D. Anderson Cancer Center.)*

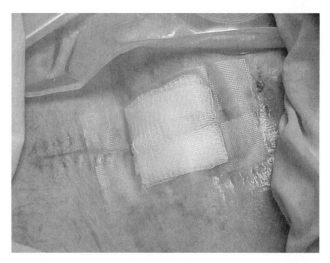

FIGURE 8-10 Gauze dressing with tape over gauze packing. *(Copyright Reid A, M. D. Anderson Cancer Center.)*

Gauze may be dry woven or nonwoven sponges and/or wraps with varying degrees of absorbency. Fabric composition includes cotton, polyester, or rayon. Gauze is available sterile or nonsterile in bulk and with or without an adhesive border.[10] Gauze is used for cleansing, packing, and covering a variety of wounds and may be impregnated with antimicrobials.

The advantages of gauze is that it debrides mechanically, has capillarity, gas permeability, fills "dead space," is conformable (especially when wet), and it is very adaptable.

The applications of gauze are for moderately to heavily exuding wounds. Gauze may be used in partial/full-thickness chronic wounds such as pressure ulcers (stages II through IV). Gauze may be used in acute wounds as a primary dressing and as a secondary dressing wrap to anchor the primary dressing (petrolatum impregnated gauze), ABD, and/or Exudry to externalized tumor wounds (Figs. 8-8, 8-9, and 8-10).

The most important limitation of gauze is that it may cause pain and damage viable tissue and cause bleeding on removal, especially when utilized in a "wet to dry" dressing method.

Fibers can remain in the wound unless it is cleansed well.

Gauze is permeable to bacteria and fluids. Its limited thermal insulation can lead to dehydration of the wound bed. It has a moderate absorption and high MVTR.[10]

▶ Impregnated dressings

"Impregnated dressings are gauzes and nonwoven sponges, ropes, and strips saturated with a solution, an emulsion, oil, or other agents or compounds. Agents most commonly used include saline, oil, zinc salts, petrolatum, Xeroform, and scarlet red."[10] Impregnated gauze is manufactured by different companies under many different names: adaptic PG Petroleum Gauze (Johnson & Johnson), Aquaphor Gauze (Smith & Nephew), Medline Petroleum Impregnated Gauze (Medline Industries, Inc.), Mesalt Sodium Chloride Impregnated Gauze (Molnlycke), Vaseline Petroleum Gauze (Kendall), Xeroform Petroleum Gauze Dressing (Alba Health LLC) (Figs. 8-11 and 8-12).

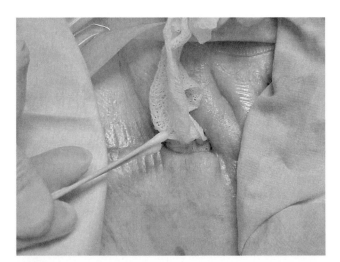

FIGURE 8-9 Gauze packing in wound. *(Copyright Reid A, M. D. Anderson Cancer Center.)*

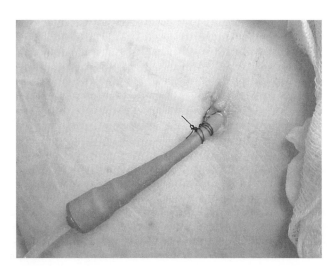

FIGURE 8-11 Erythematous tube site with drainage. *(Copyright Monge C, M. D. Anderson Cancer Center.)*

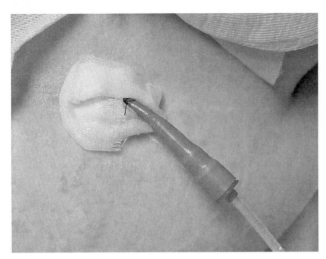

FIGURE 8-12 Petrolatum gauze used around tube site for tissue protection. *(Copyright Monge C, M. D. Anderson Cancer Center.)*

Impregnated gauzes must be used according to manufacturers' recommendations because they may be medicated. They are nonadherent and therefore less absorbent than plain gauze and require a secondary dressing. They may be used on skin donor sites, tube entry sites, and on externalized tumors as a wrap to maintain wound moisture, and protect tumor sites from dehydration and bleeding. Impregnated gauze has a moderate absorption and a moderate MVTR.[10]

Hydrogels: impregnated dressings

Impregnated gauzes and nonwoven sponges, ropes, and strips are saturated with an amorphous hydrogel. Amorphous hydrogels are formulations of water, polymer, and other ingredients with no shape, designed to donate moisture to a dry wound and to maintain a moist healing environment. The high moisture content serves to rehydrate wound tissue. These dressings are indicated for partial- and full-thickness wounds, wounds with necrosis, and deep wounds with tunneling or sinus tracts. They are available in a wide variety of sizes. Preserved products are multidose, and sterile unpreserved products are single use. The impregnated gauzes listed below are some of the most common: Aquagauze (DeRoyal), CarraGauze (Medline Industries, Inc.), Curafil Hydrogel Gauze (Tyco-Kendall), Curasol Gel Saturated Dressing (Healthpoint), Elta Hydrogel Gauze (Swiss-American Products, Inc.), PanoGauze (Sage Pharmaceuticals), Restore Hydrogel Dressing (Hollister Incorporated), Skintegrity (Medline Industries, Inc.), and SoloSite Gel Dressing (Smith & Nephew).[10]

Hydrogels: amorphous

Amorphous hydrogels are formulations of water, polymers, and other ingredients that have no shape. These dressings are designed to donate moisture to a dry wound and to maintain a moist healing environment. Their high moisture content rehydrates wound tissue. Amorphous hydrogels are indicated for partial- and full-thickness wounds, wounds with necrosis, minor burns, and tissue sequelae from radiation therapy.

Preserved products are multidose, and sterile unpreserved products are single use. They require a secondary dressing cover. The

hydrogels may be applied directly onto the wound or used to impregnate gauze prior to wound application.

The most common amorphous hydrogels are Curasol (Healthpoint), Elta Dermal Wound Gel (Swiss-American Products), IntraSite Hydrogel (Smith & Nephew), Normlgel Isotonic Saline Gel (Molnlycke), Nu-Gel Collagen Wound Gel (Johnson & Johnson), Restore Hydrogel (Hollister Incorporated), Saf-Gel (ConvaTec), Skintegrity Hydrogel (Medline Industries, Inc.), SoloSite Wound Gel (Smith & Nephew), and Woun'Dres Collagen Hydrogel (Coloplast Corp.).[10]

Hydrogels: sheets

Hydrogel sheets are three-dimensional networks of cross-linked hydrophilic polymers that are insoluble in water and swell when they interact with aqueous solutions. They are highly conformable and permeable and can absorb small amounts of drainage, depending on their composition.[10] They remain nonadhesive against the wound for easy removal and are indicated for partial- and full-thickness wounds, wounds with necrosis, minor burns, tissue sequelae from radiation therapy, and graft-versus-host disease (Figs. 8-13 and 8-14).

Hydrogel sheets are effective for use with chemotherapy patients with palmar-plantar erythrodysesthesia or hand-foot syndrome. They have a cooling effect that can reduce pain, are nonadherent, and do not harm granulating tissue.

Companies manufacturing commonly used hydrogel sheets are Vigilon (Bard Medical Division), Cool Magic (MPM Medical Inc.), NuGel (Johnson & Johnson), ClearSite (Conmed Corporation), Curagel (Tyco-Kendall), Flexigel (Smith & Nephew), and CarraDres (Medline Industries, Inc).

The advantages of using hydrogels and hydrogel-impregnated gauzes are that they form moist wound beds and provide slight thermal insulation. They are conformable and manage exudates by particle swelling.

Their limitations include dehydration of the gel and minimal absorption. The hydrogel-impregnated dressing, hydrogel, and hydrogel sheets may require secondary dressings. There may also be light exudate when using gels. There is low absorption and a moderate MVTR.[10]

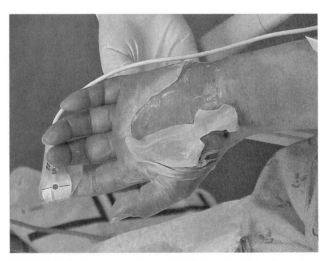

FIGURE 8-13 Graft-versus-host disease (GVHD). *(Copyright Worley C, M. D. Anderson Cancer Center.)*

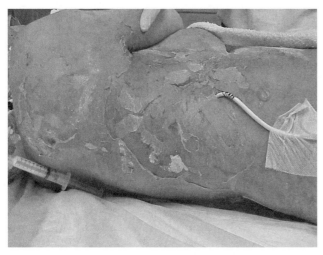

FIGURE 8-14 Graft-versus-host disease (GVHD). Standard of care for BMT patients: cleanse with warmed normal saline and rinsed out baby wipes, apply thin film of Bactroban and Vigilon (hydrogel sheet) (Bard Medical) or Cool Magic (hydrogel sheet) (MPM Medical) and secure with Kerlex, Surgiflex (for trunk), EXU-DRY (burn pad), vest or ace bandages (lower extremities) depending upon mobility and activity of patient. *(Copyright Worley C, M. D. Anderson Cancer Center.)*

▶ Cellulose wound dressings

Cellulose wound dressings are not hydrogel-impregnated dressings but are occasionally placed in the same category. They are a sterile product composed of cellulose and water and a minimal preservative. Cellulose wound dressings differ from hydrogel wound dressings in some respects. Cellulose wound dressings are primary dressings and may cover a wound, burn, or graft donor site. They are indicated as an external wound dressing for the management of superficial cuts, minor scalds, first- or second-degree burns, minor skin irritations, lacerations, and abrasions. They are intelligent wound dressings in that they absorb wound exudate while providing a moist wound environment that supports tissue hydration and autolytic debridement of necrotic tissue. The advantages of cellulose wound dressings are that a single dressing can stay on the wound for as long as 7 days, reducing time, material, and the costs associated with frequent dressing changes. This dressing is soft, flexible, and molds to the contours of the wounds, although it does require a secondary dressing such as a transparent film (Figs. 8-15, 8-16, 8-17, and 8-18).

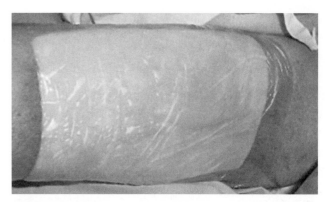

FIGURE 8-16 Application of cellulose dressing (X-Cell, Medline) on graft donor site secured with Tegaderm (transparent dressing).

Medline Industries, Inc., is the distributor and Xylos is the manufacturer.

▶ Transparent films

Transparent films are polymer membranes of varying thickness that are coated on one side with an adhesive. They are impermeable to liquid, water, and bacteria but permeable to moisture vapor and atmospheric gases. Transparency allows visualization of the wound. Transparent films are indicated for partial-thickness wounds with little or no exudate, wounds with necrosis, and as a primary and secondary dressing. They are also used to manage IV sites, donor sites, lacerations, abrasions, and second-degree burns. They reduce the friction coefficient in high-risk areas and are particularly well suited for the treatment of skin tears. Transparent films are available in a wide variety of sizes, both sterile and in bulk. They may be utilized as a secondary dressing for primary dressings such as silver-coated polyethylene mesh or nonadherent gauzes, foams, and cellulose dressings (Fig. 8-16).

The most common transparent films are made and/or distributed by the following companies: Tegaderm (3M Healthcare), OpSite (Smith & Nephew), BlisterFilm (Tyco-Kendall), Transeal (DeRoyal), Comfeel Film (Coloplast), and Arglaes Film Dressing (Medline).

Advantages listed for transparent films other than those previously enumerated are: they are low-profile, conformable, and manage exudate by MVTR.

Their limitations are: they manage very light exudate only, may tear fragile skin, provide poor thermal insulation, can be difficult to apply, incontinence may undermine adhesive, and there is a potential for skin maceration.

Transparent films have low-moderate absorption, and low, moderate, or high MVTR.[10]

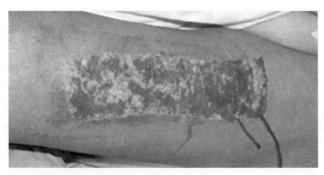

FIGURE 8-15 Graft donor site.

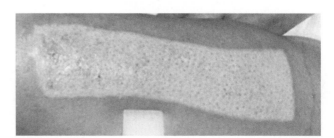

FIGURE 8-17 Results 2 weeks postoperative.

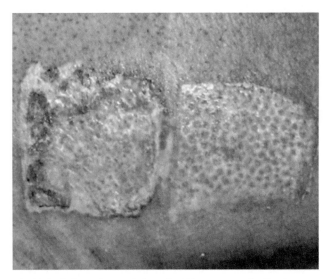

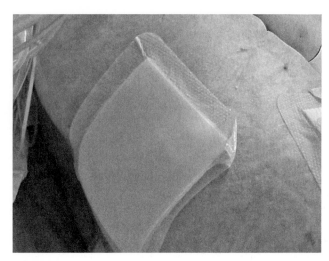

FIGURE 8-18 Comparison: graft donor sites 7 days postoperative. Xeroform dressing (left) and cellulose (X-Cell) dressing (right).

FIGURE 8-20 Thoracic chest wound dressed with Hyalofil (ConvaTec) to promote granulation, Aquacel AG (ConvaTec) to absorb drainage and curtail bioburden, with Mepilex foam dressing (Molnlycke) with silicone to prevent painful removal. *(Copyright Monge C, M. D. Anderson Cancer Center.)*

▶ Foam dressings

Foam dressings are sheets and other shapes of foamed polymer (most commonly polyurethane) with small, open cells capable of holding fluids. They may be impregnated or layered in combination with other materials such as silver, silicone, and maltodextrin. Their absorptive ability depends on thickness and composition. The area in contact with the wound surface is nonadhesive for easy removal. Foams are available with an adhesive border and/or a transparent film coating that acts as a bacterial barrier. Foams are indicated for partial- and full-thickness wounds and may be used in combination with other dressings such as gauze, amorphous gels, or topical agents.

The advantages of foam dressings are their permeability to gases, provision of thermal insulation for the wound, creation of a moist wound environment, and pain reduction.

The limitations of foam dressings are that if the foam does not have an adhesive border it may require a secondary dressing, and foam dressings can enhance wound odor (Figs. 8-19 and 8-20).

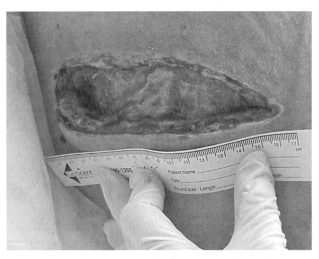

FIGURE 8-19 Thoracic chest wound. *(Copyright Monge C, M. D. Anderson Cancer Center.)*

Foam dressings are used for moderately exuding wounds, partial/full-thickness chronic wounds (pressure ulcers stages III and IV), partial-thickness burns, and acute dehisced wounds.

These dressings provide moderate absorption and a moderate to high MVTR.

Common foam products are Algidex, Polyderm, Polyderm Plus (DeRoyal), Allevyn Adhesive Dressing, Allevyn Cavity Wound Dressing, Allevyn Heel, Allevyn Island Sacral (Smith & Nephew), Ferris PolyMem Adhesive Dressing and Non-Adhesive Dressing (Ferris Mfg. Corp.), Versiva (ConvaTec), Mepilex Soft Silicone Foam, Mepilex Transfer, Mepilex Border, (Molnlycke), Tielle Hydropolymer Adhesive Dressing, and Tielle Plus Adhesive Dressing and Tielle Plus Borderless Non-Adhesive Dressing (Johnson & Johnson), Optifoam and Gentleheal (Medline Industries).[10]

▶ Composite dressings

Composite dressings are wound covers that combine physically distinct components into a single product to provide multiple functions, such as a bacterial barrier, absorption, and adhesion.

Usually they are composed of multiple layers and incorporate a semi- or nonadherent pad that covers the wound. The pad may be made of gauze, nonwoven composition, foam, or gel and can also include an adhesive border of nonwoven fabric tape or transparent film. Composite dressings can be used either as a primary or a secondary dressing for a wide variety of wounds and can be used with topical medications.

Some of the more common composite dressings are Optifoam Adhesive and Gentleheal (Medline Industries), Clear Absorbant (3M Health Care), Versiva (ConvaTec), Algidex (DeRoyal), Telfa plus Barrier Island (Tyco-Kendall), Tegaderm + Pad Transparent (3M Health Care), OpSite Composite Dressing (Smith & Nephew), CovRSite Plus (Smith & Nephew), Covaderm Plus (DeRoyal), B Braun THINSite (Swiss-American Products, Inc.), and Alldress Absorbant (Molnlycke). Advantages of composites are that they usually have a perimeter adhesive and some are bacteria resistant.

Composites have limitations and may damage fragile skin unless they contain silicone throughout the adhesive border (Fig. 8-21).

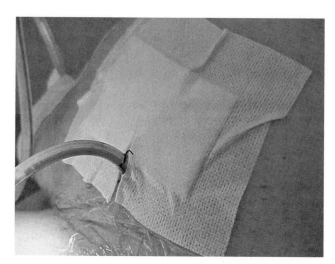

FIGURE 8-21 Composite dressing over tube site. *(Copyright Monge C, M. D. Anderson Cancer Center.)*

The applications of composite dressings are moderately exuding wounds, partial- and full-thickness chronic wounds, tube sites, and as a secondary dressing. They are moderately absorptive with a moderate MVTR.[10]

Hydrocolloids

Hydrocolloids, the oldest of the "moist wound" dressings, can be wafers, powders, or pastes composed of gelatin, pectin, or carboxymethylcellulose. The absorption capability of hydrocolloids is dependent upon thickness and composition. Wafers are self-adhering and available with or without an adhesive border and in myriad shapes and sizes.

Hydrocolloids are useful for areas that require contouring, such as heels and sacral ulcers. Hydrocolloid powders and pastes require a secondary dressing.

Common hydrocolloids are 3M Tegasorb Hydrocolloid, 3M Tegasorb Sacral Design, 3M Tegasorb Thin Hydrocolloid (Tyco-Kendall), Combiderm, DuoDERM Extra Thin DuoDERM CGF, DuoDERM Signal (ConvaTec), Exuderm LP, Exuderm Sacral (Medline Industries, Inc.), Comfeel Powder, Comfeel Paste, Comfeel Plus Pressure Relief (Coloplast Corp.), Replicare Hydrocolloid, Replicare Thin Hydrocolloid (Smith & Nephew), Restore Plus Hydrocolloid, and Restore Thin Hydrocolloid (Hollister Incorporated).

Hydrocolloids deliver moist gel to the wound bed, and they are impermeable to fluids. Other advantages are their ability to manage moderate exudate by particle swelling and to manage drainage as a function of weight. Limitations include impermeability to gases and that they may damage fragile skin.

Hydrocolloids are indicated for use in partial- and full-thickness wounds with or without necrotic tissue. They reduce friction coefficient in high-risk areas (bony prominences) and they have a low MVTR.[10]

Alginates

Alginates are nonwoven, nonadhesive pads and ribbons composed of natural polysaccharide fibers or xerogel derived from seaweed. Over time, contact with exudate causes these dressings to form a moist gel in the wound through a process of ion exchange. Alginates manage exudate by capillarity, and they are permeable to gases. Alginates must be used with a second dressing.

Commonly used alginates are AlgiSite M (Smith & Nephew), Curasorb (Tyco-Kendall), Kalginate (DeRoyal), Kaltostat (ConvaTec), Maxorb, Maxorb Extra AG (Medline Industries, Inc.), Restore (Hollister Incorporated), Seasorb (Coloplast Corp.).

The advantages to using alginates in wounds are their ability to mold to wound countour, to fill "dead space," and they are fairly easy to remove. They reduce wound pain and cause no pain upon removal.

The limitations of alginates include permeability to bacteria and fluid, occasionally producing a burning sensation upon application, soaking is required if the dressing is allowed to dry, and they should not be used on dry necrotic tissue.

The applications are for moderate to heavily exuding wounds, partial- and full-thickness chronic wounds (pressure ulcers stage III and IV), infected wounds, diabetic ulcers, venous stasis ulcers, partial-thickness burns, and skin donor sites.[10]

Antimicrobial dressings

Antimicrobial dressings (AMD) are wound covers that deliver the effects of agents, such as silver (Ag) and polyhexamethylene Biguanide (PHMB). These dressings maintain efficacy against common infectious bacteria, helping reduce the risk of infection in partial- and full-thickness wounds, over percutaneous line sites and surgical incisions, or around tracheostomies and tube sites. AMDs are available as sponges, impregnated woven gauzes, film dressings, absorptive products, island dressings, nylon fabric nonadherent barriers, or a combination of materials. The ability to handle exudate depends on the characteristics and composition of the products being used.[10]

The most common antimicrobial dressings are Algidex AG thin sheet and Algidex Ag Paste (DeRoyal), Acticoat 7 and Acticoat Burn Dressings (Smith & Nephew), Actisorb Silver 220 Antimicrobial (Johnson & Johnson), Arglaes (Medline Industries, Inc.), Contreet Adhesive Foam (Coloplast), Kerlix AMD (Tyco-Kendall), SilvaSorb Antimicrobial Silver Dressing (Medline Industries, Inc.), Silverlon Wound & Surgical Dressings, and Silverlon Wound & Burn Dressings (Argentum Medical LLC).

Antimicrobial dressings provide immediate and sustained antimicrobial activity against a broad spectrum of wound pathogens (some for as long as 7 days). The dressings provide antimicrobial activity against Methicillin-resistant *Staphylococcus aureus* (MRSA), Vancomycin-resistant *Enterococcus faecium* and *Enterococcus faecalis* (VRE), *Staphylococcus aureus (S. aureus), Pseudomonas aeruginosa, and Escherichia coli* without inducing bacterial resistance. Most silver dressings also protect against fungal infections: Candida glabrata, Candida albicans, and Candida tropicalis.

Some of the nanocrystalline silver products (Acticoat) require the use of sterile distilled water instead of normal saline for activation of the silver colloid to the silver ionic state. Other silver products do not require utilization of sterile distilled water to oxidize the metallic silver colloid to the silver ionic state (Algidex AG).

Silver products such as Acticoat are excellent for use on patients with sequelae from radiation therapy, but only after all radiation treatments are completed. Acticoat is moistened with sterile water and applied to the affected tissue and sealed with a film dressing such as Tegaderm (3M Health Care). It is left in place for 4–7 days. Epithelialization should occur within 1–2 weeks or after one to two applications (Figs. 8-22, 8-23, and 8-24).

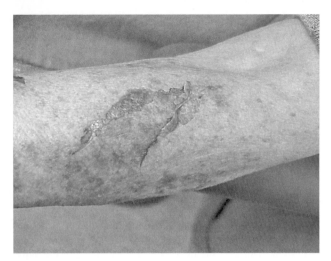

FIGURE 8-22 Dog bite/skin tear—nonadherent flap. *(Copyright Monge C, M. D. Anderson Cancer Center.)*

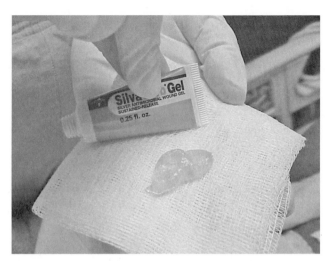

FIGURE 8-24 Silvasorb Gel (Medline) sustained release silver antimicrobial wound gel. Silver products would be utilized with dog bites to provide antimicrobial activity and reduce risk of infection. A secondary dressing such as Mepitel or Mepilex transfer should be used with patients who have friable or fragile skin. *(Copyright Monge C, M. D. Anderson Cancer Center.)*

Silver products are utilized for dog bites to provide antimicrobial activity and reduce the risk of infection.

A secondary dressing such as Mepitel or Mepilex transfer should be used with patients who have friable or fragile skin (Fig. 8-25).

Antimicrobial dressings may extend the life of absorbent secondary dressings and supply thermal insulation, particularly if the antimicrobial dressing is also an absorbent dressing. Silver products vary in MVTR: they have a high MVTR if the secondary dressing is a transparent film over a silver product or a low MVTR if the silver product is covered by a foam product with an adhesive border.[10]

▶ Biologicals and biosynthetics

Biologicals and biosynthetics are gels, solutions or semipermeable sheets derived from a natural source. A gel or solution is applied to the wound surface and covered with a dressing. A sheet may act as a membrane, remaining in place after a single application for undisturbed healing. Biologicals are indicated for partial-thickness wounds such as burns, abrasions, donor sites, skin tears, and as a temporary covering for autografts or to manage second-degree burns and pressure ulcers (Fig. 8-26).[10]

▶ Enzymes

Wound bed preparation is important so that local barriers to wound healing can be removed to reduce the bacterial burden, and to manage exudate and debridement (Table 8-2).[19]

As discussed earlier, removing all necrotic or devitalized tissue allows the depth of the wound and the condition of the tissue and surrounding structures to be assessed. Necrotic tissue can mask signs of infection and serve as a medium for bacterial proliferation. Necrotic tissue is a physical barrier to healing. Its significant support of bacterial growth can result in the production of excessive amount of proteases, which has a negative effect on healing. All debridement assessment decisions must be patient-specific and care-oriented.[19]

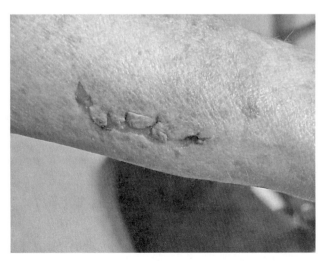

FIGURE 8-23 Dog bite/skin tear. *(Copyright Monge C, M. D. Anderson Cancer Center.)*

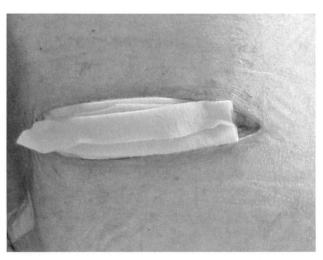

FIGURE 8-25 Aquacel AG (ConvaTec) in thoracic wound as primary dressing. *(Copyright Monge C, M. D. Anderson Cancer Center.)*

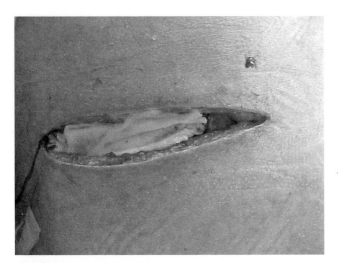

FIGURE 8-26 Hyalofil in thoracic wound used as a primary dressing. *(Copyright Monge C, M. D. Anderson Cancer Center.)*

perfusion, and skill. If successful, this strategy converts a chronic wound environment to an acute wound environment. Surgical debridement facilitates rapid wound closure in traumatic wounds, whereas it can be used to reduce infection and promote healing in chronic wounds.

Mechanical debridement. Mechanical debridement is the removal of foreign material and dead or damaged tissue by the use of physical forces. These include hydrotherapy, pulsed lavage (8–15 psi), and wet-to-dry dressings. Before using this technique considerations are that this method is nonselective, wet-dry dressings are considered by patients to be the most painful, trauma to capillaries can cause bleeding, periwound skin maceration may occur, and dressings must be changed often.

Autolytic debridement. In autolytic debridement, the wound bed utilizes phagocytic cells and proteolytic enzymes to remove debris. Although this manner of debridement is slower, it is easy to perform, produces little to no discomfort, can be performed in any practice setting (including at home), but it is contraindicated in the presence of infection.

Enzymatic debridement. In enzymatic debridement, topically applied agents stimulate the breakdown of necrotic tissue. This procedure is used in conjunction with moist wound healing, the autolytic debridement process, and antimicrobial prophylaxis. The most common topical agents are papain-urea and collagenase. The AHQR (Agency for Health Care Quality and Research)

Methods of debridement are surgical, mechanical, autolytic, and enzymatic.[20]

Surgical debridement. Surgical debridement requires a licensed/certified trained professional, analgesia/anesthesia, adequate

Table 8-2

Enzymatic Debriding Agents

Debridement Product	Panafil (Healthpoint)	Accuzyme (Healthpoint)	Collagenase Santyl (Healthpoint)
Active ingredients	Papain-enzymatic debriding agent	Papain-enzymatic debriding agent	Collagenase-enzymatic debriding agent
	Urea	Urea	
	Chlorophyllin Copper		
	Sodium Deoderizer		
Supporting science	FDA approval 1950s	FDA approval 1995	5 double blind studies
			Needed for FDA approval 1969
pH (normal wound pH is between 6 and 8)	Range 3–12	Range 3–12	Range 5–9
Dosage	Twice daily preferred	Twice daily preferred	Once daily
Indication for use	Debridement and granulation	Debridement	Debridement and granulation
Use with topical antibiotics			Studies used with Polysporin or neomycin powder with infection present in wound
Color and character of ointment	Green	Clear	Opaque
Safety and side effects	No systemic or local reactions	No system reactions	No system or local reactions noted. Only enzyme mentioned in AHCPR guidelines
Other debriment products with papain and urea	Kovia (Stratus), ethezyme (Ethex Corp.), Gladase (Smith & Nephew)		

recommends enzymatic debridement for patients who cannot tolerate surgery, reside in long-term care facilities, and/or for patients who receive care at home. Enzymatic debridement should be painless because of reduced wound trauma, easier dressing changes, although caution should be taken with infected wounds.[19]

Specific wound characteristics, avoiding damage to healthy tissue, the care setting, time constraints for wound debridement, wound bed preparation, and the skill of the clinician should be considered before using enzymatic debridement. In general, debriding agents are applicable for partial- or full-thickness chronic wounds and surgical wounds for which there is no absorption and a high MVTR. An informed clinician must make a careful and systematic assessment of each wound on a case-by-case basis. Not all wounds with nonviable tissue are candidates for debridement (e.g., dry gangrene of the extremities or ischemic wounds in general).[20]

The limitations of the listed debriding agents are that they require a prescription, are tissue-specific, involve multiple applications, need refrigeration, occasionally produce mixed results, and can be expensive. Most importantly, they can produce a transient burning sensation upon application, which may make it uncomfortable or painful for elderly patients with lower extremity wounds such as venous and arterial ulcers.

▶ Specialty absorbent dressings

Specialty absorbent dressings and garments have been uniquely designed to absorb large amounts of exudate while decreasing the risk of trauma and pain by minimizing adherence and helping to reduce friction and shearing. Specialty absorbent dressings such as EXU-DRY (Smith & Nephew) are permeable and nonocclusive and because they are available in various sizes and shapes, they can accommodate many different wound and body contours.

Specialty absorbent dressings manage drainage by osmotic action, and can be utilized in wounds with moderate to high exudate, full-thickness, chronic wounds (stage III and IV), chronic malodorous wounds, burn sites, and tube sites.

They have a high absorption rate and low-to-moderate MVTR. The advantages are they maintain superabsorbancy, reduce pain and discomfort, are easily removed from the wound bed, as a secondary dressing they extend the life of primary dressings, and they supply thermal insulation. They can also be used as primary dressings.

The limitations are that they require secondary dressings such as Kerlix wraps or adhesives when used as primary dressings and they are permeable to bacteria and fluids.

The patient's wound pictured in Figs. 8-27 and 8-28 was treated with 3M No Sting Barrier Film skin wipes, applied to all periwound tissues to protect them from maceration. A prescriptive gel, Metrogel (Galderma), was applied to the entire tumor to control odor. Silvasorb Gel (Medline) is a nonprescriptive antiseptic and may be used to control odor. The tumor was entirely covered with Vaseline gauze (Tyco/Kendall) and a Surgiflex stockinette (Acme Health Care), which was used to hold dressings in place (no tape), thereby reducing the chance of damaging the surrounding tissue.[10] The dressings were changed daily while the patient received chemotherapy and radiation therapy for his tumor.

▶ Wound fillers

Wound fillers are beads, creams, foams, gels, ointments, pads, pastes, pillows, powders, strands, or other formulations. They are nonadherent and may incorporate time-released antimicrobial agents.

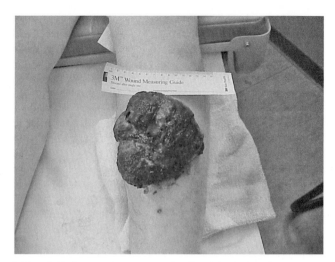

FIGURE 8-27 Sarcoma left lower extremity. *(Copyright Woodward L, M. D. Anderson Cancer Center.)*

Fillers function to maintain a moist environment and manage exudate. Wound fillers are indicated for partial- and full-thickness wounds, infected wounds, draining wounds, and deep wounds that require packing. Their capacity to absorb depends on product composition. They are not recommended for wounds with tunnels or sinus tracts. Their capacity for absorption depends on product composition.

The most common of the wound fillers are Multidex Gel or Powder (DeRoyal), Silverlon Wound Packing Strips (Argentum Medical LLC), Iodosorb Gel and Iodoflex Pad Absorbent Antimicrobial (Healthpoint), Gold Dust (Southwest Technologies, Inc.), and FlexiGel Strands Absorbent Wound Dressing (Smith & Nephew) (Fig. 8-29).

Wound fillers require a secondary dressing and may be covered with a nonadherent, nonocclusive dressing. Dry wound fillers can be applied to exuding wounds and gels to dry wounds daily or every other day. Patients do not normally complain of pain or odor with their application.[10]

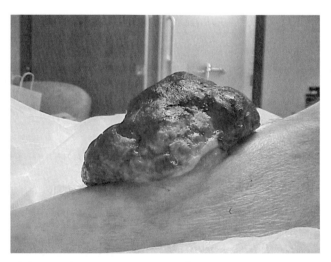

FIGURE 8-28 Sarcoma left lower extremity. *(Copyright Woodward L, M. D. Anderson Cancer Center.)*

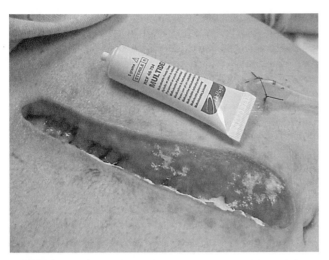

FIGURE 8-29 Multidex (DeRoyal) in thoracic chest wound on pink granulating tissue. *(Copyright Monge C, M. D. Anderson Cancer Center.)*

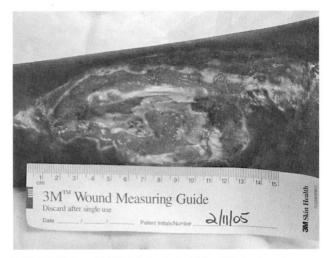

FIGURE 8-30 Date: 2/11/05. Failed graft site left leg, 30% slough, tendons exposed. *(Copyright Tayloe J, M. D. Anderson Cancer Center.)*

Negative pressure wound therapy

Negative pressure wound therapy (NPWT) can be used for wounds that are chronic, acute, dehisced, and those involving graft sites. NPWT applies subatmospheric pressure to the wound bed via a computerized therapy unit attached to an open-cell foam dressing placed in the wound and secured with an adhesive drape. The adhesive drape helps provide a semiocclusive environment that supports moist wound healing, which is the standard for wound care. The foam dressing and drape protect the wound base from environmental contaminants and other bodily fluids and reduce the risk of friction or shear, enhancing the body's ability to heal. NPWT initially removes interstitial fluid, periwound edema, which compromises the circulatory and lymphatic systems, impedes oxygen and nutrient delivery to the tissue, and supports inhibitory factors and bacterial growth. Removing this stagnant fluid allows circulation and disposal of cellular waste via the lymphatic system.[21] Studies suggest that blood flow adjacent to a wound receiving negative pressure is significantly increased, which is likely the result of decreased peripheral edema.

Studies have showed that 125 mm Hg is the optimal pressure and that this setting helps to increase blood flow level by 4 times baseline. The recommended dressing changes are at 24–48-hour intervals.

The only studies of NPWT have compared this technique to wet to moist dressings in wounds. Two recent studies have called into question NPWT's role in removing bacteria, and in some cases bacterial colonization increased. Other studies showed gram-negative bacilli in wounds treated with NPWT decreased but *S. aureus* significantly increased (Figs. 8-30, 8-31, 8-32, and 8-33).[1]

NPWTs can be effective when used in association with other treatment modalities. It is important to remember that no one method or topical or dressing can be all things to all wounds—they must all be utilized as a "piece of the wound healing pie." Each wound must be assessed individually to select the best and most efficacious painless treatment for each particular patient.[1,21]

NPWT treatment limitations include variations in patient insurance coverage, painful removal of dressings, labor intensity, clinician learning curve, requirement for monitoring by trained nurses for hospital and home use, inability to be used on fistulas connected to body cavities or organs, or for use in wounds with necrotic tissue above recommended percentages, inability for use on malignancies, osteomyelitis, or for patients with coagulation problems. Normal applications include full-thickness wounds, pressure ulcers, and dehisced surgical wounds.

NPWT has high absorption and low MVTR.

Growth factors

Growth factors are proteins (polypeptides) that occur naturally in the body and are integral to the wound-healing process. Research has determined that they stimulate cell growth and migration. Clinical efficacy has been demonstrated when they are used as an essential component of a comprehensive wound management program. They are manufactured through recombinant DNA technology.

Growth factors have received much attention in the literature in recent years. They are found in a wide array of cells. The a-granule in the platelet is known to contain high concentrations of many

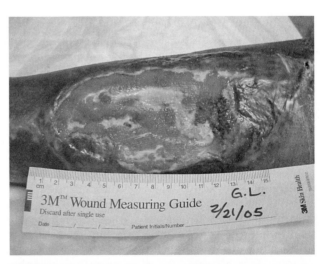

FIGURE 8-31 Date: 2/25/05. After 2 weeks of NPWT: 15% slough in granulating wound, maceration wound edges. *(Copyright Monge C, M. D. Anderson Cancer Center.)*

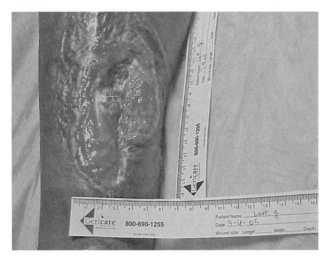

FIGURE 8-32 Date: 3/4/05. After 3 weeks of NPWT: 5% slough, hypergranulation of wound edges with no significant change in center of wound bed, maceration of wound edges. No significant change in wound size. *(Copyright Hu S, M. D. Anderson Cancer Center.)*

endogenous growth factors, including platelet-derived growth factor (PDGF), fibroblast growth factor (FGF), transforming growth factor beta (TGF-β), epidermal growth factor (EGF), insulin-like growth factor (IGF), and others. The platelet is extremely important cell because it initiates inflammation and plays a major role in the wound-healing process.[22]

Autologous platelet grafting has recently been implemented in the treatment of chronic wounds. This application is rich in growth factors; however, it differs substantially from thrombin-induced platelet releasate (TIPR) or any previous growth factor therapy. The process involves collecting blood from a patient and pheresing it to obtain a platelet-rich concentrate. A semi-solid graft is then constructed by activating the platelet concentrate with a series of reagents. The entire process takes about 20 minutes. After standard wound preparation, the graft is applied and the wound is dressed.

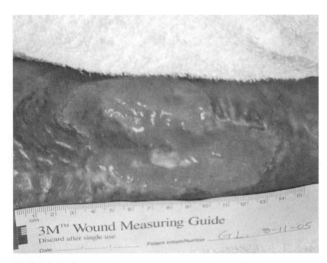

FIGURE 8-33 Date: 3/11/05. 7 days later after application of Algidex Ag (DeRoyal) thin sheet under NPWT sponge. Wound is significantly smaller, no hypergranulation of wound edges, maceration of wound edges diminished significantly, no slough noted, depth of wound at center significantly lessened. *(Copyright Hu S, M. D. Anderson Cancer Center.)*

This dressing is left intact for 5–7 days. Depending on wound progression, this process may be repeated at 2-week intervals.

Autologous platelet gel, unlike Regranex (R.W. Johnson), contains the platelet cell membrane, which is proving to be vitally important in the wound-healing process. The cell membrane contains cellular receptors that bind cytokines and growth factors, which are responsible for additional chemotactic activity as well as participating in the coagulum matrix.[22]

RADIATION SEQUELAE

Silver antimicrobial products can be used to treat desquamation caused by radiation therapy but not during therapy.

Silver antimicrobial products are used liberally in burn centers and are an effective treatment for large areas following tradiation therapy. During radiotherapy, however, the affected tissue should not be exposed to topical agents that contain metals, which includes items such as deodorants. Other products containing perfumes, talcum powders, alcohol, or dehydrating agents must not be used on irradiated tissue. The goals of treatment are skin protection, moisture, and preventing excessive transepidermal water loss (e-TEWL). Topical moisturizers minimize the patient's discomfort and protect the skin in the affected area.[23] Advanced skin care is vitally important for patients who are at risk for postradiation therapy sequelae. Excellent topical agents are the Remedy Skin Care Line (Medline Industries) and Biafine RE (OrthoNeutrogena). These products are also excellent for use on graft donor sites. Biafine can be applied up to 4 hours prior to a radiation session, and immediately after a radiation session (Figs. 8-34, 8-35, and 8-36).

When a clinician approaches a patient for dressing change(s), it is imperative to obtain a detailed history of their pain. History-taking is 70% of the requirement for making a diagnosis. The International Association for the Study of Pain (IASP) defines pain as "an unpleasant sensory and emotional experience associated with actual or potential tissue damage, or described in terms of such damage." Now considered the fifth vital sign, the presence and intensity of pain are not only a reflection of the extent of a lesion. Instead, the presence and intensity of pain and the manifestation of discomfort result from the interaction between biologic, emotional, cognitive,

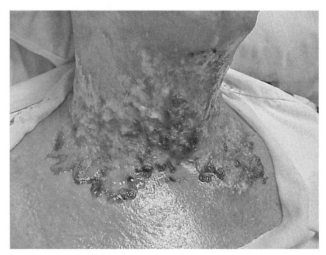

FIGURE 8-34 Date: 3/29/05. Neck and upper chest—moist desquamation postirradiation therapy session #33. *(Copyright Monge C, M. D. Anderson Cancer Center.)*

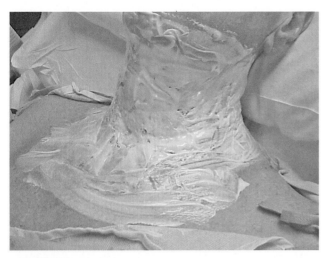

FIGURE 8-35 Date: 3/30/05. Biafine applied liberally to neck and upper chest after radiation therapy session #34. Biafine may be applied up to 4 hours prior to treatment. *(Copyright Monge C, M. D. Anderson Cancer Center.)*

and cultural factors, so that pain is always a personal and subjective experience for each patient.[2,24]

Finally, skin pain and wound care management do not exist in a vacuum: The patient must be assessed holistically and the patient/family taught to use a holistic approach.[5] Skin care and wound care products must be utilized as components of wound healing and their effects on wound care should be continually assessed and reassessed to assure uninterrupted patient-centered, evidence-based care and practice.

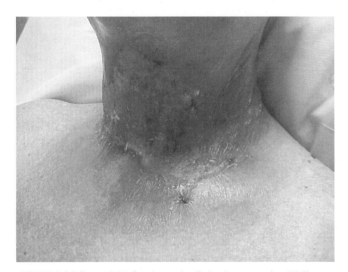

FIGURE 8-36 Date: 4/2/05. One day postirradiation therapy session #35. Note less erythema on chest; moist desquamation improved. *(Copyright Monge C, M. D. Anderson Cancer Center.)*

REFERENCES

1. Moffatt DJ, Franks PR, Hollinsworth H, et al. Pain at wound dressing changes. EWMA Position Document. 2002:1–17.
2. *Principles of Best Practice: Minimizing Pain at Wound Dressing-Related Procedures.* A Consensus Document. London: MEP Ltd; 2004.
3. Fleck C. Feed the need—advanced skin care. *Healthy Skin.* 2006;3:41–65.
4. *Physicians Guide to Advances in Wound Care.* Smith & Nephew. 2002;1:1–38.
5. Worley CA. "Why won't this wound heal?" Factors affecting wound repair. *Dermatol Nurs.* 2004;16:360–361.
6. Paustian C. Pain: nursing management. *Healthy Skin.* 2006;2:23–26.
7. Eager C. Relieving pain during dressing changes in the elderly. *Ostomy Wound Manage.* Caregiver's Corner. 2002;48(5):20–21.
8. Iowa Cancer Pain Relief Initiative. Comfort Assessment Journal. 2000.
9. Fleck C. Ethical wound management for the palliative patient. *ECPN.* 2005:38–46.
10. The Kestrel Wound Product Sourcebook. 2003;6:69–151.
11. Reddy M. Kohr R, Queen D, et al. Practical treatment of wound pain and trauma: a patient-centered approach. An overview. *Ostomy Wound Manage.* 2003;49;2–15.
12. Warshaw E, Nix D, Kula J, et al. Clinical and cost effectiveness of a cleanser protectant lotion for treatment of perineal skin breakdown in low-risk patients with incontinence. *Ostomy Wound Manage.* 2002;48:44–51.
13. Doughty D. Skin care for odor control and surface support. National Association for Continence. *Discoveries.* 2004;1:19.
14. Konya C, Sanada H, Sugama J, et al. Skin debris and micro-organisms on the periwound skin of pressure ulcers and the influence of periwound cleansing on microbial flora. *Ostomy Wound Manage.* 2005;51:50–59.
15. Gray M. Preventing and managing perineal dermatitis. A shared goal for wound and continence care. *J Wound Ostomy Continence Nurs.* 2004;31:S2–S12.
16. Fantl JA, Newman D, Colling J, et al. Urinary incontinence in adults: acute and chronic management. Clinical Practice Guideline, No 2, 1996 Update. Rockville, MD: U.S. Department of Health and Human Services. 1996;2:1–92.
17. Worley CA. Assessment and terminology: critical issues in wound care. *Dermatol Nurs.* 2004;16:451–457.
18. Moody P, Gonzales I, Cureton VY. The effect of body position and mattress type on interface pressure in quadriplegic adults: a pilot study. *Dermatol Nurs.* 2004;16:507–512.
19. Falanga V, Sibbald G. *The Science of Wound Bed Preparation.* Smith & Nephew. Module XXIII; 1–32.
20. Healthpoint Product Monograph. Papain-Urea Debriding Ointment. 1997;3–15.
21. Gupta S, Baharestani M, Baranoski S, et al. Guidelines for managing pressure ulcers with negative pressure wound therapy. *Adv Skin Wound Care.* 2005;32:1–16.
22. Dellinger RA, Britton C. Autologous Platelet Grafing Procedures: A New Approach to Healing Chronic Wounds and Comparison between Current Therapies. Presented at New Vascular Horizons and Management of Diabetic Foot & Would Healing. New Orleans. 2003.
23. Korinko A, Yurick A. Maintaining skin integrity during radiation therapy. *Am J Nurs.* 1997;97:40–44.
24. Goncalves Ml, Conceicao de Gouveia Santos VL, Andrucioli de Mattos Pimenta C, et al. Pain in chronic leg ulcers. *J W ound Ostomy Continence Nurs.* 2004;31:275–283.

PART

3

SPECIAL ISSUES IN CANCER PAIN MANAGEMENT

Ethical Issues in the Cancer Pain Patient

9

Martin L. Smith
Anne Lederman Flamm
Chad F. Slieper

INTRODUCTION

Since the 1970s, the standards of treatment and care provided by physicians and other healthcare professionals in the United States have included increased attention to patients' wishes and rights. The duty to respect patients and their autonomy now accompanies the more ancient duties of nonmaleficence ("do no harm"), beneficence ("do good"), and promoting patients' best interests. For most clinical situations and professional-patient relationships, the impact has been significant. Most notably, an ethical and legal requirement has emerged that healthcare professionals, with few exceptions such as life-threatening situations, must obtain patients' voluntary and informed consent before initiating diagnostic procedures and treatments. The doctrine of informed consent incorporates patients' right to refuse treatment, including treatments that are life-sustaining. Reflecting the importance of patient choice, professionals need skills beyond medical proficiency (e.g., communication and negotiation) to gain patients' trust and confidence in the therapeutic relationship. Occasionally, for healthcare professionals, dilemmas arise because of conflicts between or among various ethical duties and expectations regarding patient care.

Cancer pain physicians and clinicians are commensurately affected by this "age of autonomy." In routine clinical encounters, cancer pain professionals are expected to provide patients with understandable information and education, and to obtain patients' authorization before proceeding with diagnostic tests and treatments for pain and palliation. In the context of cancer pain, responsibilities to obtain informed consent and build trust (essential for any professional-patient relationship) can be complicated by the effects that patients' pain can have on their emotional and cognitive states. Occasionally, ethical dilemmas arise.

In this chapter, we present foundational concepts, methods, and strategies for thinking and acting ethically. These foundational components form a useful framework for identifying and managing ethical conflicts in any healthcare setting. We then incorporate these foundational concepts and methods to analyze three specific ethical issues arising in the management of cancer pain patients: patient nonadherence, the clinical use of placebos, and end-of-life care. Comparable to clinical training, familiarity and practice with these methods and strategies can enhance healthcare professionals' abilities to resolve ethical dilemmas arising in patient care.

BIOETHICAL FOUNDATIONS

Developments in the field of bioethics have included identification and articulation of core concepts, terms, and methods useful for analyzing and resolving clinical-ethical issues and dilemmas. We summarize here three methods of ethical analysis with their corresponding concepts and terminology that are useful for clinical practice. The methods discussed provide a foundational framework for the specific issues to be discussed in this chapter. The three methods are: principlism, consequentialism, and casuistry.

▶ The method of principlism

Principlism has its roots in the philosophical theory of deontology (*deon* meaning "duty" in Greek). When applied to clinical circumstances, deontology asserts that healthcare professionals have specific, identifiable duties that are morally and ethically right and generally should be followed. Beauchamp and Childress have identified four basic bioethical principles and duties from which, in their opinion, all other bioethical principles and duties can be derived.[1] The four principles and duties are: respect for persons, including their autonomy; beneficence; nonmaleficence; and justice. These generalized and abstract articulations of significant healthcare values are often woven into professional codes of ethics and ethics-related policies and guidelines.

There is general agreement among bioethicists that none of the four principles is absolute, that is, it must be upheld at all times in all circumstances. In fact, in many ethical dilemmas (when two or more of the principles are in conflict with one another), upholding all the principles is impossible, forcing the decision makers to choose one principle or set of principles over others. Thus, each principle or duty can be limited and conditioned by the circumstances of the case and other principles at stake.

Respect for persons and their autonomy

Respect for persons and their autonomy encompasses a wide set of concepts, including self-determination, patients' wishes, voluntariness to make one's own decisions, and privacy. In countries such as the United States where democracy has flourished, these values can have long-standing cultural and social roots. In clinical practice, respect for persons and their autonomy means that each patient should be viewed as a self-determining person who has the right to act in accord with freely chosen and informed goals, as long as those choices and their corresponding actions do not interfere with or infringe upon the choices and actions of others. Engaging patients in the educative process of informed consent,[2] respecting patients' informed refusals, honoring patients' advance directives and the decisions of their surrogates who provide substituted judgments,[3] and soliciting pediatric patients' assent and participation in health-care decisions in accord with their cognitive development[4] are all concrete formulations of respect for persons and their autonomy. The duty to respect persons and their autonomy also serves as a foundational principle from which other duties can be derived, such as veracity and confidentiality.

Veracity or truth-telling not only is a concrete manifestation of respect for patients, but it is also a prerequisite for patients to exercise their autonomy and authorize treatment through the informed consent process. Patients need honest, accurate, and understandable information in order to make healthcare choices that promote their own values and goals. Similarly, healthcare professionals demonstrate their respect for patients when they protect the confidentiality and privacy of patients' personal health information.

Nonmaleficence

The principle of nonmaleficence in health care captures the duty not to harm patients. "Above all, do no harm" is an ancient, Hippocratic expression of this basic duty. Of course, physicians and other clinicians often cause pain or discomfort, or at least expose their patients to risks of harms in the course of providing treatment or diagnostic tests. Chemotherapy, radiation therapy, and surgery can have significant side effects, toxicities, adverse events, and other risks. Even routine blood sampling for laboratory tests carries the risks of infection, bruising, and discomfort. Significant, then, to understanding the duty of nonmaleficence is consideration of the intention of the professional. Healthcare professionals who take seriously the duty to "do no harm" must not directly and intentionally harm patients, nor have harm and risk to patients as the primary and intended consequence of their actions.

Beneficence

In most clinical situations, the harm or risk of harm to patients is justified by the likelihood of benefit from the treatments or procedures. In other words, the duty of nonmaleficence can only be actualized in relationship and in proportion to the principle of beneficence, which affirms the duty to promote the health and well-being of patients. Stated more simply, the principle of beneficence requires healthcare professionals to benefit their patients and to promote patients' best interests over their own. When seeking to balance burdens and benefits, clinicians should adhere to a basic guideline of always maximizing possible benefits while minimizing possible harms. Finally, although healthcare professionals will often perceive "patient benefit" primarily in physiological categories related to good and reasonably likely medical outcomes, patients' perceptions of benefit may include not only medical outcomes but also other meaningful interests and activities (e.g., pursuing employment, maintaining relationships, participating in hobbies). Thus, a recommended treatment with a good likelihood of medical benefit (e.g., an arm amputation for a localized cancerous tumor to save a patient's life), but which will not allow a patient to continue a significant interest and activity (e.g., playing the violin), can be judged differently by the patient because of a different perception of the burden-to-benefit ratio.

Justice

The principle of justice or fairness in health care deals primarily with patient access to healthcare resources (e.g., a bed in the intensive care unit, a physician's or nurse's time and expertise, medications for pain, palliative or hospice care). The principle of justice requires that the benefits and burdens associated with healthcare delivery be distributed or allocated fairly. Ethical dilemmas of distributive justice arise frequently when resources are limited or scarce and therefore insufficient to meet the needs of everyone. The fair allocation of scarce resources requires the identification of ethically supportable criteria and their equitable application to clinical situations. For decisions affecting the distribution of and access to healthcare resources, an essential and significant (but not sufficient) criterion is the likelihood of a good medical outcome. Ultimately, the duty to act justly also requires healthcare professionals to set aside biases and discriminatory views about race, ethnicity, gender, lifestyles, or social status, and to treat similar clinical situations and cases similarly. Like respect for persons and their autonomy, the abstract principle of justice is culturally comfortable in countries like the United States, but its actualization can be complex and problematic.

▶ The method of consequentialism

The second method for thinking and acting ethically is consequentialism, which has its roots in the philosophical theory of teleology (*telos* in Greek means "ends"). Consequentialism aims to determine the rightness or wrongness of decisions and actions by calculating the positive and negative (i.e., the burdensome and beneficial) consequences or projected results of different identified options before the decisions and actions are carried out. Although healthcare decisions almost always affect patients primarily, patients are not the only ones to experience the consequences of such decisions. Patients' families and their significant others, the healthcare professionals involved, the health care institution or organization, as well as society in general can be affected by both bedside and policy-level decisions. One challenge of calculating consequences for each identified option is to be reasonably thorough in anticipating what the various outcomes will be. In many situations, experienced clinicians and healthcare teams, using their knowledge of previous cases and building on their collective wisdom, can reasonably project not only clinical consequences but also the psychological, social, spiritual, and legal results for the affected parties. An additional challenge is determining how much weight to give to each of the various positive and negative (beneficial and burdensome) consequences. In the end, if consequences can be identified, sorted into categories of burdensome and beneficial, and then weighted against each other, consequentialism requires healthcare professionals to choose and act on the option that provides more benefits, and to avoid the option that will bring the most harm.

▶ The method of casuistry

The third method for analyzing and handling ethical issues and dilemmas is casuistry.[5] Casuistry, which shares its root with the word "case," is a method of ethical analysis based on the practical judgments about the similarities and differences between cases. According to casuistry, attention must first be given to the details, specific features, and circumstances of the case or situation at hand. Then, an attempt is made to identify previous and known cases that are analogous to the new case and that had reasonably good and ethically supportable outcomes. If a previous or paradigm case can be identified for which a consensus exists as to right or wrong conduct, then the paradigm case may provide ethical guidance for the new case. In the process of identifying similarities and differences between cases, moral maxims, or rules of thumb functioning in the paradigm case are determined. Examples of such rules of thumb illuminated by casuistry and widely accepted in bioethics include the following: (1) an adult, informed patient with decisional capacity has the right to refuse treatment; (2) physicians should not be required to provide treatment that they judge to be medically inappropriate; and (3) a lesser harm can be tolerated to prevent a greater harm. For the new case, a determination must be made as to which moral maxims should guide the case and to what extent. A resolution for the case can occur through the accumulation of arguments for one option over another.

Although the term "casuistry" may be unfamiliar to clinicians, the method itself is not. In clinical practice, physicians routinely compare cases in the process of diagnosing disease. When patients present with specific sets of signs and symptoms of illness, skilled physicians are usually able to determine diagnoses because they have seen previous and similar cases or because of what they know from published literature and training. The ability to recognize similarities among clinical cases allows physicians to recommend treatment plans that have a reasonable likelihood of good medical outcomes. An effective use of this method requires healthcare professionals and medical teams to build up a kind of knowledge-based storehouse of previous ethics cases from which to draw upon when new ethical issues arise. Such a storehouse can contribute to clinicians' practical wisdom for handling appropriately their own new ethical dilemmas.

Like the two other methods described above, casuistry has its own challenges. Just as physicians can misdiagnose their patients' illnesses, those using casuistry as a practical method for ethical analysis can fail to adequately identify dissimilarities between cases and therefore choose incorrect paradigm cases. A challenge of casuistry is to pay sufficient attention to the relevant details and facts of the new case to be able to bring forth the proper moral maxims and guidance from former, analogous cases.

ETHICS RESOURCES AND PRACTICAL STRATEGIES

As is true in the clinical setting generally, one challenge of resolving ethical dilemmas in cancer pain is committing time and other resources required for the process. Practical strategies for resolving ethical problems and dilemmas demand the development of skills and familiarity with the analytic methods themselves (including, but not limited to, principlism, consequentialism, and casuistry), the assistance of experts in relevant fields, direct and consistent communication among those involved, and commitment to the task itself.[6,7]

The process of resolving bioethical dilemmas incorporates several stages. While no algorithm can account for every conflict that the care of cancer pain patients may present, we propose the following steps to promote comprehensive, thoughtful analysis and resolution.

▶ Steps in a conflict-resolution process

Fact gathering

Medical information Current and candid medical information is crucial to ethical decision-making. Does the situation call for additional information, or the expertise of a consultant? Are medical alternatives available? Ambiguous medical facts may be unavoidable, such as when a patient's source of pain cannot be identified or prognosis is unknown, but the consistency of medical information is also critical. While medical professionals may legitimately maintain divergent opinions, patients who receive conflicting opinions may need assistance in assessing which recommendation best meets their goals.

Psychosocial information Psychosocial information may be equally critical to resolving conflicts. Patients' support systems or lack thereof, financial problems, psychological or behavioral disorders, education status, and cultural or religious affiliation can dictate or influence patients' responses to recommended treatments. Thus, information about these and other psychosocial issues may enlighten the decision-making process.

"Voices" of interested parties Healthcare dilemmas always require the identification of persons ethically and legally authorized to make decisions, whether ultimate authority for a particular decision rests with a physician, patient, or surrogate. In addition, inviting participation by others whose voices may be influential to decision-making (e.g., patients' family members or friends, trusted medical consultants, legal counsel, or spiritual leaders) may inform and assist the decision-making process. Fact gathering should also explore and comprehend the dynamics and power differentials among various parties because these may affect the process of analysis and decision-making. Additionally, providing members of the healthcare team with an opportunity for their voices to be heard can ease conflicts within the team and with patients and families.

Real or potential bias Participants in the decision-making process, whether by introspection or external consideration, should identify any conflict of interest or circumstance that threatens their ability to maintain appropriate objectivity or empathy, and ensure that the potential threat is mitigated. Biases can be subtle, and all participants should be open to the possibility that some of their biases can be impacting their perspectives and the decision-making process.

Motivations and goals Direct exploration of the goals and motivations of the various participants in the bioethical dilemma may reveal information about the conflict itself. While most participants likely share the underlying goal of promoting a patient's well-being, discordance among treatment goals may be the source of an apparent conflict in values. For example, disagreements about the appropriateness of life-sustaining treatment may reflect the physician's view that palliation is the current goal, while the patient is hoping and holding out for cure. Patients' rejection of physicians' pain management recommendations may reflect their prioritization of cognitive alertness over relief of physical pain, or vice versa.

Identify and describe the conflicting principles, values, and duties

Articulating the principles, values, and duties at stake in the situation enables participants to understand that those who appear to disagree are usually motivated by laudable, albeit different, goals. Understanding the ethical issues or dilemmas in terms of conflicting principles and duties may illuminate creative options that balance or accommodate divergent values without disregarding or discounting them.

Identify paradigm cases, experiences, moral maxims, and relevant policies

Using the practical wisdom of those who have experienced the particular type of problem (e.g., medical or ancillary healthcare providers, hospital administrators, bioethicists) can inform the deliberative process as can accessing relevant published literature, case law, institutional policies, and guidelines and position statements of professional organizations. As noted above in the discussion of casuistry, precedent and paradigm cases analogous to the new situation at hand may provide insight and moral maxims facilitating resolution of the new case.

Identify options and calculate consequences

Analysis and discussion should be geared toward identifying ethically justifiable options, with openness to the perspectives of all participants in the process. Again, most options will likely require compromise or accommodation among principles, values, and duties, and those responsible for decision-making should feel that the process exposed them to all relevant considerations. As options are identified, the positive and negative consequences for the patient, family, healthcare professionals, institution, and wider society should be assessed and weighed.

Communicate ethical justifications for decision and plan of action

After the decision-makers reach consensus and conclusion, explicit communication of action plans as well as ethical justifications for their decisions promote confidence that the decisions are conscientious and optimal under the circumstances among participants in the process and others whose support is critical (e.g., family caregivers). Communication, which encompasses good written documentation of the process and conclusions in patients' medical records, also facilitates and promotes consistency in implementing the plan.

Reevaluate for self-education and reconsider as necessary

Implementation of the decision and action plan may illuminate both positive and negative aspects about the analytic process for resolving conflicts. These aspects of the process should be acknowledged to redress flaws, redirect action in the present case if necessary, educate participants, and inform future analyses.

▶ Strategies and formats for the conflict-resolution process

The process of resolving ethical dilemmas can occur in a number of formats. In some circumstances, individual physicians might successfully undertake the steps described above. Other situations might necessitate patient care conferences among healthcare professionals, patients, and their families. Still other situations may benefit from involvement of ethics consultation services or committees. Resolution may occur after an initial discussion, or require staged interventions and repeated assessments. Due to the nature of true bioethical dilemmas in which significant principles and duties conflict and the consequences of acts impact sick patients and their families and care professionals, resolution rarely brings everyone complete satisfaction, no matter what the quality of the process has been. The stakes of a true bioethical dilemma enhance the importance of a good decision-making process that gives participants confidence that the result is the best possible one.

Many factors can influence judgments in selecting a format for the analytic process. Clinical urgency is an obvious variable. For example, the need to respond to a vulnerable patient's threat to leave the hospital immediately against medical advice may allow little or no time to engage an ethics consultation service that operates using a team model. In contrast, considering how to manage an outpatient's behavior that is suspicious for drug diversion may benefit from a planned discussion among physicians, nurses, and social workers

familiar with the patient, and hospital administrators and others with expertise in chemical dependence, law, and clinical ethics.

The scope of the problem may also influence format. A patient's refusal of adequate pain management may pose a dilemma that requires open communication between the patient and physician only. However, learning that the patient is being faithful to the counsel of his religious minister, who is both a close family friend and a powerful figure in the patient's community, may convince the physician that inviting (with the patient's permission) the patient's family, the pastor, and members of the hospital ethics committee to join in discussions of the problem might promote the patient's reconsideration of his position.

Consequences of an individual patient's decision that affect a broader community might justify an intervention beyond discussion between physician and patient. For example, a patient's request for palliative sedation to redress intractable pain may be best addressed in a setting such as a family care conference that includes the patient and his extended support system. Before reaching a decision to grant the patient's request, a physician may also need to include other professionals involved in the patient's care to ensure that they are willing to participate.

Finally, the more conflictual and controversial the dilemma, the more substantial the format may need to be to maximize ethical comfort with the resolution. Implementing a request for palliative sedation may be relatively straightforward at an academic medical center with a developed and integrated palliative care program. The same request at a small community hospital with no experience in the practice may generate greater ethical concern and require a more substantial inquiry and evaluation. The same patient's request for assistance in suicide may cause alarm in both environments, suggesting the need for lengthier and deliberate analysis.

PATIENT COMPLIANCE AND ADHERENCE

Patients' compliance[8,9] or adherence to medical recommendations is both necessary and challenging in the context of cancer pain management. Poor adherence to physician-recommended regimens can contribute to ineffective cancer pain management.[10] Moreover, patients' pain and suffering is unnecessary to the extent that adherence could alleviate them. Yet studies have identified numerous barriers to patients' abilities, choices, and desires to adhere to medical recommendations related to pain management. Some significant factors in compliance include beliefs about the meaning of pain, the value and consequences of medical treatments, and the severity of pain itself.[11]

Nonadherence imposes numerous harms, the most obvious being that the patient fails to receive treatment benefits. Patients may also build resistance to otherwise effective treatments, and require more toxic medications, additional procedures, or hospital admissions as a consequence of diverging from medical advice. One estimate of the economic costs of medication nonadherence, which includes consequential hospital and nursing home admissions and lost productivity, exceeds $100 billion.[12] Nonadherence may also generate intangible harms, such as destroying patients' confidence in medical treatment and eroding providers' sense of professional integrity, morale, and commitment to caring for patients. Incidence estimates range from 15% to 93%, with an average of one-third of patients failing to adhere to a recommended therapeutic regimen.[10]

Nonadherent patients challenge several professional, ethical, and legal duties of the provider-patient relationship. Nonadherent patients' use of financial and provider resources creates an issue of justice: the concern that healthcare resources are not being distributed fairly and in proportion to need. When patients refuse to accept physicians' recommendations, commentators often describe patient autonomy as being in conflict with the physician duty of beneficence, which is grounded in both ethics and law. The principle of autonomy is also significant for healthcare professionals. Physicians traditionally have been free to choose whom they will treat, and to use their medical judgment in the determination of appropriate care. Yet, once a physician establishes a relationship with a patient, the physician must avoid abandoning the patient, which can be a legal cause of action and a violation of the duty of beneficence. Thus, treating a nonadherent patient or deciding to discontinue treatment requires a physician to balance competing ethical duties.

▶ "Divorcing" nonadherent patients

Terminating the physician-patient relationship may be justified in rare instances. Suggestions for avoiding ethical irresponsibility and legal liability for abandonment of noncompliant patients include: (1) informing the patient explicitly in advance about the terms that might result in divorce from the physician or the institution; (2) if termination will proceed, giving unequivocal written notice thereof; (3) specifying a defined grace period enabling the patient to find another physician; (4) offering assistance in finding another physician (e.g., providing a local or state referral agency); and (5) informing the patient that the physician is obligated to treat the patient for any emergent needs.[13] Because other legal constraints may exist in particular situations and jurisdictions, terminating the physician-patient relationship should be done only after receiving legal counsel.

▶ Avoiding "divorce"

Knowing legal guidelines for avoiding patient abandonment does not answer the question of *when*, ethically and professionally, termination is appropriate. Identifying ways to mitigate or minimize patients' nonadherence may preclude the need for termination. Some theories explaining nonadherence suggest strategies that might enable healthcare professionals to continue managing their patients.

Personality and psychological issues

First, patients' personalities and psychological issues can contribute to nonadherence. Patients' cognitive abilities must be considered in assessing nonadherence. When patients repeatedly forget or miss appointments or self-administration of medication, dementia or an inability to organize might be at the root of the problem. Reviewing patients' schedules and patterns of behaviors with them, or brainstorming strategies to minimize disabilities or cognitive weaknesses (e.g., use of diaries or pictorial reminders) might enhance patients' abilities to adhere to treatment regimens. Addressing more extreme personality issues, such as borderline personality disorders, might be advanced with the aid of psychiatrists or other mental health professionals. Formal assessment of decision-making capacity may be informative and is necessary when considering compulsory treatment via court order.

Patients who react negatively to authority or who are rigidly self-reliant may resent their dependence on medical professionals, and act out this personality trait by not complying with treatment recommendations.[14] Patients who are depressed or have low self-esteem might consider themselves not worthy of treatment or care. Patients who decline to participate actively in their own care, or who behave in a manner that threatens their dependent state, might

actually be expressing a desire to be cared for.[15] Physicians may be able to enhance adherence by adapting their communication style to particular patients' needs. For example, patients who resent authority figures might cooperate more fully if they perceive that they have some control of their own treatment plan. Therefore, instead of asserting medical advice, a physician might state, "I'm thinking that A, B, and C is appropriate; what do you think?" Other patients might be more receptive to receiving information stated authoritatively, and respond better to being told what to do. For patients whose nonadherent conduct reflects insecurity or dependence, a physician's assertiveness might affirm to the patient that the proposed treatment, and thereby the patient himself, is valuable and worth pursuing.

Some nonadherent patients might need to be motivated with fear of negative consequences. A written treatment contract that clearly states required behaviors and the consequences of breaches, including termination of the physician-patient relationship, may encourage adherence.[16] One consideration before embarking on an ultimatum strategy is that the promise of rewards and the threat of punishment set forth in the contract must be meaningful. Failing to fulfill a promise not only violates trust, but may exacerbate and magnify the existing problems.

Patients' decisions not to adhere to medical recommendations may reflect either their psychological need to regain some measure of control over their health and their lives,[17] or a serious denial of the reality of their illness.[18] These considerations should be explored directly with patients in the context of adherence issues. With the patient's permission, a physician could enlist third parties such as family members, friends, or a therapist or psychiatrist, to explore the patient's motivations and characteristics.

Social circumstances and health-related beliefs

Patients' social circumstances beyond their illnesses should also be considered. Illiteracy, family or work demands, inability to arrange for transportation or childcare, or lack of financial resources to pay for medications may contribute to nonadherence. Clinicians may enhance patients' abilities to achieve adherence by identifying these issues. Enlisting family members to support the patient's medical care, connecting the patient with a mentor, support group, or community social services, or referral to a social worker might be helpful.

Patients' cultural backgrounds may also impact adherence. Cultural beliefs about pain and medication influence how patients deal with pain and feel about taking analgesics.[19] Dietary restrictions or observances of religious traditions may interfere with a patient's adherence. More complicated issues, such as ongoing language barriers or different customs about caregiving responsibilities within a family, may also impede a patient's ability or willingness to adopt medical recommendations.

Patients with chronic illnesses or those who have been hospitalized for long periods may simply be overwhelmed with frustration and fatigue related to their inability to be healthy. It might be worth exploring whether a break or "holiday" from treatment is possible, or bargaining with patients to find ways for them to remain motivated for defined periods of time.[15]

Some patients have their own beliefs about the necessity of recommended treatment, or harbor concerns about the dangers or side effects of the treatment. These beliefs may not be accurate but convince the patient to disregard medical advice.[8,19] Patients may fear that analgesics cause negative effects, or they may attribute spiritual meaning to physical suffering, and elect not to adhere to pain management regimens. Making the reasons for treatment orders transparent,[20] and explicitly exploring patients' understandings of their treatments may facilitate compliance.

Reciprocally, physicians who misunderstand patients' objectives or goals might recommend therapy that patients, in order to meet their objectives, would have to refuse.[21] For example, a patient may be willing to tolerate pain rather than experience physical or mental side effects of the recommended treatment.[22] Discordance between the physician's and the patient's expectations about the relationship, or about the objectives of treatment, may yield dissatisfaction that leads to the patient's nonadherence.[21]

The physician's role

Physicians also need to think about problems deriving from their own relationship with the patient. Failures of communication are an obvious reason why patients might appear nonadherent.[23,24] Some examples of nonadherence clearly do not derive from flawed communication; directions to "Stop using cocaine while on this medicine," or "Come to your scheduled appointment" are unequivocal. But miscommunication could be the source of other forms of nonadherence (e.g., when and how much medication to take, or whether certain activities are permissible) that might be redressed with explicit clarification.

Clinicians who view a patient as noncompliant and difficult might accentuate and permit the patient's nonadherence, in the hope that the patient could more quickly be discharged. Providers caring for nonadherent patients may need to assess whether the problems are repairable, or whether transferring the patient will ameliorate the situation. Professionals should also consider whether practical problems with the healthcare delivery system are a factor. Long waits, inefficiencies, or conflicts with staff can challenge a patient's coping skills and contribute to an unwillingness to collaborate.

Accepting nonadherence

Finally, a physician may need to confront whether the patient's nonadherence reflects rationality in the face of severe illness. Mr. K was a 40-year-old patient with non-small cell lung cancer and metastases to lung and bone. He also required treatment for fibromyalgia, asthma, hypertension, and diabetes. He had completed one course of chemotherapy, but repeated instances of nonadherence resulted in his cancer now being untreatable. Mr. K had presented to the emergency center 14 times in a 3-month period for lower back and chest pain, receiving referrals to cardiology, pain management and symptom control specialists, and psychiatry. Upon each presentation, physicians learned he had not adhered to their previous recommendations for pain control and other follow-up care.

Mr. K had left home at age 14 and had spent his life on the street. He boasted of his lifestyle, which involved illegal drug and alcohol use, and seemed to glory in his self-destruction. While all of his physicians struggled to provide effective care, his pain management physicians were particularly caught between their desire to help him and their concerns about the risks their actions posed to Mr. K and to others due to his misuse of medications. Numerous interventions—care conferences, bargaining, contracts—designed to collaborate with Mr. K failed.

Mr. K had no experience with the kind of lifestyle presumed by a care plan that emphasized regular rest, nutrition, and health monitoring as well as controlled use of narcotics. Moreover, he had no external resources to support efforts to redirect the path of his life. His physicians ultimately were forced to accept that Mr. K's nonadherence

ensured his untimely and possibly painful death. As stated in a well-known article, treating "chronically self-murderous" patients requires caregivers "to recognize the limitations that such patients pose . . . and to work with diligence and compassion to preserve the denier as long as possible, just as one does with any other patient with a terminal illness."[25]

PLACEBO USE IN THE TREATMENT OF CANCER PAIN

Contemporary context, historic foundations

There may be many healthcare professionals who believe that the use of placebos in clinical practice has been discontinued and placebos are now used only in clinical research and randomized controlled trials. However, the clinical use of placebos is not simply an historic artifact, despite the fact that professional organizations have published position statements expressly prohibiting the use of placebos to assess or manage pain.[26,27] A study published in 2004 found that 60% of healthcare providers in a sample of Jerusalem-area hospitals used placebos in their practice, and of these users, 62% prescribed placebos at least once a month.[28] Thus, education and discussion about the ethics of placebo use may be necessary and relevant even in the environment of contemporary healthcare that highly values veracity, patient autonomy, and an understanding of informed consent that would preclude placebo use in most situations.

The use of placebos hearkens back to Percival's nineteenth century conception of medical ethics in which veracity must be balanced against beneficence, and if telling the truth would harm patients (according to physicians' judgments), then the truth must be withheld and physicians should instead provide a message of hope and comfort.[29] This Percivalian ethical stance reflects a paternalistic perspective in which physicians alone determine how much information patients need and what course of action needs to be taken.

Ethical analysis

When treating patients who have cancer pain, is the clinical use of placebos ever ethically justifiable? The placebo effect is well documented,[30,31] and thus the use of placebos in the clinical setting may be tempting under certain conditions when physicians judge patients' pain to be psychosomatic or when the pain has been refractory to other standard treatments. The use of placebos, however, can compromise important and accepted ethical principles and duties; specifically, the principles of veracity or truth-telling, and respect for patients and their autonomy. Both principles support the right of patients to make decisions about what will happen to their bodies in the course of medical treatment, and the violation of both principles can undermine patients' participation in the process of informed consent and their need for honest, open, and understandable information.

A proposed use of placebos is not without ethical justification; most physicians who feel compelled to use placebos may be motivated by the dual duties of beneficence and nonmaleficence, that is, wanting to benefit their patients while reducing harms and adverse side effects associated with ineffective or unnecessary medications. Further, an argument could be made that the use of placebos can contribute to physicians' duty to actualize the principle of justice, that is, more accurate diagnoses of the cause of patients' pain could lead to the use of fewer healthcare resources. In short, the use of placebos in clinical practice cannot be absolutely ruled out, but any uses of placebos judged to be ethically supportable will be extremely limited, and must fully address concerns about compromising the principles of veracity and autonomy.

As bioethics has evolved and the principles of veracity and autonomy have become more central to the analysis of ethical dilemmas in countries such as the United States where individual choice and rights are so highly valued, it is problematic to come down on the side of beneficence, nonmaleficence, and justice to the exclusion of veracity and autonomy. Veracity is central to building trust within successful physician-patient relationships.[32] Such trust is partially based on an expectation of honesty between physicians and patients; without honesty, trust can deteriorate. Actions that require deception on the part of physicians, such as prescribing placebos, can erode trust and undermine patients' relationships not only with their current physicians, but also with future physicians.

Similarly, respect for persons and their autonomy requires that professionals allow patients to make decisions about what will or will not be done to their own bodies. To facilitate the ability of patients to make healthcare decisions in an educated and informed manner, bioethics and law have asserted the doctrine of informed consent by which healthcare professionals must provide information to patients, including the disclosure of material information about a proposed treatment,[33] and engage patients in an educational process ultimately resulting in consent to a particular procedure or course of treatment. Prescribing placebos when patients believe the pills or injections received are active drugs deprives patients of material information and impedes true informed consent.

The principles of veracity and autonomy provide good reason to reject the use of placebos. There is also a legitimate argument, however, that despite concerns about placebo use, the benefits of the placebo effect may make placebo use a reasonable option for prescribing physicians.[34] In cases where no other treatment exists or is indicated for a particular condition or symptom, the use of placebos by physicians may in fact be in accordance with the principles of beneficence and nonmaleficence. In these cases, physicians must proceed carefully and deliberately to act according to accepted ethical principles while preserving any therapeutic benefit placebos may provide.

Acting ethically in the realm of placebos

As discussed above, healthcare professionals should, in general, reject the use of placebos for clinical management or assessment of particular conditions, including cancer pain, based on the principles of autonomy and veracity. However, if patients are experiencing pain symptoms for which there is no effective or indicated treatment, and the provider does not wish to lose the potential therapeutic benefit placebos might provide, physicians could ethically prescribe placebos in limited situations if specific requirements are met.

To prescribe placebos ethically, healthcare professionals must first explain clearly what a placebo is (e.g., an inert substance such as a sugar pill or a saline injection that has no proven effect on the patient's condition other than the placebo effect), and then inform patients that placebos may be used in the course of their treatment. The physician should also explain exactly what the placebo effect is and why it might be beneficial. After such explanations are provided and patients understand the information, and if patients are willing to consent to a course of treatment that may include the use of placebos, professionals will have adequately addressed concerns related to autonomy and veracity, and may ethically proceed with the use of placebos.[35] As Berkowitz and Sutton reiterate, instances of the clinical use of placebos should be rare.[35] Finally, as with all medical practice issues, physicians and other practitioners should familiarize themselves with appropriate legal considerations in their jurisdictions.

PAIN, PALLIATION, AND END-OF-LIFE CARE

A common assertion regarding end-of-life care is that too many patients die with inadequate attention to their pain and discomfort. Various reasons and barriers have been identified related to this assertion and include insufficient training of physicians in end-of-life care, inadequate resources and third-party-payer reimbursement for palliative care and hospice, misunderstandings about the likelihood of patients becoming addicted to pain medications, and uncertainty about the ethical and legal distinctions between euthanasia and palliation that may hasten death. In this section, we will provide an ethical justification for distinguishing palliation from euthanasia, and discuss the sometimes controversial practice of forgoing medically supplied or artificial nutrition and hydration (ANH) at the end of life.

The principle of double effect

The standard example used for discussing the distinction between adequate palliation and euthanasia is the administration of opioids such as morphine, sometimes in high doses, to relieve dying patients' signs and symptoms of pain and distress. Morphine can have two effects: (1) pain relief and (2) respiratory suppression. In higher doses, morphine has the possibility of occasionally and perhaps even rarely[36] hastening death or shortening life. For physicians and other clinicians who oppose euthanasia on ethical grounds or who fear legal repercussions for even the appearance of having killed their patients through the administration of morphine, a conflict of duties (i.e., an ethical dilemma) can arise. How do physicians provide adequate comfort and pain relief for dying patients while not crossing an ethical, moral, and legal boundary by directly causing patients' deaths?

In contemporary bioethics, the principle of double effect has emerged as an ethical explanation and justification for providing adequate palliation for dying patients. This principle has its origins in Roman Catholic moral theology, with significant development appearing in the writings of Thomas Aquinas (1224–1274) who addressed a variety of dilemmas facing Christians, including participation in war, deception, and cooperation in evil.[37] The traditional principle of double effect states that an action with multiple possible effects, good and bad, is morally permitted if the action: (1) is not in itself immoral; (2) is undertaken only with the intention of achieving the possible good effects, without intending the possible bad effects even though they may be foreseen; (3) does not bring about the possible good effect by means of the possible bad effect; and (4) is undertaken for a proportionally grave reason. As Sulmasy and Pelligrino note,[38] "Treating dying patients in pain with appropriate doses of morphine is generally done in a manner that satisfies the criteria of double effect." They explain:

> The use of morphine (1) is not itself immoral; (2) it is undertaken only with the intention of relieving pain, not of causing death through respiratory depression; (3) morphine does not relieve pain only if it first kills the patient; and (4) the relief of pain is a proportionally grave reason for accepting the risk of hastening death.

An additional and similar application of the principle of double effect is the occasional practice of palliative sedation.[39] In rare instances, the only recourse for treating intractable pain and discomfort is to sedate a patient to unconsciousness. Palliative sedation, while providing comfort, prevents patients from interacting with family members and healthcare professionals, and from taking food and drink by mouth. These burdens and negative consequences may be acceptable to patients in exchange for the comfort and relief that palliative sedation will bring. Palliative sedation will therefore have stronger ethical justification when the patient's or surrogate's informed consent has been obtained. Even though palliative sedation may hasten the dying of patients, it can be justified through the principle of double effect.

The principle of double effect is not without its detractors.[40] A central criterion of the principle is that the bad effect or consequence of the action is foreseen but unintended. Human intentions for a single act can be multiple, ambiguous and unclear, and even contradictory. The principle of double effect assumes almost a clearly purposeful and single-minded intention. Further, in many other spheres of life, including civil and criminal law, people are held accountable for all reasonably foreseeable consequences of their actions, not just the intended consequences (e.g., the death of a pedestrian hit by an automobile driven by someone under the influence of alcohol). Why should physicians and clinicians be exempt from a similar expectation and responsibility for foreseen but unintended consequences of their actions?

Despite these criticisms, the principle of double effect remains a recognized ethical justification for providing adequate palliation that may hasten death. On a practical level, physicians and other clinicians should administer palliative medications only in response to patients' manifestations (or reasonably anticipated manifestations) of symptoms of pain and distress. Documentation in patients' medical records should include not only the medications prescribed and administered but also the symptoms being palliated.

▶ Forgoing artificial nutrition and hydration

In the care of dying patients, ethical and clinical controversy occasionally arises when discussion turns to forgoing ANH. At the core of the controversy is the designation of ANH as either a life-supporting medical measure similar to a ventilator or dialysis, which therefore can be forgone, or an element of basic comfort and caring similar to bathing, holding, or touching patients, which therefore should always be provided. Some of the controversy surrounding the provision and discontinuation of ANH may be rooted in the human connectedness that is symbolized by and associated with familial and cultural activities of eating and drinking.[41] Both the American Medical Association[42] and the American Nurses Association[43] have published statements that assert that ANH is a medical treatment subject to the same burden-and-benefit analyses as other medical treatments that can be ethically forgone at the end of life. Because the provision of ANH is not a totally benign treatment and carries with it identifiable burdens, physicians and other clinicians should assess each patient situation individually, weighing the burdens and benefits of forgoing ANH for the specific case; educate patients and their surrogates about the risks associated with specific and proposed means for administering ANH (e.g., nasogastric tube, total parenteral nutrition through a central line, gastrostomy tube); accommodate patients' wishes as long as there will be little or no harm to the patient; and assure patients and surrogates about a commitment to comfort and palliation regardless of the decision to forgo ANH.

CONCLUSIONS

In this chapter we have presented foundational methods, concepts, and strategies, and addressed three selected ethical issues in the care of cancer pain patients. But what we have presented is only a brief summary of relevant thought and literature. Therefore, we encourage continued and ongoing bioethics education and training for cancer pain professionals.

Although bioethics is an emerging and recently organized field of interest and inquiry, the field has achieved sufficient maturity to develop resources useful for clinical-ethical application. These resources include clinical ethics journals, books, and journal articles; university and college courses; computer-based Web sites, training materials, and academic courses; national and regional conferences, workshops, and seminars; and ethics consultants and committees.

Continually enhancing knowledge, skills, and comfort in recognizing and addressing ethical issues by routinely accessing such resources should be a professional goal for physicians and other clinicians providing diagnoses, treatments, and care for cancer pain patients. Ethics-related knowledge and skills, together with an ever-present commitment to respecting patients and promoting their best interests, can foster the humanistic care of cancer pain patients.

REFERENCES

1. Beauchamp TL, Childress JF. *Principles of Biomedical Ethics*, 5th ed. New York: Oxford University Press; 2001.
2. Lidz CW, Appelbaum PS, Meisel A. Two models of implementing informed consent. *Arch Intern Med.* 1988;148:1385–1389.
3. Emanuel L, Danis M, Pearlman R, Singer P. Advance care planning as a process: structuring the discussions in practice. *J Am Geriatr Soc.* 1995;43:440–446.
4. Leikin SL. Minors' assent or dissent to medical treatment. *J Pediatr.* 1983; 102:169–176.
5. Jonsen AR. Casuistry: an alternative or complement to principles? *Kennedy Inst Ethics J.* 1995;5:237–251.
6. The American Society for Bioethics and Humanities. *Core Competencies for Health Care Ethics Consultation.* Glenview, IL; 1998.
7. Fletcher JC, Spencer EM. Ethics services in healthcare organizations. In: Fletcher JC, Lombardo PA, Marshall MF, Miller FG, eds. *Introduction to Clinical Ethics*, 2nd ed. Hagerstown, MD: University Publishing Group, Inc.; 1997:257–285.
8. Donovan JL, Blake DR. Patient non-compliance: deviance or reasoned decision-making? *Soc Sci Med.* 1992;34:507–513.
9. Holm S. What is wrong with compliance? *J Med Ethics.* 1993;19:108–110.
10. Miaskowski C, Dodd MJ, West C, et al. Lack of adherence with the analgesic regimen: a significant barrier to effective cancer pain management. *J Clin Oncol.* 2001;19:4275–4279.
11. Robinson ME, Bulcourf F, Atchison JW, et al. Compliance in pain rehabilitation: patient and provider perspectives. *Pain Med.* 2004;5:66–80.
12. Berg JS, Dischler J, Wagner DJ, et al. Medication compliance: a healthcare problem. *Ann Pharmacother.* 1993;27:S1–S24.
13. *Payton v. Weaver*, 182 Cal. Rptr. 225 (Cal. App. 1982).
14. Matthews D. The noncompliant patient. *Primary Care.* 1975;2:289–294.
15. Appelbaum PS, Roth LH. Patients who refuse treatment in medical hospitals. *JAMA.* 1983;250:1296–1301.
16. Eraker SA, Kirscht JP, Becker MH. Understanding and improving patient compliance. *Ann Intern Med.* 1984;100:258–268.
17. Conrad P. The meaning of medications: another look at compliance. *Soc Sci Med.* 1985;20:29–37.
18. Kunkel EJ, Woods CM, Rodgers C, et al. Consultations for 'maladaptive denial of illness' in patients with cancer: psychiatric disorders that result in noncompliance. *Psychooncology.* 1997;6:139–149.
19. Lai Y, Keefe FJ, Sun WZ, et al. Relationship between pain-specific beliefs and adherence to analgesic regimens in Taiwanese cancer patients: a preliminary study. *J Pain Symptom Manage.* 2002;24:415–423.

20. Brody H. Transparency: informed consent in primary care. *Hastings Cent Rep.* 1989;19:5–9.
21. Sledge WH, Feinstein AR. A clinimetric approach to the components of the patient-physician relationship. *JAMA.* 1997;278:2043–2048.
22. Weiss SC, Emanuel LL, Fairclough DL, et al. Understanding the experience of pain in terminally ill patients. *Lancet.* 2001;357:1311–1315.
23. Burgess MM. Ethical and economic aspects of noncompliance and overtreatment. *CMAJ.* 1989;141:777–780.
24. Garrity TF. Medical compliance and the clinician-patient relationship: a review. *Soc Sci Med.* 1981;15E:215–222.
25. Groves JE. Taking care of the hateful patient. *N Engl J Med.* 1978;298:883–887.
26. American Nurses Association, Oncology Nursing Society. Position statement, use of placebos for pain management in patients with cancer. http://nursingworld.org/readroom/position/social/scpain.htm, 1996. Access date: Nov 28, 2005.
27. American Society for Pain Management Nursing. Position statement, use of placebos for pain management. http://www.aspmn.org/website/pdfs/Placebos revised_2005.pdf. Access date: Nov 28, 2005.
28. Nitzan U, Lichtenberg P. Questionnaire survey on use of placebo. *Br Med J.* 2004;329:944–946.
29. Thomas WJ. Informed consent, the placebo effect, and the revenge of Thomas Percival. *J Leg Med.* 2001;22:313–348.
30. de la Fuente-Fernandez R, Stoessl AJ. The biochemical bases of the placebo effect. *Sci Eng Ethics.* 2004;10:143–150.
31. Groopman J. The biology of hope. In: Groopman J, ed. *The Anatomy of Hope.* New York: Random House Trade Paperbacks; 2005:161–190.
32. Beauchamp TL, Childress JF. *Principles of Biomedical Ethics*, 5th ed. New York: Oxford University Press; 2001:283–284.
33. Beauchamp TL, Childress JF. *Principles of Biomedical Ethics*, 5th ed. New York: Oxford University Press; 2001:79–81.
34. Markus AC. The ethics of placebo prescribing. *Mt Sinai J Med.* 2000;67:140–143.
35. Berkowitz K, Sutton T. VHA National Ethics Teleconference, Clinical Use of Placebo: An Ethics Analysis. http://www1.va.gov/vhaethics/download/Transcripts/NET.7.28.04.doc, 2004. Access date: Nov 28, 2005.
36. Fohr SA. The double effect of pain medication: separating myth from reality. *J Palliat Med.* 1998;1:315–328.
37. Garcia JLA. Double effect. In: Reich WT, ed. *Encyclopedia of Bioethics, Revised Edition.* New York: Simon & Schuster MacMillan; 1995:636.
38. Sulmasy DP, Pellegrino ED. The rule of double effect, clearing up the double talk. *Arch Intern Med.* 1999;159:545–550.
39. Rousseau P. Palliative sedation in the management of refractory symptoms. *J Support Oncol.* 2004;2:181–186.
40. Quill TE, Dresser R, Brock DW. The rule of double effect—a critique of its role in end-of-life decision making. *N Engl J Med.* 1997;337:1768–1771.
41. Slomka J. What do apple pie and motherhood have to do with feeding tubes and caring for the patient? *Arch Intern Med.* 1995;155:1258–1263.
42. Council on Ethical and Judicial Affairs, American Medical Association. Decisions near the end of life. *JAMA.* 1992;267:2229–2233.
43. American Nurses Association. Position statement, forgoing nutrition, and hydration. http://nursingworld.org/readroom/position/ethics/etnutr.htm, 1992. Access date: November 28, 2005.

Psychiatric Issues in Cancer Pain Management

Steven D. Passik
Christopher Gibson
William Breitbart
Maria L. Rotta

CHAPTER

10

INTRODUCTION

Pain is an all too common problem for cancer patients, with approximately 70% experiencing severe pain at some point in the course of their illness,[1] nearly 75% with advanced cancer having pain,[2] and 25% dying in severe pain.[3] This is a disturbing reality, especially considering the wide range of pain control treatments available to clinicians today. Effectively managing pain in patients with cancer requires a multidisciplinary approach, enlisting expertise from diverse clinical specialties, including anesthesiology, neurology, psychiatry, psychology, neurosurgery, and rehabilitation medicine.[1,4,5] The effective utilization of psychiatric interventions in the treatment of cancer patients with pain has now also become an integral part of such a comprehensive approach.[6,7] In the all too rushed and complicated world of modern medicine, we sometimes fail to see issues outside of our field of specialization. Such bias, while understandable from a human perspective, may result in our patients receiving less than optimal care. Consequently, this chapter explores the phenomenon of pain in cancer patients and its effective treatment, emphasizing both the physiological and psychological components of the pain experience and its resultant effective treatment.

PAIN IN CANCER

There is considerable variability in the prevalence of pain amongst different types of cancer. For example, whereas only 5% of leukemia patients experience pain during the course of their illness, 50%–75% of patients with tumors of the lung, gastrointestinal tract, or genitourinary system experience pain. Patients with cancers of the bone or cervix have been found to have the highest prevalence of pain, with as many as 85% experiencing significant pain during the course of their illness.[4] Despite its high prevalence, research has shown that pain is frequently underdiagnosed and inadequately treated.[1,8] Additionally, it is important to remember that pain is frequently only one of several symptoms present in cancer patients. In a survey of symptoms, patients were found to suffer from an average of three troubling physical symptoms in addition to pain.[9] A more global, multidimensional evaluation of a patient's symptom burden facilitates a more complete understanding of the impact of pain upon an individual cancer patient.

MULTIDIMENSIONAL CONCEPT OF PAIN IN CANCER

Pain, especially in advanced cancer, is not a purely nociceptive or physical experience. Rather, it involves complex aspects of human functioning, including personality, affect, cognition, behavior, and social relationships.[10] Saunders[11] provided a vivid and enlightened description of pain that results from a serious physical illness such as cancer: "total pain." This label attempts to describe the all-encompassing nature of this type of pain, which should be instructive to the treating clinician in his or her attempt to bring relief to the patient.

With this concept of "total pain" in mind, it is important to note that the use of analgesic drugs alone does not always relieve pain.[12] It has been demonstrated that psychological factors play a modest but important role in modulating pain intensity.[13] The challenge of adequately addressing the complicated and interwoven physical and psychological issues involved in pain perception is essential to developing rational and effective management strategies. The interaction among cognitive, emotional, socioenvironmental, and nociceptive aspects of pain, shown in Fig. 10-1, illustrates the multidimensional nature of pain in cancer and suggests a resultant model for effective multimodal intervention.[5] Psychosocial therapies directed primarily at psychological variables have profound impact on nociception, while somatic therapies directed at nociception have beneficial effects on the psychological aspects of pain. Ideally, such somatic and psychosocial therapies should be used simultaneously in the multidisciplinary approach to effective pain management in the cancer patient.[6]

PSYCHOLOGICAL FACTORS IN PAIN EXPERIENCE

Cancer patients confront myriad stressors during the course of their illness. Issues such as dependency, disability, disfigurement, and fear of a painful death often arise. While such fears are universal, the level of resultant psychological distress is variable and depends on medical factors, social supports, coping capacities, the patient's age and stage of life, and personality. Pain profoundly affects psychological distress in cancer patients. Psychological factors such as anxiety, depression, and the meaning of pain can magnify the cancer pain experience. Daut and Cleeland[14] showed that cancer patients who attribute a new pain to an unrelated benign cause report less interference with their activities and pleasure than cancer patients who

PATIENT NAME: _____   SSN: _____

The purpose of this Agreement is to clarify expectations and prevent misunderstandings about certain medicines I will be taking for pain management. This is to help both me and my doctor comply with the law regarding controlled prescription drugs. I understand that this Agreement is essential to the trust and confidence necessary in a doctor/patient relationship and that my doctor will treat me based on this Agreement.

I understand that if I break this Agreement, my doctor may decide to stop prescribing these pain-control medicines. In this case, my doctor may taper off the medicine (i.e., slowly decrease) over a period of several days, as necessary to avoid withdrawal symptoms. Also, a drug-dependence treatment program may be recommended.

GOALS OF OPIOID TRIAL/TREATMENT

The purpose of this medication is to increase your ability to function at work and at home. Success will be measured by your activity level, not your report of pain.

RISKS OF OPIOID TRIAL/TREATMENT

This medication has the potential to cause an addiction. Physical tolerance and dependence occurs with regular use of a narcotic, but this is different from addiction. For a person's health, safety and protection, this medication may be stopped if there is a concern about addiction.

ADDICTION BEHAVIOR

▶ A lot of time & energy focused on obtaining medication.

▶ Continuing to take medications despite being told to stop.

▶ Decline in family and/or work functioning.

▶ Loss of interest in other life activities (i.e., hobbies, social activities).

▶ Consistent misuse of medications (see below).

MISUSE OR ABUSE OF MEDICATION

▶ Taking more medication than prescribed.

▶ Use of pain medications that have not been prescribed by this program.

▶ Use of alcohol to manage pain.

▶ High number of emergency room visits seeking medication.

▶ Failing to use other recommended pain management techniques (i.e., physical therapy, relaxation techniques, TNS unit).

▶ Getting medication from more than one doctor.

▶ Using someone else's opioid medication.

▶ Reports of lost or stolen medication.

▶ Asking only for medications with a high street value.

GUIDELINES FOR OPIOID PRESCRIPTIONS

OUR RESPONSIBILITY

▶ Medication will only be prescribed by a SINGLE PROVIDER.

▶ Medication will be prescribed on a "by-the-clock" schedule.

▶ Lost or stolen prescriptions or medications will not be replaced.

▶ OPIOID MEDICATIONS WILL NOT TYPICALLY BE FILLED OVER THE PHONE.

▶ If an opioid taper is unsuccessful, medical care will be provided. Referral to facilities specializing in medication detoxification may be necessary.

FIGURE 10-1 Pain Management Guidelines – Opioid Medication Consent Form

YOUR RESPONSIBILITY

▶ A person is responsible for their medications, and needs to make sure that prescriptions are filled correctly. Therefore, they need to make certain that the pharmacy gives them the correct number prescribed.

▶ No increases in medication doses will be made without the approval of the prescribing physician.

▶ If a person takes more medication than is prescribed, they will run out of medication before being given more.

▶ Narcotic medication use questions should be made during normal business hours, Monday through Friday, 8:00 A.M. to 4 P.M.

▶ Patients are expected to be on time for all appointments, including those not related to refills of medications. You will be asked to come in for an appointment before a medication is to be refilled at times.

INFORMED CONSENT

▶ I will communicate fully with my doctor about the character and intensity of my pain, the effect of the pain on my daily life, side effects, and how well the medicine is helping to relieve the pain.

▶ I may be asked to bring unused medications to clinic with me for a "pill count" to ensure that I am using the medication as prescribed.

▶ I consent to submit to a blood or urine test if requested by my doctor to determine my compliance with my program of pain control medicine.

▶ I will not use any illegal controlled substances, including marijuana, cocaine, etc., as these will interact poorly with my pain medications.

▶ I will not share, sell or trade my medication with anyone as these are dangerous to use when not under a doctor's care.

▶ I will not attempt to obtain any pain medicines, including opioid pain medicines, stimulants, or anti-anxiety medicines from any other doctor.

▶ I authorize the doctor and my pharmacy to cooperate fully with any city, state or federal law enforcement agency, including this state's Board of Pharmacy, in the investigation of any possible misuse, sale, or other diversion of my pain medicine. I authorize my doctor to provide a copy of this Agreement to my pharmacy. I agree to waive any applicable or right of privacy or confidentiality with respect to these authorizations.

If these guidelines are not met you may be discharged from the program.

I, the undersigned, agree that the above guidelines have been explained to me, and that my questions and concerns regarding this treatment have been adequately answered. I agree to comply with the above guidelines. I have a copy of this document.

Signed: _____   Date:_____

Physician/Clinician: _____   Date:_____

Witness: _____   Date:_____

FIGURE 10-1 (*Continued*)

believe their pain signifies progression of disease. Spiegel and Bloom[15] found, for example, that women with metastatic breast cancer experience more intense pain if they believe their pain represents spread of their cancer, and if they are depressed. Beliefs about the meaning of pain and the presence of a mood disturbance are often better predictors of level of pain than is the site of metastasis.

In an attempt to define the potential relationships between pain and psychosocial variables, Padilla et al.[16] found pain-related quality of life variables in three domains: (1) physical well-being; (2) psychological well-being consisting of affective factors, cognitive factors, spiritual factors, communication, coping, and meaning of pain or cancer; and (3) interpersonal well-being focusing on social support or role functioning. The perception of significant impairment in activities of daily living has been associated with increased pain intensity.[17] Measures of emotional disturbance have been reported to be predictors of pain in late stages of cancer.[18] For example, cancer patients with less anxiety and depression are less likely to report

pain.[19] Patients with cancer who report negative thoughts about their personal or social competence report increased pain intensity and emotional distress.[17] Similarly, in a prospective study of cancer patients it was found that maladaptive coping strategies, lower levels of self-efficacy, and distress specific to a treatment or disease progression were modest but significant predictors of pain intensity.[13]

All too frequently, however, psychological variables are proposed to explain continued pain or lack of response to therapy when, in fact, medical factors have not been adequately appreciated. Often, the psychiatrist or psychologist is the last clinician to consult on a patient with pain. Such a situation is quite unfortunate, but is changing as we come to appreciate the impact of psychological variables on pain. Psychological distress in terminally ill patients with pain must initially be assumed to be the consequence of uncontrolled pain. Personality factors may be quite distorted by the presence of pain, and relief of pain often results in the disappearance of a perceived psychiatric disorder.[8,20]

PSYCHIATRIC DISORDERS AND PAIN IN THE CANCER PATIENT

There is an increased frequency of psychiatric disorders found in cancer patients with pain, a fact which the treating clinician should remain sensitive to. In a study examining the prevalence of psychiatric disorders in cancer patients, of the patients who received a psychiatric diagnosis (see Table 10-1), 39% reported significant pain, whereas only 19% without a psychiatric diagnosis reported significant pain.[21] The psychiatric disorders seen in cancer patients with pain include primarily adjustment disorder with depressed or anxious mood (69%) and major depression (15%).[22,23]

Cancer patients with advanced disease are a particularly vulnerable group. The incidence of pain, depression, and delirium increases with greater debilitation and advanced stages of illness.[24] Approximately 25% of all cancer patients experience severe depressive symptoms, with the prevalence increasing to 77% in those with advanced illness. The prevalence of organic mental disorders (delirium) among cancer patients requiring psychiatric consultation has been found to range from 25% to 40%, and to be as high as 85% during the terminal stages of illness.[25] Narcotic analgesics, such as meperidine, levorphanol, and morphine sulfate, can cause confusional states, particularly in the elderly and terminally ill.[26]

Epidural spinal cord compression (ESCC) is a relatively common neurologic complication of advanced systemic cancers that is observed in 5%–10% of patients with cancer and can often result in severe pain. These patients are routinely treated with a combination therapy of high-dose dexamethasone and radiotherapy. Patients who receive this high-dose regimen are exposed to as much as 96 mg a day of dexamethasone for as long as a week, and continue on a tapering course for up to 3 or 4 weeks. Stiefel et al.[27] described psychiatric complications seen in cancer patients undergoing such treatment for ESCC. Twenty-two percent of patients with ESCC were diagnosed with a major depressive syndrome compared to 4% in the comparison group. In addition, delirium was significantly more common in the dexamethasone-treated patients with ESCC.

Table 10-1	
Sample Behaviors That Are More or Less Likely to Be Indicative of Abuse/Diverson	
Probably Less Predictive of Abuse/Diverson	Probably More Predictive of Abuse/Diverson
Drug hoarding during periods of reduced symptoms	Prescription forgery
Acquisition of similar drugs from other medical sources	Concurrent abuse of related illicit drugs
Aggressive complaining about the need for higher doses	Recurrent prescription losses
Unapproved use of the drug to treat another symptom	Selling prescription drugs
Unsanctioned dose escalation one or two times	Multiple unsanctioned dose escalations
Reporting psychic effects not intended by the clinician	Stealing or borrowing another patient's drugs
Requesting specific drugs	Obtaining prescription drugs from nonmedical sources

Of those patients, 24% were diagnosed with delirium during the course of treatment compared to 10% in the control group.

CANCER PAIN AND SUICIDE

Uncontrolled pain is a major factor in suicide and suicidal ideation in cancer patients.[28] Cancer is perceived by the public as an extremely painful disease compared with other medical conditions. For example, one study in Wisconsin revealed that 69% of the public agreed that cancer pain could cause a person to consider suicide.[29] Most suicides observed among patients with cancer had severe pain, which was often inadequately controlled or tolerated poorly.[30] Although relatively few cancer patients commit suicide, they are at increased risk.[29,31] Patients with advanced illness are at highest risk and are the most likely to have the complications of pain, depression, delirium, and deficit symptoms. Psychiatric disorders are frequently present in hospitalized cancer patients who attempt suicide. A review of the psychiatric consultation data at Memorial Sloan-Kettering Cancer Center (MSKCC) showed that one-third of cancer patients who were seen for evaluation of suicide risk received a diagnosis of major depression; approximately 20% met criteria for delirium and more than 50% were diagnosed with an adjustment disorder.[28]

Thoughts of suicide probably occur quite frequently, particularly in the setting of advanced illness,[32] and seem to act as a safety valve for feelings often expressed by patients, such as "If it gets too bad, I always have a way out." It has been our experience working with terminally ill pain patients that once a trusting and safe relationship is developed, patients almost universally reveal that they have occasionally had periods of time during which thoughts of suicide were persistent. Such ideation is most commonly experienced as a means of escaping the threat of being overwhelmed by pain. However, several published reports suggest that suicidal ideation is relatively infrequent in cancer and is limited to those who are significantly depressed. Silberfarb et al.[33] found that only 3 of 146 breast cancer patients had suicidal thoughts, whereas none of the 100 cancer patients interviewed in a Finnish study expressed suicidal thoughts.[34] A study conducted in Winnipeg, Canada, revealed that only 10 of 44 terminally ill cancer patients were suicidal or desired an early death, and all 10 were suffering from clinical depression.[35] At MSKCC, suicide risk evaluation accounted for 8.6% of psychiatric consultations, usually requested by staff in response to patients verbalizing suicidal wishes.[28] In the 71 cancer patients who had suicidal ideation with serious intent, significant pain was a factor in only 30% of cases. In striking contrast, virtually all 71 suicidal cancer patients had a psychiatric disorder (mood disturbance or organic mental disorder) at the time of evaluation.[28]

The role of cancer pain in suicidal ideation in 185 cancer pain patients of the MSKCC Pain and Psychiatry Services has been examined.[36] Results indicated that suicidal ideation occurred in 17% of the study population. The majority reported suicidal ideation, but no intent to act. Interestingly, in this population of cancer patients who all had significant pain, suicidal ideation was not directly related to pain intensity but was strongly related to degree of depression and mood disturbance. Pain was related to suicidal ideation indirectly in that patients' perception of poor pain relief was associated with suicidal ideation. Perceptions of pain relief may have more to do with aspects of hopelessness than pain itself. Pain plays an important role in vulnerability to suicide; however, associated psychological distress and mood disturbance seem to be essential cofactors in raising the risk of suicide in cancer patients. Pain has adverse effects on patients' quality of life and sense of control and impairs the family's ability to provide support. Factors, other than pain, such as mood disturbance, delirium, loss of control, and hopelessness contribute to cancer suicide risk.[30]

INADEQUATE PAIN MANAGEMENT: ASSESSMENT ISSUES IN THE TREATMENT OF PAIN

Recent studies suggest that pain in cancer is still being undertreated.[37] Inadequate management of pain is often due to the inability to properly assess pain in all of its dimensions.[1,3,6] All too frequently, psychological variables are proposed to explain continued pain or lack of response to therapy, when in fact medical factors have not been adequately appreciated. Other causes of inadequate pain management include lack of knowledge of current pharmaco- or psychotherapeutic approaches, focus on prolonging life rather than alleviating suffering, lack of communication between doctor and patient, limited expectations of patients to achieve pain relief, limited capacity of patients impaired by organic mental disorders to communicate, unavailability of narcotics, doctors' fears of causing respiratory depression, and, most importantly, doctors' fears of amplifying addiction and substance abuse. In advanced cancer, several factors have been noted to predict the undermanagement of pain, including discrepancy between physician and patient in judging the severity of pain, the presence of pain that physicians did not attribute to cancer, better performance status, age 70 years or older, and female gender.[37]

Fear of addiction affects compliance and physician management of narcotic analgesics, leading to the undermedication of pain in cancer patients.[3,5,38,39] Studies of the patterns of chronic narcotic analgesic use in patients with cancer have demonstrated that, although tolerance and physical dependence are common, addiction (psychological dependence) is rare and almost never occurs in an individual without a history of drug abuse prior to cancer illness.[40] Escalation of narcotic analgesic use by cancer patients is usually due to progression of cancer or the development of tolerance. Tolerance means that a larger dose of narcotic analgesic is required to maintain an original analgesic effect. Physical dependence is characterized by the onset of signs and symptoms of withdrawal if the narcotic is suddenly stopped or a narcotic antagonist is administered. Tolerance usually occurs in association with physical dependence but does not imply psychological dependence or addiction, is not equivalent to physical dependence or addiction, and is a behavioral pattern of compulsive drug abuse characterized by a craving for the drug and overwhelming involvement in obtaining and using it for effects other than pain relief. The cancer pain patient with a history of intravenous (IV) opioid abuse presents an often unnecessarily difficult management problem. Macaluso et al.[39] reported on their experience in managing cancer pain in such a population. Of 468 inpatient cancer pain consultations, only eight (1.7%) had a history of IV drug abuse, but none had been actively abusing drugs in the previous year. All eight of these patients had inadequate pain control and more than half were intentionally undermedicated because of concern by staff that drug abuse was active or would recur. Adequate pain control was ultimately achieved in these patients by using appropriate analgesic dosages and intensive staff education.

The risk of inducing respiratory depression is too often overestimated and can limit appropriate use of narcotic analgesics for pain and symptom control. Bruera et al.[41] demonstrated that in a population of terminally ill cancer patients with respiratory failure and dyspnea, administration of subcutaneous morphine actually improved dyspnea without causing a significant deterioration in respiratory function. The adequacy of cancer pain management can be influenced by the lack of concordance between patient ratings or complaints of their pain and those made by caregivers. Persistent cancer pain is often ascribed to a psychological cause when it does not respond to treatment attempts. In our clinical experience, patients who report their pain as *severe* are quite likely to be viewed as having a psychological contribution to their complaints. Staff members' ability to empathize with a patient's pain complaint may be limited by the intensity of the pain complaint. Grossman et al.[42] found that while there is a high degree of concordance between patient and caregiver ratings of patient pain intensity at the low and moderate levels, this concordance breaks down at high levels. Thus, a clinician's ability to assess a patient's level of pain becomes unreliable once a patient's report of pain intensity rises above 7 on a visual analog rating scale of 0 to 10. Physicians must be educated as to the limitations of their ability to objectively assess the severity of a subjective pain experience. Additionally, patient education is often a useful intervention in such cases. Patients are more likely to be believed and adequately treated if they are taught to request pain relief in a nonhysterical, business-like fashion.

PSYCHIATRIC MANAGEMENT OF PAIN IN ADVANCED DISEASE

Optimal treatment of pain associated with advanced disease is multimodal and includes pharmacologic, psychotherapeutic, cognitive-behavioral, anesthetic, neurostimulatory, and rehabilitative approaches. Psychiatric participation in pain management involves the use of psychotherapeutic, cognitive-behavioral, and psychopharmacologic interventions, usually in combination, that are described below.

▶ Psychotherapy and pain

The goals of psychotherapy for medically ill patients with pain are to provide support, knowledge, and skills (Table 10-2). Utilizing short-

---

Table 10-2

Basic Principles for Prescribing Controlled Substances to Patients with Advanced Illness and Issues of Addiction

Choose an opioid based on around-the-clock dosing

Choose long-acting agents when possible

As much as possible, limit or eliminate the use of short-acting or "breakthrough" doses

Use nonopioid adjuvants when possible and monitor for compliance with those medications

Use nondrug adjuvants whenever possible (i.e., relaxation techniques, distraction, biofeedback, TNS, communication about thoughts and feelings of pain)

If necessary, limit the amount of medication given at any one time (i.e., write prescriptions for a few days' worth or a weeks' worth of medication at a time)

Utilize pill counts and urine toxicology screens as necessary

If compliance is suspect or poor, refer to an addictions specialist

term supportive psychotherapy focused on the crisis created by the medical illness, the therapist provides emotional support, continuity, information, and assists in adaptation. The therapist has a role in emphasizing past strengths, supporting previously successful coping strategies, and teaching new coping skills such as relaxation, cognitive coping, use of analgesics, self-observation, documentation, assertiveness, and communication skills. Communication skills are of paramount importance for both patient and family, particularly in regard to pain and analgesic issues. The patient and family are the unit of concern, and need a more general, long-term, supportive relationship within the healthcare system in addition to specific psychological approaches dealing with pain and dying, that a psychiatrist, psychologist, social worker, chaplain, or nurse can provide.

Psychotherapy with the dying patient in pain consists of active listening with supportive verbal interventions and occasional interpretations.[43] Despite the seriousness of the patient's plight, it is not necessary for the psychiatrist or psychologist to appear overly solemn or emotionally restrained. Often, it is only the psychotherapist, of all the patient's caregivers, who is comfortable enough to converse lightheartedly and allow the patient to talk about his life and experiences, rather than focus solely on impending death. The dying patient who wishes to talk or ask questions about death and pain and suffering should be allowed to do so freely, with the therapist maintaining an interested, interactive stance. It is not uncommon for the dying patient to benefit from pastoral counseling. If a chaplaincy service is available, it should be offered to the patient and family. As the dying process progresses, psychotherapy with the patient may be limited by cognitive and speech deficits. At this point, the focus of supportive psychotherapeutic interventions shifts primarily to the family. In our experience, a very common issue for family members at this point is the level of alertness of the patient. Attempts to control pain are often accompanied by sedation that can limit communication between patient and family. This can sometimes become a source of conflict, with some family members disagreeing amongst themselves or with the patient about what constitutes an appropriate balance between comfort and alertness. It can be helpful for the physician to clarify the patient's preferences as they relate to these issues early so that conflict can be avoided and work related to bereavement can begin.

Group interventions with individual patients (even in advanced stages of disease), spouses, couples, and families are a powerful means of sharing experiences and identifying successful coping strategies. The limitations of using group interventions for patients with advanced disease are primarily pragmatic. The patient must be physically comfortable enough to participate and have the cognitive capacity to be aware of group discussion. It is often helpful for family members to attend support groups during the terminal phases of the patient's illness. Passik et al.[44] have worked with spouses of brain tumor patients in a psychoeducational group that has included spouses at all phases of the patient's illness. They have demonstrated how bereavement issues are often a focus of such interventions from the time of diagnosis. The group members have benefit from one another's support until the family member's death. The leaders have been impressed by the increased quality of patient care that can be given at home by a spouse (including pain management and all forms of nursing care) when such support is utilized.

Psychotherapeutic interventions that have multiple foci may be most useful. A prospective study of cancer pain showed that cognitive-behavioral and psychoeducational techniques based upon increasing support, self-efficacy, and providing education may prove to be helpful in assisting patients in dealing with increased pain.[45]

Results of an evaluation of patients with cancer pain indicate that psychological and social variables are significant predictors of pain. More specifically, distress specific to the illness, self-efficacy, and coping styles were predictors of increased pain.

Utilizing psychotherapy to diminish symptoms of anxiety and depression, factors that can intensify pain, has beneficial effects on the cancer pain experience. Spiegel and Bloom[46] demonstrated, in a controlled randomized prospective study, the effect of both supportive group therapy for metastatic breast cancer patients in general and, in particular, the effect of hypnotic pain control exercises. Their support group focused not on interpersonal processes or self-exploration, but rather on a series of themes related to the practical and existential problems of living with cancer. Patients were divided into two treatment groups and a control group. The treatment patients experienced significantly less pain than the control patients. Those in the group that included a self-hypnosis exercise subgroup showed a slight increase, and the control group showed a large increase in pain.

While psychotherapy in the cancer pain setting is primarily non-analytical and focuses on current issues, exploration of reactions to cancer often involve insights into earlier, more pervasive life issues. Some patients consequently choose to pursue an exploratory form of psychotherapy during extended illness-free periods or survivorship.

▶ Cognitive-behavioral techniques

Cognitive and behavioral techniques can be useful adjuncts in cancer pain management. These techniques include passive relaxation combined with mental imagery, cognitive distraction or focusing, progressive muscle relaxation, biofeedback, hypnosis, and music therapy.[20,47–49] The goal of treatment is to guide patients toward a sense of having control over their pain. Some techniques are primarily cognitive in nature, focusing on perceptual and thought processes, whereas others are directed at modifying patterns of behavior that help cancer patients cope with pain. Behavioral techniques for pain control seek to modify physiologic pain reactions, respondent pain behaviors, and operant pain behaviors.

Cognitive techniques for coping with pain are aimed primarily at reducing the intensity and distress that are part of the pain experience. These include modification of thoughts the patient has about pain or psychological distress, introduction of adaptive coping strategies, and instruction in relaxation techniques. Cognitive modification (cognitive restructuring) is an approach derived from cognitive therapy for depression or anxiety and is based on how one interprets events and bodily sensations. It is assumed that patients have dysfunctional automatic thoughts that are consistent with underlying assumptions and beliefs, and that this mechanism is operative in the cancer pain setting. In cancer pain populations, negative thoughts about pain have been shown to be significantly related to pain intensity, degree of psychological distress, and level of interference in functional activities.[17] By identifying and challenging dysfunctional automatic thoughts and underlying beliefs, a more rational response to pain can occur by restructuring or modifying thought processes.[47] Examples of automatic thoughts that reportedly worsen the pain experience are "The intensity of my pain will never diminish" or "Because my pain limits my activities, I am completely helpless." Patients can be taught to recognize and interrupt such thoughts and proceed to develop a view of the pain experience as time-limited and themselves as functional despite having periods of time during which their ability to function entirely normally is limited.

Although cognitive restructuring can be a useful technique in the earlier stages of cancer, the goals of this approach change in the palliative care context. In this setting, the goal is not necessarily to change the patient's maladaptive thoughts but rather to utilize techniques designed to diminish frustration, anxiety, and anger. Helping patients to employ adaptive coping strategies, that is, avoiding catastrophizing and encouraging increased problem-solving skills can be helpful at this stage of illness.[50–52]

Aside from modifying dysfunctional thoughts and attitudes, self-monitoring is the most fundamental behavioral technique. Developing the ability to monitor one's behavior allows a person to become aware of their dysfunctional reactions to the pain experience and to learn to control these reactions. Systematic desensitization is useful in extinguishing anticipatory anxiety that leads to avoidant behaviors and in remobilizing inactive patients. Graded task assignment is essentially systematic desensitization as it is applied to patients who are encouraged to take small, gradual steps, allowing them to perform activities more readily. Contingency management is a method of reinforcing *well* behaviors only, thus modifying dysfunctional operant pain behaviors associated with secondary gain.[48,49]

Cognitive-behavioral interventions that are useful in the setting of advanced illness include techniques such as supplying preparatory information, self-monitoring, systematic desensitization, and methods of distraction and relaxation.[53] Most often, techniques such as hypnosis, biofeedback, or systematic desensitization utilize cognitive and behavioral elements together, such as muscular relaxation and cognitive distraction.

▶ Patient selection for cognitive-behavioral interventions for pain

Many cancer patients fear that focusing on their pain could distract their physicians from treating the underlying causes of their disease. Consequently, they are highly motivated to learn and practice cognitive-behavioral techniques, which are often effective not only for pain control, but in restoring a sense of self-control, personal efficacy, and active participation in their care. It is important to note that these techniques must not be used as a substitute for appropriate analgesic management of pain, but rather as part of a comprehensive multimodal approach. The lack of side effects of these techniques makes them attractive in the palliative care setting as a supplement to complicated medication regimens. A caveat is that the successful use of these techniques should never lead to the erroneous conclusion that a patient's pain was of psychogenic origin and, as such, not *real*. The mechanisms by which these cognitive and behavioral techniques relieve pain are not known; however, they all seem to share the elements of relaxation and distraction. Distraction or redirection of attention helps reduce awareness of pain, and relaxation reduces the muscle tension and sympathetic arousal triggered by pain.[48]

Most patients with advanced illness and pain are appropriate candidates for useful application of these techniques; the clinician, however, should take into account the intensity of pain and the mental clarity of the patient. Ideal candidates have mild to moderate pain and can expect benefit, whereas patients with severe pain can expect limited benefit from psychological interventions unless somatic therapies can lower the level of pain to some degree. Confusional states interfere dramatically with a patient's ability to focus attention, and thus limit the usefulness of these techniques.[49] Occasionally, these techniques can be modified for mildly cognitively impaired patients. In this setting, the therapist often takes a more active role by orienting the patient, creating a safe and secure environment, and evoking a conditioned response to the therapist's voice or presence.

Barriers to engaging patients in cognitive-behavioral therapies can be divided into physician/nurse-based barriers and patient-based barriers. The healthcare provider who works with patients with advanced illness may have particular difficulty in becoming comfortable with the use of behavioral therapies. Pharmacotherapy is highly effective in the management of pain and seems simpler and easier to use by physicians than labor-intensive and time-consuming nonpharmacologic interventions. Physicians and nurses have concerns about the practice of behavioral interventions such as "What if the patient laughs, doesn't buy it?" or "It seems too theatrical, unscientific, nonmedical; too New Age!" Overcoming such obstacles will be greatly rewarded. It is imperative that physicians working with patients with advanced illness be aware of the effective nonpharmacologic interventions for pain that are available, and be able to make appropriate referrals to practitioners who can provide such interventions.

Patients themselves sometimes question the utility of behavioral therapies, asking "How can breathing take away my pain?" They may be put off by the word "hypnosis" and its connotations. Hypnosis, as patients conceptualize it, is often associated with powerful and magical properties, and some patients are frightened at the prospect of giving up control or being under the influence of someone else. It is generally best to introduce behavioral interventions only after rapport has been established with a patient and they have been engaged in a therapeutic alliance with us. Some patients may benefit from a discussion about the theoretical basis of these interventions, although it is important to stress that understanding why a technique works is not as important as using a technique that works. Apprehensions must be validated and discussed. It is imperative for patients to feel in control of the process at all times and be reassured that they can stop an intervention at any time.

GENERAL INSTRUCTIONS

A general approach to incorporating cognitive-behavioral interventions into the care of patients with advanced illness and pain involves (1) assessing the presenting symptom(s), (2) choosing an appropriate cognitive-behavioral strategy, and (3) properly preparing the patient and the setting.

The main purpose of conducting a cognitive-behavioral assessment of pain is to determine which, if any, behavioral interventions are indicated.[49] One must initially engage the patient and establish a therapeutic alliance. A history of the pain symptom must be taken, including previous efforts to treat the patient's pain, and data regarding the nature of the pain and its impact on the patient and their family should be collected.

The assessment process can lead to various behavioral interventions. Choosing the appropriate behavioral strategy involves taking into consideration the patient's medical condition, physical and cognitive limitations, time constraints, and other practical matters. For instance, patients with cognitive impairment or delirium will probably be unable to keep a pain diary or employ techniques that involve cognitive manipulation.

▶ Relaxation techniques

Several techniques can be used to achieve a mental and physical state of relaxation. Muscular tension, autonomic arousal, and mental distress exacerbate pain.[48,49] Specific relaxation techniques include

(1) passive relaxation focusing attention on sensations of warmth and decreased tension in various parts of the body, (2) progressive muscle relaxation involving active tensing and relaxing of muscles, and (3) meditation. Other techniques that employ both relaxation and cognitive techniques include hypnosis, biofeedback, and music therapy. These are discussed later in this chapter.

Passive relaxation, focused breathing, and passive muscle relaxation exercises involve focusing attention systematically on one's breathing, on sensations of warmth and relaxation, or release of muscular tension in various body parts. Verbal suggestions and imagery help promote relaxation. Muscle relaxation is an important component of the relaxation response and can augment the benefits of simple focused breathing exercises, leading to a deeper experience of relaxation and self-control.

Progressive or active muscle relaxation involves actively tensing and relaxing various muscle groups in the body, focusing attention on the sensations of tension and relaxation. Clinically, in the hospital setting, relaxation is most commonly achieved through a combination of focused breathing and progressive muscle relaxation exercises. Once patients are in a relaxed state, imagery techniques can be used to induce deeper relaxation and facilitate distraction from or manipulation of various cancer-related symptoms.

The following script is a generic relaxation exercise, utilizing passive relaxation or focused breathing, that is based on and integrates the work of Erickson,[54] Benson,[55] and others.[49]

SCRIPT FOR PASSIVE RELAXATION (FOCUSED BREATHING)

"Why don't you begin by finding a comfortable position. It could be in a bed or in a chair. Slowly allow your body to unwind and just let it go. That's it. I wonder if you can allow your body to become as calm as possible . . . just let it go, just let your body sink into that bed (or chair) . . . feel free to move or shift around in any way that your body needs to, to find that comfortable position. You need not try very hard, simply and easily allow yourself to follow the sound of my voice as you allow your body to find itself a safe, comfortable position to relax in."

"If you like, (patient's name here), you can gently allow your eyes to close, just let the lids cover your eyes . . . allow your eyes to sink back deeply into their sockets . . . that's it, just let them go, falling back gently and deeply into their sockets as your lids begin to feel heavier and heavier. As you allow your head to fall back deeply into the pillow, feeling the weight of your head sinking into the pillow as you breath out, just breath out, one big breath. Slowly, if you can begin to turn your attention to your breathing. Notice your breath for a few moments, how much air you take in, how much air you let out, and just breathe evenly and naturally, and with the sound of my voice I wonder if you can begin to take in more air, breathing in and out, in and out, that's it, gradually breathing in and out . . . in and out . . . breathing in calmness and quietness, breathing out tiredness and frustration, that's it . . . let it go, it's not important to you now . . . breathing in quietness and control, breathing out fear and tension . . . breathing in and out . . . in and out . . . you can enjoy breathing in this relaxed way for as long as you need to. You are peaceful now as you continue to observe your even and steady breathing that is allowing you to feel gentle and calm, breathing that is allowing you to feel a gentle calm, that's it, breathing relaxation in and tension out . . . in and out . . . breathing in quietness and control, breathing out tiredness and tension . . . that's it (patient's name here) as you

continue to notice the quietness and stillness of your body, why don't you take a few quiet moments to experience this process more fully."

It may be helpful for the clinician to mark the end of an exercise by increasing the pace, raising the volume of voice, and shifting position. Additionally, it is helpful for the clinician to both pace and model for the patient. This includes positioning yourself as similarly to the patient as possible (e.g., closing eyes, assuming a position of relaxation, and breathing at the same rate). If the patient exhibits any visible anxiety or agitation, this can be briefly explored verbally, and then, if appropriate, the exercise can be continued.

SCRIPT FOR ACTIVE OR PROGRESSIVE MUSCLE RELAXATION

This exercise involves the patient actively tensing and then relaxing specific body parts. As with focused breathing, it may be helpful if the clinician paces and models for the patient when using this technique.

"Now, I wonder if you can tense up every muscle in your body . . . that's it, squeeze in the muscles . . . hold it, and then just let it go . . . once more, tense up your muscles . . . make them very tight and tense, hold it, hold it . . . and then breath out, and let your muscles relax, just let them go . . . Now, as your body begins to feel more and more relaxed, clench your jaw, squeeze it tight, clench it and then let it go . . . now open your mouth wide, as wide as it will go, stick out your tongue, stick it way out, hold it and then let it go. Feel your head becoming more and more relaxed, as it sinks down into the pillow, allowing all the tension and tightness to drift out of it . . . Now, I wonder if you can lift up your shoulders, lift them up, up to your ears, hold them there, squeezing them tightly, squeeze, and then let them drop down, just let them go . . . and then once more lift them up . . . hold it . . . then let them go . . . as you feel all the tightness and tension in your shoulders begin to drain away . . . Now, I wonder if you can clench your hands into a fist, make a tight fist as your whole arm tightens, tense your arms as you squeeze in your fingers tighter and tighter . . . and now just let them go, once more now make a fist, a tight fist, hold it, and then let it go."

As with passive muscle relaxation, the clinician guides the patient through the exercise, requesting the patient to tense and release specific muscles in a progressive order.

IMAGERY/DISTRACTION TECHNIQUES

Clinically, relaxation techniques are most helpful in managing pain when combined with distracting or pleasant imagery. The use of distraction or focusing involves control over the focus of attention and can be used to make the patient less aware of noxious stimuli.[56] One can employ imaginative inattention by picturing oneself on a beach. Mental distraction can be used and is similar to the practice of counting sheep to aid sleep. Keeping oneself busy is a form of behavioral distraction. Imagery, that is, using one's imagination while in a relaxed state, can be used to transform pain into a warm or cold sensation. One can also imaginatively transform the context of pain, that is, imagining oneself in battle on the football field instead of the hospital bed. Disassociated somatization can be employed by some patients whereby they imagine that a painful body part is no longer part of their body.[5,6,47,49] It is important to note that not every patient finds these techniques acceptable, and the therapist must try out a number of approaches to determine which are consistent with the patient's style.

Imagery (often referred to as guided imagery) is most effective when the specific image to be used is obtained from the patient. The clinician may ask the patient to close his or her eyes and think of a place, an activity, or an experience where the patient felt most safe and secure. The clinician may provide suggestions for the patient such as a favorite beach scene, or a room in a house, or riding a bicycle in a state park. Once the patient identifies the scene, the clinician may ask the patient to elaborate upon the scene, asking for specific details such as the temperature, season, time of day, type of ocean (calm or with big waves), and other descriptors. The clinician then utilizes this information and describes an image for the patient in detail. The skill is for the clinician to be as flexible and as creative as possible, and to elaborate upon the scene, utilizing all aspects of the senses and bodily sensations such as "feel the sun's rays that touch your skin, allow your skin to feel warm and tingly all over . . ." or " breathe in the fresh, clear air, allow it to fill your lungs with its freshness . . . " or "feel the fresh dew of the grass under your feet." The clinician can focus on "aromas in the garden" or the "sounds of birds singing," always reminding the patient to breathe evenly and steadily as he or she feels more and more relaxed and more and more in control. If possible, the clinician should avoid volunteering an image or scene for the patient if the clinician is unaware of the association or meaning the image may have for the patient. For example, a patient may have a fear of the water, and therefore a beach scene may invoke feelings of fear and loss of control.

▶ Script for using pleasant distracting imagery

"Once you are in a comfortable position, I wonder if you can continue lying there with your eyes closed, continuing to breathe in and out . . . in and out to the sound of my voice. Let your mind wander . . . just let it go . . . and if any unwanted thoughts come into your mind, you can allow them to pass out as easily as they came in . . . You don't need them now . . . they are not important to you now. You have the ability to control your thoughts. You have the ability to be in control."

The clinician now begins to describe a specific image in detail as originally suggested by the patient.

"Slowly, I wonder if you can allow your mind to travel . . . to travel far away to your favorite beach. The beach that you have many fond memories of. I wonder if you can imagine that it's almost the end of the day and the beach is deserted . . . and the sun, while setting, is still warm, as it beats down . . . and makes your skin feel tingly and warm all over. As you begin to walk on the sand, you can feel the granules underneath your feet. Step evenly and steadily along the sand. As you look around, you can see the different colors in the sky. You can see for miles off into the distance and you feel exhilarated and free because no one is around you. You are alone and in control. As you walk closer to the edge of the ocean the sand is becoming a little damp and you can feel the dampness underneath your feet—it feels refreshing. As you continue walking, you may notice a few odds and ends on the sand maybe something that the ocean brought in . . . some shells perhaps. They may be broken from being knocked against the rocks . . . or there may be a few bits of seaweed or some jellyfish. You stop to notice them as you walk past . . . marveling at the wonders of nature. As you get to the edge of the ocean, you can feel the tiny little ripples of water washing over your feet . . . bouncing over your feet making you feel light and fresh. The water is warm—it soothes your feet. Washing back and forth . . . back and forth. As you keep walking you see your rubber raft. This is your old dependable rubber raft. You get to the raft and you secure it in your hands and lie down on it letting your whole body sink into the raft—just let it go . . . that's it. Slowly you kick off as the raft begins to take you away. The ocean is very calm and very gentle. Your whole body begins to unwind and sink deeper and deeper into the raft as you feel more and more relaxed. This raft allows you to drift off . . . and underneath you can feel the ripples of the ocean . . . rocking back and forth . . . back and forth as you continue to float away evenly and gently. You can become aware of the sun beating down on your skin. You are aware of the sounds around you—you can hear the ocean washing against the rocks as the waves rock back and forth . . . back and forth. You can hear the gulls crying in the distance. There is a very tiny protected bay that you are floating away in. It is a very calm and peaceful time of day, and you are feeling more and more relaxed. You are in control now . . . and as you continue to float away, all your troubles and problems wash right out of you. They're not important to you now. You don't need them now. What's important is that your whole body, from the tip of your toes all the way up to the top of your head, is relaxed and calm in this very safe and private place that is your own. You can continue to lie here as you rock back and forth . . . back and forth for as long as you need to."

"When you are ready, you can slowly readjust yourself to the sound of my voice and I am going to count slowly backward from 10 and with each count backward, you can become more and more familiar with where you are. Perhaps when I get to number 5 you may want to open your eyes or you can keep them closed for as long as you need to. Ten, nine . . . —become aware of the sounds around you . . . eight, seven . . . become aware of the temperature of the room—how does it feel? How does your body feel? . . . six, five . . . —you can open your eyes now if you want to or you can keep them closed . . . four, three, two, one. You can stay in this relaxed position for as long as you need to. When you feel ready you may slowly prepare to sit up."

▶ Hypnosis

Hypnosis can be a useful adjunct in the management of cancer pain.[46,56–59] In a controlled trial comparing hypnosis with cognitive-behavioral therapy in relieving mucositis following a bone marrow transplant, patients utilizing hypnosis reported a significant reduction in pain compared to patients who used cognitive-behavioral techniques.[45] The hypnotic trance is essentially a state of heightened and focused concentration, and thus it can be used to manipulate the perception of pain. The depth of hypnotizability may determine the effectiveness as well as the strategies employed during hypnosis. One-third of cancer patients are not hypnotizable, and it is recommended that other techniques be used with them. Of the two-thirds of patients who are identified as being less, moderately, and highly hypnotizable, three principles underlie the use of hypnosis in controlling pain[60]: (1) use self-hypnosis; (2) relax, do not fight the pain; and (3) use a mental filter to ease the hurt in pain. Patients who are moderately and highly hypnotizable can often alter sensations in a painful area by changing temperature sensation or experiencing tingling. Less hypnotizable patients can often utilize an alternative focus by concentrating on a sensation in a nonaffected body part or on a mental image of a pleasant scene. The main disadvantage of hypnosis for cancer patients is that the technique frequently requires more attentional capacity than these patients generally have.

▶ Biofeedback

Fotopoulos et al.[61] noted significant pain relief in a group of cancer patients who were taught electromyographic (EMG) and electroencephalographic (EEG) biofeedback-assisted relaxation. Only 2 of 17 were able to maintain analgesia after the treatment ended. A lack of generalization of effect can be a problem with biofeedback techniques. Although physical condition may make a prolonged training period impossible, especially for the terminally ill, most cancer patients can often utilize EMG and temperature biofeedback techniques for learning relaxation-assisted pain control.[48]

MUSIC, AROMA, AND ART THERAPIES

Munro and Mount[62] have written extensively on the use of music therapy with cancer patients, documenting clinical examples and suggesting mechanisms of action. Music can often capture the focus of attention like no other stimulus, offers patients a new form of expression, and helps patients distract themselves from their perception of pain, while expressing themselves in meaningful ways.[63]

Aromas have been shown to have innate relaxing and stimulating qualities. Our colleagues at Memorial Hospital have recently begun to explore the use of aroma therapy for the treatment of procedure-related anxiety (i.e., anxiety related to magnetic resonance imaging [MRI] scans). Utilizing the scent, heliotropin, Manne et al.[64] reported that two-thirds of the patients found the scent especially pleasant and reported much less anxiety than those who were not exposed to the scent during MRI. As a general relaxation technique, aroma therapy may have an application for pain management, but this is as yet unstudied.

Art therapy allows the less verbally skilled adult or children to express the fears and concerns that they have in a more comfortable fashion. The creative experience can be used as both an important means of providing support and as an avenue for providing patients with psychological insights into their experience.[65]

PSYCHOTROPIC ADJUVANT ANALGESICS FOR PAIN IN THE PATIENT WITH ADVANCED ILLNESS

In addition to the psychotherapeutic interventions described above, the patient with advanced disease and pain has much to gain from the appropriate and maximal utilization of psychotropic drugs. Psychotropic drugs, particularly the tricyclic antidepressants (TCAs), are useful as adjuvant analgesics in the pharmacologic management of cancer pain and neuropathic pain. These medications are not only effective in managing symptoms of anxiety, depression, insomnia, or delirium that commonly complicate the course of advanced disease in patients with cancer or acquired immunodeficiency syndrome (AIDS) who are in pain, they also potentiate the analgesic effects of the opioid drugs and have innate analgesic properties of their own.[66]

▶ Antidepressants

The current literature supports the use of antidepressants as adjuvant analgesic agents in the management of a wide variety of chronic pain syndromes, including cancer pain.[67–74] While clinically useful as adjuvant analgesics in managing AIDS-related pain (e.g., human immunodeficiency virus [HIV] neuropathies), there are no published controlled clinical trials of antidepressants as analgesics.[75,76] Amitriptyline is the most studied tricyclic antidepressant, whose effectiveness as an analgesic has been proved in a large number of clinical trials, addressing a wide variety of chronic pains.[77–81] Other TCAs that have been shown to have efficacy as analgesics include imipramine,[82–84] desipramine,[85,86] nortriptyline,[87] clomipramine,[88,89]

and doxepin.[90] In a placebo-controlled, double-blind study of imipramine in chronic cancer pain, Walsh[91] demonstrated that imipramine had analgesic effects independently from its mood effects, and was a potent coanalgesic when used with morphine. In general, the TCAs are used as adjuvant analgesics for treating cancer pain, potentiating the effects of opioid analgesics, and are rarely used as the primary analgesic.[72,91,92] Ventafridda et al.[72] reviewed a multicenter clinical experience with antidepressant agents (trazodone and amitriptyline) in the treatment of chronic cancer pain that included a deafferentation of neuropathic pain component. Almost all of the patients were already receiving weak or strong opioids and experienced improved pain control. A subsequent randomized double-blind study showed that amitriptyline and trazodone had similar therapeutic analgesic efficacy profiles.[72] Magni et al.[73] reviewed the use of antidepressants in Italian cancer centers and found that a wide range of antidepressants were used for a variety of cancer pain syndromes, with amitriptyline being the most commonly prescribed for various types of cancer pain. In nearly all cases, antidepressants were used in association with opioids. There is evidence that there may be subgroups of patients who respond differentially to tricyclics, so if amitriptyline fails to alleviate pain, another tricyclic should be tried.[93] The TCAs are effective as adjuvants in cancer pain through a number of mechanisms that include (1) antidepressant activity,[67] (2) potentiation or enhancement of opioid analgesia,[92,94,95] and (3) direct analgesic effects.[96]

The heterocyclic and noncyclic antidepressant drugs such as trazodone, mianserin, maprotiline, and the newer serotinin-specific reuptake inhibitors fluoxetine and paroxetine may also be useful as adjuvant analgesics for cancer patients with pain; however, clinical trials of their efficacy as analgesics have been equivocal.[97–101] Several case reports suggest fluoxetine may be a useful adjuvant analgesic in the management of headache,[102] fibrositis,[103] and diabetic neuropathy.[104] In a recent clinical trial, fluoxetine was shown to be no better than placebo as an analgesic in painful diabetic neuropathy.[105] Paroxetine is the first serotonin-specific reuptake inhibitor shown to be a highly effective analgesic in the treatment of neuropathic pain,[106] and may be a useful addition to our armamentarium of adjuvant analgesics for cancer pain. Newer antidepressants such as sertraline, venlafaxine, and nefazodone may also eventually prove to be clinically useful as adjuvant analgesics. Nefazodone, for instance, has been shown to potentiate opioid analgesics in an animal model.[107] It is becoming increasingly clear that many antidepressants have analgesic properties. Although there is no definite indication that any one drug is more effective than the others, the most experience has been with amitriptyline, which remains the antidepressant of choice. The therapeutic analgesic effects of amitriptyline are apparently correlated with serum levels, just as the antidepressant effects are, and analgesic treatment failure is due to low serum levels.[77,78,108] A high-dose regimen of up to 150 mg of amitriptyline or greater is suggested.[80,190] As to the time course of onset of analgesia with antidepressants, there appears to be a biphasic process that occurs with immediate or early analgesic effects that occur within hours or days,[89,92,96] and later, longer analgesic effects that peak over a 4–6-week period.[77–79]

Treatment should be initiated with a small dose of amitriptyline, for instance, 10–25 mg at bedtime, especially in debilitated patients, and increased slowly by 10–25 mg every 2–4 days working toward a dose of 150 mg. Pain and side effects should be frequently assessed and the dose escalated to 150 mg until a beneficial therapeutic effect has been achieved. Achieving a maximal effect as an adjuvant analgesic may require using the drug for 2–6 weeks. Serum levels of antidepressant drugs, when available, can also help assure that therapeutic serum levels of drug are being realized. Pain and depression in cancer patients often respond to lower doses (25–100 mg) of antidepressants than are usually required for physically healthy individuals (100–300 mg), most likely because of impaired metabolism of these drugs. The choice of drug often depends on the patient's side-effect profile, medical problems, the nature of depressive symptoms, if present, and past response to specific antidepressants. Sedating drugs like amitriptyline are helpful when insomnia complicates the presence of pain and depression suffered by a cancer patient. Anticholinergic properties of some of these drugs should also be kept in mind. Occasionally, in patients who have a limited analgesic response to a tricyclic agent, potentiation of analgesia can be accomplished with the addition of lithium.[110]

Monoamine oxidase inhibitors (MAOIs) are also minimally useful in the cancer setting because of dietary restriction and potentially dangerous interactions between MAOIs and narcotics such as meperidine. Among the available MAOI drugs, phenelzine has been shown to have adjuvant analgesic properties in patients with atypical facial pain and migraine.[111,112]

Psychostimulants

The psychostimulants, dextroamphetamine, and methylphenidate, are useful antidepressant agents prescribed selectively for medically ill cancer patients with depression.[113,114] Psychostimulants are also useful in diminishing excessive sedation secondary to narcoic analgesics, and are potent adjuvant analgesics. Bruera et al.[115–117] demonstrated that a regimen of 10 mg methylphenidate with breakfast and 5 mg with lunch significantly decreased sedation and potentiated the analgesic effect of narcotics in patients with cancer pain. Dextroamphetamine has also been reported to have additive analgesic effects when used with morphine for postoperative pain.[118] In relatively low doses, psychostimulants stimulate appetite, promote a sense of well-being, and improve feelings of weakness and fatigue in cancer patients. Treatment with dextroamphetamine or methylphenidate usually begins with a dose of 2.5 mg at 8:00 AM and at noon. The dosage is slowly increased over several days until a desired effect is achieved or side effects (overstimulation, anxiety, insomnia, paranoia, confusion) intervene. Typically, a dose greater than 30 mg/day is not necessary although occasionally patients require up to 60 mg/day. Patients usually are maintained on methylphenidate for 1–2 months, and approximately two-thirds will be able to be withdrawn from methylphenidate without a recurrence of depressive symptoms. Those who do recur can be maintained on a psychostimulant for up to 1 year without significant abuse problems. Tolerance will develop and adjusting the dose may be necessary. A strategy we have found useful in treating cancer pain associated with depression is to start a psychostimulant (starting dose of 2.5 mg of methylphenidate at 8:00 AM and noon), and then to add a tricyclic antidepressant after several days to help prolong and potentiate the short effect of the stimulant. Pemoline is a unique alternative psychostimulant that is chemically unrelated to amphetamine, but may have similar usefulness as an antidepressant and adjuvant analgesic in cancer patients.[119] Advantages of pemoline as a psychostimulant in cancer pain patients include the lack of abuse potential, the lack of federal regulation through special triplicate prescriptions, mild sympathomimetic effects, and the fact that it comes in a chewable tablet form that can be absorbed through the buccal mucosa and thus can be used by cancer patients who have difficulty swallowing or who have intestinal obstruction. In our clinical experience, pemoline is as effective as methylphenidate or

dextroamphetamine in the treatment of depressive symptoms, and in countering the sedating effects of opioid analgesics. There are no studies of pemoline's capacity to potentiate the analgesic properties of opioids. Pemoline can be started at a dose of 18.75 mg in the morning and at noon, and increased gradually over days. Typically, patients require 75 mg a day or less. Pemoline should be used with caution in patients with liver impairment, and liver function tests should be monitored periodically with longer-term treatment.[120]

Neuroleptics

Methotrimeprazine is a phenothiazine that is equianalgesic to morphine, has none of the opioid effects on gut motility, and probably produces analgesia through alpha-adrenergic blockade.[121] In patients who are opioid-tolerant, it provides an alternative approach in providing analgesia by a nonopioid mechanism. It is a dopamine blocker and so has antiemetic as well an anxiolytic effects. Methotrimeprazine can produce sedation and hypotension and should be given cautiously by slow IV infusion. Other phenothiazines such as chlorpromazine and prochlorperazine (Compazine) are useful as antiemetics in cancer patients, but probably have limited use as analgesics.[122] Fluphenazine in combination with TCAs has been shown to be helpful for treating neuropathic pain.[88] Haloperidol is the drug of choice in the management of delirium or psychoses in cancer patients, and has clinical usefulness as a coanalgesic for cancer pain.[122] Pimozide (Orap), a butyrophenone, has been shown to be effective as an analgesic in the management of trigeminal neuralgia, at doses of 4–12 mg/day.[123]

Anxiolytics

Hydroxyzine is a mild anxiolytic with sedating and analgesic properties that are useful for the anxious cancer patient with pain.[124,125] This antihistamine also has antiemetic activity. One hundred milligrams of parenteral hydroxyzine has analgesic activity similar to 8 mg of morphine, and has additive analgesic effects when combined with morphine. Benzodiazepines have not been believed to possess direct analgesic properties, although they are potent anxiolytics and anticonvulsants.[126] Some authors have suggested that their anticonvulsant properties make some benzodiazepine drugs useful in the management of neuropathic pain. Recently, Fernandez et al.[127] showed that alprazolam, a unique benzodiazepine with mild antidepressant properties, was a helpful adjuvant analgesic in cancer patients with phantom limb pain or deafferentation (neuropathic) pain. Clonazepam (Klonopin) may also be useful in the management of lancinating neuropathic pains in the cancer setting, and has been reported to be an effective analgesic for patients with trigeminal neuralgia, headache, and posttraumatic neuralgia.[128,129] With the use of IV midazolam in a patient-controlled dosage regimen, neither postoperative morphine requirements nor the patient's perception of pain were reduced.[130]

Substance abuse issues

Particularly problematic is the management of pain in patients that are actively abusing IV drugs.[75] Such active drug use, in particular IV opiate abuse, poses several pain treatment difficulties, including (1) high tolerance to narcotic analgesics, (2) drug-seeking and manipulative behavior, and (3) lack of compliance and/or reliability of patient history. Unfortunately, the patient's subjective report is often the best or only indication of the presence and intensity of pain as well as the degree of pain relief achieved by an intervention. Physicians who believe they are being manipulated by drug-seeking individuals are hesitant to use narcotic analgesics in appropriate dosages for adequate control of pain, often leading to undermedication. Most clinicians experienced in working with this addictive patient population recommend clear and direct limit setting. While that is an important aspect of such care, it is certainly not the entire answer for providing effective pain relief to cancer patients who also have substance abuse issues.

Incidence of substance abuse

Although relatively few studies have been conducted to evaluate the epidemiology of substance abuse in patients with advanced illness, substance use disorders appear to be relatively rare within the tertiary care cancer population and among those with other advanced diseases. Findings of a review of consultations performed by Psychiatry Services at MSKCC revealed that requests for management of issues related to substance abuse comprised only 3% of consultations.[131,132]

While the incidence of substance use disorders is much lower in patients with advanced disease than that in society at large, this may not be truly representative of the actual overall prevalence of substance abuse within the advanced illness spectrum. Factor such as institutional biases or a tendency for patients' underreporting this problem in tertiary-care hospitals may be reflective of the relatively low prevalence of substance abuse among patients with advanced illnesses. Social forces may also inhibit patients' reporting of drug use behavior. For example, many drug abusers are of lower socioeconomic standing and feel alienated from the healthcare system, and therefore may not seek treatment in tertiary-care centers. Furthermore, those who are treated in these centers may not acknowledge drug abuse for fear of stigmatization.[131–133]

Risks in patients with histories of substance abuse

There is a lack of information regarding the risk of abuse or addiction during or subsequent to the therapeutic administration of potentially abusable drugs to medically ill patients with a current or remote history of abuse or addiction.[132] The possibility of successful long-term opioid therapy in patients with cancer or chronic nonmalignant pain has been suggested by anecdotal reports, particularly if the abuse or addiction is remote.[134–136]

Since it is commonly accepted that the likelihood of aberrant drug-related behavior occurring during treatment for medical illness will be greater for those with a remote or current history of substance abuse, it is reasonable to consider the possibility of abuse behaviors occurring when utilizing different therapies. For example, while no clinical evidence exists to support the position that the use of short-acting drugs or the parenteral route is more likely to cause questionable drug-related behaviors than other therapeutic strategies, it may be prudent to avoid such therapies in patients with histories of drug abuse.[132] A basic set of principles pertaining to prescribing controlled substances to this patient population is presented in Table 10-2.

Clinicians should remember that essentially any drug that acts upon the central nervous system or any route of administration has the potential to be abused. Therefore, a more comprehensive approach that recognizes the biological, chemical, social, and psychiatric aspects is necessary in effectively managing patients with substance abuse histories. Utilizing such a strategy will extend beyond merely avoiding certain drugs or routes of administration, it will also afford practical means to manage risk during cancer treatment.[132]

Clinical management of patients with substance use issues

Patients who are actively abusing alcohol or other drugs typically present the most challenging issues to pain management clinicians, particularly when the abuse complicates managing their pain effectively.[137] Patients may become caught in a cycle in which pain functions as a barrier to seeking treatment for addiction and with addiction sometimes complicating treatment for chronic pain.[138] Secondarily, the undertreated pain of drug abusing patients can lead to an increased risk of bingeing with prescription medications and or other substances.[137]

The following guidelines can be beneficial whether the patient is actively abusing drugs or has a history of substance abuse. The principles outlined can be used by clinicians to structure, control, and monitor addiction-related behaviors during pain treatment.[139]

▶ General guidelines

Recommendations for the long-term administration of potentially abusable drugs, such as opioids, to patients with a history of substance abuse are based exclusively on clinical experience. Research is needed to ascertain the most effective strategies and to empirically identify patient subgroups that may be most responsive to specific approaches. The following guidelines broadly reflect the types of interventions that might be considered in this clinical context.[131,139]

▶ Multidisciplinary approach

Pain and symptom management is often complicated by various medical, psychosocial, and administrative issues in the population of advanced patients with a substance use disorder. The most effective team may include a physician with expertise in pain/palliative care, nurses, social workers and, when possible, a mental healthcare provider with expertise in the area of addiction medicine.[131,139]

▶ Assessment of substance use history

In an effort to not offend, threaten, or anger patients, clinicians often avoid asking patients about drug abuse and they also expect patients to frequently not answer truthfully. However, obtaining a detailed history of duration, frequency, and desired effect of drug use is vital. Adopting a nonjudgmental position and communicating in an empathetic and truthful manner is the best strategy when taking patients' substance abuse histories.[133,139]

In anticipating defensiveness on the part of the patient, it can be helpful for clinicians to mention that patients often misrepresent their drug use for logical reasons, such as stigmatization, mistrust of the interviewer, or concerns regarding fears of undertreatment. It is also wise for clinicians to explain that in an effort to keep the patient as comfortable as possible by preventing withdrawal states and prescribing sufficient medication for pain and symptom control, an accurate account of drug use is necessary.[133,139]

Using a careful, graduated style of interview can be beneficial in slowly introducing the assessment of drug abuse. This approach begins with broad and general inquires regarding the role of drugs in the patient's life, such as caffeine and nicotine, and gradually proceeds to more specific questions regarding illegal drugs. This interview style can also assist in discerning any coexisting psychiatric disorders, which can significantly contribute to aberrant drug-taking behavior. Once identified, treatment of comorbid psychiatric disorders can greatly enhance management strategies and decrease the risk of relapse.[133,139]

Set realistic goals for therapy

The rate of recurrence for drug abuse and addiction is high. The stress associated with advanced illness and the easy availability of centrally acting drugs increase this risk. Therefore, total prevention of relapse may be impossible in this type of setting. Gaining an understanding that compliance and abstinence are not realistic goals may decrease conflicts with staff members in terms of management goals. Instead, the goals might be perceived as the creation of a structure for therapy that includes ample social/emotional support and limit-setting to control the harm done by relapse.[133,139]

Some subgroups of patients may be unable to comply with the requirements of oncology therapy due to severe substance use disorders and comorbid psychiatric diagnoses. In these instances, clinicians must modify limits on various occasions and endeavor to develop a greater variety and intensity of supports. This may necessitate frequent team meetings and consultations with other clinicians. However, pertinent expectations must be clarified and therapy that is not successful should be modified.[133,139]

EVALUATING AND TREATING COMORBID PHYCHIATRIC DISORDERS

This chapter has stressed the overall impact of psychiatric disorders on pain management. It should be noted that there is an extremely high comorbidity of personality disorders, depression, and anxiety disorders in alcoholics and other patients with substance abuse histories.[140] The treatment of depression and anxiety can increase patient comfort and decrease the risk of relapse or aberrant drug-taking.[133,139]

Prevent or minimize withdrawal symptoms

Since many patients with drug abuse histories utilize multiple drugs, it is necessary to conduct a complete drug-use history to prepare for the possibility of withdrawal reactions. Delayed abstinence syndromes, such as may occur after abuse of some benzodiazepine drugs, are particularly diagnostically challenging.[133,139]

Consider the therapeutic impact of tolerance

Patients who are active substance abusers may be tolerant to drugs administered for therapy, which will make pain management more difficult. The magnitude of such tolerance is never known. Therefore, it is best to begin with a conservative dose of therapeutic drug and then rapidly titrate the dose with frequent reassessments until the patient is comfortable.[132,136]

Apply pharmacological principles to treating pain

Widely accepted guidelines for cancer pain management must be utilized to optimize long-term opioid therapy (AHCPRM, 1994; APS, 1992). These guidelines stress the importance of patient self-reporting as the basis for dosing, individualization of therapy to identify a favorable equilibrium between efficacy and side effects, and the value of monitoring over time.[139] They also are strongly indicative of the concurrent treatment of side effects as the basis for enhancing the balance between both analgesia and adverse effects.[141]

Individualization of the dose without regard to the patient's size, which is the most important guideline for long-term opioid therapy, can be difficult in populations with substance abuse histories.[139] Although it may be appropriate to use care in prescribing potentially abusable drugs to these populations, deciding to forego the guideline of dose individualization without regard to absolute dose may increase the risk of undertreatment.[142] Aberrant drug-related behaviors may develop in response to unrelieved pain. Although these behaviors might be best understood as pseudoaddiction, the incidence of such behaviors serves to verify clinicians' fears and encourages greater prudence in prescribing practices.[139]

Another common misconception surrounds the use of methadone. Clinicians who manage patients with substance abuse histories must be familiar with the pharmacology of methadone due to its dual role as a treatment for opioid addiction and as an analgesic.[143,144] Methadone impedes withdrawal for significantly longer periods of time than it relieves pain. That is, abstinence can be prevented and opioid cravings lessened with a single dose, whereas most patients typically require a minimum of three doses daily to obtain sustained analgesia. Although patients who are receiving methadone maintenance as treatment for opioid addiction can be given methadone as an analgesic beyond the guidelines of the addiction treatment program, this usually necessitates a substantial modification in therapy, including dose escalation and multiple daily doses.[133,139]

From a pharmacological stance, the management of such a change does not pose difficult issues, it can however create substantial stress for the patient and clinicians involved in the treatment of the addiction disorder. Because the drug has been classified as addiction therapy, as opposed to pain therapy, some patients express disbelief about the analgesic efficacy of methadone. Others wish to continue the morning dose for addiction even if treatment throughout the remainder of the day uses the same drug at an equivalent or higher dose. Some clinicians who work at methadone clinics are willing to continue to be involved and prescribe opioids, outside the program, and others wish to relinquish such care.[138]

Selecting appropriate drugs and route of administration for the symptom and setting

Administering long-acting analgesics in sufficient amounts to control symptoms may minimize the number of rescue doses needed, lessen cravings, and decrease the risk of abuse of prescribed medications, given the possible difficulty of using short-acting formulations in patients with substance abuse histories. Rather than being overly concerned about the choice of drug or route of administration, prescribing of opioids and other potentially abusable drugs should be carried out in a setting of limits and guidelines.[133,139]

Recognizing specific drug abuse behaviors

To monitor the development of aberrant drug-taking behaviors, patients who are prescribed potentially abusable drugs must be evaluated over time. This is particularly true for patients who have a remote or current history of drug abuse, including alcohol abuse. Should a high level of concern exist regarding such behaviors, frequent visits and regular assessments of significant others who can contribute information about the patient's drug use may be required. It may also be necessary to have patients who have been actively abusing drugs in the recent past to submit urine specimens for regular screening of illicit or licit but unprescribed drugs to promote early recognition of aberrant drug-related behaviors. In informing the patient of this approach, it should be explained as a method of monitoring that can reassure the clinician and provide a foundation for aggressive symptom-oriented treatment, thus enhancing the therapeutic alliance with the patient.[133,139]

Utilize nondrug approaches as appropriate

Many nondrug approaches can be utilized to assist patients in coping with chronic pain in advanced illness. Such educational interventions may include relaxation techniques, ways of thinking and describing the experience of pain, and methods of communicating physical and emotional distress to staff members (see Table 10-2), and are described in more detail earlier in this chapter. While nondrug interventions may be helpful adjuvants to management, they should not be perceived as substitutes for drugs targeted at treating pain, or at other physical or psychological symptoms.[133,139]

Inpatient management plan

When designing an inpatient management plan for an actively abusing patient with advanced illness, it is helpful to utilize structured treatment guidelines. While the applicability of these guidelines may vary from setting to setting, they provide a set of strategies that can ensure the safety of the patient and staff, control of the patient's manipulative behaviors, allow for the supervision of illicit drug use, enhance the appropriate use of medications for pain and symptom control, and communicate an understanding of pain and substance abuse management.[133,139]

Under certain circumstances, such as actively abusing patients who are scheduled for surgery, patients should be admitted several days in advance when possible to allow for the stabilization of the drug regimen. This time can also be utilized to avoid withdrawal and provide an opportunity to assess whether modifications to the established plan are necessary.[133,139]

Once established, the structured treatment plan for managing active abuse must proceed conscientiously. In an effort to assess and manage symptoms, frequent bedside visits are usually necessary. It is also important to avoid drug withdrawal and, to the extent possible, prescribed drugs for symptom control should be administered on a regularly scheduled basis (see Table 10-2). This helps to eliminate repetitive encounters between the patient and staff members that center on the desire to obtain drugs.[133,139]

Treatment management plans must be designed to represent the treating clinician's assessment of the severity of drug abuse. Open and honest communication between the clinician and patient that stresses the necessity for having established guidelines is in the best interest of the patient and is often helpful in confronting the problem and avoiding untoward sequelae associated with the drug abuse. However, in cases where patients are unable to follow these guidelines, despite repeated interventions from the staff, discharge should be considered. Clinicians should discuss the decision to discharge a patient with hospital staff and administration, while considering the ethical and legal ramifications of this action.[133,139]

Outpatient management plan

Alternative guidelines may be utilized in the management of the actively abusing patient with advanced illness who is being treated on an outpatient basis. In some instances, the treatment plan can be coordinated with referral to a drug rehabilitation program. However, patients who are facing end-of-life issues may have difficulty participating in such programs. Several interventions may prove useful for this population. For example, utilizing written agreements that clearly state the roles of the team members and the rules and expectations for the patient is helpful when structuring outpatient treatment. While using the patient's behaviors as the basis for the level of restrictions, graded agreements should be enforced that clearly state the consequences of aberrant drug use.[133,139] A sample contract for the initiation of opioid therapy is provided in Fig. 10-1. This template can be modified and structured to fit individual practices and clinics, but is a good general format for outlining the responsibilities of the patient and the provider.

In addition to the use of contracts, the clinician should consider referring the patient to a 12-step program with the stipulation that attendance be documented for ongoing prescription purposes. The clinician may wish to contact the patient's sponsor in an effort to disclose the patient's illness and to state that medication is required in the treatment of the illness. This contact will also assist in decreasing the risk of the stigmatization of the patient as being noncompliant with the ideals of the 12-step program.[133,139] Finally, periodic urine toxicology screens should be performed for most patients to encourage compliance and detect the concurrent use of illicit substances. This practice, as well as how positive screens will be managed, should be clearly explained to the patient at the beginning of outpatient therapy. A response to a positive screen generally involves increasing the guidelines for continued treatment, such as more frequent visits and smaller quantities of prescribed drugs.[133,139]

REFERENCES

1. Foley KM. The treatment of cancer pain. *N Engl J Med.* 1985;313:84–95.
2. Bonica JJ. Cancer pain. In: Bonica JJ, ed. *The Management of Pain.* 2nd ed. Philadelphia, PA: Lea & Febiger; 1990:400–460.
3. Twycross RG, Lack SA. *Symptom Control in Far Advanced Cancer: Pain Relief.* London: Pitman Brooks; 1983.
4. Foley KM. Pain syndromes in patients with cancer. In: Bonica JJ, Ventafridda V, eds. *Advances in Pain Research and Therapy,* vol. 2. New York: Raven Press; 1979.
5. Breitbart W, Holland J. Psychiatric aspects of cancer pain. In: Foley KM, Bonica JJ, Ventafridda V, eds. *Advances in Pain Research and Therapy,* vol. 16. New York: Raven Press; 1990:73–87.
6. Breitbart W. Psychiatric management of cancer pain. *Cancer.* 1989;63: 2336–2342.
7. Massie MJ, Holland JC. The cancer patient with pain: psychiatric complications and their management. *J Pain Symptom Manage.* 1992;7(2): 99–109.
8. Marks RM, Sachar EJ. Undertreatment of medical inpatients with narcotic analgesics. *Ann Intern Med.* 1973;78:173–181.
9. Grond S, Zech D, Diefenbach C, et al. Prevalence and pattern of symptoms in patients with cancer pain: a prospective evaluation of 1635 cancer patients referred to a pain clinic. *J Pain Symptom Manage.* 1994;9:372–382.
10. Stiefel F. Psychosocial aspects of cancer pain. *Support Care Cancer.* 1993;1:130–134.
11. Saunders CM. *The Management of Terminal Illness.* Londres: Hospital Medicine Publications;1967.
12. Hanks G W. Opioid-responsive and opioid non-responsive pain in cancer. *Br Med Bull.* 1991;47:718–731.
13. Syrjala KL, Chapko ME. Evidence for a biopsychosocial model of cancer treatment-related pain. *Pain.* 1995;61:69–79.
14. Daut RL, Cleeland CS. The prevalence and severity of pain in cancer. *Cancer.* 1982;50:1913–1918.
15. Spiegel D, Bloom JR. Pain in metastatic breast cancer. *Cancer.* 1983;52:341–345.
16. Padilla G, Ferrell B, Grant M, et al. Defining the content domain of quality of life for cancer patients with pain. *Cancer Nurs.* 1990;13:108–115.
17. Payne D. *Cognition in Cancer Pain.* 1995. Unpublished dissertation.
18. McKegney FP, Bailey LR, Yates JW. Prediction and management of pain in patients with advanced cancer. *Gen Hosp Psychiatry.* 1981;3:95–101.
19. Bond MR, Pearson IB. Psychological aspects of pain in women with advanced cancer of the cervix. *J Psychosom Res.* 1969;13:13–19.
20. Cleeland CS. Pain control in cancer. In: Brain MC, Carbone PP, eds. *Current Therapy in Hematology-Oncology.* Philadelphia: BC Decker; 1988:255–259. Current Therapy Series.
21. Derogatis LR, Morrow GR, Fetting J, et al. The prevalence of psychiatric disorders among cancer patients. *JAMA.* 1983;249:751–757.

22. Ahles TA, Blanchard EB, Ruckdeschel JC. The multidimensional nature of cancer-related pain. *Pain.* 1983;17:277–288.

23. Woodforde JM, Fielding JR. Pain and cancer. *J Psychosom Res.* 1970;14: 365–370.

24. Bukberg J, Penman D, Holland JC. Depression in hospitalized cancer patients. *Psychosom Med.* 1984;46:199–212.

25. Massie MJ, Holland J, Glass E. Delirium in terminally ill cancer patients. *Am J Psychiatry.* 1983;140:1048–1050.

26. Bruera E, Macmillan K, Hanson J, et al. The cognitive effects of the administration of narcotic analgesics in patients with cancer pain. *Pain.* 1989;39:13–16.

27. Stiefel FC, Breitbart W, Holland JC. Corticosteroids in cancer: neuropsychiatric complications. *Cancer Invest.* 1989;7:479–491.

28. Breitbart W. Suicide in cancer patients. *Oncology.* 1987;1:49–55.

29. Levin DN, Cleeland CS, Dar R. Public attitudes toward cancer pain. *Cancer.* 1985;56:2337–2339.

30. Bolund C. Suicide and cancer: II. Medical and care factors in suicide by cancer patients in Sweden. 1973–1976. *J Psychosoc Oncol.* 1985;3:17–30.

31. Farberow NL, Schneidman ES, Leonard CV. Suicide among general medical and surgical hospital patients with malignant neoplasms. *Med Bull Vet Adm.* 1963;MB-9;1–11.

32. Massie MJ, Gagnon P, Holland JC. Depression and suicide in patients with cancer. *J Pain Symptom Manage.* 1994;9:325–340.

33. Silberfarb PM, Manrer LH, Crouthamel CS. Psychological aspects of neoplastic disease I. Functional status of breast cancer patients during different treatment regimens. *Am J Psychiatry.* 1980;137:450–455.

34. Achte KA, Vanhkonen ML. Cancer and the psychology. *Omega.* 1971;2: 46–56.

35. Brown JH, Henteleff P, Barakat S, et al. Is it normal for terminally ill patients to desire death? *Am J Psychiatry.* 1986;143:208–211.

36. Saltzburg D, Breitbart W, Fishman B, et al. The relationship of pain and depression to suicidal ideation in cancer patients (abstract). ASCO Annual Meeting; May 21–23, 1989; San Francisco.

37. Cleeland CS, Gonin R, Hatfield AK, et al. Pain and its treatment in outpatients with metastatic cancer. *N Engl J Med.* 1994;330:592–596.

38. Charap AD. The knowledge, attitudes, and experience of medical personnel treating pain in the terminally ill. *Mt Sinai J Med.* 1978;45: 561–580.

39. Macaluso C, Weinberg D, Foley KM. Opioid abuse and misuse in a cancer pain population (abstract). Second International Congress on Cancer Pain; July 14–17, 1988; Rye, New York.

40. Kanner RM, Foley KM. Patterns of narcotic use in a cancer pain clinic. *Ann NY Acad Sci.* 1981;362:161–172.

41. Bruera E, Macmillan K, Pither J, et al. Effects of morphine on the dyspnea of terminal cancer patients. *J Pain Symptom Manage.* 1990;5: 341–344.

42. Grossman SA, Sheidler VR, Swedeen K, et al. Correlations of patient and caregiver ratings of cancer pain. *J Pain Symptom Manage.* 1991;6:53–57.

43. Cassem NH. The dying patient. In: Cassem NH, Stern TA, Rosenbaum JF, Jellinek MS, eds. *Massachusetts General Hospital Handbook of General Hospital Psychiatry.* 4th ed. St. Louis: Mosby-Year Book, Inc.; 1997.

44. Passik S, Horowitz S, Malkin M, Gargan R. A psychoeducational support program for spouses of brain tumor patients (abstract). Symposium on New Trends in the Psychological Support of the Cancer Patient. American Psychiatric Association Annual Meeting; May 7–12, 1991; New Orleans, LA.

45. SyrajalaKL, Cummings C, Donaldson GW. Hypnosis or cognitive behavioral training for the reduction of pain and nausea during cancer treatment: a controlled trial. *Pain.* 1992;48:137–146.

46. Spiegel D, Bloom JR. Group therapy and hypnosis reduce metastatic breast carcinoma pain. *Psychosom Med.* 1983;45:333–339.

47. Fishman B, Loscalzo M. Cognitive-behavioral interventions in the management of cancer pain: principles and applications. *Med Clin North Am.* 1987;71:271–287.

48. Cleeland CS. Nonpharmacologic management of cancer pain. *J Pain Symptom Manage.* 1987;2:S23–S28.

49. Loscalzo M, Jacobsen PB. Practical behavioral approaches to the effective management of pain and distress. *J Psychosoc Oncol.* 1990;8:139–169.

50. Turk DC, Fernandez E. On the putative uniqueness of cancer pain: do psychological principles apply? *Behav Res Ther.* 1990;28:1–13.

51. Fishman B. The treatment of suffering in patients with cancer pain. In: Foley K, Bonica J, Ventafridda V, eds. *Advances in Pain Research and Therapy,* vol 16. New York: Raven Press Ltd.; 1990:301–316.

52. Jensen MP, Turner JA, Romano JM, et al. Coping with chronic pain: a critical review of the literature. *Pain.* 1991;47:249–283.

53. Breitbart W, Holland JC. Psychiatric complications of cancer. In: Brain MC, Carbone PP, eds. *Current Therapy in Hematology Oncology-3.* Toronto and Philadelphia: B.C. Decker Inc.; 1988:268–274.

54. Erickson MH. Hypnosis in painful terminal illness. *J Ark Med Soc.* 1959;56:67–71.

55. Benson H. *The Relaxation Response.* New York: William Morrow; 1975.

56. Spiegel D. The use of hypnosis in controlling cancer pain. *CA Cancer J Clin.* 1985;35:221–231.

57. Redd WB, Reeves JL, Storm FK, Minagawa RY. Hypnosis in the control of pain during hyperthermia treatment of cancer. In: Bonica JJ, ed. *Advances in Pain Research and Theory,* vol. 5. New York: Raven Press Ltd.; 1982:857–861.

58. Barber J, Gitelson J. Cancer pain: psychological management using hypnosis. *CA Cancer J Clin.* 1980;30:130–136.

59. Levitan A, The use of hypnosis with cancer patients. *Psychiatr Med.* 1992;10:119–131.

60. Broome ME, Lillis PP, McGahee TW, et al. The use of distraction and imagery with children during painful procedures. *Oncol Nurs Forum.* 1992;19:499–502.

61. Fotopoulos SS, Graham C, Cook MR. Psychophysiologic control of cancer pain. In: Bonica JJ, Ventafridda V, eds. *Advances in Pain Research and Therapy,* vol 2. New York: Raven Press Ltd.; 1979.

62. Munro S, Mount B. Music therapy in palliative care. *Can Med Assoc J.* 1978;119:1029–1034.

63. Schroeder-Sheker T. Music for the dying: a personal account of the new field of music thanatology—history, theories, and clinical narratives. *J Holist Nurs.* 1994;12(1):83–99.

64. Manne S, Redd W, Jacobsen P, Georgiades I. Aroma for treatment of anxiety during MRI scans (abstract). Symposium on New Trends in the Psychological Support of the Cancer Patient. American Psychiatric Association Annual Meeting; May 7–12, 1991; New Orleans, LA.

65. Connell C. Art therapy as a part of palliative care programs. *Palliat Med.* 1992;6:18–25.

66. Breitbart W. Psychotropic adjuvant analgesic drugs for cancer pain. *J Pain Symptom Manage.* 1989;4(Suppl. 3):2,4.

67. France RD. The future for antidepressants: treatment of pain. *Psychopathology.* 1987;20:99–113.

68. Getto CJ, Sorkness CA, Howell T. Issues in drug management. Part I. Antidepressants and chronic nonmalignant pain: a review. *J Pain Symptom Manage.* 1987;2:9–18.

69. Walsh TD. Antidepressants and chronic pain. *Clin Neuropharmacol.* 1983;6:271–295.

70. Walsh TD. Adjuvant analgesic therapy in cancer pain. In: Foley KM, ed. *Advances in Pain Research and Therapy,* vol. 16, Second International Congress on Cancer Pain. New York: Raven Press Ld.; 1990:155–165.

71. Butler S. Present status of tricyclic antidepressants in chronic pain therapy. In: Benedetti C, ed. *Advances in Pain Research and Therapy,* vol. 7. New York: Raven Press Ltd.; 1986:173–196.

72. Ventafridda V, Bonezzi C, Caraceni A, et al. Antidepressants for cancer pain and other painful syndromes with deafferentation component: comparison of amitriptyline and trazodone. *Ital J Neurol Sci.* 1987;8: 579–587.

73. Magni G, Arsie D, De Leo D. Antidepressants in the treatment of cancer pain. A survey in Italy. *Pain.* 1987;29:347–353.

74. Onghena P, Van Houdenhove B. Antidepressant-induced analgesia in chronic non-malignant pain: a meta-analysis of 39 placebo-controlled studies. *Pain.* 1992;49:205–219.

75. W. Breitbart W, Patt R. Pain management in the patient with AIDS. *Pain Manag.* 1994;2:391.

76. Lefkowitz M, Breitbart W. Chronic pain and AIDS. *Innov Pain Med.* 1992;36:2–3,18.

77. Max MB, Culnane M, Schafer SC, et al. Amitriptyline relieves diabetic neuropathy pain in patients with normal or depressed mood. *Neurology.* 1987;37:589–596.

78. Max MB, Schafer SC, Culnane M, et al. Amitriptyline, but not lorazepam, relieves postherpetic neuralgia. *Neurology.* 1988;38: 1427–1432.

79. Pilowsky I, Hallett EC, Bassett DL, et al. A controlled study of amitriptyline in the treatment of chronic pain. *Pain.* 1982;14:169–179.

80. Sharav Y, Singer E, Schmidt E, et al. The analgesic effect of amitriptyline on chronic facial pain. *Pain.* 1987;31:199–209.

81. Watson CP, Evans RJ, Reed K, et al. Amitriptyline versus placebo in post herpetic neuralgia. *Neurology.* 1982;32:671–673.

82. Kvinesdal B, Molin J, Froland A, et al. Imipramine treatment of painful diabetic neuropathy. *JAMA.* 1984;251:1727–1730.

83. Young RJ, Clarke BF. Pain relief in diabetic neuropathy: the effectiveness of imipramine and related drugs. *Diabetic Med.* 1985;2:363–366.

84. Sindrup SH, Ejlertsen B, Froland A, et al. Imipramine treatment in diabetic neuropathy: relief of subjective symptoms without changes in peripheral and autonomic nerve function. *Eur J Clin Pharmacol.* 1989; 37:151–153.

85. Max MB, Kishore-Kumar R, Schafer SC, et al. Efficacy of desipramine in painful diabetic neuropathy: a placebo-controlled trial. *Pain.* 1991;45:3–9.

86. Gordon NC, Heller PH, Gear RW, et al. Temporal factors in the enhancement of morphine analgesic by desipramine. *Pain.* 1993;53: 273–276.

87. Gomez-Perez FJ, Rull JA, Dies H, et al. Nortriptyline and fluphenazine in the symptomatic treatment of diabetic neuropathy. A double-blind cross-over study. *Pain.* 1985;23:395–400.

88. Langohr HD, Stohr M, Petruch F. An open and double-blind cross-over study on the efficacy of clomipramine (Anafranil) in patients with painful mono- and polyneuropathies. *Eur Neurol.* 1982;21:309–317.

89. Tiegno M, Pagnoni B, Calmi A, et al. Clomipramine compared with pentazocine as a unique treatment in postoperative pain. *Int J Clin Pharmacol Res.* 1987;7:141–143.

90. Hameroff SR, Cork RC, Scherer K, et al. Doxepin effects on chronic pain, depression and plasma opioids. *J Clin Psychiatry.* 1982;43:22–27.

91. Walsh TD. Controlled study of imipramine and morphine in chronic pain due to advanced cancer (abstract). ASCO May 4–6, Los Angeles, 1986.

92. Botney M, Fields HL. Amitriptyline potentiates morphine analgesia by direct action on the central nervous system. *Ann Neurol.* 1983;13: 160–164.

93. Watson CP, Chipman M, Reed K, et al. Amitriptyline versus maprotiline in postherpetic neuralgia: a randomized, double-blind, crossover trial. *Pain.* 1992;48:29–36.

94. Malseed RT, Goldstein FJ. Enhancement of morphine analgesia by tricyclic antidepressants. *Neuropharmacology.* 1979;18:827–829.

95. Ventafridda V, Bianchi M, Ripamonti C, et al. Studies on the effects of antidepressant drugs on the antinociceptive action of morphine and on plasma morphine in rat and man. *Pain.* 1990;43:155–162.

96. Spiegel K, Kalb R, Pasternak GW. Analgesic activity of tricyclic antidepressants. *Ann Neurol.* 1983;13:462–465.

97. Davidoff G, Guarracini M, Roth E, et al. Trazodone hydrochloride in the treatment of dysesthetic pain in traumatic myelopathy: a randomized, double-blind, placebo-controlled study. *Pain.* 1987;29:151–161.

98. Costa D, Mogos I, Toma T. Efficacy and safety of mianserin in the treatment of depression of woman with cancer. *Acta Psychiatr Scand Suppl.* 1985;320:85–92.

99. Eberhard G, von Knorring L, Nilsson HL, et al. A double-blind randomized study of clomipramine versus maprotiline in patients with idiopathic pain syndromes. *Neuropsychobiology.* 1988;19:25–34.

100. Feighner JP. A comparative trial of fluoxetine and amitriptyline in patients with major depressive disorder. *J Clin Psychiatry.* 1985;46:369–372.

101. Hynes MD, Lochner MA, Bemis KG, et al. Fluoxetine, a selective inhibitor of serotonin uptake, potentiates morphine analgesia without altering its discriminative stimulus properties or affinity for opioid receptors. *Life Sci.* 1985;36:2317–2323.

102. Diamond S, Frietag FG. The use of fluoxetine in the treatment of headache. *Clin J Pain.* 1989;5:200–201.

103. Geller SA. Treatment of fibrositis with fluoxetine hydrochloride (Prozac). *Am J Med.* 1989;87:594–595.

104. Theesen KA, Marsh WR. Relief of diabetic neuropathy with fluoxetine. *DICP.* 1989;23:572–574.

105. Max MB, Lynch SA, Muir J, et al. Effects of desipramine, amitriptyline, and fluoxetine on pain in diabetic neuropathy. *N Engl J Med.* 1992;326:1250–1256.

106. Sindrup SH, Gram LF, Brosen K, et al. The selective serotonin reuptake inhibitor paroxetine is effective in the treatment of diabetic neuropathy symptoms. *Pain.* 1990;42:135–144.

107. Pick CG, Paul D, Eison MS, et al. Potentiation of opioid analgesia by the antidepressant nefazodone. *Eur J Pharmacol.* 1992;211:375–381.

108. McQuay H, Carroll D, Glynn C. Dose-response for analgesic effect of amitriptyline in chronic pain. *Anaesthesia.* 1993;48:281–285.

109. Watson CP, Evans RJ. A comparative trial of amitriptyline and zimelidine in post-herpetic neuralgia. *Pain.* 1985;23:387–394.

110. Tyler MA. Treatment of the painful shoulder syndrome with amitriptyline and lithium carbonate. *Can Med Assoc J.* 1974;111(2):137–140.

111. Lascelles RG. Atypical facial pain and depression. *Br J Psychiatry.* 1966;112:651–659.

112. Anthony M, Lance JW. Monoamine oxidase inhibition in the treatment of migraine. *Arch Neurol.* 1969;21:263–268.

113. Fernandez F, Adams F, Holmes VF, et al. Methylphenidate for depressive disorders in cancer patients. An alternative to standard antidepressants. *Psychosomatics.* 1987;28:455–461.

114. Kaufmann MW, Murray GB, Cassem NH. Use of psychostimulants in medically ill depressed patients. *Psychosomatics.* 1982;23:817–819.

115. Bruera E, Chadwick S, Brenneis C, et al. Methylphenidate associated with narcotics for the treatment of cancer pain. *Cancer Treat Rep.* 1987;71:67–70.

116. Bruera E, Brenneis C, Paterson AH, et al. Use of methylphenidate as an adjuvant to narcotic analgesics in patients with advanced cancer. *J Pain Symptom Manage.*t 1989;4:3–6.

117. Bruera E, Fainsinger R, MacEachern T, et al. The use of methylphenidate in patients with incident cancer pain receiving regular opiates: a preliminary report. *Pain.* 1992;50:75–77.

118. Forrest WH Jr, Brown BW, Jr, Brown CR, et al. Dextroamphetamine with morphine for the treatment of postoperative pain. *N Engl J Med.* 1977;296:712–715.

119. Breitbart W, Mermelstein H. Pemoline. An alternative psychostimulant in the management of depressive disorders in cancer patients. *Psychosomatics.* 1992;33:352–356.

120. Nehra A, Mullick F, Ishak KG, et al. Pemoline-associated hepatic injury. *Gastroenterology.* 1990;99:1517–1519.

121. Beaver WT, Wallenstein SL, Houde RW, et al. A comparison of the analgesic effects of methotrimeprazine and morphine in patients with cancer. *Clin Pharmacol Ther.* 1966;7:436–446.

122. Maltbie AA, Cavenar JO, Jr, Sullivan JL, et al. Analgesia and haloperidol: a hypothesis. *J Clin Psychiatry.* 1979;40:323–326.

123. Lechin F, van der Dijs B, Lechin ME, et al. Pimozide therapy for trigeminal neuralgia. *Arch Neurol.* 1989;46:960–963.

124. Beaver WT, Feise G. Comparison of the analgesic effects of morphine, hydroxyzine and their combination in patients with post-operative pain. In: Bonica JJ, Albe-Fessard D, eds. *Advances in Pain Research and Therapy.* New York: Raven Press; 1976;533–557.

125. Rumore MM, Schlichting DA. Clinical efficacy of antihistamines as analgesics. *Pain.* 1986;25:7–22.

126. Coda BA, Mackie A, Hill HF. Influence of alprazolam on opioid analgesia and side effects during steady-state morphine infusions. *Pain.* 1992;50:309–316.

127. Fernandez F, Adams F, Holmes VF. Analgesic effect of alprazolam in patients with chronic, organic pain of malignant origin. *J Clin Psychopharmacol.* 1987;7:167–169.

128. Caccia MR. Clonazepam in facial neuralgia and cluster headache. Clinical and electrophysiological study. *Eur Neurol.* 1975;13:560–563.

129. Swerdlow M, Cundill JG. Anticonvulsant drugs used in the treatment of lancinating pain. A comparison. *Anaesthesia.* 1981;36:1129–1132.

130. Egan KJ, Ready LB, Nessly M, et al. Self administration of midazolam for postoperative anxiety: a double blinded study. *Pain.* 1992;49:3–8.

131. Passik SD, Portenoy RK, Ricketts PL. Substance abuse issues in cancer patients. Part 1: Prevalence and diagnosis. *Oncology.* 1998a;12:517–521.

132. Passik SD, Portenoy RK. Substance abuse issues in palliative care. In: Berger A, Portenoy RK, Weissman DE, eds. *Principles and Practice of Supportive Oncology.* Philadelphia, PA: Lippincott-Raven Publishers; 1998:513–529.

133. Passik SD, Portenoy RK. Substance abuse disorders. In: Holland JC, ed. *Psycho-oncology.* New York, NY: Oxford University Press; 1998b: 576–586.

134. Dunbar SA, Katz NP. Chronic opioid therapy for nonmalignant pain in patients with a history of substance abuse: report of 20 cases. *J Pain Symptom Manage.* 1996;11:163–171.

135. Gonzales GR, Coyle N. Treatment of cancer pain in a former opioid abuser: fears of the patient and staff and their influences on care. *J Pain Symptom Manage.* 1992;7:246–249.

136. Macaluso C, Weinberg D, Foley KM. Opioid abuse and misuse in a cancer pain population [abstract]. *J Pain Symptom Manage.* 1988;3: S24–S31.

137. Kemp C. Managing chronic pain in patients with advanced disease and substance-related disorders. *Home Healthc Nurse.* 1996;14:255–261.

138. Savage SR. Addiction in the treatment of pain: significance, recognition, and management. *J Pain Symptom Manage.* 1993;8:265–278.

139. Passik SD, Portenoy RK, Ricketts PL. Substance abuse issues in cancer patients. Part 2: Evaluation and treatment. *Oncology.* 1998b;12: 729–734.

140. Khantzian EJ, Treece C. DSM-III psychiatric diagnosis of narcotic addicts. Recent findings. *Arch Gen Psychiatry.* 1985;42:1067–1071.

141. Portenoy RK. Management of common opioid side effects during long-term therapy of cancer pain. *Ann Acad Med Singapore.* 1994;23:160–170.

142. Breitbart W, Rosenfeld BD, Passik SD, et al. The undertreatment of pain in ambulatory AIDS patients. *Pain.* 1996;65:243–249.

143. Fainsinger R, Schoeller T, Bruera E. Methadone in the management of cancer pain: a review. *Pain.* 1993;52:137–147.

144. Lowinson JH, Marion IJ, Joseph H, Dole VP. Methadone maintenance. In: Lowinson JH, Ruiz P, Millman RB, eds. *Substance Abuse: A Comprehensive Textbook.* 2nd ed. Baltimore, MD: Williams & Wilkins; 1992:550–561.

Chronic Pain in the Cured Cancer Patient

CHAPTER

11

Allen W. Burton
Gilbert J. Fanciullo
Ralph D. Beasley

INTRODUCTION

The overall state of cancer pain care has improved over the past two decades through the widespread use of traditional therapies. While agreement exists regarding the best strategies for assessment and treatment of most cancer pain syndromes, little consensus exists about the treatment of chronic pain in the cancer survivor. Improved cancer therapy has led to increasing life expectancy and cure rates in most types of cancers; in some tumor types long-term survival has increased dramatically. The American Cancer Society has stated a goal in the coming decade of making cancer into a chronic disease state, much along the lines of rheumatologic diseases, in which long-term control is possible, even in the absence of a traditional "cure." A recent report from the Institute of Medicine (IOM) is titled "From Cancer Patient to Cancer Survivor: Lost in Transition."[1] This report points out that the number of cancer survivors in the United States has more than tripled to approximately 10 million people during the past 30 years. The authors also note that although survival rates are increasing, no one knows at what cost to the health and well-being of the survivors. More than 6 million cancer survivors are over age 65, creating a huge challenge to the Medicare system, while in the under age 65 set more than 10% of survivors are uninsured. While most survivors return to work, 20% will have work limitations up to 5 years later. It is clear that there are numerous challenges presented by this growing patient population, with chronic pain among them.

Opioid-based strategies like the World Health Organization (WHO) pain ladder have been validated in the treatment of active cancer pain syndromes, whereas the use of chronic opioid treatment in the treatment of chronic pain remains controversial. Chronic pain in cancer survivors is a poorly studied and understood entity. Incidence, prevalence, and basic epidemiologic data are, with a few exceptions, lacking. Only within the last decade has attention been directed toward the identification and treatment of chronic pain syndromes in cancer survivors.

The goals of this chapter are to provide an overview of the prevalence and types of chronic pain occurring in cancer patients as a direct consequence of their cancer or cancer treatment to help providers recognize these syndromes and their presentations. Further, therapeutic insights are presented that may help providers decrease the occurrence of chronic pain in cancer survivors. The most commonly known surgery, chemotherapy, and radiation therapy-associated chronic pain syndromes will be described.

EPIDEMIOLOGY OF CHRONIC PAIN IN CANCER SURVIVORS

People with cancer suffer from a variety of symptoms at all stages of their disease including after effective eradication of the cancer. A total of 1.4 million Americans were newly diagnosed with cancer in 2004, approximately 4000 per day.[2] In the same year, 564,000 U.S. deaths were attributed to cancer, about 22% of all deaths. It is estimated that more than 10 million individuals in the U.S. are living with cancer at the present time, around 3% of the population. The prevalence of pain at the time of cancer diagnosis and early in the course of disease is estimated to be 50%, increasing to 75% in advanced stages. The prevalence of chronic pain in cured cancer patients is less well studied, but some data exist.

Posttreatment pain syndromes may stem from chemotherapy, radiation therapy, or surgery. Post chemotherapy painful peripheral neuropathy is well described with the use of vincristine, platinum, taxanes, thalidomide, bortezomib, and some other agents. Radiation neural damage and pain may surface decades after radiotherapy completion, confounding the diagnosis in some cases. Finally, postsurgical pain syndromes come in many varieties, including postmastectomy, postamputation, postthoracotomy, and other chronic pain states (Table 11-1). The prevalence of chronic pain in breast cancer survivors is estimated to be at least 50%.[3] The prevalence of phantom limb pain (PLP) after amputation is estimated to be between 7% and 72% depending on the "cutoff" points applied to evaluate the pain severity.[4] Long-term severe pain after thoracotomy may have a prevalence as high as 50%.[5] The incidence of pain following treatment for head and neck cancer may be as high as 50%, with more than 50% disabled 1 year after diagnosis highly correlated to pain scores.[6–8] Perkins and Kehlet identified several risk factors that predispose surgical patients to chronic pain (Table 11-2).[8] Many of these "predisposing factors" for chronic pain are oncologic in nature, including preexisting pain, repeat surgery, psychological vulnerability, radiation, chemotherapy, and finally depression and anxiety.

"Existential consequences of unrelieved cancer pain" have been well reported.[10] Fear that postsurvival pain may be a dire prognostic indicator and other factors may lead to underreporting of pain by cancer survivors. Chronic pain after cancer treatment is an underappreciated problem that occurs commonly in a population of patients less likely to spontaneously seek treatment because they are afraid that the pain may represent recurrence of their cancer. The types of pain that occur are often complex, difficult to diagnose,

Table 11-1

Incidence of Developing Chronic Postoperative Pain by Type of Surgery

Type of Surgery	Reported Incidence of Chronic Pain
Limb amputation	30%–80%
Thoracotomy	22%–70%
Cholecystectomy	3%–56%
Inguinal hernia	0%–37%

Source: Modified from Perkins FM, Kehlet H. Chronic pain as an outcome of surgery. *Anesthesiology.* 2000;93:1123–1133.[9]

may be myalgic or neuropathic, and might be less responsive than somatic pain to usual treatments. Radiation plexopathy may occur up to 20 years after cancer treatment that occurred so long ago but may be unrecognized as an etiology by many providers.[8] Detailed knowledge of painful conditions that can occur in survivors is necessary to optimize treatment and this understanding may be absent even among oncologists and pain specialists.

GENERAL PRINCIPLES OF TREATING CHRONIC PAIN

Chronic pain in survivors may occur as a consequence of severe, poorly controlled acute cancer pain. Patients who endure severe, inadequately controlled pain during the acute treatment phase of their disease are more likely to develop chronic pain later on. This is not unique to cancer pain patients but is known to occur in pain patients in general.[11] Every effort should be made to control pain well at the time of diagnosis, after surgery, during chemotherapy, and radiation treatment. Good acute pain control *may* reduce the incidence of chronic pain in cancer survivors.[12]

Psychological factors influence chronic pain in patients cured of cancer.[13] The expression and ability to cope with pain heavily impact the magnitude of debility caused by the chronic painful condition. Patients who use active coping strategies report less chronic pain than those who use passive strategies. Active strategies are an attempt by the patient to control pain and to continue to function in spite of pain, while passive strategies involve relinquishing the control of pain entirely to others. Catastrophizing is a tendency to

Table 11-2

Factors which Predict Chronic Pain Postoperatively

Preoperative factors: chronic preoperative pain >1 month duration; repeated surgery; psychological traits including passive coping skills; worker's compensation claims

Intraoperative factors: type of surgery, risk of nerve trauma

Postoperative factors: severe pain poorly controlled; radiation therapy to the area; chemotherapy; anxiety

Source: Modified from Perkins FM, Kehlet H. Chronic pain as an outcome of surgery. *Anesthesiology.* 2000;93:1123–1133.

ruminate on and exaggerate the threat of pain and to adopt a helpless orientation to pain. Patients who have this personality trait report a greater intensity of pain and have a predilection for developing *chronic* pain even before they experience pain.[14] Early institution of behavioral medicine strategies in the treatment of both acute and chronic cancer pain may result in an improved quality of life for survivors. Extrapolation from the chronic pain literature reveals effectiveness of the use of so-called *cognitive-behavioral* psychological therapies to help chronic pain patients retain control of their pain and functionality.[15] Promotion of wellness behaviors and the use of physical therapy and physical medicine techniques early in cancer recovery may help to diminish the intensity and incidence of chronic pain in long-term survivors.

The distinction between acute cancer-related pain and chronic pain is rarely entirely clear. Many patients will suffer repeated bouts of acute pain, during chemotherapy cycles, for example, or perioperatively. Some of these acute episodes may linger on to become subacute, lasting for some months, or ultimately lasting longer in the case of the chronic pain syndromes. Siddall and Cousins has argued for the definition *persistent pain* for pain lasting longer than 3 months, to allow adequate time for the expected healing phase. Siddall and Cousins has further argued that this persistent pain represents a disease state unto itself with unique nervous system pathophysiology and treatment strategies.[11] Recognition of specific chronic pain syndromes in various cancer survivor groups, with aggressive, appropriate treatment may help to improve quality of life in this growing patient population.

It is imperative to develop a mechanism-based diagnosis and treatment approach to the treatment of such complex patients. Distinguishing between neuropathic and nociceptive pain, visceral and somatic pain, bone pain, spontaneous and evoked pain, incident pain, voiding pain, allodynic pain, and understanding temporal and activity-related patterns can help optimize selection and timing of appropriate remedies. Whereas the typical patient response to acute pain, including reducing activity and splinting the affected area, is adaptive and helpful, this same response to chronic pain does not allow an optimal outcome. Chronic pain patients typically gradually avoid activity, becoming progressively deconditioned, and enter a cycle of inactivity, reduced socialization, altered sleep-wake cycles, and medication misuse, all termed *maladaptive behaviors.*[16]

Lastly, the same interdisciplinary treatment paradigms that apply to all chronic pain patients apply to cancer survivors.[17] Attention not just to pain and other symptoms, but including social, emotional, and spiritual issues will result in improved quality of life and outcome measures. The therapeutic focus in chronic pain shifts to a management and adaptive coping strategy rather than a continual search for the cure of the pain. The proper balance of interventional measures, pharmacological treatments, behavioral interventions, and physical medicine approaches will produce the best outcome. Cancer survivors may be deconditioned following their treatment. Reconditioning measures, physical and occupational medicine referrals, and/or personal training regimens should always be considered as part of the treatment plan. These patients may suffer from addictive disorders as do many chronic pain patients and this should not be overlooked in cancer survivors.[18] There may be social impediments to treatment such as lack of prescription coverage or health insurance. These factors are not unique to cancer survivors, nor should they be unnoticed in treating cancer survivors for chronic pain. Providers should recognize their own strengths and weaknesses and involve other specialists such as chaplains, social workers, psychologists, occupational and physical therapists, vocational rehabilitation counselors, spiritual advisors, and family members

Table 11-3

Characteristics of "Chronic Pain Patients and Behaviors" versus "Wellness Behaviors/Chronic Pain Recovery"

Chronic Pain Patients and Behaviors

▶ Demanding, angry, passive-dependent personality traits

▶ Limited insight into self-defeating behavior patterns

▶ Facial grimacing, moaning, crying, blaming

▶ Focus on pain, catastrophizing

Wellness Behaviors/Chronic Pain Recovery

▶ Takes responsibility for own actions

▶ Sets realistic goals, exercises regularly, positive attitude

▶ Practices pain-reducing techniques and coping strategies

▶ Seeks out support, including family, religious, or community groups

Source: Adapted from Buse D, Loder E, McAlary P. Chronic pain rehabilitation. Pain management rounds. 2005;2:1–6. Accessed at www.painmanagementrounds.org on November 27, 2005.[20]

whenever needed and possible. Organized centers for multidisciplinary care of chronic pain have shown benefit versus single discipline treatment in a recent meta-analysis by Flor and others.[19,20] These centers combine medical management of pain and symptoms with physical, occupational, and vocational therapies. Additionally, group educational sessions are integrated to promote wellness behaviors and family dynamics are also addressed (see Table 11-3). This multidisciplinary approach to chronic pain management uses medications and the aforementioned techniques to permit functional restoration. This treatment strategy will serve the patient with chronic cancer pain well, keeping in mind unique aspects of post-cancer syndromes. For example, when a patient with chronic cancer pain has a significant pain exacerbation, one must consider the possibility of recurrent cancer.[21]

CHRONIC PAIN SECONDARY TO TREATMENT FOR CANCER

Most chronic pain in cancer survivors is a consequence of cancer treatment. Survival is the principle goal in cancer treatment and the prevalence of chronic pain, disfigurement, or other adverse treatment-related effects in survivors may be either underappreciated or considered a recognized and subordinate risk in the quest for survival by both providers and patients.[22] Survival accompanied by suffering and a poor quality of life, however, is not the intended goal. Many chronic pain treatment strategies can be employed to optimize the quality of life and functionality of the cancer survivor. In the following sections, specific treatment-related pain syndromes are identified with epidemiologic data, prevention strategies, and specific treatment options where they exist.

SURGERY

Chronic pain is a potential consequence of any surgery.[9] Interestingly, surgical informed consent often overlooks this issue. The magnitude of chronic postoperative pain has only recently been clarified. In a

survey of all chronic pain patients in the United Kingdom, surgery was the second most common etiology of chronic pain (with degenerative diseases being the most common cause).[23] Predictors of the development of chronic postoperative pain include preoperative pain, repeat surgery, psychological vulnerability (including personality disorders and neuroticism), nerve damage, and previous chemotherapy or radiation therapy (Table 11-2). Depression and anxiety are well-known to amplify painful symptoms and complaints.

Chronic pain after common surgical cancer treatments are reviewed.

▶ **Breast surgery**

Chronic pain after breast surgery is seen in as many as 50% of mastectomy patients. Postmastectomy pain syndrome has been well described, and Jung et al. characterized four distinct types of chronic postmastectomy pain, including phantom breast pain, intercostobrachial neuralgia, neuroma pain (including scar pain), and other nerve injury pains (including long thoracic and thoracodorsal).[24] Pain can be present in the arm, neck, shoulder, axilla, chest wall, or breast. Paresthesia, dysesthesia, allodynia, hyperalgesia, and loss of shoulder function have all been reported. Pain in the breast region in women who have had modified radical mastectomy as well as breast-conserving surgical treatment with axillary node dissection has been reported to be present in 39% of survivors by one investigator with 8% of patients reporting pain that interfered considerably with their daily life.[25] In the same study, 36% of women reported pain in the ipsilateral arm 30 months after surgery and 8% had pain that interfered considerably in their daily life. Perkins and Kehlet have reviewed the subject of chronic pain as an outcome of surgery and have concluded that 50% of women suffer pain 1 year after surgery for breast cancer, and that moderate to severe pain is reported by 10%.[9]

Choice of surgical procedure and technique influence the occurrence of chronic pain. While intuitively, providers may believe that breast-conserving treatment results in a decreased incidence of chronic pain when compared to modified radical mastectomy, this has not been shown to be true and, in fact, there is some evidence that breast-conserving surgery with axillary node dissection may result in a higher incidence of chronic pain.[26] This is likely related to increased use of chemotherapy and radiotherapy in patients undergoing more conservative resection. In addition, women who have a breast prosthesis implanted may also have a higher incidence of chronic pain.

Sensory abnormalities in the intercostobrachial nerve distribution have been reported by 61% of women in whom the nerve was preserved and 80% of women for whom the nerve sparing procedure was not utilized. Twenty-five to fifty percent of these women with sensory changes developed intercostobrachial neuralgia. Extent of axillary dissection correlates directly with increased incidence of pain, and axillary dissection increases the likelihood of arm problems in general as well as psychological distress.[27]

Tasmuth et al. have shown that an increased incidence of chronic posttreatment pain in breast cancer patients is related to the intensity of acute postoperative pain, the type of operation, involvement of regional lymph nodes, and radiotherapy.[25] The severity of acute postoperative pain is in fact the best predictor of chronic pain in breast cancer survivors. While increased postoperative pain may be related to the prevalence of underrecognized neuropathic pain and less skilled postoperative pain management, it is also related to prevalence of depression and anxiety in patients undergoing surgery, surgical technique (traction and nerve sparing procedures), and postoperative complications such as bleeding or infection. Whether or not the presence of preoperative pain is a predictor of chronic pain in patients undergoing breast surgery for cancer is an unresolved question. An additional question is whether the use of regional anesthetic nerve block techniques perioperatively could favorably impact the incidence of long-term pain.

Postoperative radiation therapy is a risk factor for pain in both the breast and arm. Keramopoulos and colleagues showed a correlation between axillary radiation and the incidence of chronic arm pain.[28]

The general prognosis for prediction of persistence of pain in the breast area within the first postoperative year is one of gradually decreasing pain. Postoperative pain in the breast area is likely to gradually diminish for up to 1 year following surgery. However, postoperative neuropathic pain in the form of phantom breast pain and/or arm pain is usually much more chronic and problematic.[3] Recently, the preemptive use of antineuropathic pain medications (gabapentin and mexiletine) has been investigated in the setting of mastectomy with promising, but preliminary results.[29,30]

In summary, the incidence of chronic pain after breast surgery may be as high as 50% with up to 10% of women complaining of moderate to severe chronic pain. Predictors of chronic pain after surgery include poorly controlled postoperative pain, extent of axillary dissection, radiation therapy, and overall psychological state.

Thoracotomy

The etiology of postthoracotomy pain is likely due to intercostal nerve injury and difficulty controlling acute pain immediately postoperatively.[12] The presence of preoperative pain or emotional distress in patients undergoing thoracotomy has not been shown to be predictive of postoperative chronic pain.

Intraoperative factors may be important in predicting the incidence of chronic pain after thoracotomy. While studies are somewhat contradictory and of mostly moderate quality, there does seem to be a decreased incidence of chronic pain in patients undergoing video-assisted thoracoscopic surgery when compared to open thoracotomy and perhaps a decreased incidence of chronic pain in patients undergoing anterolateral versus posterolateral open thoracotomy.[5] Preoperatively initiated epidural analgesia is more effective at decreasing the incidence (and severity) of chronic pain than postoperative epidural analgesia or intravenous patient-controlled intravenous analgesia.[31,32]

The natural history of postthoracotomy pain is of severe immediate discomfort with a gradual improvement over months following surgery. The prevalence of pain at 3 months after surgery is 80% and decreases to 60% at 1 year, reporting pain significant enough for analgesic use.[33] Chronic pain after thoracotomy may have an incidence as high as 50% with up to half of these patients reporting moderate to severe pain.[34] Optimal therapies for this chronic chest wall pain remain speculative and include medical management, intercostal nerve blockade, and other blocks, but recent work has included development of a rat model of postthoracotomy pain, allowing critical evaluation of numerous treatment strategies.[35]

Limb amputation

The incidence of PLP after amputation varies from 7% to 72% depending on the cut points applied for pain.[4] Phantom sensations, phantom pain, and stump pain are common phenomena seen in the postamputation period. Phantom sensation is present in nearly all amputees with a subset reporting pain.

Risk factors predisposing for chronic PLP include preamputation pain, female gender, severe postoperative pain, a poorly fitting prosthesis, and a more proximal amputation. Approximately two-thirds of patients with PLP also suffer from stump pain. There may be a higher incidence of PLP after amputation for cancer than for noncancer causes. The use of chemotherapy increases the incidence of PLP.[36] The presence of PLP decreases during the first year after surgery, but pain present after this time is likely to persist unchanged indefinitely. The complex interplay of pain and disability with regard to PLP has been carefully evaluated by Borsje and colleagues.[4] The strongest correlation for ongoing impaired function was the level of the amputation, closely followed by severe stump pain and significant phantom sensation. An interesting finding was a negative correlation between *frequency* of phantom pain and impairment, indicating that if phantom pain was experienced more frequently it did not result in more impairment because of it. The authors hypothesize that subjects who experience phantom pain frequently learn coping strategies, whereas the *infrequent* phantom pain patient experiences more impairment even with less overall pain, due to the lack of being used to it.

Head and neck cancer

Treatment for head and neck cancer usually involves surgery, radiation, and chemotherapy treatments. These therapies typically cause severe side effects such as facial deformity, speech and swallowing difficulties, and chronic pain in the oral cavity, neck, face, or shoulder. The incidence of chronic pain approaches 40% at 1 year and 15% at 5 years, with 50% of patients diagnosed with head and neck cancer taking medical disability 1 year post-diagnosis highly correlated with ongoing pain scores.[6–8,37]

The accessory nerve and the nerves of the superficial cervical plexus are commonly injured and can cause typical and identifiable neuropathic pain syndromes. Detailed follow-up examination of 153 patients 1 year following neck dissection surgery with or without radiotherapy revealed the following morbidity: the incidence of neck pain was 33%, shoulder pain 37%, myofascial pain 46%, with associated loss of sensation 65%.[7] The optimal treatment of these chronic post head and neck cancer surgery symptoms remains speculative, but some pilot research is focused on the use of early postoperative physical therapy techniques to prevent chronic shoulder pain syndromes.[38]

RADIOTHERAPY

As noted above, radiotherapy used as an adjunctive therapy in breast cancer or head and neck cancer increases the incidence of chronic pain. Radiation toxicity is generally divided into early and late effects. Early or acute effects, including nausea, skin reactions, diarrhea, and neutropenia usually are self-limited. Late effects, including connective tissue fibrosis, neural damage, and secondary malignancies can occur long after completion of radiotherapy.[39] A recent large retrospective cohort study revealed an association between previous pelvic radiation and hip fractures, with an increase in lifetime fracture rate from 17% (control) to 27% (radiation group).[40] Radiation therapy is a risk factor for pain in both the breast and arm in women treated for breast cancer presumably due to connective tissue fibrosis and neural damage.[41,42] Radiation-induced brachial plexopathy is a well-defined clinical entity known to occur after radiotherapy for the treatment of breast carcinoma.[43] There is a considerable range in estimates of incidence, which is likely due to inconsistencies of dosage, technique, and concurrent chemotherapies. However, the incidence of disabling painful brachial plexopathy is approximately between 1% and 5%, and mild plexopathy may occur in up to 9% of women undergoing radiotherapy for breast cancer.[42] There is no specific clinical presentation of radiation-induced plexopathy that can distinguish this syndrome from tumor recurrence as a cause of plexopathy with great accuracy, but tumor recurrence tends to involve the lower trunks of the plexus and radiation tends to involve C5, C6, or C7 roots. Imaging such as magnetic resonance imaging (MRI) or positron emission tomography-computed tomography (PET-CT) may help distinguish tumor recurrence from neural damage syndromes. Nerve conduction studies are normal in roughly 10% of patients with radiation-induced brachial plexopathy.[43,44]

The onset of symptoms ranges from 6 months to 20 years and most patients develop symptoms within 3 years with a median time to onset of 1.5 years. Initial presentation can be dysesthesia, pain, or weakness progressing to pain and global limb weakness often progressing to a flaccid arm.[42] In one study of 33 patients with radiation-induced brachial plexopathy, the authors reported that 17 patients required opioids for treatment of their pain and suggested early institution of opioid treatment. These authors also reported that 3 of 33 patients had a good response to chemical sympathectomy. Once onset of plexopathy occurred, progression was often inexorable and led to loss of useful hand function in a time range of 6 weeks to 5 years. Two patients who underwent amputation as a treatment for brachial plexus pain suffered from phantom limb pain afterward. A single patient (out of 33) had spontaneous remission of pain after 2 years.[42]

Generally, toxicities are felt to be more prevalent with *short-course* radiotherapy techniques, which utilize higher doses per fraction, although recent work is calling this dogma into question noting significant toxicities with standard, more fractionated techniques administered over 6 weeks.[39] Frequency and size of each treatment (fraction) has been shown not to affect the occurrence of brachial plexopathy, but *high-dose* techniques are strongly associated with an increased incidence of brachial plexopathy. Numerous confounders exist when attempting to attribute late toxicities to radiotherapy, as more techniques now combine chemotherapy, surgery, and radiation. Thus, some have advocated the terminology *treatment-related toxicity* versus assigning the etiology to a specific modality.[38,45]

Pelvic pain after radiotherapy may be due to pelvic insufficiency fracture, enteritis, visceral dysfunction, or neural damage.[46] Chronic pelvic pain has been reported as a consequence of prostate brachytherapy. Wallner and colleagues have reported three patients who developed painful urination within 1 month after brachytherapy whose pain persisted longer than 3 years.[47] Brachytherapy-related dysuria is thought to typically resolve within 6–24 months after implantation.[48] Twenty percent of patients receiving brachytherapy have been reported to complain of dysuria 1 year after treatment.[49] These patients describe pain either localized to the prostate or diffusely throughout the urinary tract or pelvis that is either only present during urination or is exacerbated during urination. Many authors have speculated that they believe postradiation pelvic pain syndromes are underreported.

Radiation myelopathy is defined as injury to the spinal cord by ionizing radiation. Generally paresthesia, especially abnormalities in thermesthesia and algesthesia, and muscle weakness, which begins in the legs, are the earliest symptoms and signs. Symptoms such as gait disturbance, hemiplegia, and transverse signs may ensue. Radiation myelopathy may present with pain or dysesthesia at or below the level of injury.[45]

Late postradiation chronic pain syndromes have an onset greatly delayed from the radiotherapy—often by many years. Thus, clinicians should be aware of this syndrome so that appropriate treatment can commence. As noted above, an electromyogram (EMG) study will reveal characteristic changes solidifying the diagnosis. Recent research has focused on limiting radiation-induced toxicities either through alteration of the treatment protocols or coadministration of various protective agents.[39]

CHEMOTHERAPY

Painful peripheral neuropathy is frequently a dose-limiting side effect of certain chemotherapeutic regimens. Mild chemotherapy-induced peripheral neuropathy is commonly seen during chemotherapeutic cycles, with these agents leading to a reduced dose or elimination of the offending agent in subsequent courses.[50] Typically, this neuropathic pain will then resolve with or without symptomatic treatment. However, in a small number of patients, the neuropathy does not resolve and may continue to be intensely painful chronically. Prevalence during treatment varies from agent to agent, with the intensity of treatment (dose intensity and cumulative dose), other concurrent therapies such as surgery and radiotherapy, and the use of combination chemotherapy. Estimates of prevalence range from 4% to 76% during chemotherapy treatment.[51,52] Preexisting nerve damage such as neuropathy caused by diabetes, alcoholism, inherited neuropathy, or paraneoplastic syndrome may increase the incidence and severity of chemotherapy-induced peripheral neuropathy.

Commonly used current neurotoxic agents include paclitaxel, docetaxel, vincristine, cisplatin, oxiliplatin, thalidomide, and bortezomib. There is an increased incidence of neurotoxicity if two or more neurotoxic agents are combined. These neuropathies are generally sensory and nonpainful. Painful chronic neuropathic pain as a direct consequence of chemotherapy appears to be less common. Treatments currently include all antineuropathic pain medications, physical medicine techniques including desensitization therapy, and in refractory cases interventional pain therapies such as spinal cord stimulation.[53] Ongoing research efforts are focused on mechanisms of neural injury to ultimately lead to protective or preventative strategies.[54,55]

Lastly, chemotherapeutic toxicity may be attributable to corticosteroids that are coadministered in many chemotherapeutic protocols; in some cases such as myeloma, the corticosteroid is an integral chemotherapeutic agent.

Osteonecrosis is a well-described complication of steroid use. Morbidity is related to progressive joint damage, often leading to decreased range of motion, pain with movement, and arthritis. Weight-bearing joints are most commonly involved and the disease often requires joint replacement to restore function and relieve pain. The shoulder, elbow, wrist, hand, and vertebral bodies can also be involved. Osteonecrosis typically develops within 3 years of steroid treatment.

Osteonecrosis or avascular necrosis may occur as a complication of either intermittent or continuous corticosteroid treatment. It most commonly involves the femoral head and presents with pain in the hip, thigh, or knee that is worse with movement, with or without localized tenderness. Humeral head disease presents similarly with pain in the shoulder, upper arm, or elbow. It may occur in any bone in the body. Focal osteonecrosis may mimic boney tumor and may result from steroid therapy as well as radiation and chemotherapy.

There is little correlation between the degree of bone involvement and the intensity of associated pain. Physician awareness of the incidence and severity of this complication is low and a uniform diagnostic approach is not used. Fifty-five percent of adult patients treated for lymphoblastic disease developed avascular necrosis that was disabling a mean of $3^{1}/_{2}$ years after treatment.[56] Nonspecific bone pain first occurred in five of nine adult males during reintensification block of chemotherapy containing high doses of dexamethasone. Mattano and colleagues found a 14% risk of developing osteonecrosis following multiple, prolonged courses of corticosteroids in children aged 10–20 who were treated for acute lymphoblastic leukemia.[57] Children less than 10 years of age had a risk of only 0.9% in the same study. These authors hypothesize that the maturing bones of adolescents may be more susceptible to the development of osteonecrosis.

MISCELLANEOUS POSTCANCER PAIN SYNDROMES

Numerous types of chronic pain conditions are seen more commonly in debilitated patient groups, including the elderly or chronically ill patients. Cancer patients are at high risk for the development of acute herpes zoster and postherpetic neuralgia (PHN).[58] Acute herpes zoster or shingles occurs most commonly in the thoracic dermatomes and in the ophthalmic division of the trigeminal nerve. The highest risk group of cancer patients is those with hematological malignancies, and the incidence of acute herpes zoster in patients with Hodgkin's disease is between 20% and 50%. Zoster occurs more commonly in patients receiving chemotherapy and radiotherapy and typically occurs within 1 year in patients receiving radiotherapy and 1 month in patients receiving chemotherapy. The frequency of occurrence in patients receiving bone marrow transplant is approximately 30%.[58] PHN is persistence of pain of some variable period of time, usually beyond 3–6 months, and occurs in as many as 15% of patients with acute herpes zoster. There is an increasing incidence of PHN after acute herpes zoster in patients with increased age and in those with increased severity of pain during the acute infection. Up to 50% of patients over the age of 50 may develop PHN. Aggressive treatment with antiviral agents, as well as of pain during the acute disease, may help to diminish the occurrence of PHN. This topic is nicely covered in Chap. 7 on neuropathic pain.

SUMMARY

Numerous distinct cancer treatment-related chronic pain syndromes exist as outlined in the chapter. The exact prevalence of these syndromes is unknown, but most certainly it is a significant health issue as cancer survival continues to improve. The recent IOM report points out the challenge inherent in long-term care of cancer patients facing multiple sequelae of their disease and treatment.[1]

Optimal treatment of the cancer survivor with chronic pain is an evolving clinical story borrowing current best practices from the chronic noncancer pain arena. Areas of ongoing research include defining the magnitude of these chronic pain syndromes, uncovering mechanisms of chronic pain, and preventative strategies. Newer, minimally invasive surgical approaches and different radiation and chemotherapeutic protocols will hopefully decrease the development of chronic painful conditions. Lastly, there is evidence that optimal treatment of acutely painful conditions may lower the incidence of chronic pain. Also, careful attention to the patients' emotional and psychological state is imperative as part of pain treatment to assist in optimal coping with the pain.

REFERENCES

1. From Cancer Patient to Cancer Survivor: Lost in Transition. Institute of Medicine of the National Academies Report, Nov 7, 2005. Accessed online at http://www.iom.edu/report.asp?id=30869 on November 10, 2005.
2. Cancer Facts and Figures 2004. American Cancer Society, Atlanta, GA, 2004, p. 10. Accessed online at http://www.cancer.org/downloads/STT/CAFF_finalPWSecured.pdf on October 25, 2005.
3. Tasmuth T, von Smitten K, Hietanen P, et al. Pain and other symptoms after different treatment modalities of breast cancer. Ann Oncol. 1995;6:453–459.
4. Borsje S, Bosmans JC, Van Der Schans CP, et al. Phantom pain: a sensitivity analysis. Disabil Rehabil. 2004;26:905–910.
5. Rogers ML, Duffy JP. Surgical aspects of chronic post-thoracotomy pain. Eur J Cardiothorac Surg. 2000;18:711–716.
6. Taylor JC, Terrell JE, Ronis DL, et al. Disability in patients with head and neck cancer. Arch Otolaryngol Head Neck Surg. 2004;130:764–769.
7. van Wilgen CP, Dijkstra PU, van der Laan BF, et al. Morbidity of the neck after head and neck cancer therapy. Head Neck. 2004;26:785–791.
8. Evensen JF, Bjordal K, Knutsen BH, et al. Side effects and quality of life after inadvertent radiation overdosage in brachytherapy of head-and-neck cancer. Int J Radiat Oncol Biol Phys. 2002;52:944–952.
9. Perkins FM, Kehlet H. Chronic pain as an outcome of surgery. Anesthesiology. 2000;93:1123–1133.
10. Strang P. Existential consequences of unrelieved cancer pain. Palliat Med. 1997;11:299–305.
11. Siddall PJ, Cousins MJ. Persistent pain as a disease entity: implications for clinical management. Anesth Analg. 2004;99:510–520.
12. Katz J, Jackson M, Kavanagh BP, et al. Acute pain after thoracic surgery predicts long-term post-thoracotomy pain. Clin J Pain. 1996;12:50–55.
13. Bishop SR, Warr D. Coping, catastrophizing and chronic pain in breast cancer. J Behav Med. 2003;26:265–281.
14. Novy D, Berry MP, Palmer JL, et al. Somatic symptoms in patients with chronic non-cancer related and cancer-related pain. J Pain Symptom Manage. 2005;29:603–612.
15. Linton SJ, Boersma K, Jansson M, et al. The effects of cognitive-behavioral and physical therapy preventive interventions on pain-related sick leave: a randomized controlled trial. Clin J Pain. 2005;21:109–119.
16. McCraken LM, Eccleston C. Coping or acceptance: what to do about chronic pain. Pain. 2003;105:197–204.
17. Robbins H, Gatchel RJ, Noe C, et al. A prospective one-year outcome study of interdisciplinary chronic pain management: compromising its efficacy by managed care policies. Anesth Analg. 2003;97:156–162.
18. Passik SD, Kirsh KL. Managing pain in patients with aberrant drug-taking behaviors. J Support Oncol. 2005;3:83–86.
19. Flor H, Fydich T, Turk DC. Efficacy of multidisciplinary pain treatment centers: a meta-analytic review. Pain. 1992;49:221–230.
20. Buse D, Loder E, McAlary P. Chronic pain rehabilitation. Pain management rounds. 2005;2:1–6. Accessed at www.painmanagementrounds.org on November 27, 2005.
21. Gonzales GR, Elliott KJ, Portenoy RK, Foley KM. The impact of a comprehensive evaluation in the management of cancer pain. Pain. 1991;47(2):141–144.
22. List MA, Rutherford JL, Stracks J, et al. Prioritizing treatment outcomes: head and neck cancer patients versus nonpatients. Head Neck. 2004;26:163–170.
23. Crombie IK, Davies HT, Macrae WA. Cut and thrust: antecedent surgery and trauma among patients attending a chronic pain clinic. Pain. 1998;76:167–171.
24. Jung BF, Ahrendt GM, Oaklander AL, et al. Neuropathic pain following breast cancer surgery: proposed classification and research update. Pain. 2003;104:1–13.
25. Tasmuth T, Kataja M, Blomqvist C, et al. Treatment-related factors predisposing to chronic pain in patients with breast cancer—a multivariate approach. Acta Oncol. 1997;36:625–630.

26. Wallace MS, Wallace AM, Lee J. Pain after breast surgery: a survey of 282 women. *Pain.* 1996;66:195–205.

27. Maunsell E, Brisson J, Deschenes L. Arm problems and psychological distress after surgery for breast cancer. *Can J Surg.* 1993;36:315–320.

28. Keramopoulos A, Tsionou C, Minaretzis D. Arm morbidity following treatment of breast cancer with total axillary dissection: a multivariated approach. *Oncology.* 1993;50:445–449.

29. Dirks J, Fredensborg BB, Christensen D, et al. A randomized study of the effects of single-dose gabapentin versus placebo on postoperative pain and morphine consumption after mastectomy. *Anesthesiology.* 2002;97:560–564.

30. Fassoulaki A, Patris K, Sarantopoulos C, et al. The analgesic effect of gabapentin and mexiletine after breast surgery for cancer. *Anesth Analg.* 2002;95:985–991.

31. Obata H, Saito S, Fujita N, et al. Epidural block with mepivacaine before surgery reduces long-term post-thoracotomy pain. *Can J Anaesth.* 1999;46:1127–1132.

32. Senturk M, Ozcan PE, Talu GK, et al. The effects of three different analgesia techniques on long-term postthoracotomy pain. *Anesth Analg.* 2002;94:11–15.

33. Perttunen K, Tasmuth T, Kalso E. Chronic pain after thoracic surgery: a follow up study. *Acta Anaesthesiol Scand.* 1999;43:463–467.

34. Kalso E, Perttunen K, Kaasinen S. Pain after thoracic surgery. *Acta Anaesthesiol Scand.* 1992;36:96–100.

35. Buvanendran A, Kroin JS, Kerns JM, et al. Characterization of a new animal model for evaluation of persistant postthoracotomy pain. *Anesth Analg.* 2004;99:1453–1460.

36. Smith J, Thompson JM. Phantom limb pain and chemotherapy in pediatric amputees. *Mayo Clin Proc.* 1995;70:357–364.

37. Gellrich NC, Schramm A, Bockmann R, et al. Follow-up in patients with oral cancer. *J Oral Maxillofac Surg.* 2002;60:380–386.

38. McNeely ML, Paliament M, Courneya KS, et al. A pilot study of a randomized controlled trial to evaluate the effects of progressive resistance exercise training on shoulder dysfunction caused by spinal accessory neurapraxia/neurectomy in head and neck cancer survivors. *Head Neck.* 2004;26:518–530.

39. Small W, Jr, Kachnic L. Postradiotherapy pelvic fractures: cause for concern or opportunity for future research? *JAMA.* 2005;294:2635–2637.

40. Baxter NN, Habermann EB, Tepper JE, et al. Risk of pelvic fractures in older women following pelvic irradiation. *JAMA.* 2005;294:2587–2593.

41. Olsen NK, Pfeiffer P, Johannsen L, et al. Radiation induced brachial plexopathy: neurological follow-up in 161 recurrence-free breast cancer patients. *Int J Radiat Oncol Biol Phys.* 1993;26:43–49.

42. Fathers E, Thrush D, Huson SM, et al. Radiation-induced brachial plexopathy in women treated for carcinoma of the breast. *Clin Rehabil.* 2002;16:160–165.

43. Harper CM, Jr, Thomas JE, Cascino TL, et al. Distinction between neoplastic and radiation-induced brachial plexopathy, with emphasis on the role of EMG. *Neurology.* 1989;39:502–506.

44. Kori SH, Foley KM, Posner JB. Brachial plexus lesions in patients with cancer: 100 cases. *Neurology.* 1981;31:45–50.

45. Whelan TJ, Levine M, Julian J, et al. The effects of radiation therapy on quality of life of women with breast carcinoma: results of a randomized trial. *Cancer.* 2000;88;2260–2266.

46. Ogino I, Okamoto N, Ono Y, et al. Pelvic insufficiency fractures in postmenopausal woman with advanced cervical cancer treated by radiotherapy. *Radiother Oncol.* 2003;68:61–67.

47. Wallner K, Elliott K, Merrick G, et al. Chronic pelvic pain following prostate brachytherapy: a case report. *Brachytherapy.* 2004;3:153–158.

48. Merrick GS, Butler WM, Wallner KE, et al. Dysuria after permanent prostate brachytherapy. *Int J Radiat Oncol Biol Phys.* 2003;55:979–985.

49. Kleinberg L, Wallner K, Roy J, et al. Treatment-related symptoms during the first year following 125I prostate implantation. *Int J Radiation Oncol Biol Phys.* 1994;28:985–990.

50. Dougherty PM, Cata JP, Cordella JV, et al. Taxol-induced sensory disturbance is characterized by preferential impairment of myelinated fiber function in cancer patients. *Pain.* 2004;109:132–142.

51. Chaudhry V, Rowinsky EK, Sartorius SE, et al. Peripheral neuropathy from taxol and cisplatin combination chemotherapy: clinical and electrophysiological studies. *Ann Neurol.* 1994;35:304–344.

52. Andre T, Boni C, Mounedji-Boudiaf L, et al. Oxiliplatin, fluorouracil, and leucovorin as adjuvant treatment for colon cancer. *New Engl J Med.* 2004;350:2343–2351.

53. Cata JP, Cordella JV, Burton AW, et al. Spinal cord stimulation relieves chemotherapy-induced pain: a clinical case report. *J Pain Symptom Manage.* 2004;27:72–78.

54. Weng HR, Cordella JV, Dougherty PM. Changes in sensory processing in the spinal dorsal horn accompany vincristine-induced hyperalgesia and allodynia. *Pain.* 2003;103:131–138.

55. Cata JP, Weng HR, Dougherty PM. Cyclooxygenase inhibitors and thalidomide ameliorate vincristine-induced hyperalgesia in rats. *Cancer Chemother Pharmacol.* 2004;54:391–397.

56. Chan-Lam D, Prentice AG, Copplestone JA, et al. Avascular necrosis of bone following intensified steroid therapy for acute lymphoblastic leukemia and high-grade malignant lymphoma. *Br J Haematol.* 1994;86:227–230.

57. Mattano LA, Jr, Sather HN, Trigg ME, et al. Osteonecrosis as a complication of treating acute lymphoblastic leukemia in children: a report from the Children's Cancer Group. *J Clin Oncol.* 2000;18:3262–3272.

58. Modi S. Pereira J. Mackey JR. The cancer patient with chronic pain due to herpes zoster. *Curr Rev Pain.* 2000;4:429–436.

Cultural and Family Issues

CHAPTER

12

Donald R. Nicholas
Stefanía Ægisdóttir
Theresa Kruczek

"It is more important to know what sort of a patient has a disease, than what sort of disease a patient has."

Sir William Osler, 1911[1]

The assessment, treatment, and ongoing management of cancer pain are influenced by the cultural context in which they occur,[2] while the family serves as the primary organizing structure for cultural experience.[3] Understanding the multicultural and familial context in which cancer pain management is provided can result in improved health outcomes.[4] However, in an era when professional guidelines, clinical standards, and meta-analyses are typically the most reputable sources for developing evidence-based approaches to health care, current research efforts on cultural and family issues in cancer pain management are not directed at specific clinical questions.[5] Very little research has been focused on issues surrounding culture, family, and cancer pain. However, some classic theoretical models have been formulated to explain the roles of culture and family in health care[6–9] that guide our clinical recommendations. Therefore, we have reviewed the available literature, looking for clinically relevant information, and have organized it in a logical and accessible format.

This chapter has two major parts. Part one provides introductory information on culture, family theory, barriers to pain management, and patient and family caregiver research. Each section is preceded by a bulleted summary of the major point(s) extracted from the literature. Part two provides recommendations for the provision of culturally competent, family-based, cancer pain management.

INTRODUCTION

Culturally competent health care requires an understanding of basic definitions, concepts, and a number of foundational principles.

Table 12-1 presents definitions and concepts relevant to culture. In addition, the following are offered as foundational principles of cultural competence.

Principle 1. Culture has a wide-ranging influence on daily events. Social interactions, communication patterns, attitudes, beliefs, and behaviors are all influenced by culture. Awareness of one's own culture and cultural biases is important, but not easy.[3] As the analogy states, "it's a little like teaching fish about water."

Principle 2. Many cancer care professionals provide services within a diverse, multicultural environment at present, and nearly all others will be doing so in the near future. As the population of North America becomes increasingly diverse,[11] the accepted paradigm of health care is undergoing change and resources are being directed at confronting and altering healthcare disparities.[12] Racial and ethnic minorities are continuing to grow and represent increasingly larger percentages of the overall U.S. population.

Principle 3. Moving beyond an ethnocentric view of the world is an initial step in providing culturally competent health care and eliminating any ethnocentric bias in patient care. Ethnocentrism, or belief in the superiority of one's own racial/ethnic group, results in bias. Bias is present when perception and judgment of differences are viewed as "good," "bad," or "different."[3]

Principle 4. Stereotyping can influence clinical decision-making and contribute to racial/ethnic healthcare disparities. Stereotyping, defined as the process by which people use social categories (e.g., race, sex) to acquire, process, and recall information about others[12] is a universal phenomenon. It results from the need to understand, predict, and make sense of a very complex social world. In a recent report of the Institute of Medicine (IOM), it was hypothesized that "people tend to categorize others into social groups because of the complexity of the social environment and our limited cognitive resources to organize and manage this complexity."[12]

Principle 5. Understanding *the unique within the similar* is essential in avoiding the bias inherent in stereotyping. Cultures differ from other cultures and, yet, unique individual differences within a cultural group remain.[13] Individual, universal (etic), and group (emic) experience from personal identity. As members of the same species, individuals share many similarities that are *universal* to all human beings. Similar anatomic structures and physiologic processes and universal life experiences such as birth, death, love, and grief are examples. At the *group* level, persons are born into a cultural context with certain beliefs, values, mores, and social practices. As a result of factors such as race, gender, ethnicity, socioeconomic status (SES), geography, and religion, persons come to belong to various cultural groups. At the *individual* level persons have certain unique, nonshared life experiences that also influence personal identity.[13] Recognizing the *unique within the similar* involves an appreciation of the diversity inherent in combinations of universal, group, and individual life experiences.

Principle 6. "It is crucial to recognize that patient-doctor interactions are transactions between explanatory models. These transactions often involve major discrepancies in cognitive content as well as therapeutic values, expectations, and goals".[14] Discrepancies between explanatory models are related to differences in the concepts of disease and illness. *Disease*, often defined as the pathophysiologic abnormalities in specific bodily or organ systems, is a construct used by conventional biomedicine and is focused on a single, pathogenic etiology (usually seeking a reductionistic, single cause), course, and treatments. *Illness* refers to the human experience

Table 12-1

Terms and Concepts Relevant to Culture

Culture

The belief systems and value orientations, shared by a group of people, that influence customs, norms, practices, and social institutions (e.g., family).[10]

Race

No consensual definition. Historically viewed predominantly as a biologically based concept, but more recently viewed as socially constructed, rather than biologically determined. Thus, race can be defined as a category to which persons (self- or other defined) assign individuals on the basis of shared ancestry and more or less distinctive physical characteristics.[10] A recent U.S. census included five categories: (1) White, (2) Black or African American, (3) American Indian & Alaska Native, (4) Asian, Native Hawaiian, & other Pacific Islander, and (5) other race.[11]

Ethnicity

No consensual definition. Variously defined as a group of people who share social and cultural characteristics (beliefs, values, behaviors, rituals, history) and an accompanying sense of belonging, or "the acceptance of the group mores and practices of one's culture of origin".[10]

Multiculturalism/Diversity

These terms have often been used interchangeably. They include various aspects of one's identity such as race, ethnicity, gender, socioeconomic status, sexual orientation, disability, education, religious/spiritual orientation, and so forth. The resulting multiple identities that emerge from the interaction of these variables emphasize the importance of awareness of both the heterogeneity within racial/ethnic groups as well as the homogeneity across groups.[10]

Ethnocentrism

The belief in the superiority of one's own ethnic group.

Emic

Culturally specific. This term has been used to describe the importance of emphasizing cultural differences and the necessity for developing interventions that are specifically tailored to the cultural context of a particular racial/ethnic group.

Etic

Universal, or widely generalizable. Etic approaches or interventions are those that are universal and applicable to multiple groups of people. Thus, treatments may or may not always be etic.

Minority

No consensual definition. Minority groups refer to the five categories for "racial" groups as defined in the recent U.S. census and the two categories for "ethnic" groups (Hispanic/Latino or Not Hispanic/Latino).[11] "Minority" status is acknowledged to be relative and is continually changing (e.g., in some communities White, European Americans are minorities).

Discrimination

Differences in care that result from biases, prejudices, stereotyping, and uncertainty in clinical communication and decision-making.[12]

Health Care Disparities

Racial or ethnic differences in the quality of health care that are not due to access-related factors or clinical need, preferences, and appropriateness of intervention.[12]

Stereotyping

The process by which people use social categories (e.g., race, sex) in acquiring, processing, and recalling information about others.[12] Stereotyping tends to result in bias.

---

of the disease. Illness experiences include a patient's ideas, expectations, and emotional reactions to symptoms and related worries or concerns about daily functioning. A single disease can thus result in many illness experiences and both disease and illness are influenced by culture. It is not surprising then, that when patient and provider are from different cultural groups, the likelihood of each of them approaching health care from different explanatory models is heightened.[14]

Principle 7. Culturally competent cancer pain management will benefit by considering both the universal (etic) and the culturally specific (emic) aspects of care. Pain perception of experimentally induced pain seems to be universally experienced (an etic consideration). However, other research has determined some significant differences in drug metabolism, side effects, dosing requirements, and therapeutic response[15] across different racial/ethnic groups (an emic consideration). Educational interventions tailored to the needs and world view of specific ethnic and racial groups are more effective than those designed for the general population,[16] and there have been many calls for more investigations of emic approaches to pain management.[17–20]

FAMILIES AND THE CANCER EXPERIENCE

Families are the primary organizing structure of cultural experience[3] and family systems theory is the predominant theoretical model for understanding how families function.

Table 12-2 presents definitions and key family system principles. Family systems theory views the family as a coherent whole formed by individual family members and consisting of subsystems such as the marital dyad, sibling relationships, parent-child relationships, and cross-generational relationships. These relational subsystems, along with family rules, roles, and boundaries can be understood as *structural components* (like anatomy) of the family system. Decisions about family roles are strongly influenced by culture and members have different roles. In health care, family members may assume various roles, such as patient advocate, care provider, trusted companion, and/or surrogate decision-maker.[21] For example, the female spouse of a male patient or the adult daughter of an elderly patient are most likely to assume the role of primary caregiver for cancer pain patients.[22] As more outpatient cancer care occurs in the home, understanding family roles becomes important in planning patient care. Family rules are also influenced by culture. For example, being taught not to complain of pain is a family rule in some Hispanic/Latino families.[19]

These structural components exist along with related *functional components* (like physiology), which represent the forces of change within the family system. Two primary and opposing system forces influence the family system. One emphasizes growth, development, and change and the other emphasizes stability, order, and constancy. The first involves developmental change across the normal family life cycle.[23] Typical developmental challenges and transitions across various life stages occur as families move from (1) new couple, to (2) family with young children, (3) family with adolescents, (4) family "launching" children, and (5) family in later life. These are expected changes. Unexpected or nonnormative changes are also encountered (e.g., diagnosis of cancer) requiring change and adaptation. The second force involves the family system's desire to maintain stability and order. Forces of change are resisted as the system seeks homeostasis, balance, order, and stability. These two forces (i.e., growth, development, and change vs. stability, order, and constancy) are in constant interaction with one another and require balance for the family to function effectively. Functional and dysfunctional family

---

Table 12-2

Family Systems Definitions and Key Principles

System—A whole, comprised of a set of parts or subsystems whose unique properties emerge out of the interactions among the parts.

Family System—General systems theory as applied to family functioning. The family system is a coherent whole, maintained by the mutual interaction among family members. The family system is best understood by studying the whole rather than its individual members.

Family Subsystems—Subsets of the larger family system. Specifically, relational patterns among various combinations of family members such as the couple (as partners & coparents), parent-child, sibling, and cross-generational. Culture has a significant influence on the patterns of relationships in family subsystems.

Family Rules—The governing principles that underlie the beliefs, attitudes, and behaviors of family members. Often unspoken and assumed. Strongly influenced by culture.

Family Roles—The expected behaviors of an individual within the family system. Strongly influenced by culture and socially defined gender and generational roles.

Family Boundaries—The barriers between subsystems within the family used to protect the integrity, autonomy, and safety of different subsystems. Barriers include expression of emotions, thoughts, and decision-making processes.

System Forces—Two competing sources of influence on the family system.

Change and Development—Sources of influence that (a) move the family system through normal, family life cycle development (e.g., childbirth, adolescence, "empty nest") and/or (b) require the family system to adapt and change (e.g., cancer).

Stability and Order—Sources of influence that serve to maintain homeostasis, to maintain the familiar, seek constancy, consistency, and predictability.

Patterns of Family Functioning—The influence of these two system forces results in patterns of family functioning.

"Healthy" or "Resilient"—The two system forces are well balanced and the adaptive mechanisms of the system function well.

"Rigid"—Stability and order are overemphasized, relative to those of change and growth. Adjustive or regulatory mechanisms function to resist change; the family system becomes "stuck."

"Chaotic"—Change and development are overemphasized relative to those of stability and order. Adjustive or regulatory mechanisms fail to maintain sufficient stability and order; the family system becomes "out of control."

Adaptive Mechanisms—Family processes that occur in response to change, that enhance the likelihood of continued, effective family functioning.

Role Flexibility—Family members' ability to adapt by adopting new family roles that meet the demands of current life situations.

Rule Flexibility—Family members' willingness to become aware of, examine, and challenge family rules that may no longer be functional, given the tasks of adaptation (e.g., pain management).

Maintenance of Boundaries—Family members' efforts to maintain functional boundaries between family subsystems, to protect the integrity, autonomy, and safety of subsystems and individual members.

Clear, Open, and Honest Communication—An individual family member's verbal and nonverbal communicated message, and the resulting other family member's perception of that message, are the information processing components that collectively make up family communication. Communication is the primary mechanism for implementing the other adaptive mechanisms.

Source: Adapted from Veach TA, Nicholas DR, Barton MA.[23]

systems are determined by the degree of balance between these two forces. When the forces of stability and order are overemphasized, relative to those of change and growth, the family is often viewed as "rigid" or "fragile." Change is resisted. Stability, order, and predictability are fiercely maintained, and family adaptation, is poor. The family may appear "stuck." Conversely, when the forces of change and growth are overemphasized relative to those of stability and order, the family is viewed as "chaotic" or "disorganized". The family system lacks the ability to provide order, stability, and constancy in the face of change. There is little predictability in family routine, relationships suffer, and the overall family system appears "out of control." When these two competing forces are well balanced, however, the family system is viewed as "healthy" or "resilient."

"Healthy" or resilient family functioning involves the use of three primary adaptive mechanisms: role flexibility, rule flexibility, and maintenance of boundaries, all of which are achieved by open, clear, and honest communication.

When a family is faced with cancer, and related tasks such as pain management, the processes by which the family responds to the necessary changes are defined as their adaptive mechanisms. Families will have many and varied adaptive mechanisms that will be influenced by culture and context. While variability in family adaptation to the challenges of cancer is expected, some general statement can be made about "healthy" family adaptation. Three mechanisms help adaptation. They include (1) increased role flexibility, (2) enhanced awareness and alteration of maladaptive family rules, and (3) maintenance of functional boundaries. A fourth principle, clear, open, and honest communication is the process by which these adaptive mechanisms are achieved. An individual family member's verbal and nonverbal message and other family member's perception of that message are the information processing components that collectively make up family communication. Resilient families show clear, organized communication patterns that result in accurate or clear perceptions, empathy and support for each other, adaptive problem-solving, and flexible implementation of family rules and roles, while maintaining healthy family boundaries. Rigid families, with maladaptive mechanisms, show unclear or distorted communication patterns that result in misperception, misunderstanding, faulty assumptions, poor support, and maladaptive problem solving. In the rigid family system, resistance to change might lead to avoidance, denial, and disengagement from the healthcare system. In the chaotic, disorganized family system, family members may avoid attempts at communication or breach generational boundaries. This lack of communication may result in misperception, misunderstanding, faulty assumptions, poor support, and maladaptive problem solving. Chaos may prevail, as usual family rules, roles, and boundaries seem to "disintegrate" in the face of the additional stressors and tasks of cancer. Knowledge and sensitivity to the many burdens of the family caregiver are essential. In addition, physicians can promote "healthy" family functioning by conducting family meetings that model clear, open, and honest communication.[24]

BARRIERS TO EFFECTIVE PAIN CONTROL

Racial and ethnic disparities in cancer pain management are the result of a variety of barriers to effective care. Many of these barriers are related to issues of culture and family.

Historically, cancer-related pain has been inadequately recognized and treated both in majority and minority populations.[17] Despite the ability of available treatments to provide satisfactory relief for nearly 90% of all cancer-related pain syndromes, as many as 45% of early stage cancer patients, and 75% of advanced stage patients continue to experience some pain.[25] In the Eastern Cooperative Oncology Group (ECOG) minority outpatient pain study[17] of 1997, 77% of racial/ethnic minority outpatients reported disease-related pain or took analgesics. Forty-one percent rated their pain as severe and 65% did not receive the amount of analgesics recommended by the World Health Organization (WHO), compared to 50% of nonminority patients. In a similar study[26] from 2000, some improvements in analgesic prescribing practices were noted, yet about 28% of the Hispanic and 31% of the African American cancer patients received analgesics of insufficient strength to match their self-reported pain levels and 65% continued to report episodes of severe pain. In a large study[27] of more than 13,000 elderly (over 65 years old) nursing home residents, diagnosed with cancer, more than one in four who reported experiencing daily pain (26%) received no analgesic medication at all. Of these elderly patients, African Americans compared to Whites, were 63% more likely to receive no analgesics. Inadequate care might be related to the lack of availability of opioids in predominantly non-White neighborhood pharmacies.[28] Table 12-3 presents a list of cultural and family-related barriers to cancer pain management, some of which are hypothesized barriers, as suggested in a recent IOM report.[12]

Clinical uncertainty under complex, time-pressured, decision-making situations is one hypothesized barrier leading to the undertreatment of cancer pain. Such uncertainty is likely to be greater when the encounter is between a patient and provider who are of different ethnicities or races. Stereotyping may be a part of the decision-making process.[12]

One hypothesized explanation for inadequate care is the clinical uncertainty that can occur in complex medical decision-making.[12] Physicians operate "with prior beliefs about the likelihood of their patient's conditions, *priors* that will be different according to age, gender, SES, and possibly race/ethnicity"[12] (p.167). Healthcare decisions are a combination of these priors plus information obtained during the clinical encounter. The relative weight given to these two sources of information is dependent upon the strength of the evidence, which in turn, is influenced by the perceived quality (i.e., accuracy, ability to understand) of the information obtained. Quality of information varies within the clinical encounter, particularly because of barriers such as linguistic differences between provider and patient, lack of time, reluctance to report pain, cultural attitudes such as stoicism, and other factors. The dependability of information obtained from a patient of a different cultural group may be judged by the provider to be less convincing, and thus it is given less weight. In the face of this less convincing evidence greater emphasis is placed on priors, which are preconceptions driven by age, gender, SES, and beliefs about the likelihood of the occurrence of a given illness in a given patient. For example, since the expression of pain symptoms is thought to differ among different cultural groups,[8,29] a healthcare provider whose cultural identification differs from the patient (or who is unfamiliar with the pain expressions of different cultural groups) may not perceive the expression of pain symptoms in his or her patient. Patients from a culture that differs from their provider may receive disparate treatment, unlike patients whose culture is the same as the provider. The providers' prior beliefs could influence their clinical decision-making process. A critical question to address is if such priors are factual and accurate, or if they are influenced by stereotyping, another barrier to effective pain control.[12]

Table 12-3

Cultural and Family-Related Barriers to Effective Cancer Pain Management

Healthcare System Level

  *,†Lack of adequate staff time[26]

  *,†Lack of access to a wide range of analgesics[26]

  ‡Insufficient availability of opioid analgesics in non-White neighborhood pharmacies[28]

  ¶Language barriers[12]

  ¶Fragmented healthcare systems[12]

  ¶Lack of availability and access[12]

  ¶Referral patterns and access to specialty care[12]

Healthcare Provider Level

  Inadequate pain assessment[25,26]

  ¶Clinical uncertainty[12]

  ¶Healthcare provider's prejudice or bias[12]

  ¶Stereotyping[12]

Patient and Family Level

  †Patient's reluctance to report pain[26]

    Desire to be "good" patient[25]

    Fear that pain means worsening disease[26]

  †Belief in stoicism[18]

  †Concerns about possible addiction to opioids[18]

  †Difficulties in communication with providers[18]

  †Nonadherence to regimen (e.g., "as needed" rather than "around the clock")[26]

  ¶Patient preferences[12]

    Greater satisfaction with provider of same

    race/ethnicity

    Mistrust and experiences of discrimination

    Refusal of recommended treatment

*A higher percentage of healthcare professionals treating minority patients reported these barriers than professionals treating nonminorities.
†The minorities in these studies are nearly all African American and Hispanic cancer patients.
‡Noncancer patient study (predominant minority neighborhood pharmacies).
¶Hypothesized variable in racial/ethnic disparities, no data specifically from studies of cancer patients.

In stereotyping, people use social categories such as race and gender to acquire, process, and recall information about others.[12] If clinical decision-making heuristics (priors) include stereotyped considerations of patient characteristics, stereotyping, and its inherent bias, can influence treatment recommendations. The case below illustrates this decision-making process.

A 45-year-old Hispanic/Latino male patient and a 45-year-old White male patient each suffer with back pain, which is attributable to bone metastases. At the time of presentation, neither patient had received opioid analgesics. Both underwent a pain assessment as a part of the clinical encounter. In both cases, the physician, who is a White male, has the same prior beliefs about the likelihood of both patients experiencing significant pain from bone metastases. In the clinical interview with the White male patient, the White male physician is able to understand the patient's expressions of pain. These behaviors include grimacing, mild moaning during the clinical examination, and an accurate verbal explanation in English of the characteristics of the pain (i.e., persistently throbbing, worse with movement). When given a *pain thermometer* to view and asked to rate his pain, the White male responds, "About a 6 when lying still, and then an 8 when I try to move." The White male physician is easily able to comprehend the patient's explanation. However, given his own prior beliefs about this patient's bone metastases, the physician actually anticipated a lower pain rating of about 4 or 5. Yet, he has no reason to assume the patient is not providing honest and accurate information, and draws the conclusion that the patient requires a stronger analgesic dosage than originally anticipated.

In the clinical encounter between the Hispanic/Latino male patient and the White male physician, the same examination is performed, but the physician observes fewer pain behaviors than expressed by the White patient. Culturally, Hispanic males react with stoicism, hiding verbal behaviors such as grimacing or moaning, and avoiding limping when moving. Given his limited understanding of English (and the lack of availability of an interpreter), the Hispanic patient doesn't completely understand the pain thermometer. Concomitantly, he wants to be perceived as a "good patient," so being compliant, simply points to a number roughly in the middle of the scale. Given his time constraints, the busy White male physician is uncertain about the accuracy of the patient's self-report of pain on the pain thermometer, but can't afford to take more time to explain or to ask further questions. He thus concludes that the patient has an overall pain rating of mild to moderate pain and prescribes an analgesic dosage that is of a lower strength than he prescribed for the White male patient.

PAIN CONTROL AND FAMILY CAREGIVERS

Research on roles of the patient and family caregiver(s) in cancer pain management has been limited. The studies that do exist, however, identified patient and family attitudinal, knowledge and skills deficits; tested interventions designed to improve cancer pain management in nonminority families; and investigated the influence of culture on quality of life and cancer pain management.

The knowledge and skills deficits found in cancer pain patients and family caregivers include not understanding the pharmacology of analgesics; not understanding the concepts of addiction, tolerance, and physical dependence; not knowing how to assess and evaluate pain, nor how to administer pain medications; and not knowing about nonpharmacologic methods of pain control. Attitudinal confounds are fears of addiction intermingled with various beliefs about pain expression (e.g., stoicism vs. expression of pain).[30,31] The reader is referred to two reviews that summarize patient and family caregiver intervention studies.[30,31] The interventions tested vary considerably in type, content, and duration. Some investigators took an etic approach, in which all participants received general and identical information, operating under the assumption that certain deficits are universal,[32] while others used a more individualized, tailored strategy, in which deficits were first identified and then information was tailored to the specific needs of the patient and his/her family.[33] Although a need for such studies has been noted,[18–20] no emic intervention studies were identified. Studies that were tailored to the needs of patient and family resulted in increased knowledge, more helpful attitudes, and improved skills, which resulted in improved pain management.[34]

A limited number of studies with small sample sizes looked at the influence of culture on the family experiencing cancer pain.[19,20,35] Two of these were based on qualitative interviews of Hispanic patients and families by Spanish-speaking nurses.[19,35] Those studies found that culture influences quality of life and pain management. Identified themes regarding cancer pain management emanated from various attitudes, including being taught not to complain of pain, taught to believe in God and live a God-fearing life, a belief in the use of folk healers, and that pain medication should not be taken until the pain is at its worst. Other themes include the importance of family, and the importance of receiving advice from family, neighbors, and pharmacists. It was shown that stoicism influenced the Hispanic patients' willingness to verbally express pain so that they tended to rely on a number of nonpharmacologic methods of pain control. In addition, a study of 350 cancer pain patients and families,[20] from three racial/ethnic groups (231 Whites, 60 African Americans, 59 Hispanics) found disparities among the three groups in knowledge about pain and pain experiences. Hispanics scored significantly lower on overall knowledge and beliefs about pain than Whites and African Americans. Hispanic patients also reported higher pain severity and intensity scores than Whites. While these findings provide suggestions about ethnic differences in experiencing pain, their conclusions were limited by significant differences in related demographic variables (e.g., education, time since pain onset) that may have interacted with race and ethnicity.

CULTURALLY COMPETENT, FAMILY-BASED CANCER PAIN MANAGEMENT

The remainder of this chapter focuses on the provision of culturally competent care. Cultural competence, which is a developmental process, has been defined as *a set of congruent behaviors, attitudes, and policies that come together in a system, agency, or among professionals and enables that system, agency, or those professionals to work effectively in cross-cultural situations.*[36]

Federal organizations developed guidelines for cultural competence, which are focused both on providers and healthcare organizations. The U.S. Department of Health and Human Services (USDHHS), Office of Minority Health (2001) developed national standards for culturally and linguistically appropriate services (CLAS).[37] These 14 CLAS standards focus on culturally competent care (standards 1 through 3), language access services (4 through 7), and organizational support (8 through 14).[38] Consistent with the CLAS standards, the Health Resources and Service Administration (HRSA) of USDHHS identified nine critical domains for further study.[39] These domains encompass healthcare providers' values and attitudes, healthcare providers' cultural sensitivity, culturally competent communication, policies and procedures facilitating culturally competent care within organizations, training and staff development, facility characteristics, capacity and infrastructure providing equal access to health care, culturally sensitive interventions and treatment models, family and community participation, and activities used to monitor, evaluate, and conduct research to increase cultural competence.

The culturally competent provider (CCP) is aware of, and knowledgeable about how culture influences access to, and the use and effectiveness of healthcare resources. The CCP uses this awareness and knowledge to provide culturally appropriate intervention strategies and serves as an advocate for policies and procedures that promote culturally competent healthcare organizations.

Table 12-4 provides characteristics of a culturally competent healthcare provider and organization. Part one of the table shows the development of increasing competence; first in awareness, then knowledge, and finally skills as they apply to self, others, and intervention strategies.[40] Part two describes organizational policies and procedures, as set forth in the CLAS standards and the HRSA domains of cultural competence. Healthcare providers can evaluate their own level of cultural competence with the help of self-assessment tools[42,43] and the study of cross-cultural case examples.[44,45]

The CCP recognizes that his or her personal experience, values, and cultural attitudes can influence the provision of patient care.[46]

For instance, a provider who values stoicism over an overt expression of pain may judge a patient who expresses pain loudly and overtly as exaggerating, or inappropriately seeking care. Conversely, the quiet, stoic patient may be judged as being cooperative and courageous. Consequently, an awareness of how one's personal experiences, biases, and values influence patient care is essential.

The CCP considers a range of cultural and family variables in trying to understand patient and family health beliefs and practices.

Table 12-5 provides a list of cultural and family variables to consider when trying to understand cultural group differences.

Narayan[47] devised questions that can be asked to enhance a provider's general understanding of the culture of a patient and his or her family. These are presented in Table 12-6. For instance, do the patient and family value individual identity, autonomy, and individual decision-making, with open and direct communication that emphasizes the patient's rights? Or, do they value the family or group identity, reliance on others, with a preference for a more subtle, indirect communication style that emphasizes the family over the individual in matters pertaining to decision-making and the right to know? Do the patient and family believe in a reductionistic, biomedical model of disease with its emphasis on mind/body dualism, and causes of diseases as best explained by observable, measurable, pathogens? Or, do they subscribe to a holistic philosophy of mind/body/spirit as one entity, in which diseases are caused by disharmony or imbalance in various aspects of life? Do they insist on a very active, involved, continuously informed role, or do they prefer a less active and less informed role?

Conclusion 1. The provision of culturally competent, family-based cancer pain management is a time-intensive and complex healthcare task.

Completing a comprehensive pain assessment,[48] including evaluation of pain intensity, location, onset, duration, frequency, and quality, along with past medical history, physical examination, recent laboratory and imaging studies, and an assessment of potential risk factors for undertreatment of pain, is time-intensive. Providing culturally competent care that avoids stereotyping in a milieu that favors arriving at complex clinical decisions under the constraints associated with not having enough time, requires collaboration and consultation with various healthcare professionals. In addition to the primary team of palliative care specialists, oncologists, and oncology nurses, other team members may include anesthesiologists, neurologists, psychologists, social workers, physical therapists, psychiatrists, bilingual staff, interpreters, chaplains, family therapists, and others.[22,48] As evidence of this growing need, grassroots

Table 12-4

Characteristics of a Culturally Competent Provider and Healthcare Organization

	Awareness	Knowledge	Skills
Awareness of Own Cultural Values and Biases	**Culturally competent providers:** Recognize that cultural self-awareness and sensitivity to one's own cultural heritage is essential and are aware of how their own cultural background and experiences influence attitudes, values, and judgment about behavior	**Culturally competent providers:** Have specific knowledge about their own racial and cultural heritage and how it personally and professionally affects their definition of and biases about appropriate behavior	**Culturally competent providers:** Seek out educational, consultative, and training experiences to improve their understanding and effectiveness in working with culturally different populations Recognize the limits of their competencies and (a) seek consultation, (b) seek further training or education, (c) refer to more qualified individuals or resources, or (d) engage in a combination of these
Awareness of Patients' Belief Systems and Values	Are aware of the stereotypes and "priors" that they may hold toward other racial and ethnic minority groups that may prove detrimental to the patient relationship. They are willing to contrast their own beliefs and attitudes with those of their culturally different patients in a non-judgmental fashion	Possess specific knowledge and information about the particular group with which they work. They are aware of the life experiences, cultural heritage, and historic background of their culturally different patients. Can distinguish cultural differences and expectations regarding role and responsibility in family, participation of family in decision making, appropriate family members to be involved when seeking health care, and culturally acceptable means of expressing emotion	Should familiarize themselves with relevant research and the latest findings regarding disparities in health care that affect various ethnic and racial groups. They should actively seek out educational experiences that enrich their knowledge, understanding, and cross-cultural skills for more effective health care delivery
Culturally Appropriate Intervention Strategies	Respect patients' religious and spiritual beliefs and values, including attributions and taboos, because they affect psychosocial functioning and expressions of distress and pain Respect indigenous helping practices and respect help-giving networks within diverse communities Value bilingualism and do not view another language as an impediment to health care	Have a clear and explicit knowledge and understanding of the generic characteristics of communication style and how it may differ between various cultural groups Are aware of institutional barriers that prevent minorities from using healthcare services and help-seeking patterns of different cultural groups Have knowledge of the potential bias in assessment instruments and use procedures and interpret findings in a way that recognizes the cultural and linguistic characteristics of the patients Have knowledge of family structures, hierarchies, values, and beliefs from various cultural perspectives. They are knowledgeable about the community where a particular cultural group may reside and the resources in the community Should be aware of relevant discriminatory practices at the social and the community level that may be affecting the psychosocial welfare of the population being served Are aware of legal issues that affect various communities and populations	Are able to engage in a variety of verbal and non-verbal helping responses Are not averse to seeking consultation with traditional healers or religious and spiritual leaders and practitioners in the treatment of culturally different patients when appropriate Take responsibility for interacting in the language requested by the patient and, if not feasible, seek a translator with cultural knowledge and appropriate professional background or refer to a knowledgeable and competent bilingual provider Have training and expertise in the use of traditional assessment instruments. They not only understand the technical aspects of the instruments, but are also aware of their cultural limitations

Table 12-4

Characteristics of a Culturally Competent Provider and Healthcare Organization (*Continued*)

	Language Access Services	Accessibility of Services	Organization Support for Cultural Competence
Organization Policies & Procedures	**Culturally competent organization:** Provides language assistance services, including bilingual staff and interpreter services, at no cost to patients with limited English proficiency at all points of contact, in a timely manner during all hours of operation Provides to patients in their preferred language both verbal offers and written notices informing them of the right to receive language assistance services Assures the competence of language assistance to limited English-proficient patients by interpreters and bilingual staff. Family and friends should not be used to provide interpretation (except on request by patient) Makes available easily understood patient-related materials and posts signage in the language of the commonly encountered group and/or groups represented in the service area	**Culturally competent organization:** Can address the needs of different cultures by developing service models that are adapted to the cultural-specific needs of the population residing in the service area Develops participatory, collaborative partnership with communities and utilizes a variety of formal and informal mechanisms to facilitate community and patient/consumer involvement in designing and implementing CLAS-related activities Ensures that conflict and grievance resolution processes are culturally and linguistically sensitive and capable of identifying, preventing, and resolving cross-cultural conflicts of complaints by patients/consumers Regularly makes available to the public information about the progress and successful innovations in implementing the CLAS standards and provides public notice in the communities about the availability of this information	**Culturally competent organization:** Recruits, retains, and promotes a diverse staff and leadership that are representative of the demographic characteristics of the service area Ensures that staff receives ongoing education and training in culturally and linguistically appropriate services Develops, implements, and promotes written strategic plan that outlines clear goals, policies, operational plans and management accountability/oversight mechanisms to provide culturally and linguistically appropriate services Engages in ongoing self-assessment of activities initiated to enhance cultural competence. This may include assessment of organization, services, consumer needs, and satisfaction, as well as promoting research designed to increase and disseminate new knowledge on cultural competence Ensures that data on patients' race, ethnicity, and spoken and written language are collected in health records, integrated into the organization's management information systems, and periodically updated Maintains current demographic, cultural, and epidemiologic profile of the community as well as a needs assessment to accurately plan for and implement services that respond to the cultural and linguistic characteristics of the service area

Source: Adapted and compiled from U.S. Department of Health and Human Services, Office of Public Health and Science, Office of Minority Health;[33] U.S. Department of Health and Human Services (DHHS), Health Resources and Service Administration (HRSA);[39] Arredondo P, Toporek R, Brown S, et al.;[40] Sue DW, Arrendondo P, McDavis RJ;[41] Thobaden M.[38]

Table 12-5

Contrasting Health Beliefs, Values, and Practices

Individualism	Collectivism
Personal identity	Group/family identity
Independence	Interdependence
Self-reliant	Relies on others
Competition	Cooperation
Time Orientation	
Future-oriented	Present-oriented
Punctuality	Flexibility
Attitudes toward Aging Elderly	
Youth/beauty	Age/wisdom
Communication Patterns	
Open, direct, forthright	Subtle, indirect
"Truth telling"	"Better not to know"
Individual rights	Group/family rights
Patient right to know	Family right to know
Patient right to privacy	Family right to decide
Etiology of Disease	
Reductionism	Holism
Body/mind dualism	Body/mind/spirit as one
Measurable pathogens	Imbalance, disharmony
Patient/Family Role	
Active	Passive

Table 12-6

Questions to Elicit and Understand Pain Explanatory Models

Diagnosis
  What do you call your pain?
  Do you have a name for it?
Onset
  When did you start having this pain?
  Why do you think it started when it did?
Cause
  What do you think caused your pain?
  What might others (e.g., family) think caused your pain?
Severity
  How severe is your pain?
  How would you rate your pain?
Impact on Functioning
  What are the main problems your pain has caused you?
Treatment
  How have you treated the pain?
  How does your family think the pain should be treated?
  How do you think the pain should be treated?
Prognosis
  How long do you think the pain will last?
  What are the most important results you hope to receive from the treatment?

Source: Adapted from Narayan;[47] Kleinman et al.[14]

initiatives are being promoted to improve cancer pain knowledge among a wide variety of healthcare professions, while also encouraging interdisciplinary care.[49]

Appropriate referral patterns are especially important for providing family-based care. Identifying patients and families who are at increased risk for inadequate treatment of cancer pain is essential. Identifying these individuals in a timely fashion and intervening in appropriate ways is optimal. Clinical practice guidelines[48] have identified minorities, cultural factors, and communication barriers as risk factors for undertreatment of pain. The CLAS standards[37] mandate accessible language assistance services by bilingual staff and/or interpreters for patients and families with limited English proficiency. Families who are facing significant, nonnormative changes and whose adaptive mechanisms are dysfunctional may benefit from referrals to mental health professionals. Furthermore, families exhibiting poor communication or other signs of "chaos" or "rigidity" may benefit from seeing a psychologist, family therapist, or other mental health professional with experience in psychosocial oncology.

Recommendation 1. Culturally competent, family-based care requires interdisciplinary care.[22,48]

Conclusion 2. Assessment and management of cancer pain is influenced by patient-provider communication barriers, originating from different explanatory models.

As previously noted, "patient-doctor interactions are transactions between explanatory models."[14] Patient and family explanatory models are typically illness-focused and emphasize (1) a common understanding of cause, severity, and prognosis, (2) fears and worries about being ill, (3) the effect of the illness on day-to-day functioning, and (4) expectations, hopes about treatment outcome. Conversely, many provider explanatory models are disease-focused with an emphasis on logical, deductive reasoning to determine diagnosis, a reductionistic, pathophysiologic understanding of cause, severity and prognosis, and expectations about treatment course, side effects, or complications. Many previously identified patient-provider communication barriers represent clashes between explanatory models (see Tables 12-3 and 12-5). These and other barriers to cancer pain management are more likely to be adequately addressed when differences in the explanatory models of patients and providers are recognized.

An individual patient may not be the best choice for articulating an explanatory model. Family members may help. Many families have an identified member who is often seen as particularly savvy in negotiating the healthcare system, and is often viewed within the family as the best choice for understanding and communicating with providers.[19] Patient-family communication problems can also exist and caution is warranted when language barriers exist. In the absence of a qualified interpreter, a bilingual family member may help, but there is a risk of family dynamics influencing the communication process. Table 12-6 provides a list of questions that can be helpful for eliciting and understanding patient explanatory models.[14,47] Once elicited, recognized differences can be clarified and discrepancies reduced.

> Recommendation 2. Recognize, elicit, and clarify discrepancies between patient and provider explanatory models. Involve families in the process.

> Conclusion 3. Assessment and management of cancer pain is influenced by patient-family differences in perception.

Family caregivers tend to overestimate patient pain severity.[21] This is particularly true when the patient seems to be relatively stoic or when both patient and family report high levels of pain-related distress.[50] Observing a loved one's expressions of pain, often communicated nonverbally, heightens both caregiver distress and their perception of pain intensity.[22]

Healthcare providers can help facilitate good patient-family caregiver communication and avoid such misunderstandings. Discussing the disparities in observations of pain between the patient and family member, concerns related to existential suffering, and explaining the additional distress family caregivers experience from observing a loved one's pain might be beneficial, while also communicating empathy for the family caregiver's experience. Understanding that their perception of their family member's pain might also be greater than the patient's perception can be somewhat reassuring.

> Recommendation 3. Facilitate good family communication. Recognize and acknowledge differences in family perception. Explain that these differences are common. When family adaptive mechanisms are inadequate, refer the family to appropriate mental health professionals.

> Conclusion 4. Assessment and management of cancer pain is influenced by culturally influenced expressions of pain behaviors: stoic/emotive, nonverbal style, and acceptability of help-seeking.[46]

Pain behaviors are overt, observable actions associated with the covert perception of pain. Verbal expression of discomfort such as moaning/groaning and nonverbal expressions such as limping, bracing, avoidance of activity, and facial grimacing are examples of pain behaviors. Affective expression of pain can range on a continuum from stoic to emotive. Davidhizar and Giger[46] reviewed the literature related to pain among culturally diverse patients. They discuss studies that investigated differences in verbal expression of pain across different racial/ethnic groups.[8] In a classic study of Black, Irish, Jewish, Italian, and Puerto Rican patients[29] it was found that Black, Italian, and Jewish patients were most similar in regards to stoicism, expressiveness of pain, and the effect on daily functioning. Others found that Italians tend to be highly expressive of pain. Garro[51] stated that Jewish and Italian patients were more expressive and more likely to ask for assistance when in pain than other White patients. It has also been noted that Hispanic families often encourage stoicism.[19] In addition to differences among groups, there are also many individual differences within cultural groups.

In some cultures, asking for help is considered rude and disrespectful. For instance, Chinese patients might be hesitant to ask for pain medicine since the request might be seen as disrespectful of the provider's expertise. The underlying thought process is that if pain medication was necessary, it would be given. Additionally, expressing and acknowledging pain may be considered an act of weakness[8,51] or loss of face. In one study[18] more than 80% of African American and Hispanic cancer patients reported that they wait until their pain severity is a 10 on a 10-point rating scale before they ask for help.

Verbal and nonverbal communication of pain varies between cultures. For some, nonverbal pain behaviors (e.g., moaning, groaning, facial grimaces) are considered a sufficient means of communication and verbalization is not needed. Hispanic, American Indian, Black, and White individuals were found to have similar descriptions of pain intensity.[52] Individuals from these cultural groups used the term "pain" to describe the most intense pain and the term "ache" for the least intense. Narayan[47] highlights the importance of a cultural assessment as a routine part of home health care.

> Recommendation 4. Include cultural assessment of pain behaviors as part of a comprehensive pain assessment. Note and record styles of affective expression (stoic vs. emotive), help-seeking, and nonverbal expression of pain behaviors.

> Conclusion 5. Accurate and culturally sensitive pain assessment is critical to good cancer pain management.

Three of the four conclusions noted above are related to poor communication. Poor communication may occur between the patient and the provider due to different explanatory models or to cultural differences in expression of pain behaviors. Poor communication about pain can also occur between patients and their family (e.g., pain intensity, distress, or knowledge/attitudes). All highlight the critical role that communication plays in culturally competent, cancer pain management. Along with training programs for residents, fellows, and practicing oncologists, valid and reliable pain assessment procedures can reduce the effects of communication barriers on cancer pain assessment and management.

Both unidimensional and multidimensional pain assessment instruments have been recommended.[46] Unidimensional self-report instruments include Numeric Rating Scales (NRS), Verbal Descriptor Scales (VDS), Visual Analog Scales (VAS), and Faces Scales. In NRS, patients are asked to rate the severity of their pain on a scale from 0 to 5 or 0 to 10, with extremes labeled as "no pain" and "worst possible pain." Such scales have been translated into Chinese, French, German, Greek, Hawaiian, Hebrew, the Philippine language, Italian, Japanese, Korean, Pakistan, Polish, Russian, Samoan, Spanish, Tagalog, Tongan, and Vietnamese.[53] The validity of the 0–10 NRS has been established.[54] Such scales can also be administered verbally, if a patient is unable to respond in writing. VDS are similar, but have word descriptors rather than numbers. In this instrument, words describing pain are presented in a vertical format (none, mild, moderate, severe, very severe). VAS use a single, 10-cm line, typically presented horizontally, with descriptors "no pain" and "pain as bad as it possibly could be" on each end. Patients are instructed to place a mark on the line that indicates the severity of their pain. Hispanic patients have been found to prefer VDS over other standardized instruments. Yet Palos[55] suggested that Hispanic persons preferred open-ended questions to the use of standardized measures. In a study of the VAS with a sample of Chinese patients, they reported a preference for a vertical line over horizontal,[56] consistent with the reading of the Chinese characters in a vertically downward orientation. Faces Scales[57,58] are Likert scales of faces showing varying degrees of pain. Respondents (e.g., children) indicate the face that best portrays their pain experience. Ratings on this instrument correlated with scores on an observational rating tool, demonstrating concurrent validity.[57] A high degree of correlation between the NRS, VDS, and VAS scales has been noted.[59]

The most widely cited multidimensional scale is the Brief Pain Inventory (BPI).[60] In its short form, it is a 9-item self-report questionnaire designed to evaluate the location, quality, and impact pain has had on a patient's life. It has been translated into Vietnamese,

Chinese, the Philippine language, and French.[53] It has been found to be a reliable measure of pain in Singapore,[61] U.S., China, Philippines, and France.[62] Furthermore, the BPI has been found to have a similar two-factor structure in several countries: pain severity and pain interference.[61]

> **Recommendation 5. Use culturally/linguistically valid and reliable assessment tools.[46]**

> **Conclusion 6. A few studies have found differences in some drug-related factors (dosing, metabolism, and side effects) across racial/ethnic groups.[15]**

Differences in drug-related factors such as metabolism, dosing requirements, side effects, and therapeutic response, have been found across racial or ethnic groups.[15] For example, Chinese patients required lower dosages of benzodiazepines, tricyclic medications, atropine, and propranolol than White patients.[46] When the reactions to morphine in White and Chinese patients were compared, White patients reported less pain but more gastrointestinal side effects. While it is important to be knowledgeable about potential between-group differences on reaction to medication, it is equally important to consider within-group differences (i.e., heterogeneity within racial/cultural groups), and recognize that ultimately all patient care is provided on an individual basis.

> **Recommendation 6. Utilize knowledge of biologic variations among diverse cultural groups.[46]**

> **Conclusion 7. A few intervention programs, with nonminority patients, have increased knowledge and changed the behavior of patients and family caregivers, resulting in improved pain management.**

Intervention programs have varied considerably in type, content, and duration.[63] They have ranged from one, brief counseling session by an oncology nurse[64] to a series of six weekly sessions among oncology nurses, patients, and their family caregiver, provided both at home and via telephone.[65,66] Patient populations have varied, but none were identified that targeted specific racial and ethnic groups and provided tailored, emic educational approaches.

A randomized controlled trial of a psychoeducational intervention for 212 mixed-type (predominantly breast, prostate, and lung) cancer patients, all experiencing metastatic bone pain, demonstrated improved patient knowledge, increased use of opioid analgesics, and decreased pain intensity.[65] This 6-week intervention consisted of (1) educational information tailored to specific patient and family knowledge and attitude deficits, (2) patient/family skill building by use of nurse coaching, and (3) ongoing, interactive nursing support.[66] At the present time, given the lack of controlled trials of cancer pain management programs tailored to the specific needs of racial/ethnic groups, interventions should include components identified as effective in nonminority populations with future studies investigating emic adaptations to specific cultural contexts. At present, the PRO-SELF: Pain Control Program is a good, etic psychoeducational program from which to model emic programs.[65,66]

> **Recommendation 7. Provide comprehensive patient and family-based educational programs targeted at specific knowledge, attitude, and skill deficits.**

> **Conclusion 8. Most etic intervention programs have included similar knowledge, and attitudinal and skill components.**

A number of similar patient and family caregiver knowledge, and attitudinal and skill deficits have been identified. Tailored

approaches that begin with an assessment of deficits appear to do better than those that only include general educational information.[34] Emic psychoeducational approaches that include components focused on knowledge, attitudes, and specific skills that change pain management behaviors are needed. Most etic approaches[22,65,66] have included knowledge components focused on the pharmacology of analgesics; concepts of addiction, tolerance, and physical dependence; and opioid side effects such as constipation and respiratory effects. Attitudinal components have focused on fears of addiction and beliefs about pain expression (e.g., stoic vs. emotive). Skill-building components have focused on the assessment and evaluation of pain (e.g., use of self-report tools), effective administration of pain medicines (e.g., "round the clock" vs. "as needed") and the use of nonpharmacologic methods of pain control (e.g., heat/cold, massage, positioning, relaxation).

A limited number of studies[19,20,35] have investigated the influence of culture on pain management and the quality of life of cancer pain patients and family caregivers. However, no randomized trials have been completed.

The utilization of currently available etic approaches with various racial/ethnic groups requires the incorporation of emic modifications into the intervention program. For instance, it appears that an emic modification for some Hispanic families should include discussions about stoicism, help seeking, and the importance of early identification of pain (ratings of 2–4, rather than 8–10) for effective pain management. Emic modifications also require accurate translation of all materials into appropriate languages and/or the use of competent bilingual staff or interpreters.

> **Recommendation 8. At present, utilize etic approaches to cancer pain management by including what is already known about patient and family caregiver knowledge, attitude, and skill deficits, while continuing to investigate emic modifications.**

In conclusion, the effective management of cancer pain is influenced by the cultural context in which it occurs,[2] while the family serves as the organizing structure for cultural experience.[3] Therefore, understanding the cultural and familial context in which cancer pain management is provided is essential for providing adequate care.

REFERENCES

1. Dubois RJ. *Mirage of Health: Utopias, Progress and Biological Change.* New Brunswick, NJ: Rutgers University Press; 1987.
2. Paice JA, O'Donnell JF. The cultural experience of cancer pain. In: Moore RJ, Spiegel D, eds. *Cancer, Culture, and Communication.* New York, NY: Kluwer Academic/Plenum Publishers; 2004:187–219.
3. Moore RJ, Butow P. Culture and oncology: Impact of context effects. In: Moore RJ, Spiegel D, eds. *Cancer, Culture, and Communication.* New York, NY: Kluwer Academic/Plenum Publishers; 2004:15–54.
4. Di Blasi Z, Harkness E, Ernst E, et al. Influence of context effects on health outcomes: a systematic review. *Lancet.* 2001;357:757–762.
5. Goudas L, Carr DB, Bloch R, et al. Management of cancer pain. Evidence Report/Technology Assessment No. 35 (prepared by the New England Medical Center Evidence-based Practice Center under Contract No 290-97-0019). AHRQ Publication No. 02-E002, Rockville, MD: Agency for Healthcare Research and Quality. October 2001.
6. Engel GL. The need for a new medical model: a challenge for biomedicine. *Science.* 1977;196:129–136.
7. Kleinman A. *The Illness Narratives: Suffering, Healing and the Human Condition.* New York: Basic Books; 1989.
8. Zborowski M. *People in Pain.* San Francisco, CA: Jossey-Bass; 1969.
9. Bates MS. Ethnicity and pain: a biocultural model. *Soc Sci Med.* 1987; 24(1):47–50.

10. American Psychological Association. Guidelines on multicultural education, training, research, practice, and organizational change for psychologists. *Amer Psychol*. 2003;58:377–402.

11. Grieca EM, Cassidy RC. *Overview of race and Hispanic origin: Census 2000 brief*. U.S. Census Bureau website, 2001. Available at http://www.census.gov and then use search terms *race and Hispanic origin*. Accessed December 10, 2005.

12. Smedley BD, Stith AY, Nelson AR, eds. *Unequal Treatment: Confronting Racial and Ethnic Disparities in Health Care*. Institute of Medicine (U.S.) Committee on Understanding and Eliminating Racial and Ethnic Disparities in Health Care. Washington, DC: National Academies Press; 2003.

13. Sue DW. Multidimensional facets of cultural competence. *Couns Psychol*. 2001;29:790–821.

14. Kleinman A, Eisenberg L, Good B. Culture, illness, and care: clinical lessons from anthropologic and cross-cultural research. *Ann Intern Med*. 1978;88:251–258.

15. Johnson JA. Influence of race or ethnicity on pharmacokinetics of drugs. *J Pharm Sci*. 1997;86:1328–1333.

16. Kalichman SC, Kelly JA, Hunter TL, et al. Culturally tailored HIV-AIDS risk-reduction messages targeted to African-American urban women: impact on risk sensitization and risk reduction. *J Consult Clin Psychol*. 1993;61:291–295.

17. Cleeland CS, Gonin R, Baez L, et al. Pain and treatment of pain in minority patients with cancer: the Eastern Cooperative Oncology Group Minority Outpatient Study. *Ann Intern Med*.1997;127:813–816.

18. Anderson KO, Richman SP, Hurley J, et al. Cancer pain management among underserved minority outpatients: perceived needs and barriers to optimal control. *Cancer*. 2002;94:2295–2304.

19. Juarez G, Ferrell B, Borneman T. Influence of culture on cancer pain management in Hispanic patients. *Cancer Pract*. 1998;6:262–269.

20. Juarez G, Ferrell B, Borneman T. Cultural considerations in education for cancer pain management. *J Cancer Educ*. 1999;14:168–173.

21. Levine C, Zuckerman C. The trouble with families: toward an ethic of accommodation. *Ann Intern Med*. 1999;130:148–152.

22. Ferrell B. Pain observed: the experience of pain from the family caregiver's perspective. *Clin Geriatr Med*. 2001;17:595–609.

23. Veach TA, Nicholas DR, Barton MA. *Cancer and the Family Life Cycle*: *A Practitioner's Guide*. New York: Brunner/Routledge; 2002.

24. Rabow MW, Hauser JM, Adams J. Supporting family caregivers at the end of life. *JAMA*. 2003;291(4):483–491.

25. Pargeon KL, Hailey BJ. Barriers to effective cancer pain management: a review of the literature. *J Pain Symptom Manage*. 1999;18:358–368.

26. Anderson KO, Mendoza TR, Valero V, et al. Minority cancer patients and their providers: pain management attitudes and practices. *Cancer*. 2000;88:1929–1938.

27. Bernabei R, Gambassi G, Lapane K, et al. Management of pain in elderly patients with cancer. SAGE Study Group. Systematic assessment of geriatric drug use via epidemiology. *JAMA*. 1998;279:1877–1882.

28. Morrison RS, Wallenstein S, Natale DK, et al. "We don't carry that"—Failure of pharmacies in predominantly nonwhite neighborhoods to stock opioid analgesics. *New Engl J Med*. 2001;342:1023–1026.

29. Lipton JA, Marbach JJ. Ethnicity and the pain experience. *Soc Sci Med*. 1984;17:1279–1298.

30. Ferrell BR, Schneider C. Experiences and management of cancer pain at home. *Cancer Nurs*. 1988;11:84–90.

31. Yeager KA, Miaskowski C, Dibble SL, Wallhagan M. Differences in pain knowledge in cancer patients with and without pain. *Cancer Pract*. 1997;5:39–45.

32. Glajchen M, Moul JW. Teleconferencing as a method of educating men about managing advanced prostate cancer and pain. *J Pain Symptom Manage*. 1996;14:73–87.

33. de Wit R, van Dam F, Zandbelt L, et al. A pain education program for chronic cancer pain patients: follow-up results from a randomized controlled trial. *Pain*. 1997;73:55–69.

34. Miaskowski C. Pain management. In: Given C, ed. *Evidence-Based Cancer Care and Prevention: Behavioral Interventions*. New York, NY: Springer Pub. Co., 2003:274–291.

35. Juarez G, Ferrell B, Borneman T. Perceptions of quality of life in Hispanic patients with cancer. *Cancer Pract*. 1998;6:318–324.

36. Cross TL, Bazron BJ, Dennis KW, Isaacs MR. *Toward a Culturally Competent System of Care*, vol. 1. NIMH, Child and Adolescent Service System Program (CASSP) Technical Assistance Center, Georgetown University Child Development Center; 1999.

37. U.S. Department of Health and Human Services, Office of Public Health and Science, Office of Minority Health. National standards for culturally and linguistically appropriate services (CLAS). Available at http://www.omhrc.gov/templates/browse.aspx?lvl=2&lvllD=15. Accessed September 24, 2006.

38. Thobaden M. Culturally competent health care: the national standards on culturally and linguistically appropriate services. *Home Health Care Manage Pract*. 2003;15:454–455.

39. U.S. Department of Health and Human Services (DHHS), Health Resources and Service Administration (HRSA). Section II: Conceptualizing Cultural Competence and Identifying Critical Domains. Available at http://www.hrsa.gov/culturalcompetense/measures/sectionii.htm. Accessed September 24, 2006.

40. Arredondo P, Toporek R, Brown SP, et al. Operationalization of the multicultural counseling competencies. *J Multicult Couns Devel*. 1996;24:42–78.

41. Sue DW, Arredondo P, McDavis RJ. Multicultural counseling competencies and standards: A call to the profession. *J Couns Dev*.1992;70: 477–486.

42. Dozier KJ, Juarez G, Nambayan AG, et al. *Multicultural Tool Kit*. Oncology Nurse Society. Available at http://www.ons.org/clinical/Treatment/Toolkit.shtml. Accessed February 13, 2005.

43. U.S. Department of Health and Human Services (DHHS), Office of Minority Health (OMH). A family physician's practical guide to culturally competent care. http://www.omhrc.gov/templates/content.aspx?ID=2805&lvl=2&lvllD=12. Accessed September 24, 2006.

44. Kagawa-Singer M, Blackhall LJ. Negotiating cross-cultural issues at the end of life. *JAMA*. 2001;286(23):2993–3001.

45. Crawley LM, Marshall PA, Lo B, Koenig BA. Strategies for culturally effective end of life care. *Ann Intern Med*. 2002;136(9):673–679.

46. Davidhizar R, Giger JN. A review of the literature on care of clients in pain who are culturally diverse. *Int Nurs Rev*. 2004;51:47–55.

47. Narayan MC. Six steps toward cultural competence: a clinician's guide. *Home Health Care Manage Prac*. 2001;14:40–48.

48. National Comprehensive Cancer Centers. *Cancer Pain Clinical Practice Guideline* (Version 1), 2004. Available at http://www.nccn.org/professionals/ physician_gls/f_guidelines.asp under Guidelines for Supportive Care. Accessed December 10, 2005.

49. American Alliance of Cancer Pain Initiatives. Available at: http://www.aacpi.wisc.edu/. Accessed May 23, 2005.

50. Redinbaugh EM, Baum A, DeMoss C, et al. Factors associated with the accuracy of family caregiver estimates of patient pain. *J Pain Symptom Manage*. 2002;23:31–38.

51. Garro LC. Culture, pain and cancer. *J Palliat Care*. 1990;6:34–44.

52. Gaston-Johansson F, Albert M, Fagan E, Zimmerman L. Similarities in pain descriptions of four different ethnic-culture groups. *J Pain Symptom Manage*. 1990;5:94–100.

53. McCaffery M, Pasero, C. *Pain: Clinical Manual*. St. Louis, MO: Mosby; 1999.

54. Jensen M, Karoly P. Self-report scales and procedures for assessing pain in adults. In: Turk DC, Melzack R, eds. *Handbook of Pain Assessment*, 2nd ed.. New York, NY: Guilford Press; 2001:15–34.

55. Palos G. Culture and pain assessment in Hispanic patients. In: Payne R, Patt RB, Hill CS, eds. *Assessment and Treatment of Cancer Pain* (Progress in Pain Research and Management). Seattle: IASP Press; 1998:35–47.

56. Aun C, Lam YM, Collett B. Evaluation of the use of visual analogue scale in Chinese patients. *Pain*. 1986;25:215–221.

57. LeBaron S, Zeltzer L. Assessment of acute pain and anxiety in children and adolescents by self-reports, observer reports, and a behavior checklist. *J Consult Clin Psychol*. 1984;52:729–738.

58. Kuttner L, Lepage T. Face scales for the assessment of pediatric pain: critical review. *Can J Behav Sci*. 1989;21:198–209.

59. Jensen MP, Karoly P, Braver S. The measurement of clinical pain intensity: a comparison of six methods. *Pain*. 1986;27:117–126.

60. Daut RL, Cleeland CS, Flanery RC. Development of the Wisconsin Brief Pain Questionnaire to assess pain in cancer and other diseases. *Pain*. 1983;17:197–210.

61. Cleeland CS, Ryan KM. Pain assessment: global use of the Brief Pain Inventory. *Ann Acad Med Singapore.* 1994;23:129–138.

62. Cleeland CS, Nakamura Y, Mendoza TR, et al. Dimensions of the impact of cancer pain in a four country sample: new information from multidimensional scaling. *Pain.* 1996;67:267–273.

63. Allard P, Maunsell E, Labbe J, Dorval M. Educational interventions to improve cancer pain control: a systematic review. *J Palliat Med.* 2001;4:191–203.

64. Rimer B, Levy MH, Keintz MK, et al. Enhancing cancer pain control regimens through patient education. *Patient Educ Couns.* 1987;10:267–277.

65. Miaskowski C, Dodd M, West C, et al. Randomized clinical trial of the effectiveness of a self-care intervention to improve cancer pain management. *J Clin Oncol.* 2004;22:1713–1720.

66. West CM, Dodd MJ, Paul SM, et al. The PRO-SELF(c): Pain Control Program—an effective approach for cancer pain management. *Oncol Nurs Forum.* 2003;30:65–73.

Spiritual Care of the Cancer Pain Patient

CHAPTER

13

Lois Ramondetta
David R. Jenkins

INTRODUCTION

Palliative care denotes an interdisciplinary team approach to the needs of the dying patient. These needs include psychosocial, spiritual, and physical needs pertaining to nearing the end of life.[1] Pain and suffering are two of the most difficult aspects to manage during this critical time. Pain is caused by body experiences resulting from physical illness, whereas suffering is the response to that pain, experienced by both by the patient and palliative care team. Spiritual needs at the end of life have been recognized by the theological and medical communities, but these needs can be widely defined and subject to diverse interpretation. Spirituality becomes an increasingly pressing issue when existential needs at the end of life are unmet and unexpressed. Spirituality, in these cases, can contribute to suffering rather than fostering serenity and peace of mind at the end of life. This chapter focuses on the varying definitions of spiritual suffering, methods of assessing spiritual suffering, and techniques that can be used to address and heal the spiritual suffering of patients and caregivers.

Suffering and spiritual pain have historically been described in various religious texts and traditions. However, as the field of psychotherapy has evolved, especially with the work of Victor Frankl,[2] a secular aspect to suffering and spiritual pain has evolved along with it. This more modern understanding of spiritual suffering includes the concept of moral suffering and "man's search for meaning" as well as formulating individual responses to the events of life and death. For the purposes of this chapter, spiritual suffering and interventions pertaining to spiritual suffering are primarily discussed in terms of a crisis of meaning or *existential suffering*. For some, existential meaning pertains to one's family; for others it is primarily about a relationship with God in terms of being deserving of life and the hereafter; or it is about professionalism and morality; and for some it is about enlightenment. Thus, at M. D. Anderson we believe the key to effective palliating or cloaking spiritual suffering is to first identify its root cause in each affected individual. This process involves identifying physical, psychological, and psychiatric patient characteristics as well as any existential, spiritual, and family influences that may contribute to the peace of mind or the lack thereof in the terminally ill patient.[3] In our institution, we approach this challenge differentially. Our first level of approach is that of the primary oncology nurse and physician. At the discretion of the primary physician or the request of the patient, recognizing spiritual pain can be dealt with primarily by this team. The problem can also be addressed with the help of one or all of four or five departments within the institution. These departments include psychiatry, palliative care, chaplaincy, the wellness center, and potentially the department of biomedical ethics. What is absolute is that recognizing the spiritual aspects of cancer care is an integral part of the intent and mission of the institution in dealing with dying patients. We know that physical healing is only part of the cancer treatment process.

WHY SHOULD WE ASK PATIENTS ABOUT SPIRITUAL SUFFERING?

Murray et al. showed that regardless of an individual patient's "religious" beliefs or their absence, spiritual concerns such as need for love, meaning, purpose, and transcendence are important to patients with inoperable lung cancer and to end-stage cardiac patients.[4] Tang et al. reported that statistically significant predictors of quality of life at the end of life included living with the caregiver, spirituality as measured by the Spiritual Well Being Scale (SWBS), and presence of social support.[5] Patients who did not live with their caregivers, those who possessed a greater degree of spirituality, and those who had more social support had a significantly better quality of life.

Emotional, existential, and spiritual factors have been associated with refractory pain syndromes, which obviously impact quality of life.[6,7] Meaning "involves the conviction that one is fulfilling a unique role and purpose in a life that is a gift; a life that comes with a responsibility to live up to one's full potential as a human being and, in so doing, being able to achieve a sense of peace, contentment, or even transcendence through connectedness with something greater than one's self."[8] Using the FACI SWBS, Brady et al., found that cancer patients who reported a high degree of meaning in their lives were able to tolerate severe physical symptoms to a greater degree than patients who reported lower scores on the meaning/peace subscale.[9] Spiritual well-being and finding meaning in life can protect against depression, hopelessness, and desire for hastened death among terminally ill cancer patients.[10–13] In fact, in several studies, religiosity seemed to have a negligible association with depression compared with the impact of the existential aspect of spirituality.

Frankl suggested that suffering offered an opportunity for personal growth. Others have described suffering brought on by cancer as a "critical juncture in the illness-wellness trajectory."[14] The potential outcomes of such a "crisis of being" are growth or, potentially, demoralization. Clearly, fostering the benefits of such personal growth opportunities is an essential aspect of palliative care that cannot be ignored.

Thus, the reasons to include assessment of spiritual-existential suffering in the dying patient are obvious. The question to be addressed, however, is whether there are interventions that can be used to improve spiritual well-being and whether or not such interventions will reverse suffering.

SPIRITUALITY DEFINED

Definitions of spirituality range from E.B. Tylor's "belief in spiritual beings" to Rudolf Otto's "idea of the holy."[15,16] Burkhardt and Nagai-Jacobson[17] describe spirituality as "the essence of our being which permeates our living in relationship, infuses our unfolding awareness of who and what we are, our purpose in being, and inner resources, and shapes our life journey." In 1971, the White House Council on Aging defined spiritual concerns as "the human need to deal with sociocultural deprivation, anxieties and fears, death and dying, personality integration, self-image, personal dignity, social alienation, and philosophy of life."[18] More recently, the National Cancer Institute recognized the need to define spirituality, suggesting that "spirituality is generally recognized as encompassing experiential aspects, whether related to engaging in these practices, or to a general sense of peace and connectedness."[19]

Spirituality is "a vital life principle, which integrated other aspects of the person and is an essential ingredient in interpersonal relationships and bonding."[20] Importantly, spirituality has relational qualities to those involved in the care of one with terminal illness. Cancer threatens relationships. The anticipation of dying evokes loneliness, sadness and fear, hopelessness, abandonment, punishment, anger (self, others, God); these concerns may relate to past, present, or future as described in *The Oxford English Dictionary*.[20]

There are many relational levels of spirituality. One is that of an individual person in relation to the world, to God, to other humans, to nature, and to himself or herself. But, in addition, there is a relational spirituality in the medical world. Medical professionals are particularly interested in writing about this subject. The unique relationship that develops between such a caregiver and a terminally ill patient lends itself to a special type of spiritual solidarity. When a caregiver addresses the issues of suffering with a patient, an entirely new spiritual relationship is created. For some patients it may be dependent on their relationship with a higher power, in which they might view God as working through the hands of the caregivers. This interpretation can render peace of mind to those who feel they have lost control of their fate. In other cases, the relationship may be grounded in the caregiver and the patient recognizing the élan vital together as they experience the terminal illness through each other's eyes. At other times, the relatedness between a dying patient and a medical caregiver becomes a transcendent form of radical empathy or solidarity. *Radical empathy* in the healing relationship, as defined here, refers to intersubjective space in which intra- and interindividual differences are melded into one field of feeling and experience."[21]

DEFINING RELIGION AND SPIRITUAL SUFFERING

Religion is often defined as an organization that provides a framework, both theological and communal, within which answers to spiritual questions through a specific set of beliefs and practices are provided. What and where then is the intersection between religion and medicine? Barnes argues, "Spirituality and religion intersect with medicine at the juncture of suffering."[22] His observations are not far from anthropologist Clifford Geertz's suggestions that what religions do, transculturally, is to "make suffering sufferable."[23] Religions define suffering in different ways. Qualitative differences in pain intensity experienced by patients may be ascribed to cultural, ethnic, and religious differences.[24]

In monotheistic religions, suffering is often associated with the concept of sin and human failing.[25] In the Old Testament, for example, one explanation is that suffering is seen as punishment for a person's sin or wrongdoing: "No harm befalls the righteous, but the wicked have their fill of misfortune (Proverbs 12:21)." In the New Testament, physical suffering is also sometimes considered to be a consequence of sin or, possibly, a venue for spiritual growth leading to salvation. "Therefore, since Christ suffered in his body, arm yourselves also with the same attitude, because he who has suffered in his body is done with sin" (1 Peter 4:1). Death, in the Islamic faith, is viewed as a natural occurrence and as part of the philosophy that present life should be lived as a preparation for the life to come. The suffering accompanying illness and death are passageways within the journey of life leading toward the eventual return to Allah.[26] In many Eastern religions, suffering results from humankind's lack of understanding, or lack of enlightenment. Hindus believe that all suffering is due to one's own past actions, in this or in a previous life.[26] Buddhists believe that life is suffering, and enlightenment occurs when one experiences pain without suffering by letting go of impediments such as attachment and desire.[26] Whatever the source of suffering and death may be—human failure or human "blindness"—religions offer to their members hope of being able to overcome suffering and death through their individual credos.[26]

In an Israeli study, religious belief was positively correlated with "psychosocial well-being and negatively related to psychological distress only for the religious and secular identity sub samples." Interestingly, this study also showed that "meaning in life but not social support nor fear of death" accounted for both correlations.[27] Others have suggested that belief in an afterlife is associated with lower levels of end-of-life despair. However, belief in an afterlife has not been associated with the presence of depression or anxiety. In one study, 72% of Catholic, 64% of Protestant, and 46% of Jewish participants believed in an afterlife.[28]

Although religious differences may account for a fair amount of differences in the interpretation of suffering, so may gender and race. Women and African Americans (AA) report higher levels of personal religiousness and more religious involvement. Dunn et al. noted that AA used more religious coping strategies to manage pain to a greater degree than the Caucasian sample.[29] Pargament suggested that due to the lack of access to resources and power, older people, AAs, and women may rely on religion (an accessible resource) in time of crisis.[30] Harrison showed that religious involvement plays a significant role in affecting pain in AA patients with sickle cell disease.[31] Reasons may include church providing social support, a supportive context for coping, and a framework for managing existential issues.

WHAT IS SPIRITUAL SUFFERING?

Dame Cicely Saunders, the mother of the hospice movement, described the intense suffering experienced by dying patients as encompassing physical, social, psychological, and spiritual pain. What is clear is that spiritual pain can be addressed even when physical cure is not possible. "The realization that life is likely to end soon may well give rise to feelings of the unfairness of what is happening, and at much of what has gone before, and above all a desolate feeling of meaninglessness. Here lies, I believe, the essence of spiritual pain."[1] Certainly, suffering can be the result of the cancer experience but also, in turn, suffering can affect the experience of having cancer itself. Cancer may evoke such values as fighting, bargaining, endurance, or punishment. Cancer evokes a human response to a terminal illness so that one asks, "What is the meaning of this disease?" "What is my meaning if I am to die?" "How should I respond to this challenge?" and for some, "What have I done to deserve this?" Or, worse yet, "I deserve this." Pain control can be linked to such feelings of anger, fear, abandonment, personal loss, negative memories, depression, and interpersonal conflicts and may consequently result in psychosocial spiritual pain amplification. Existential or spiritual suffering can contribute to increased physical pain expression.[32] As stated the source of spiritual pain is primarily related to a "disturbance in the individual's connectedness with the events and relationships considered 'normal' to their stage and circumstance in life."[33,34] However, the degree of pain is subjective and can only be "assessed by the individual in relation to their life space." For some it can be "suffering without meaning,"[2] a loss of sense of self or of previous identity, lost activity and independence or dignity, felt anger at God, a sense of betrayal that leads to a disruption in one's faith system, a fear of punishment or guilt, a need for reconciliation/forgiveness, or for others, unfulfilled hopes and achievements. Negative religious coping has been shown to be positively associated with distress and depression and negatively associated with physical and emotional well-being.[35] These positive and negative emotional states are related to spiritual well being in this context. The Griffith model is useful for pastoral care in the context of health care. In this model, the human responses to the dynamic tensions are seen as "existential crisis states."[36] They suggest: "Each existential crisis state is itself one half of a couplet of emotional postures: despair versus hope, meaningless versus purpose." They continue: "Despair, meaningless, helplessness, isolation, resentment, and sorrow each represent a retreat from a purposeful activity, a readiness to quit responding to challenges whether they be mental or physical ones. These are states of breakdown in which coping actions become chaotic and ineffective. As such, they constitute states of vulnerability to illness."[36] Hiltner, for example, uses the human experience of anxiety as an indicator or sign that one is experiencing the tension inherent in existential states, as well as underlying theological themes (i.e., judgment and grace). Anxiety, when reflected upon, becomes one way for human beings to acknowledge the inherent tension and seek ways to cope or even transcend the apparent dilemma represented by the couplet.

Moadel et al.[37] surveyed 248 cancer patients, asking them what their most important needs were. Of them 51% said they needed help overcoming fears, 41% needed help finding hope, 40% needed to find meaning in life, 43% needed help to find peace of mind, and 39% needed help in finding spiritual resources.[37] If we contextualize the concept of spiritual suffering to a need for finding meaning in life, whether that means through a relationship with a higher power, one's children and family, or the love of nature and art, then the concept of "spirituality and medicine" and the possibility of healing intervention is much more fathomable. All these factors contribute to end-of-life despair or, simply put, to emotional distress.[3] However, before addressing spiritual suffering such emotional, mental contributors must be distinguished from other psychological conditions that have established therapies. These include depression, delirium, anxiety, and familial discord, marked by demoralization-hopelessness,

attitudes of pessimism, helplessness, personal failure, loss of drive or motivation, social isolation, and persistence for more than 2 weeks in the absence of another identified psychiatric disorder.[38]

Do all people have spiritual pain, and should this be addressed on all hospital admissions? Most individuals do not want to think about death. We suspect this is true for many clinicians who experience their own emotional spiritual and existential distress through patient encounters. That withstanding, most people experience or explore existential issues only when faced with an existential crisis such as the loss of control that may lead to one's death, for example, cancer, or for Viktor Frankl, the time spent in a concentration camp. Furthermore, patients also experience differing levels of distress throughout their cancer journey. For many, cancer has become a chronic disease where death is often the known outcome and in most cases, timing of death can be estimated. However, this impending "doom" although stressfull may give patients and physicians the opportunity to explore and come to peace (hopefully) with existential issues.

MEASURING SPIRITUAL SUFFERING

Recognizing spiritual suffering can be difficult. The patient might be suffering from insomnia, social withdrawal, noncompliance, anguish, complicated inconsolable reactions to loss, hopelessness, fear, and conflict with family and hospital staff.[39] Physical pain might be chronic and out of proportion to a known physical cause. Millspaugh hypothesized that spiritual pain or suffering can be quantified by a mathematical formula wherein the components are not physically measurable[40] (see Fig. 13-1). The concept emphasizes, that the larger the numerator the larger the degree of pain, and the larger the denominator the more minimal the spiritual pain.[40] However, measuring spiritual suffering, as with defining spiritual suffering, to date depends upon a subjective interpretation.

What is extremely pertinent in Millspaugh's formula is his incorporation of the strength of relationships into the definition. As per Millspaugh, spirituality is defined by relationship; however there are five aspects of relationship: (1) to self, (2) to other, (3) to the Holy, (4) to the environment, and (5) to evil. Herein lies the difficulty, defining the weight of relationships in the definition of spirituality. The conundrum is that for each individual there may not be a focus on or even recognition of the importance of all five types of relationships. Some of these relationships will be more important than others (depending on the person) and some will even be nonexistent. More importantly, spiritual needs change over time as a result of changing relationships, awareness of death, and one's internal sense of control.[40]

What is probably most significant in the exploration and ability to measure spiritual pain is the need to develop a pertinent vocabulary. One approach has been to directly inventory various descriptive terms qualitatively. Such inventories have included words like

$$\frac{[(\text{Awareness of death} + \text{Loss of relationships} + \text{Loss of self})}{\text{Life affirming and transcending purpose} + \text{Internal sense of control}}$$

FIGURE 13-1 Measuring spiritual suffering.

What gives meaning to your life?

What gives meaning to your patient's life?

Do you ask why is this happening to me?

How will I be remembered?

How can I be forgiving?

FIGURE 13-2 Questions to help caregivers address spiritual suffering.

Spiritual Belief System

Personal Spirituality

Integration in Spiritual Community

Ritualized Practices

Implications for Medical Care

Terminal Events Planning

FIGURE 13-4 The SPIRIT questionnaire uses the mnemonic SPIRIT.[53]

hopelessness, meaning, demoralization, dignity, will to live, unfairness, guilt, vulnerability, abandonment, punishment, suicidal ideations, and euthanasia.[41,42] As the understanding of spiritual suffering remains somewhat vague and individualized, the more terms one could use to question patients or could recognize when listening to patients, the greater chance one has of identifying on the important issues. What is clear is that the meaning of suffering differs from person to person and it is important for the caregiver to avoid religious clichés and religion-specific language to avoid alienating the patient.

Some spiritual inventories are designed to assess importance of spirituality in one's life, whereas other inventories attempt to assess the degree and nature of the spiritual crisis. A thorough review can be found in *The Handbook of Religion and Health*.[43] None are universally employed. Spirituality surveys usually ask about the role spirituality plays in one's life[44] or the frequency of spiritual experiences,[45,46] or on the other end of the spectrum, they focus on the fear of death and end-of-life despair.[47,48] Few are perfect for any one patient. The University of Maryland School of Medicine[49] developed the following sets of questions to help caregivers address spiritual suffering (Fig. 13-2).

Other approaches are more general and query, "Do you have any spiritual or religious concerns at this point?" or "Are there spiritual resources or is there a religious community that could be a help to you at this time?" Dr. Puchalski[50] has developed a questionnaire (F.I.C.A.) that may work well for caregivers who are not accustomed to asking such personal questions. This questionnaire provides a novice with a starting point for such discussions (Fig. 13-3). The questionnaire, however, generally provides only a superficial evaluation. Once a patient's belief system is evaluated, one might then go on to ask, "Do you believe in karma? Do you believe in fate?" and then deal with questions of forgiveness. Speck suggested asking the question "Do you have a way of making sense of the things that happen to you?"[51,52] In another tool designed by Maugans et al[53], we find a more detailed assessment. The SPIRIT questionnaire uses the mnemonic SPIRIT [53] (Fig. 13-4).

Regardless of what method is used, the bottom line is that if a caregiver is not comfortable with questions pertaining to spirituality, perhaps because he or she has spiritual crises of his or her own, then the assessment method will be less effective because the caregiver is not able to listen impartially to a patient's responses. We would call this extrinsic spiritual care. In this schema, the patient's spirituality is viewed as his or her own and from an outsider's viewpoint. However, comfort comes with repetition, and asking a patient how he or she feels about spiritual matters can ultimately lead to a reconfiguration of one's own belief system. Without taking the conversation to a deeper level, any questionnaire might only serve as a conduit for collecting information. The true value of the information collection process depends on what happens to the patient and caregiver afterward both as individuals and as a team.

What is missing from many assessment tools is the assessment of the honesty in the relationship between the caregiver and patient. Without honesty and a willingness on the part of each participant to approach questions of mortality and meaning, the core issues translating to spiritual suffering will be missed. Such a survey may be able to be designed but as of yet has not.

At M. D. Anderson, our physician and nursing approach to this issue is as diverse as our patient population. As per Joint Commission on Accreditation of Healthcare Organizations (JHACO) requirements, there are simple questions about spiritual well-being on our patient intake form. They are "I have spiritual concerns" and "I would like to talk with a chaplain." M. D. Anderson physicians and nurses, when informally surveyed, had difficulty answering the question "Do you address spiritual pain?" because of the lack of a universal definition of spiritual pain. Some physicians reported that when they see a patient struggling with "why" questions and existential issues they may make reference to the fact that some people find strength in their faith and then move the conversation in such a direction if so directed by the patient. Others validate the patients' stated beliefs as they arise or simply assess patient coping skills. A very helpful approach by one physician was stated as: "I address it only very superficially and limit my discussion to always encouraging the importance of spirituality as it pertains to maintaining hope and strength as the patients battle their disease." Others use a validated assessment tool such as the FACT.[54] Most providers, however, have developed their own way of assessing spiritual suffering—one that they are comfortable with. A psychiatric nurse at M. D. Anderson, Phyddy Kettler, RN, CNS, LMFT, LPC Advanced Practice

F.I.C.A.

Faith: What is your faith or belief?

Importance and influence: Is it important in your life?

Community: Are you part of a spiritual or religious community?

Address: How would you like me to address these issues in your health care?

FIGURE 13-3 Questionnaire providing a starting point for discussions.[50]

What is your theory about what causes cancer?

As you contemplate your death, what feelings and thoughts come to mind?

How do you define "hope" for yourself?

How does one live, really live, one day at a time?

Is there an afterlife?

FIGURE 13-5 Existential questions.

Nurse, Psychiatry, seems to be the most structured in her approach. She asks specific existential questions and then depending on the answers designs specific interventions (Fig. 13-5).

M. D. Anderson Chaplaincy uses a specific spiritual pain vocabulary to help patients make their own spiritual self-assessment (Fig. 13-6). If one or more markings are placed by the patient to the left side of the listed continuums, it is suggested to the patient or family member that spiritual support may be beneficial. This approach may be beneficial to helping patients identify spiritual themes and concerns, which they can then discuss with a chaplain.

Working in a major cancer center such as M. D. Anderson has many advantages. In such a place, treating cancer is a shared passion and there are specialists of many kinds, chaplains, social workers, case managers, psychiatrists, child life specialists, pain as well as cancer treatment specialists. As a result, multidisciplinary care is the treatment approach from the beginning, starting with

**ASSESSMENT INFORMATION: INITIAL Pt. SCREEN [ ]
FOLLOW-UP VISIT [ ] Date:_____ Time_____**

X—Non-verified Spiritual Needs—spiritual needs perceived by chaplain; unable to verify with patient.

0—No Spiritual Care—Spiritual care offered; patient expressed no need for spiritual care.

1—Spiritual Support—Spiritual care provided; patient expressed no emergent spiritual needs.

2—Spiritual Concerns—
Mild expressions:
A: Anxiety
B: Grief
C: Pain
D: Fatigue
E: _____

3—Spiritual Distress—
Marked expressions:
A: Mod./Severe anxiety
B: Grief
C: Pain
F: Fatigue
E: Anger
H: Ethical dilemma

4—Spiritual Despair—
Marked expressions:
A: Social withdrawal
B: Loss of belief
C: _____

1. Despair   –2 –1 0 1 2 Hopeful

2. Broken   –2 –1 0 1 2 Whole

3. Dread   –2 –1 0 1 2 Courage

4. Alienated   –2 –1 0 1 2 Connected

5. Meaningless –2 –1 0 1 2 Meaningful

6. Guilt/Shame –2 –1 0 1 2 Accepted

7. Helpless   –2 –1 0 1 2

FIGURE 13-6 Spiritual inventory.

the diagnosis of cancer and continuing throughout the trajectory of the illness. More recently has been recognition of the benefits of instituting a palliative care approach early in the cancer patient's disease course.

Regardless of which methods have been validated or are used, personal experiences with cancer patients validates the following statement: "Assessment of spiritual pain will have to depend at least as much upon the spirituality of the caregiver, and upon their capacity for contemplation, for close listening to narrative, for intuition, and for discernment, as it will upon the results of any neatly developed questionnaire."[55] Although methods teaching "how to break bad news" might be helpful, this approach is biased toward healthcare providers who are receptive to the empathy and compassion required to truly deliver complete care that includes a spiritual dimension. As a patient and friend once said, "All of your doctors want you to get well, but some of them are better at it than others." This is true not only of oncologic care but also of spiritual care. A very important role of the physician is to recognize his or her limitations so as to best help the patient.

INTERVENTIONS

It has been written that "Interventions suggest doing, rather than being and imply that the care given is superior to the client." Spiritual care, however, more frequently involves a way of being (rather than doing), and this approach requires a symmetric relationship between the patient and his or her nurse, physician, caregiver, family member.[56]

The M. D. Anderson palliative care team follows The National Consensus Project for Quality Palliative Care,[57] which includes recommendations on the spiritual, religious, and existential aspects of care. To summarize, our interdisciplinary team includes professionals with skills in assessing and responding to these issues. There is ongoing exploration of spiritual and existential concerns, although not necessarily assessed by every member of the team or in exactly the same manner. Before even addressing spiritual pain, physical pain must first be addressed. A basic assessment is used to identify the patient's religion or spiritual preferences. Assessment may lead to the discovery of personal crises of integrity or identity, body-mind spirit disjunction, challenged relationships with God, or a lack of sense of belonging. When appropriate, pastoral care is offered and cultural sensitivity is always the goal. M. D. Anderson chaplains represent a wide range of faiths and spiritual beliefs, and are specifically trained to work with cancer patients and their families. Every effort is made to support the practice of religious rituals. Psychiatric help is also requested when specific treatable diagnoses are identified. Furthermore, there are many alternative approaches, including yoga and meditation, which may address the discord between mind and body and spirit. The M. D. Anderson Place of Wellness is a complementary therapy facility for all cancer patients and their caregivers, offering a wide range of programs that focus on healing the mind, body, and spirit (for more information on The Place of Wellness, see Chap. 14).

The palliative care team includes a social worker, chaplain, and nurse therapist as integral members of this team, demonstrating the importance of interdisciplinary care. Social workers at M. D. Anderson do comprehensive grief assessments to identify areas of need, A nondenominational chaplain works with patients of all faiths and cultures to support and guide their own spiritual journey, helping them review their lives and find meaning and closure.

Prayer, ritual, music, journal writing, and meditation are some of the tools offered to patients.[58] It has become increasingly clear that physical pain has many domains and that treatment with pharmacotherapy, especially in the case of spiritual pain, is unlikely to be 100% of the solution.

Characterizing a spiritual intervention depends upon who is intervening and who is receiving the intervention. For a chaplain, specifically dealing with religiously-based existential questions may be in order, whereas for psychotherapists, investigating and applying aspects of depression, demoralization, and a meaning-based therapy, such as Logotherapy, may be appropriate. For physicians and nursing staff, development of trust and pain control may be the most important factors. That said, there is no intervention that all specialties agree upon except for simply listening and validating the needs of the terminal patient. Burton, for example, suggests that resolution of spiritual pain involves any or all of the following features: support (including listening); space (a degree of privacy); freedom to speak honestly, question, and pray; expressions of reassurance and assurance that he or she is loved; and lastly, opportunities for forgiveness and reconciliation.[55] Intervention may start with the acknowledgement of spiritual pain by helping the patient express distress in words or writing rather than by describing physical symptoms. This approach can help to sort out and illuminate the cause of a patient's distress.

Nurses surveyed in 1998 listed 10 most frequently used spiritual interventions. They reported the following: referral to spiritual care experts, applying prayer, the importance of listening and validating a patient's feelings, assuming a necessary nonjudgmental attitude, the need to instill hope, clarifying values, using touch, and referral to community resources when appropriate.[59] Although many different approaches are used, not only with different patients but also by different types of caregivers, the goals are usually similar. The main goal in alleviating spiritual pain is to renew meaning, and possibly rework the patient's faith system when appropriate, with the aim of redirecting philosophic focus toward seeking fulfillment in daily life, illness notwithstanding. Renewed hope, whether that be hope for cure or hope for a peaceful death, and achieving some degree of closure through reconciliation, leaving a legacy, readjusting goals, or finding forgiveness is also important, Renewing hope involves identifying one's emotions and finding a balance between emotions of fear and hope to arrive at a state where there can be peace of mind. First and foremost, this requires a secure, trusting relationship in a peaceful environment between the patient and the caregiver. It is imperative that a caregiver recognizes a relationship that is not conducive to such honesty and refers the patient elsewhere when appropriate. There has to be a good fit between the patient and his or her human resource for attaining spiritual satisfaction. Spiritual solidarity requires companionship, which implies openness, empathic listening, compassion, and suffering within the context of caring for those who are ill and on a level playing ground where the most common bond between the patient and the caregiver is their mutual humanity.

Establishing such a relationship requires the not so simple skill of listening. Theodore Reik referred to it as "Listening with the Third Ear." The simple interest one shows to one's patient through listening and through one's attentive presence can increase a patient's sense of self worth. Such an opportunity can arise with the request for a patient to tell his or her (illness) story, then for the listener to echo and validate his or her experiences, ask questions and make observations about recurring themes. The goal is to (1) identify and express spiritual-emotional-existential distress, (2) reduce symptom

expression, (3) understand the patient's experience, (4) normalize the patient's experience, (5) attach emotions to an identifiable cause, and (6) potentially bring life to a graceful close.[38] The UNIPAC handbooks suggest the following simple questions to help a patient who might need to reframe their situation: "How would you respond if you were well and another family member were dying? If you were writing the story of your life, can you imagine an ending that might leave the reader sad, but with a sense that you had achieved a sense of fullness and completion."[60]

McClain-Jacobson[28] suggests that separating religious interventions from interventions designed to promote a sense of meaning and peace may have a much broader application. For example, UNIPAC identified the developmental tasks of dying patients.[60] UNIPAC discusses developing a renewed sense of personhood and meaning, bringing closure to personal and community relationships, bringing closure to worldly affairs, accepting the finality of life, surrendering to the transcendent, concentrating on adjusting to circumstances, finding ways of making sense, letting go of previous roles, borrowing strength from others, opening themselves to the love of others, and developing transpersonal meanings. For a caregiver to be effective he or she must first recognize his or her own convictions, ambivalence, or hostility to religious and spiritual issues. This may help enable a caregiver to show respect for others' beliefs, while supporting their personal integrity, and validating another's voice in a time of distress.

Psychotherapy may be the best approach for patients with advanced cancer who need to find meaning in their experience.[61,62] Early palliative measures, family support, effective coping strategies, and religious belief systems may influence the way patients with advanced cancer deal with existential concerns.[38] The benefits of psychotherapy in treating a crisis of meaning have been well described. Probably best known is Logotherapy, which means therapy through meaning. This system was originally described by Dr. Victor Frankl,[63] and has continued through work by Dr. Breitbart.[64] This form of existential psychotherapy/ analysis incorporates many factors, with a focus on finding meaning in the future: (1) the capacity for self-awareness and the potential to continually grow, (2) freedom and responsibility through taking ownership of one's life, (3) the need for centering, (4) the need for others, (5) the search for meaning in face of the changing challenges of life, (6) anxiety as a condition of living, (7) trying to see this search as a source for growth, and (8) lastly, awareness of death and nonbeing.[64] Existential psychotherapy encourages patients to seriously explore their past, present, and future in terms of meaningful choices and the experiences that created and to continue to generate their story.[61,62] Self-transcendence therapy, one aspect of Frankl's Logotherapy, relies upon the inherent human trait of being able to connect with that which is greater than oneself and a human desire to find meaning in life. This approach requires an understanding of oneself as one's boundaries are expanded to include the transcendent.[60] Studies using these techniques in women with breast cancer, as well as men with prostate cancer have demonstrated a correlation with a sense of well-being and mental health, although the data are weak.[61,65–67]

Group therapy that focuses on exploring an existential form of psychotherapy uses discussion, didactics, and experiential exercise. These techniques are directed toward exploring specific themes related to finding meaning in the context of having advanced cancer. The group nature of this type of therapy creates an environment that fosters communal support during this exploratory period. Furthermore, meaning-centered therapy can incorporate assessment and interventions in the form of dignity therapy as defined by Chochinov[68] and Kissane[69]. The subject of the Kissane study, the demoralization syndrome, is described as a triad of hopelessness, loss of meaning, and desire for death. Identifying ways to prevent this syndrome can significantly decrease the number of patients who might otherwise suffer spiritual pain. The five dimensions of this distinct syndrome, distinct from depression, encompass: (1) loss of meaning, (2) dysphoria, (3) disheartenment, (4) helplessness, and (5) a sense of failure.

Not many randomized studies have explored the value psychotherapy based interventions. However, a meta-analysis published in 2002 concluded that psychological intervention strategies were unable to improve cancer patient outcomes vis-à-vis state of mind.[70] A study by Chan[71] arrived at the same conclusion. Interestingly, however, this study excluded patients who were "too ill to participate," thereby possibly excluding those who most needed intervention or those who should have received intervention earlier in the cancer trajectory. These investigators provided patients with psychoeducation and supportive care, stress management, crisis counseling, relaxation, pain and distress management via cognitive behavioral therapy.[71] This study was limited by its lack of focus on meaning and by its patient cohort who were all under the age of 50 with early stage tumors, and almost all of whom reported a lack of any formal religious beliefs.

Narrative writing, also known as expressive writing, has had mixed results in clinical trials. Smyth et al. evaluated the benefits of writing about emotionally traumatic experiences and reported clinically relevant changes in the physical status of patients with asthma and rheumatoid arthritis.[72] Stanton et al. conducted a randomized trial in patients with early-stage breast cancer and compared those who wrote about their deepest thoughts and feelings regarding their experience with breast cancer versus those who wrote about nonemotional topics. Although the effects on psychological outcomes varied, the breast cancer patients who had an opportunity for emotional expression had a lesser number of medical visits for cancer-related morbidities than the other cohort of patients.[73] In 2002, another study randomized renal cell patients to emotional or neutral writing. Patients in the emotional writing arm demonstrated improved sleep and less daytime dysfunction.[74] The study was limited by the inability to measure "dose", or clarify frequency and form, for example, directed versus free-form writing, which made it difficult to determine the objective benefits of such interventions despite observed subjective improvement.

Reminiscence as therapy involves remembering the past by recounting one's life story, which helps integrate the past and present.[75] To apply reminiscence therapy, the caregiver might have the patient explain the details of a photo album as a life review while at the same time helping the patient to recognize their contributions to their lives. Others incorporate the transcription of a taped autobiography, also called a life review,[76] as a gift for those who are left behind.

Chaplaincy at M. D. Anderson has addressed many of the aspects of intervention through preoperative surgical prayer groups, centering prayer, and centering meditative instruction. There are also support groups that are specific to discrete tumor types, which are led by the chaplaincy department. Some support groups focus specifically on finding meaning in the cancer journey. The pastoral caregiver tries to access a patient's anxiety, a possible symptom of spiritual crisis, by carefully listening for existential theme(s) within the patient's story, as well as by noting the affective energy associated with the patient's anxiety. The most effective goal is to help empower the patient to recognize, acknowledge, and work with his

or her anxiety in a timely, reflective manner with the goal of achieving a healthy life style and deepened spiritual life.

Rousseau has presented a particularly excellent approach for treating spiritual pain. The caregiver initially concentrates on controlling physical symptoms and providing a supportive presence and then encourages life review to assist the patient in recognizing purpose, value, and meaning. Time is spent exploring guilt, remorse, forgiveness, reconciliation, and facilitating religious expression. Realistic goals are set and meditative practices focusing on healing rather than cure are encouraged.[7] In this approach, refractory existential suffering is distinguished from other treatable emotional/psychiatric disorders. Rousseau proposed the following clinical guidelines to identify refractory existential suffering. After a diagnosis of terminal illness or an active do-not-resuscitate (DNR) order, of all palliative treatments have been exhausted. Senior palliative caregivers should be consulted. A psychological and spiritual assessment should then be completed. If nutritional or intravenous support are an issue initiate discussions regarding quality of life versus the benefits/burdens of treatment. With informed consent one might then consider trial of sedation for 24–48 hours. The goal of this last attempt at sedation is to break the patient's cycle of anxiety and distress. If temporary sedation does not alleviate suffering, sedation can be maintained, but not increased as long as the patient experiences no discomfort and distress.[7]

EXAMPLES—CASE HISTORIES

CJ was a 38-year-old AA female with a controlled seizure disorder and stage II cervical cancer. She was initially treated with standard therapy, including chemotherapy and radiation. Her initial treatment course was difficult and required multiple admissions for nausea and vomiting due to her limited ability to understand and follow recommended supportive therapy guidelines. She was compliant to the best of her ability given her limited access to transportation and inadequate social support system. Approximately 1 year after completing therapy, CJ experienced increasing gastrointestinal distress as a result of a radiation-induced small bowel stricture, which necessitated an extensive small bowel resection and reanastomosis. During this time she lost 20 lb and suffered from pain and cramping. She often asked, "Why is this happening to me, especially when I have done all that I was told to do?" Her medical situation worsened shortly after surgery. She developed an inoperable enterocutaneous fistula associated with continued pain and need for total parenteral nutrition. Her life for the next few years was complicated by multiple hospital admissions for radiation-related cystitis and proctitis as well as nausea, vomiting, and pain associated with the fistula. Her distress was both physical and existential. She wondered out loud if she had done something to deserve the situation. Some members of CJ's care team internalized her pain and found themselves praying for "the serenity to accept the things I cannot change."

Over the next few years CJ developed very intimate and supportive relationships not only with her primary physician, but also with the nursing staff, and the patients she met in the hospital common areas. Compared to her world outside the hospital, where she found herself feeling out of place and of limited importance, she had now formed a world where her presence was known and loved and where she knew others had a viscerally felt compassion for her situation. In this way she developed a meaning to her life and through this she gathered strength to face her terrible circumstances, to stop asking why and, in the end, to find peace of mind in recognizing when quality had left her life. Through her trust in her "hospital family" she spoke her mind like she had probably never done before. Near the end of her life, during a defining family-caregiver meeting, CJ was able to tell her family and care team with a courageous, decisive voice that she wished to stop all supplemental nutrition. Although there were tears, she had a wonderful serenity that also flowed to all who loved her.

As cancer patients share their experiences with chaplains, they often reflect upon their journeys through the use of metaphors. "Janet," an out-of-town breast cancer patient in her forties, came to the hospital for treatment. Anxious and crying, she described her treatment plan as a "roller-coaster ride." For Janet, some days were filled with hope for remission, while on other days she found herself deep in despair for her health and future. When her cancer failed to respond to treatment, she felt angry with God. "I felt I was working as hard as possible to fight this disease, and God was not helping in the fight." The chaplain heard her plea and normalized her anger as justifiable. The chaplain helped enable Janet with her struggle and with maintaining hope by providing assurance of God's love and abiding presence. The chaplain also invited Janet to explore ways by which to live courageously, inviting her to share her thoughts about what kept her going in the midst of her chronic disease. By doing so, together Janet and the chaplain sought different ways that Janet could cope creatively from the position of a human being who was on a life-and-death "roller-coaster ride."

CAREGIVER SPIRITUAL SUFFERING

Caring for the dying forces a caregiver to eventually ask difficult questions of himself or herself: Who am I as a person/physician in the face of another's suffering?

Compassion equates to some degree of suffering on the part of the caregiver. Those who have experienced the intensity of relationships with the terminally ill are at high risk for burnout, also called "career adversity syndrome," "an erosion of the soul," and "a deterioration of values, dignity, spirit, and will."[77] The rate of burnout in oncologists in the United States is greater than 60%.[78] Furthermore, burnout has been associated with self-reported suboptimal patient care.[79] Burnout occurs in both young and old physicians in the range of 40% in academic practice to as many as 60% in private practice. It can lead to emotional exhaustion and decreased effectiveness, and specifically, can express itself in absenteeism, cynicism, depression, anxiety, substance abuse, divorce, and disillusionment.[79] Interestingly, some have suggested that surgeons may be particularly at risk for burnout due to the: (1) high-stakes nature of surgical interventions, (2) the intimate nature of the relationship with the patient, (3) the drastically different postsurgical emotional sequelae, for example, the rush of success and the devastation of failure, and (4) the tradition of emotional detachment from patients in surgery.[80] Scripted "end-of-life" talks do not work for caregivers who have not come to terms with their own mortality. UNIPAC[60] describes a process of surrender that the caregiver must also engage in. It includes engaging in a deeper search for meaning, the willingness to learn from the struggles of one's patients coming to terms with their fate, the need to trust deeper intuition, to let go of the need to control the outcome of difficult situations, along with fostering dependence not only on medical knowledge but also the humanities to help relieve pain of any type. Applying UNIPAC's LET GO process, the caregiver may also discover a "renewed sense of

---

UNIPAC discusses: LET GO

Listen to the patient's story

Encourage the search for meaning

Tell of your concern and acknowledge the pain of loss

Generate hope whenever possible

Own your limitations and refer when appropriate

FIGURE 13-7 Figure 13-7 UNIPAC's LET GO.

purpose, value, self-worth, meaning, and hope that may lead to spiritual healing" (Fig. 13-7).

Our sense of personal integrity may be threatened as we find ourselves confused between the role of torturer and healer as we watch the pain of another, but are unable to help. Caring for the suffering patient may eventually erode the caregiver's sense of wholeness and self-esteem, so that the caregiver experiences spiritual and moral suffering. Caregivers may ultimately wonder why they are doing the work that they do, and experience a sense of frustration, anxiety, and anger. Such emotions can erode relationships within the medical treatment team as well as potentially seep into one's family life outside the hospital.

Moral distress may be an aspect of spiritual suffering that concentrates within the caregiver. An obstacle to caregiver compassion toward terminally ill patients is fear. Engulfing fear, loss of control, a feeling that one is "in too deep" can interfere with healthy compassion and lead to "compassion fatigue." Furthermore, as many individuals caring for the terminally ill well know, anguish is contagious; fear of confronting our own mortal vulnerability in a process of countertransference exposes the professional to personal distress, creating a downward spiral that threatens the well-being of the caregiver and ultimately the patients.

Maintaining a healthy compassion and healthy spiritual solidarity may decrease burnout, allowing the caregiver to find spiritual growth in tandem with the patient's healing. The relational context of compassion as well as its asymmetrical and vulnerable aspects are all important in the context of embracing spiritual suffering. Recognizing the power of this relationship is an aspect of assessing and treating spiritual suffering that has not yet been fully explored. Indeed, it is important to recall the words of John Donne (1572–1631): "No man is an island, entire of itself; every man is a piece of the continent, a part of the main; any man's death diminishes me, because I am involved in mankind . . . and therefore never send to know for whom the bell tolls; it tolls for thee."

Specific methods that can be used to reduce burnout-related stress have been explored by physicians. Many of the strategies involve aspects of connecting with meaning in life, not unlike the strategies used to deal with illness-related distress in dying patients. These approaches include fostering relationships, hobbies, exercise, and religious and spiritual practices. Some physicians have found meditation designed to increase awareness and reflection helpful for identifying values and promoting personal well-being.[81] Five primary wellness promotion practices have been reported in caregivers surveys and include relationships, religion or spirituality, self-care, work, and philosophical approaches to life.[82]

There is some evidence that educating medical students in compassion, philosophical values and meaning, and personal wellness during medical school may increase empathy and personal wellness in medical practice.[83] Humanity training and the application of narrative medicine for medical trainees may also help caregivers to find meaning in their work. Perhaps expanding understanding of the palliative care team as an aspect of the interdisciplinary care, not just for the patient, but for the health of the caregiver will help highlight the need for caregiver assistance, such a team can be an additional resource for the caregiver by its role in absorbing some of the excess burden of caring without forcing the primary team to abandon the patient or its role in disease management.[58]

Disciplined spiritual practices can increase the caregiver's capacity to transcend difficult working realities by keeping them in perspective. Spiritual disciplines access inner resources for giving and receiving, finding personally satisfying meanings in existence, and coping with the exigencies in life. In this sense, spiritual disciplines run the gamut from physical exercise, reading, and art and poetry to meditation and prayer."[60]

CONCLUSION

Identifying and addressing issues related to meaning and faith are integral aspects of palliative care for patients facing a terminal illness. Because this is a new field, definitions are still somewhat vague, although a vocabulary is beginning to emerge. There are few universally accepted intake tools and therapies. Screening for existential and spiritual distress is dependent on the experience of the healthcare worker. Healthcare workers should be aware of their own limitations, have strategies in place that they can use to understand and handle their own emotions, and be comfortable that they can endure such encounters with a good level of comfort. In fact, the fear of psychic discomfort can prevent even the initial step, which is to listen and thus fear can prevent the cristential growth of both the patient and the caregiver.

Key to all spiritual assessments and to spiritual palliative care is not having the answer to the questions that have been in existence for centuries but to listen and witness. "Skillful spiritual intervention entails being equipped to ask questions and make observations that will encourage the patient to explore the issues and come to their own conclusions."[34] As physicians, it is important to reflect and come to some of our own conclusions, journeying further into this area of unknown with each patient encounter, each time healing a part of ourselves while providing improved care to our patients. Furthermore, such an opportunity to witness the patient's journey is an opportunity for our own growth not only as caregivers but also as human beings.

REFERENCES

1. Saunders C. The founding philosophy. In: Saunders C, Summers D, Teller N, eds.. *Hospice: the Living Idea*. London: Edward Arnold; 1981.
2. Frankl V. The suffering person in search of meaning. Osterr Krankenpflegez. 1982;35:10–12.
3. Strasser F, Walker P, Bruera E. Palliative pain management: when both pain and suffering hurt. *J Palliat Care*. 2005;21:69–79.
4. Murray SA, Kendall M, Boyd K, et al. Exploring the spiritual needs of people dying of lung cancer of heart failure: a prospective qualitative interview study of patients and their careers. *Palliat Med*. 2004;18:39–45.
5. Tang WR, Aaronson LS, Forbes SA. Quality of life in hospice patients with terminal illness. *West J Nurs Res*. 2004;26:113–128.
6. Zaza C, Baine N. Cancer pain and psychosocial factors: a critical review of the literature. *J Pain Symptom Manage*. 2002;24:526–542.
7. Rousseau P. Existential suffering and palliative sedation: a brief commentary with a proposal for clinical guidelines. *Am J Hosp Palliat Care*. 2001;18:151–153.
8. Breitbart W. Reframing hope: meaning-centered care for patients near the end of life. Interview by Karen S. Heller. *J Palliat Med*. 2003;6:979–988.
9. Bussing A, Ostermann T, Matthiessen PF. Role of religion and spirituality in medical patients: confirmatory results with the SpREUK questionnaire. *Health Qual Life Outcomes*. 2005;3:10.
10. Breitbart W, Rosenfeld B, Pessin H, et al. Depression, hopelessness, and desire for hastened death in terminally ill patients with cancer. *JAMA*. 2000;284:2907–2911.
11. Fehring RJ, Miller JF, Shaw C. Spiritual well-being, religiosity, hope, depression, and other mood states in elderly people coping with cancer. *Oncol Nurs Forum*. 1997;24:663–671.
12. Nelson CJ, Rosenfeld B, Breitbart W, et al. Spirituality, religion, and depression in the terminally ill. *Psychosomatics*. 2002;43:213–220.
13. McClain CS, Rosenfeld B, Breitbart W. Effect of spiritual well-being on end-of-life despair in terminally-ill cancer patients. *Lancet*. 2003;361:1603–1607.
14. Manning-Walsh J. Spiritual struggle. Effect on quality of life and life satisfaction in women with breast cancer. *J Holist Nurs*. 2005;23:120–140.
15. Primitive culture. In: Tylor EB, Smith CH, eds. *The Academy* (15), 1972.
16. Rudolf Otto. The idea of the Holy. In: Trans J, Harvey W, eds. 2nd ed. New York: Oxford University Press; 1923.
17. Burkhardt MA, Nagai-Jacobson MG. Reawakening spirit in clinical practice. *J Holist Nurs*. 1994;12:9–21.
18. White House Council on Aging. Special White House Conference Edition. In: Seeber JW, Ellor JW, Kimble MA, McFadden SH, eds. *CARS Chronicle* The Center for Aging, Religion, & Spirituality Chronicle, 1995; Summer.
19. Spirituality in Cancer Care. *Health Professional Version, National Cancer Institute* 2003.
20. *The Oxford English Dictionary*, 2nd ed., Oxford University Press; 1989.
21. Lonenz JM. Of Addiction and Spirituality, reviewed by Janet M. Lorenz. Morgan & Merle Jordan eds. http://www.metanexus.net/metanexus_online/show_article.asp?7745
22. Barnes LL, Plotinikoff GA, Fox K, Pendleton S. Spirituality, religion, and pediatrics: intersecting worlds of healing. *Pediatrics*. 2000;106:S899–S908.
23. The Interpretation of Culture. Selected essays. In: Clifford Geertz, ed., New York: Basic Book Publication; 1973.
24. Zbarowski MJ. *Social Issues*. 1952, Speile.
25. Bosch F, Banos JE. Religious beliefs of patients and caregivers as a barrier to the pharmacologic control of cancer pain. *Clin Pharmacol Ther*. 2002;72:107–111.
26. Sheiner EK, Sheiner E, Shoham-Vardi I, et al. Ethnic differences influence care giver's estimates of pain during labor. *Pain*. 1999;81:299–305.
27. Vilchinsky N, Kravetz S. How are religious belief and behavior good for you? An investigation of mediators relating religion to mental health in a sample of Israeli Jewish students. *J Sci Study Relig*. 2005;44:459–471.
28. McClain-Jacobson C, Rosenfeld B, Kosinski A, et al. Belief in an afterlife, spiritual well-being and end-of-life despair in patients with advanced cancer. *Gen Hosp Psychiatry*. 2004;26:484–486.
29. Dunn KS, Horgas AL. Religious and nonreligious coping in older adults experiencing chronic pain. *Pain Manag Nurs*. 2004;5:19–28.
30. Pargament KI, Smith BW, Koenig HG, et al. Patterns of positive and negative religious coping with major life stressors. *J Sci Study Religion*. 1998;37:710–724.
31. Harrison MO, Edwards CL, Koenig HG, et al. Religiosity/spirituality and pain in patients with sickle cell disease. *J Nerv Ment Dis*. 2005;193:250–257.
32. Syrjala KL, Donaldson GW, Davis MW, et al. Relaxation and imagery and cognitive-behavioral training reduce pain during cancer treatment: a controlled clinical trial. *Pain*. 1995;63:189–198.
33. McGrath P. Reflections on serious illness as spiritual journey by survivors of hematological malignancies. *Eur J Cancer Care*. 2004;13:227–237.
34. Otis-Green S, Sherman R, Perez M, et al. An integrated psychosocial-spiritual model for cancer pain management. *Cancer Pract*. 2002;10: S58–S65.
35. Hills J, Paice JA, Cameron JR, et al. Spirituality and distress in palliative care consultation. *J Palliat Med*. 2005;8:782–788.
36. Griffith JL, Griffith ME. *Encountering the Sacred in Psychotherapy: How to Talk with People About Their Spiritual Lives*. New York: The Guildford Press; 2002.
37. Moadel A, Morgan C, Fatone A, et al. Seeking meaning and hope: self-reported spiritual existential needs among an ethnically-diverse cancer patient population. *Psychooncology*. 1999;8:378–385.

38. Blinderman CD, Cherny NI. Existential issues do not necessarily result in existential suffering: lessons from cancer patients in Israel. *Palliat Med.* 2005;19:371–380.

39. Hay MW. Principles in building spiritual assessment tools. *Am J Hosp Palliat Care.* 1989;6:25–31.

40. Millspaugh CD. Assessment and response to spiritual pain: Part I. *J Palliat Med.* 2005;8:919–923.

41. Musi M. Creating a language for "spiritual pain": why not to speak and think in terms of "spiritual suffering"? *Support Care Cancer.* 2003;11: 378–379.

42. McGrath P. Creating a language for "spiritual pain" through research: a beginning. *Support Care Cancer.* 2002;10:637–646.

43. Koenig HG, McCullough ME, Larson DB. Handbook of Religion and Health. New York: Oxford University Press; Oxford, NY, 2001.

44. Sherman A, Plante T, Simonton S, et al. A multidimensional measure of religious involvement for cancer patients: the Duke Religious Index. *Support Care Cancer.* 2000;8:102–109.

45. Peterman A, Fitchett G, Brady M, et al. Measuring spiritual well-being in people with cancer: the functional assessment of chronic illness therapy-spiritual well-being scale (FACIT-SP). *Ann Behav Med.* 2002;24: 49–58.

46. Underwood LG, Teresi JA. The daily spiritual experience scale: Development, theoretical description, reliability, exploratory factor analysis and preliminary construct validity using health-related data. *Ann Behav Med.* 2002;24(1):22–23.

47. Robinson P, Wood K. Fear of death and physical illness: a personal construct approach. In: Epting F, Neimeyer R, eds. *Personal Meanings of Death.* Washington: Hemisphere Publishing Company; 1984:213–228.

48. Herth K. Development and refinement of an instrument to measure hope. *Sch Inq Nurs Pract.* 1991;5:39–51.

49. University of Maryland School of Medicine. Spirituality and palliative care. Update: July 17, 2002. http://cancer-research.umaryland.edu/spirituality.htm.

50. Puchalski C. Spiritual Assessment Tool. Innovations in End-of-life Care. 1999;1:1–2. http://www2.edc.org/lastacts/archives/archivesNov99/assesstool.asp.

51. Speck P. Spiritual Pain. Hospice Education Institute; 1985:1–6. http://www.hospiceworld.org/book/spiritual-pain.htm.

52. Speck P. *The Nature of Non-Physical Pain.* Edinburgh: Churchill Livingstone, 2001.

53. Maugans TA. The SPIRITual History. *Arch Fam Med.* 1996;5:11–16.

54. Peterman AH, Fichett G, Brady MJ, et al. Measuring spiritual well-being in people with cancer: the functional assessment of chronic illness therapy—Spiritual Well-being Scale (FACIT-Sp). *Ann Behav Med.* 2002;24:49–58.

55. Burton R. Spiritual pain: a brief overview and an initial response within the Christian tradition. *J Pastoral Care Counsel.* 2003;57:437–446.

56. Taylor E. *Spiritual Care, Nursing Theory, Research, and Practice.* River, NJ: Prentice Hall; 2002.

57. National Consensus Project for Quality Palliative Care. Clinical practice guidelines for quality palliative care. *Kans Nurse.* 2004;79:16–20.

58. Fisch MJ. Principles of palliative care. In: Kantarjian H, Wolff RA, Koller CA, eds. *M. D. Anderson Manual of Medical Oncology.* New York: McGraw-Hill Medical Publishing Division; 2006.

59. Sellers SC, Haag BA. Spiritual nursing interventions. *J Holist Nurs.* 1998; 16:338–354.

60. Storey P, Knight CF. UNIPAC two: alleviating psychological and spiritual pain in the terminally ill. In: Storey P, Knight CF, eds. *Hospice/Palliative Care Training for Physicians.* New York: Mary Ann Liebert; 1997.

61. Breitbart W. Spirituality and meaning in supportive care: spirituality- and meaning-centered group psychotherapy interventions in advanced cancer. *Support Care Cancer.* 2001;10:272–280.

62. Breitbart W, Gibson C, Poppito SR, et al. Psychotherapeutic interventions at the end of life: a focus on meaning and spirituality. *Can J Psychiatry.* 2004;49:366–372.

63. Frankl VE. *Doctor and the Soul.* Peter Smith; Bantam Books, N.Y., 1967.

64. Noguchi W, Morita S, Ohno T, et al. Spiritual needs in cancer patients and spiritual care based on logotherapy. *Support Care Cancer.* 2006;14:65–70.

65. Chin-A-Loy SS, Fernsler JL. Self-transcendence in older men attending a prostate cancer support group. *Cancer Nurs.* 1998;21:358–363.

66. Coward D. Facilitation of self-transcendence in a breast cancer support group. *Oncol Nurs Forum.* 1998;25:75–84.

67. Coward D. Self-transcendence and emotional well being in women with advanced breast cancer. *Oncol Nurs Forum.* 1991;18:857–863.

68. Chochinov HM, Hack T, Hassard T, et al. Dignity therapy: a novel psychotherapeutic intervention for patients near the end of life. *J Clin Oncol.* 2005;23:5520–5525.

69. Clarke DM, Kissane DW. Demoralization: its phenomenology and importance. *Aust N Z J Psychiatry.* 2002;36:733–742.

70. Newell SA, Sanson-Fisher RW, Savolainen NJ. Systematic review of psychological therapies for cancer patients: overview and recommendations for future research. *J Natl Cancer Inst.* 2002;94:558–584.

71. Chan YM, Lee PW, Fong DY, et al. Effect of individual psychological intervention in Chinese women with gynecologic malignancy: a randomized controlled trial. *J Clin Oncol.* 2005;23:4913–4924.

72. Smyth JM, Stone AA, Hurewitz A, et al. Effects of writing about stressful experiences on symptom reduction in patients with asthma or rheumatoid arthritis: a randomized trial. *JAMA.* 1999;281:1304–1309.

73. Stanton AL, Danoff-Burg S, Sworowski LA, et al. Randomized, controlled trial of written emotional expression and benefit finding in breast cancer patients. *J Clin Oncol.* 2002;20:4160–4168.

74. de Moor C, Sterner J, Hall M, et al. A pilot study of the effects of expressive writing on psychological and behavioral adjustment in patients enrolled in a Phase II trial of vaccine therapy for metastatic renal cell carcinoma. *Health Psychol.* 2002;21:615–619.

75. Kaye P. Notes on symptom control in hospice and palliative care. Hospice Education Institute. http://www.hospiceworld.org/book/spiritual-pain.htm.

76. Lichter I, Mooney J, Boyd M. Biography as therapy. *Palliat Med.* 1993;7: 133–137.

77. Kaufmann M. Physician burnout: part II. Personal factors in burnout prevention and health maintenance. *Ont Med Rev.* 2002.

78. Allegra CJ, Hall R, Yothers G. Prevalence of burnout in the U.S. oncology community: results of a 2003 survey. *J Oncol Pract.* 2005;1:140–148.

79. Shanafelt TD, Bradley K, Wipf JE, et al. Burnout and self-reported patient care in an internal medicine residency program. *Ann Intern Med.* 2002;136:358–367.

80. Hinshaw DB. Spiritual issues in surgical palliative care. *Surg Clin North Am.* 2005;85:257–272.

81. Shanafelt TD, Sloan JA, Habermann TM. The well being of physicians. *Am J Med.* 2003;114:513–519.

82. Weiner EL, Swain GR, Wolf B, et al. A qualitative study of physicians' own wellness-promotion practices. *West J Med.* 2001;174:19–23.

83. DiLalla LF, Hull SK, Dorsey JK, et al. Effect of gender, age, and relevant course work on attitudes toward empathy, patient spirituality, and physician wellness. *Teach Learn Med.* 2004;16:165–170.

Use of Complementary and Alternative Medicine in Oncology

Joann Aaron

INTRODUCTION

Doctor-patient communication and information exchange are of paramount importance in cancer treatment. Complementary and alternative medicine (CAM) has become an increasingly significant arena of communication and a metaphor for the support of patients with cancer, with as many as 50%–83% of cancer patients reporting taking at least one type of CAM therapy.[1] Accordingly, it is important for physicians and other healthcare providers to understand the psychological and clinical benefits that may accrue to patients who practice CAM. This is particularly true because the widespread use of CAM by cancer patients is likely to increase, particularly as insurance benefits expand to cover its frequently high cost and as more objective data are garnered from evidence-based clinical trials. The experience in Washington State, for example, suggests that a substantial number of insured cancer patients use alternative providers if they are given the choice.[2] The popularity of CAM is an international phenomenon. The prevalence of CAM use is estimated at 25% among residents of the United Kingdom, 50% among German, French, and Australian populations, and 42%–69% among residents of the United States.[3]

WHAT IS COMPLEMENTARY AND ALTERNATIVE MEDICINE?

While CAM is used along with standard medical treatments, alternative medicine is used in lieu of standard medical treatments and neither of these is an integral part of conventional medicine. Integrative medicine is, on the other hand, a total approach to care that involves the patient's mind, body, and spirit and combines standard medicine with CAM practices that have the most potential benefit. CAM practices are grouped within five major domains: (1) alternative or whole medical systems; (2) mind-body interventions; (3) biologically-based treatments; (4) energy therapies; and (5) manipulative and body-based methods.[4]

▶ Whole medical systems

Whole medical systems are total systems of theory and practice, which have evolved independently from or parallel to allopathic (conventional) medicine. Major Western whole medical systems include homeopathy and naturopathy, among others. Other systems include traditional Chinese medicine (TCM) and Ayurvedic medicine,

one of India's traditional systems of medicine. TCM is a complete system of healing that dates back to 200 BC.[5] In the TCM worldview, the body is a delicate balance of two opposing and inseparable forces: yin and yang. Yin represents the cold, slow, or passive principle, whereas yang represents the hot, excited, or active principle. Among the major assumptions in TCM are that health is achieved by maintaining the body in a "balanced state," and that disease is due to an internal imbalance of yin and yang. This imbalance leads to blockage in the flow of Qi (or vital energy) and of blood along pathways known as meridians. TCM practitioners typically use herbs, acupuncture, and massage to help unblock Qi and blood in patients in an attempt to bring the body back into harmony and wellness. There are three main therapeutic modalities: (1) acupuncture[5] and moxibustion[6-8] (moxibustion is the application of heat from the burning of the herb moxa at the acupuncture point); (2) Chinese Materia Medica (the catalogue of natural products used in TCM; (3) massage and manipulation.[4]

Acupuncture is widely practiced in TCM for various health conditions, including treating cancer pain.[5,9-12] Preclinical studies have documented acupuncture's effects, but they have not been able to fully explain how acupuncture works within the framework of the Western system of medicine. Acupuncture putatively produces its effects by conducting electromagnetic signals at a greater-than-normal rate, thus aiding the activity of pain-killing biochemicals, such as endorphins, and immune system cells at specific sites in the body. In addition, acupuncture may alter brain chemistry by changing the release of neurotransmitters and neurohormones and affecting the parts of the central nervous system related to sensation and involuntary body functions, such as immune reactions and processes by which blood pressure, blood flow, and body temperature are regulated.[4]

Ayurveda, whose literal meaning is "the science of life," is a natural healing system developed in India.[13-15] This comprehensive system of medicine places equal emphasis on the body, mind, and spirit, and strives to restore the innate harmony of the individual. Some of the primary Ayurvedic treatments include diet, exercise, meditation, herbs, massage, exposure to sunlight, and controlled breathing.

Naturopathy is a system of healing, originating from Europe, that views disease as a manifestation of alterations in the processes by which the body naturally heals itself. It emphasizes health restoration as well as disease treatment. Six principles form the basis of naturopathic practice in North America: (1) the healing power of nature; (2) identification and treatment of the cause of disease;

(3) the concept of "first do no harm"; (4) the doctor as teacher; (5) treatment of the whole person; and (6) prevention. The core modalities supporting these principles include diet modification and nutritional supplements, herbal medicine, acupuncture and Chinese medicine, hydrotherapy, massage and joint manipulation, and lifestyle counseling. Treatment protocols combine what the practitioner deems to be the most suitable therapies for each patient. To date, no research studies on naturopathy as a complete system of medicine have been published.[4,16–20]

Homeopathic medicine is a somewhat controversial CAM alternative medical system.[21–24] The underlying belief of homeopathic medicine is that "like cures like," meaning that small, highly diluted quantities of medicinal substances are given to cure symptoms, when the same substances, given in higher or more concentrated doses, would actually cause those symptoms.

Mind-body medicine

Mind-body interventions are among the most widely used CAM practices.[25] Mind-body medicine focuses on interactions among the brain, mind, body, and behavior, and the powerful ways in which emotional, mental, social, spiritual, and behavioral factors can directly affect health. Its fundamental approach respects and enhances each person's capacity for self-knowledge and self-care, and it emphasizes techniques that are grounded in this approach.[4] Mind-body medicine typically focuses on intervention strategies that are thought to promote health, such as relaxation, hypnosis, visual imagery, meditation, yoga, biofeedback, tai chi, Qigong, cognitive-behavioral therapies, group support, autogenic training, and spirituality. The field views illness as an opportunity for personal growth and transformation, and healthcare providers as catalysts and guides in this process. Mind-body interventions have also been applied to various types of pain. Some of these interventions are discussed further along in this chapter. Clinical trials indicate that these interventions may be a particularly effective adjunct in the management of arthritis, with reductions in pain maintained for as long as 4 years as well as reductions in the number of physician visits. When applied to more general acute and chronic pain management, headache, and low-back pain, mind-body interventions demonstrate some benefit, although results vary based on the patient population and type of intervention studied.[4]

Evidence from multiple studies with various types of cancer patients suggests that mind-body interventions can improve mood, quality of life, and coping, as well as ameliorate disease- and treatment-related symptoms, such as chemotherapy-induced nausea, vomiting, and pain. Some studies have suggested that mind-body interventions can alter various immune parameters, but it is unclear whether these alterations are of sufficient magnitude to have an impact on disease progression or prognosis.[4,26–28]

Neurochemical and anatomical foundations may exist for some of the effects of mind-body approaches. Evidence from randomized controlled trials and, in many cases, systematic reviews of the literature, suggest that: (1) mechanisms may exist by which the brain and central nervous system influence immune, endocrine, and autonomic functioning, which is known to have an impact on health; (2) multicomponent mind-body interventions that include some combination of stress management, coping skills training, cognitive-behavioral interventions, and relaxation therapy may be appropriate adjunctive treatments for coronary artery disease and certain pain-related disorders, such as arthritis; (3) multimodal mind-body approaches, such as cognitive-behavioral therapy, particularly when combined with an educational/informational component, can be effective adjuncts in the management of a variety of chronic conditions; (4) an array of mind-body therapies (e.g., imagery, hypnosis, relaxation), when employed presurgically, may improve recovery time and reduce pain following surgical procedures.[4]

Energy medicine

Practitioners of energy medicine believe that illness results from disturbances of subtle energies (the biofield).[4,29] Energy medicine is a domain in CAM that deals with energy fields of two types: (1) veritable, which can be measured, and (2) putative, which have yet to be measured. The veritable energies employ mechanical vibrations (such as sound) and electromagnetic forces, including visible light, magnetism, monochromatic radiation (such as laser beams), and rays from other parts of the electromagnetic spectrum. They involve the use of specific, measurable wavelengths and frequencies to treat patients. Therapies involving putative energy fields are based on the concept that human beings are infused with a subtle form of energy.[29] Vital energy is believed to flow throughout the material human body, but it has not been unequivocally measured by means of conventional instrumentation. Nonetheless, therapists claim that they can work with this subtle energy, see it with their own eyes, and use it to effect changes in the physical body and influence health. These approaches are among the most controversial of CAM practices because neither the external energy fields nor their therapeutic effects have been demonstrated convincingly by any biophysical means.[29]

Examples of practices involving putative energy fields[4,29–36] include (1) Reiki[37] and Johrei, both of Japanese origin; (2) Qigong, a Chinese practice; (3) healing touch,[38–40] in which the therapist is purported to identify imbalances and correct a client's energy by passing his or her hands over the patient; (4) intercessory prayer, in which a person intercedes through prayer on behalf of another.[41,42]

Numerous other practices have evolved over the years to promote or maintain the balance of vital energy fields in the body. Examples of these modalities include therapeutic touch, vortex healing, and polarity therapy. All of these modalities involve movement of the practitioner's hands over the patient's body to become attuned to the condition of the patient, with the idea that by so doing, the practitioner is able to strengthen and reorient the patient's energies.[29]

Many small studies of therapeutic touch have suggested its effectiveness in a wide variety of conditions, including wound healing, osteoarthritis, migraine headaches, and anxiety in burn patients.[30,38,40]

Proponents of energy field therapies also claim that some of these therapies can act across long distances.

Manipulative and body-based practices

Manipulative and body-based practices focus primarily on the structures and systems of the body, including the bones and joints, the soft tissues, and the circulatory and lymphatic systems.

Under the umbrella of manipulative and body-based practices is a heterogeneous group of CAM interventions and therapies. Some of the body-based practices are defined as follows:

Alexander technique: Patient education/guidance to improve posture and movement, and to use muscles efficiently.[43–45]

Bowen technique: Gentle massage of muscles and tendons over acupuncture and reflex points.[46]

Chiropractic manipulation: Adjustments of the joints of the spine, as well as other joints and muscles.[47]

Craniosacral therapy: Form of massage using gentle pressure on the plates of the patient's skull.

Feldenkrais method: Group classes and hands-on lessons designed to improve the coordination of the whole person in comfortable, effective, and intelligent movement.[44]

Massage therapy: Assortment of techniques involving manipulation of the soft tissues of the body through pressure and movement.[4,48–51]

Osteopathic manipulation: Manipulation of the joints combined with physical therapy and instruction in proper posture.

Reflexology: Method of foot (and sometimes hand) massage in which pressure is applied to "reflex" zones mapped out on the feet (or hands).[4,52–54]

Rolfing: Deep tissue massage (also called structural integration).[4]

Trager bodywork: Slight rocking and shaking of the patient's trunk and limbs in a rhythmic fashion.[55]

Tui Na: Application of pressure with the fingers and thumb, and manipulation of specific points on the body (acupoints).[56]

▶ Biologically-based practices

In 2002, sales of dietary supplements increased to an estimated $18.7 billion per year, with herbs/botanical supplements accounting for an estimated $4.3 billion in sales.[57,58] The CAM domain of biologically based practices includes botanicals, animal-derived extracts, vitamins, minerals, fatty acids, amino acids, proteins, prebiotics and probiotics, whole diets, and functional foods. Dietary supplements are a subset of this CAM domain. The "dietary ingredients" in these products include vitamins, minerals, herbs or other botanicals, amino acids, and substances such as enzymes, organ tissues, glandulars, and metabolites. Dietary supplements can be extracts or concentrates, and can occur in many forms, such as tablets, capsules, soft gels, gel-caps, liquids, or powders. Interest in and use of dietary supplements has grown considerably in the past two decades. A primary reason that consumers use herbal supplements is to promote overall health and wellness, but supplements are also used to improve performance and energy, to treat and prevent illnesses (e.g., cold and flu), and to alleviate depression. In contrast to dietary supplements, functional foods are components of the usual diet that may have biologically active components (e.g., polyphenols, phytoestrogens, fish oils, carotenoids) that may provide health benefits beyond basic nutrition. Examples of functional foods include soy, nuts, chocolate, and cranberries. These foods' bioactive constituents are appearing with increasing frequency as ingredients in dietary supplements.[57] Table 14-1 lists some of the supplements that have a putative role in cancer prevention and treatment.

WHY DO PATIENTS VALUE CAM?

Oncologists have become increasingly aware that many of their patients are involved with CAM, yet few oncologists talk about these therapies with patients.[3] Similarly, patients often don't discuss their use of CAM with their physicians. In a study conducted at M. D. Anderson Cancer Center, more than 99% of the participants had heard of CAM and more than 80% had used at least one CAM therapy. Prevalence of use was highest for spiritual practices, vitamins and herbs, and movement and physical therapies.[3] In view of its widespread part of the healing culture and use, it is important for physicians to understand how to talk to their patients about CAM,

and to do so effectively it is helpful to understand the meaning and value of CAM for patients.

The value of CAM for many patients centers upon embracing a holistic point of view, a pragmatic perspective, perceived safety of the methods, and a sense of participating in one's own care.[59] Overall, the patient-practitioner relationship and explanatory frameworks provided by CAM are frequently perceived as important components of the therapeutic process, irrespective of treatment efficacy.[60] Importantly, most patients don't eschew allopathic medicine when they engage in CAM. In one study, all the participants viewed their relationship with the CAM practitioner as an important component of the therapeutic process.[60] The therapeutic relationship is valued by patients as an important source of social support, a relationship in which patients have the opportunity to discuss concerns and worries with a practitioner skilled in active listening, as a relationship of trust, and as a relationship of equals.[60] In one study cancer patients reported that their most common reasons for using CAM were a desire to feel hopeful, their belief that these approaches are nontoxic, and their desire for more control in making decisions about their medical care. Most patients expected CAM to improve their quality of life, boost their immune system, prolong life, relieve symptoms, and cure their disease.[3] Other factors of importance to patients are the concept of links between different levels of the body, perceptions of CAM as natural and traditional, as a form of treatment without concerns over iatrogenic effects associated with orthodox medicine or the side effects of treatment along with limited effectiveness of standard medical practice.[60] Additional key attractors of CAM are the strong emphasis given to the psychological processes underlying treatment effects, linkage with evidence of the body's capacity to self-heal, a sense of reduced dependence on external or unnatural factors, an improvement in primary and secondary symptoms, increased energy levels, increased levels of relaxation, providing an additional means of coping with specific health problems and wider life stressors, and a feeling that participants were able to take control over their health.[60] Restoring physical and psychosocial balance was considered to be an important treatment outcome.[60] Specific reasons why people with cancer choose CAM are to help cope with the side effects of cancer treatments, such as nausea, pain, and fatigue; to comfort themselves and ease the worries of cancer treatment and related stress; to feel that they are doing something more to help with their own care; and to try to treat or cure their cancer.

HOW TO TALK TO PATIENTS ABOUT CAM?

The communication gap that separates patient practices vis-à-vis CAM from physician awareness needs to be bridged, particularly because of the increasingly widespread use of complementary therapies by patients.[1,61] In one study, the major barriers to successful communication between physicians and patients regarding CAM usage were the physicians' indifference or opposition toward CAM use, their emphasis on scientific evidence, and patients' anticipation of a negative response from their physicians.[1] These barriers can be related to more general barriers to effective patient-physician communication. The reasons for this disjuncture are varied: insufficient communication training, poor multidisciplinary communication, lack of support, stress/depression/anxiety, lack of satisfaction, emotional burnout, insufficient ethics consideration, insufficient time, and countertransferences issues.[62–64] In addition to these crucial factors, the language of evidence-based medicine, which is particularly

Table 14-1

Herbs and Supplements that have a Putative Role in Cancer Prevention and Treatment

Herbs & Supplements	Cancer Prevention	Cancer Treatment
Curcumin	Curcumin, the yellow pigment and active component of turmeric (Curcuma longa), exhibits chemopreventive and growth inhibitory activity against several tumor cell lines.[94] This spice is consumed in the diet in quantities up to 4 g/adult/day in some countries, which also appear to have low incidence rates of colorectal cancer. Curcumin has been shown to inhibit tumor formation in the skin, forestomach, duodenum, and colon of mice and in the tongue, colon, mammary glands, and sebaceous glands of rats. Mechanisms by which curcumin causes cancer chemoprevention are thought to involve antioxidation, inhibition of kinases, interference with the activity of transcription factors, and suppression of expression of the enzyme COX-2.[94]	
Soy	Several large population studies have asked women about their eating habits, and reported higher soy intake (such as dietary tofu) to be associated with a decreased risk of developing breast cancer. However, this type of research (retrospective, case-control, epidemiologic) can only be considered preliminary, because people who choose to eat soy may also partake in other lifestyle decisions that may lower the risk of cancer. These other habits, rather than soy, could theoretically be the cause of the benefits seen in these studies (e.g., lower fat intake, more frequent exercise, lack of smoking). Controlled human trials are necessary before a firm conclusion can be drawn.	Genistein, an isoflavone found in soy, has been found in laboratory and animal studies to possess anticancer effects, such as blocking new blood vessel growth (antiangiogenesis), acting as a tyrosine kinase inhibitor (a mechanism of many new cancer treatments), or causing cancer cell death (apoptosis). In contrast, genistein has also been reported to *increase* the growth of pancreas tumor cells in laboratory research. None of these effects has been adequately assessed in humans.
	Theoretical concerns have been raised that soy may actually *increase* the risk of breast cancer because of the presence in soy of "phytoestrogens" (plant-based compounds with weak estrogen-like properties), such as isoflavones. This remains an area of controversy. Recently, some scientists have theorized that isoflavones may reduce the risk of cancer by blocking estrogen effects in the body, based on laboratory studies showing isoflavones to partially block (noncompetitively inhibit) estrogen receptors. In fact, early research suggests that soy isoflavones do not have the same effects on the body as estrogens, such as increasing the thickening of the uterus lining (endometrium). Genistein has been found in laboratory and animal studies to have other anticancer effects, such as blocking new blood vessel growth (antiangiogenesis), acting as a tyrosine kinase inhibitor (a mechanism of many new cancer treatments), or causing cancer cell death (apoptosis).	In the past, theoretical concerns have been raised that soy may increase the risk of hormone-sensitive cancers (e.g., breast, ovarian, endometrial/uterine) because of the presence in soy of "phytoestrogens" (plant-based compounds with weak estrogen-like properties), such as isoflavones like genistein. This remains an area of controversy. Recently, some scientists have suggested that isoflavones may actually reduce the risk of hormone-sensitive cancers by blocking estrogen effects in the body, based on laboratory studies showing isoflavones to partially block (noncompetitively inhibit) estrogen receptors. Preliminary human research suggests that soy isoflavones do not have the same effects on the body as estrogens, such as increasing the thickening of the uterus lining (endometrium).
	Until better research is available, it remains unclear if dietary soy or soy isoflavone supplements increase or decrease the risk of developing breast cancer.	Until reliable human research is available, it remains unclear if dietary soy or soy isoflavone supplements are beneficial, harmful, or neutral in people with various types of cancer.
Selenium	The role of selenium in cancer prevention has been the subject of recent study and debate. Initial evidence from the Nutritional Prevention of Cancer (NPC) trial suggests that selenium supplementation reduces the risk of prostate cancer among men with normal baseline PSA (prostate-specific antigen) levels, and low selenium blood levels. However, in this study selenium did not reduce the risk of lung, colorectal, or basal cell carcinoma of the skin, and actually *increased* the risk of squamous cell skin carcinoma. The ongoing Selenium and Vitamin E Cancer Prevention Trial (SELECT) aims to definitively address the role of selenium in prostate cancer prevention.	

Table 14-1

Herbs and Supplements that have a Putative Role in Cancer Prevention and Treatment *(continued)*

Herbs & Supplements	Cancer Prevention	Cancer Treatment
	Initial evidence has suggested that selenium supplementation reduces the risk of developing prostate cancer in men with normal baseline PSA (prostate-specific antigen) levels, and low selenium blood levels. This is the subject of large well-designed studies, including the Nutritional Prevention of Cancer Trial (NPC), and the ongoing Selenium and Vitamin E Cancer Prevention Trial (SELECT), as well as prior population and case control studies.	
	The NPC was conducted in 1312 Americans, and reported that 200 mcg of daily selenium reduces the overall incidence of prostate cancer, although these protective effects only occurred in men with baseline PSA levels less than or equal to 4 ng/mL, and those with low baseline blood selenium levels (<123.2 ng/mL). The NPC trial was primarily designed to measure the development of nonmelanoma skin cancers, not other types of cancers, and therefore these prostate cancer results cannot be considered definitive. To settle this question, further study is underway: The SELECT trial is in progress, with a goal to include 32,400 men with serum PSA levels less than or equal to 4 ng/mL. SELECT was started in 2001, with results expected in 2013.	
	Laboratory studies have reported several potential mechanisms for selenium's beneficial effects in prostate cancer, including decrease in androgen receptors and PSA production, antioxidant effects, angiogenesis inhibition, or apoptosis.	
	It is not known if selenium is helpful in men who already have been diagnosed with prostate cancer to prevent progression or recurrence of disease. It does appear that selenium may not be beneficial in those with elevated PSA levels, or with normal/high selenium levels. It remains unclear whether men at risk (or all men) should have their serum selenium values measured; results of the SELECT study may provide additional guidance. There is evidence that low selenium levels are associated with an increased risk of prostate cancer, and several mechanisms for the beneficial effects of selenium supplementation have been suggested.	
	In the NPC trial, no benefits were seen in reducing the risk of colorectal or lung cancers. Although an overall reduction in cancer risk was observed, it is not clear which specific types of cancer besides prostate cancer prevention may benefit.	
Green tea	Several large population-based studies have been undertaken to examine the possible association between green tea consumption and cancer incidence. Cancers of the digestive system (stomach, colon, rectum, pancreas, and esophagus) have primarily been tracked. The risk of prostate cancer, cervical cancer and breast cancer in women has also been studied. Although much of this research suggests cancer-protective properties of habitual green tea consumption, some studies have not observed significant benefits. In studies that have shown benefits, it is not clear if other lifestyle choices of people who drink tea may actually be the beneficial factors. If there is a benefit, it may be small and require large amounts of daily consumption (several cups per day). At this time, the scientific evidence remains indeterminate.	

(Continued)

Table 14-1

Herbs and Supplements that have a Putative Role in Cancer Prevention and Treatment *(continued)*

Herbs & Supplements	Cancer Prevention	Cancer Treatment
	Laboratory and animal studies report that components of tea, such as polyphenols, have antioxidant/free radical scavenging properties and may possess various effects against tumor cells (such as angiogenesis inhibition, hydrogen peroxide generation, or induction of apoptosis). Preliminary data show that drinking 4 cups/day of decaffeinated green or black tea may decrease the amount of DNA damage in heavy smokers. Limited human study reports lower estrogen levels in women drinking green tea, proposed as possibly beneficial in estrogen-receptor positive breast cancers. However, other animal and laboratory research suggests that components of green tea may actually be carcinogenic, although effects in humans are not clear. Based on preliminary data, theanine, a specific glutamate derivative in green tea, may reduce the adverse reactions caused to the heart and liver by the prescription cancer drug doxorubicin. Further research is needed to confirm these results. Overall, the relationship of green tea consumption and human cancer remains inconclusive. Evidence from a controlled trial of sufficient size and duration is needed before a recommendation can be made in this area.	
Coenzyme Q		Several studies in women with breast cancer report reduced levels of CoQ10 in diseased breast tissue or blood. It has been suggested by some researchers that raising CoQ10 levels with supplements might be helpful. However, it is not clear if CoQ10 is beneficial in these patients, or if the low levels of CoQ10 may actually be a part of the body's natural response to cancer, helping to fight disease. Supplementation with CoQ10 has not been proven to reduce cancer, and has not been compared to other forms of treatment for breast cancer.
Fish oil	Several population (epidemiologic) studies report that dietary omega-3 fatty acids or fish oil may reduce the risk of developing breast, colon, or prostate cancer. Randomized controlled trials are necessary before a clear conclusion can be drawn.	
Vitamin E	Vitamin E has been suggested as a possible therapy for the prevention or treatment of breast cancer. Published studies have included measurement of vitamin E levels, laboratory experiments, and population studies. Evidence remains inconclusive, and no clear conclusion can be drawn at this time.	There is no reliable scientific evidence that vitamin E is effective as a treatment for any specific type of cancer. There is preliminary evidence of possible benefits of long-term vitamin E supplementation to reduce the risk of mortality in bladder cancer patients, although additional research is necessary before a clear conclusion can be reached.

Table 14-1

Herbs and Supplements that have a Putative Role in Cancer Prevention and Treatment (continued)

Herbs & Supplements	Cancer Prevention	Cancer Treatment
		Caution is merited in people undergoing treatment with chemotherapy or radiation, because it has been proposed that the use of high-dose antioxidants may actually reduce the anticancer effects of these therapies. This remains an area of controversy and studies have produced variable results. Patients interested in using high-dose antioxidants such as vitamin E during chemotherapy or radiation should discuss this decision with their medical oncologist or radiation oncologist. Like other antioxidants, vitamin E has been suggested as a therapy to prevent complications due to chemotherapy, such as nerve damage (neuropathy). There is some evidence of benefits, for example when used with cisplatin. However, caution is merited, because it is not known if the use of high-dose antioxidants during chemotherapy may actually reduce the anticancer effects of some chemotherapy agents or radiation therapy. This remains an area of controversy, and patients interested in using antioxidants during chemotherapy should discuss this decision with their oncologist.
Beta-carotene	While diets high in fruits and vegetables rich in beta-carotene have been shown to potentially reduce the incidence of certain cancers, results from randomized controlled trials with oral supplements do not support this claim.	There is some concern that beta-carotene metabolites with pharmacological activity can accumulate and potentially have cancer causing (carcinogenic) effects. A higher, statistically significant incidence of lung cancer in male smokers who took beta-carotene supplements has been discovered. Beta-carotene/vitamin A supplements may have an adverse effect on the incidence of lung cancer and on the risk of death in smokers and asbestos exposed people or in those who ingest significant amounts of alcohol. In addition, high-dose antioxidants theoretically may interfere with the activity of some chemotherapy drugs or radiation therapy. Therefore, individuals undergoing cancer treatment should speak with their oncologist if they are taking or considering the use of high-dose antioxidants. Beta-carotene in the amounts normally found in food does not appear to have this adverse effect.
Folate (folic acid)	Preliminary evidence surrounding the use of folate seems promising for decreasing the risk of breast, cervical, and gastrointestinal cancer. However, currently there is insufficient evidence available to recommend folate supplementation for any type of cancer prevention or treatment. Please follow the advice of a qualified healthcare provider in this area.	

Source: The information in this table, with the exception of the information on curcumin, can be found at the Natural Standard Web site.[58]

confusing to some patients, is lodged in statistics and objective data. This lingo has no particular personal applicability for many patients and it is difficult for them to relate to this framework. Importantly, the failure of physicians to communicate effectively with patients on CAM topics may result in a loss of trust within the therapeutic relationship.[65] Poor communication can also diminish patient autonomy and self-efficacy and possibly interfere with the self-healing response. Furthermore, patients may select harmful, useless, or ineffective and costly nonconventional therapies when effective ones may exist.[65] For these varied reasons, physicians should raise the question of CAM use with their patients and devise a mutually acceptable plan of usage that is appropriate for each stage of cancer and to other medical care, from prevention to postacute care and follow-up. An important hurdle to overcome is the apparent inconsistency in the perception of CAM between patients and physicians.[1] The need to appreciate the patient's perspective is paramount and may require a change in how physicians view the needs of their patients with cancer. It has been suggested that to help cancer patients be truly informed and autonomous, what is needed is to (1) identify the patient's beliefs, fears, hopes, and expectations; (2) learn what conventional treatments have been tried, have failed, or have been rejected because of safety, quality of life, cost, or other issues; (3) make sure the patient understands prognostic factors associated with the stage of the disease and also understands the potential benefit of conventional therapy as well as its potential harm; (4) acknowledge the patient's spiritual and religious values and beliefs, including his/her view about the end of life, and seek to understand how these impact healthcare choices; (5) discover what levels of support the patient relies on from family, community, faith community, and friends.[65] Frank, nonjudgmental discussion with the patient is necessary to inform the patient effectively about the known risks and benefits of the various supplements available to them. Another approach to discussing CAM with patients is to follow the "four Ps." That is, to (1) Protect—involving the safety of the therapy; (2) Permit—not oppose CAM therapies that are safe even if their efficacy has not been conclusively proven; (3) Promote Proven Practices—if rigorous research shows that a CAM product of procedure is safe and effective, try it and help make it responsibly available; and (4) Partnership—work as a team with patients and their complementary therapists.[59]

CANCER PAIN AND CAM

Almost all patients diagnosed with cancer experience pain, which is related either to their disease or to its treatment. Despite the availability of effective analgesic medication for pain management, many patients experience uncontrolled pain in the course of their treatment.[66–68] Because conventional treatments do not always satisfactorily relieve these symptoms, and some patients may not be able to tolerate their side effects, standard therapies are sometimes combined with the best complementary modalities, which defines the practice of "integrative medicine."

However, the paucity of randomized controlled trials, of a heterogenous patient population across studies, and the resultant lack of an evidence base, have made it difficult to evaluate the utility of complementary and integrative therapies for treating cancer pain. This ambiguity exists even though more than two-thirds of Americans with chronic pain are now using complementary and alternative therapies,[54,69] and recent research suggests that these therapies have positive results on symptoms in oncology patients.[54]

The growing interest in complementary and integrative therapies is reflected in an extensive body of literature that examines the benefits of cognitive-behavioral interventions for managing acute and chronic pain,[67,70,71] although most studies of pain in cancer patients have examined the benefits of behavioral interventions to manage acute pain.

▶ Psychosocial interventions

Recent publications have examined the benefits of psychosocial interventions for managing cancer pain. One meta-analysis found moderate efficacy for psychosocial interventions in managing pain.[72] Specifically, the use of relaxation-based interventions (e.g., progressive muscle relaxation alone or with guided imagery, or hypnosis) was associated with a modest to large effect on pain outcomes.[73–77] Hypnosis and multicomponent cognitive-behavioral interventions that include progressive muscle relaxation, relaxation training, and cognitive restructuring also have been found to be useful in managing cancer-related pain.[73–75,78]

▶ Mind-body techniques and pain

Complementary therapies, including massage, acupuncture, imagery/ hypnosis, and relaxation training, have been studied in clinical trials for pain and distress associated with lumbar puncture, catheter placement, bone marrow aspiration, endoscopy, and skin and breast biopsy.[79] Patients can be taught how to use some interventions, including self-hypnosis, guided imagery, and relaxation techniques, which can be used before and during painful or stressful procedures, chemotherapy, or radiation therapy. Patients who are anxious or fearful about pending procedures or who need an enhanced sense of control may be considered for these interventions.[79]

Most studies show beneficial effects for complementary therapies in ameliorating procedural pain.[79] One example is a study that compared oral mucositis pain levels in a total of 94 cancer patients in four groups receiving bone marrow transplants. The four groups were (1) treatment as usual control, (2) therapist support, (3) relaxation and imagery training, and (4) training in a package of cognitive-behavioral coping skills, which included relaxation and imagery. The results showed that patients who received either relaxation and imagery alone or patients who received the combination of cognitive-behavioral coping skills reported less pain than patients in the other two groups.[78]

The clinical setting is an important consideration in determining whether or not a complementary modality to prevent or relieve pain is appropriate. Although procedural pain can often be relieved with various alternative therapies, cancer pain often comes from the invasion of tissue by tumor or its pressure on nerves. In the acute setting, complementary therapies alone do not provide adequate pain control and are impractical, as using them typically requires multiple evaluations and interventions over a short period of time. After the acute phase of pain management, emphasis shifts to sustaining pain relief, controlling symptoms to minimize side effects, and to psychosocial issues and in these settings complementary modalities have been shown to have some utility.[79]

▶ Massage therapy and cancer pain

Massage therapy or reflexology (foot massage) may be beneficial for patients with chronic cancer pain and is increasingly available in hospital programs.[4] Reduction of pain and anxiety has been demonstrated in randomized, controlled trials and also has been demonstrated in the largest cancer data set reported. This intervention is safe when given by properly trained massage therapists.[79] Indeed, massage is progressively more used for symptom relief in patients with cancer. Approximately 20% of U.S. cancer patients seek massage therapy, and approximately 70% of UK hospices offer it. Massage is included in treatment guidelines such as those of the National Comprehensive Cancer Network, which recommends consideration of massage for refractory cancer pain. Research supports such recommendations. Several trials suggest that massage can reduce pain in cancer patients at varying stages of disease. In one relatively large study, 87 hospitalized cancer patients were randomized to massage therapy or to control on a crossover basis. Pain and anxiety scores fell by approximately 40% during massage compared with little or no change during control sessions. Massage therapy was superior to control against anxiety, nausea, fatigue, and general well-being in a randomized study of patients awaiting bone marrow transplantation.[80]

The efficacy of massage therapy is largely supported by evidence from small randomized trials. However, one study at Memorial Sloan-Kettering Cancer Center examined the outcome of using massage therapy in a large group of patients in which 1290 patients were treated over a 3-year period. Patients reported symptom severity pre- and postmassage therapy using 0–10 rating scales of pain, fatigue, stress/anxiety, nausea, depression, and "others." Changes in symptom scores and the modifying effects of patient status (in- or outpatient) and type of massage were analyzed. Symptom scores were reduced by approximately 50%, even for patients reporting high baseline scores. Specifically, the pain results ($N = 1284$ evaluable) were baseline = 3.6 (2.9); posttreatment = 1.9 (2.2); change = 1.7 (2); improvement = 40.2% (40.9). Pain results for patients rating pain at 4 or higher at baseline, the traditional threshold for considering a symptom at least as of moderate severity, were $N = 625$ with a 47.8% improvement in pain.[80] Outpatients improved about 10% more than inpatients. Benefits persisted, with outpatients experiencing no return toward baseline scores throughout the duration of 48 hours of follow-up. These data indicate that massage therapy is associated with substantive improvement in cancer patients' symptom scores.[80]

In a randomized, prospective, 2-year period, crossover intervention study, the authors tested the effects of therapeutic massage (MT) and healing touch (HT), compared to presence alone or standard care for inducing relaxation and reducing symptoms in 230 subjects. MT and HT lowered blood pressure, respiratory rate (RR), and heart rate (HR). MT lowered anxiety and HT lowered fatigue, and both lowered total mood disturbance. Pain ratings were lower after MT and HT, with 4-week nonsteroidal anti-inflammatory drug use less during MT. There were no effects on nausea. Presence reduced RR and HR but did not differ from standard care on any measure of pain, nausea, mood states, anxiety, or fatigue. The authors concluded that MT and HT are more effective than presence alone or standard care in reducing pain, mood disturbance, and fatigue in patients receiving cancer chemotherapy.[50]

Acupuncture and cancer pain

Much of the research into acupuncture focuses on diverse pain problems. There is clear evidence that needle acupuncture is efficacious for adult postoperative and chemotherapy nausea and vomiting, and probably for the nausea of pregnancy. There is substantiation of efficacy for postoperative dental pain. Other studies demonstrate pain relief for pain conditions such as menstrual cramps, tennis elbow, and fibromyalgia. Combined, these data suggest that acupuncture may have a more general effect on pain. However, other studies did not find efficacy for acupuncture in pain. Nevertheless,

one of the important advantages of acupuncture is that the incidence of adverse effects with its use is substantially lower than that of many drugs or other accepted medical procedures used for the same conditions.[9]

One focus of attention has been the role of endogenous opioids in acupuncture analgesia. Considerable evidence supports the claim that opioid peptides are released during acupuncture, and that the analgesic effects of acupuncture are at least partially explained by their actions. The fact that opioid antagonists such as naloxone hydrochloride reverse the analgesic effects of acupuncture further strengthens this hypothesis. Stimulation by acupuncture may also activate the hypothalamus and the pituitary gland, resulting in a broad spectrum of systemic effects. Alteration in the secretion of neurotransmitters and neurohormones and changes in the regulation of blood flow, both centrally and peripherally, have been documented. There is also proof of alterations in immune functions produced by acupuncture. Specifically which of these and other physiological changes mediate clinical effects remains unclear.[9,11]

Despite some promising findings, controversy over the utility of acupuncture for cancer pain continues, with some groups reporting success in ameliorating cancer pain. Alimi et al. found an observed reduction in pain intensity measured on the visual analog scale, which demonstrated a clear benefit from auricular acupuncture for cancer patients with pain, despite having been treated with a stable analgesic regimen,[81] although others reported no proven benefit.[11] Further research into this modality will be required before consensus regarding its utility can be realized.

Reflexology and cancer pain

Reflexology is a complementary therapeutic modality that has been used in an attempt to diminish cancer pain. Reflexology is a systematic application of pressure to specific reflex points on the feet (or hands) whose intention is to promote physiologic homeostasis. Working from the premise that reflex areas in the foot or hand are linked to principal organs and glands via energy zones, the application of pressure to these areas is presumed to release congestion and promote the flow of energy.

Thirty-six oncology inpatients participated in a third pilot study investigating the effects of foot reflexology in which equianalgesic dosing was calculated. Foot reflexology demonstrated a positive immediate effect for patients with metastatic cancer who reported pain, although there was no statistically significant effect at 3 or at 24 hours after intervention.[82]

In another study, 23 patients with breast or lung cancer received one 30-minute reflexology treatment and one 30-minute interval of standard care in a crossover design. Eleven breast cancer patients showed a significantly greater decrease in pain following foot reflexology than in response to usual care ($M = -0.41, SD = 0.71, p = 0.048$).[54]

Education and cancer pain

Educational interventions have been found to be effective, with decreased pain reported, greater knowledge about pain and analgesic medications, and in increasing the appropriate use of analgesic medications.[83–88] For example, Oliver and colleagues[85] showed that patients who received a 20-minute individualized education and coaching session reported lower pain levels 2 weeks later than patients who received standardized education on controlling pain delivered by a health educator. Finally, several randomized trials suggest that supportive expressive psychotherapy that included the use of relaxation training skills and self-hypnosis is useful for managing pain.[89,90]

A WELLNESS PROGRAM AT M. D. ANDERSON CANCER CENTER

The Place of Wellness at the University of Texas M. D. Anderson Cancer Center[91] is one example of how integrative medicine is being utilized in major cancer centers. The philosophy at M. D. Anderson is that physical healing is one part of total wellness. The Place of Wellness has created an environment where individuals with cancer can enhance their quality of life through programs that complement medical care and focus on the mind, body, and spirit.

The Place of Wellness offers more than 75 complementary therapy programs, most of which are free. These programs complement mainstream care to manage cancer-related symptoms, relieve stress, and enhance quality of life. The Place of Wellness is open to anyone touched by cancer, their family members and caregivers, whether or not they were treated at M. D. Anderson. No physician referral is required.

▶ Education programs

Education programs are integral to the Place of Wellness. These are detailed below:

Touch Therapy for Caregivers, Family, Friends, and Loved Ones. Participants are taught how to help their loved one through the cancer experience by learning the hands-on practice of several gentle touch massage techniques, how and when to use massage, and the benefits and precautions of massage for patients with cancer.

"Chemobrain"—Is it Real? Cancer patients often experience cognitive impairments from a combination of factors: the cancer itself, treatment side effects, other medications, and medical complications. These changes can reveal themselves as memory loss, decreased ability to multitask, and lack of sustained attention. This program teaches techniques that can be used to address these effects.

Weight Management Class. A monthly weight management class is aimed at patients desiring to achieve/maintain a healthier weight.

Reiki. This is an ancient Japanese hands-on healing method. Reiki is a controversial form of alternative medicine, which was popularized during the early twentieth century by Mikao Usui (*usui mikao* 臼井甕男) in Japan. Practitioners use a technique similar to the laying on of hands in which they claim that they act as channels for Reiki energy—which flows through their palms to specific parts of the body in order to facilitate healing. Scientific studies have not confirmed the existence of this specific Reiki energy, yet some patients report feeling various subjective and objective sensations: heat, cold, pressure, and so forth. While Reiki is comparatively rare in Japan today, it flourishes in the West and has gained a small following worldwide. Many scientists, healthcare workers, and others dispute the effectiveness of Reiki, claiming that it does not facilitate healing beyond that expected from the placebo effect.[92]

Healing Touch for Self and Others. This energy-based therapeutic approach to healing uses touch to influence the body's energy, and is thought to affect one's physical, mental, and spiritual health.

▶ Expressive arts

Creating a Lifebook. This program teaches the skills needed to organize a personal memory album, which celebrates the patient's life. Materials are supplied to first-time participants.

Journaling: The Healing Power of Story. This program focuses on the healing power of accessing stories from the patient's life and writing about them in a noncritical atmosphere. Each class is self-contained and offers different material as a springboard for memory.

▶ Meditation and prayer

Introduction to Centering Prayer. This ancient prayer practice is open to people of all faiths, beliefs, and denominations, and prepares its followers to receive the gift of God's presence, traditionally called *contemplative prayer*. It consists of responding to the Spirit of Christ by consenting to God's presence and action within. It furthers the development of contemplative prayer by quieting our faculties to cooperate with the gift of God's presence. Centering prayer facilitates the movement from more active modes of prayer—verbal, mental, or affective prayer—into a receptive prayer of resting in God. It emphasizes prayer as a personal relationship with God. At the same time, it is a discipline to foster and serve this relationship by a regular, daily practice of prayer. It is Trinitarian in its source, Christ-centered in its focus, and ecclesial in its effects; that is, it builds communities of faith.

Inner Joy: Meditation Techniques. The goal of this program is promoting relaxation and stress relief to its practitioners.

Meditation for Stress Relief. Teaches how to still the mind and achieve valuable rest, which can lead to decreased anxiety, and increased emotional stability through Transcendental Meditation.

The Art of Living. Participants are introduced to the ancient practices of yoga, meditation, and rhythms of breath. These are combined in ways to nourish all levels of body, mind, and spirit.

The Road Less Traveled: Cancer Path and Spiritual Journey. This is a group of fellow travelers on the path who join together in an open-ended discussion and exploration of cancer as a spiritual crossroads.

Tibetan Meditation. Teaches the participants how to access a deeper awareness through connecting the mind, body, and heart, and find one's "home." Participants learn to connect the mind and the breath in a good balance of relaxation, to bring peace and a release of tension.

▶ Movement

Pilates. The Pilates method is a physical fitness system that was developed in the early twentieth century by Joseph Pilates who called the method *The Art of Contrology*, which refers to the way the method encourages the use of the mind to *control* the muscles. It is an exercise program that focuses on the core postural muscles that help keep the body balanced and are essential to providing support for the spine. In particular, Pilates exercises teach awareness of neutral alignment of the spine and strengthening the deep postural muscles that support this alignment, which are important to help alleviate and prevent back pain. Pilates practitioners use their own bodies as "weights" in training, to build strength and flexibility; this is targeted without a focus on high-powered cardiovascular exercise. Today, Pilates is used in the rehabilitation process by many physical therapists.[92]

Chi Kung (Qigong). This ancient Chinese system of self-care uses meditation, breathing exercises, and gentle movements to promote deep relaxation, stress reduction, and energy balance. The philosophy of Qigong shares key concepts with TCM: (1)

the system of Qi channels, or meridians, that courses throughout the body; (2) the principle of yin-yang or "dynamic opposites" in the way the body functions; (3) the Five-Element relationship of organ systems.[93] *Tai Chi* is a soft and gentle exercise of the mind and body accomplished through mindful awareness and continuous fluid movement. It is a Chinese system of slow meditative physical exercise designed for relaxation and balance and health.

Yoga (Hatha/Restorative). These yogic exercises (popular in the West) combine difficult postures (which force the mind to withdraw from the outside world) with controlled breathing.

Awareness Through Movement. Through movement, patients learn how to improve their capacity to function in daily life and learn how the whole body cooperates in any movement.

Relaxation and Stress Management

Aromatherapy and Self-Massage. Consists of simple massage techniques to use on oneself or a partner and identifies which essential oils have therapeutic and healing uses to fit the needs of the patient. A comprehensive guide is given to participants along with aroma samples. Aromatherapy is the use of essential oils and other aromatic compounds from plants to affect someone's mood or health. The word was coined in the 1920s by the French chemist René Maurice Gattefossé.

The main branches of aromatherapy include home aromatherapy (self-treatment, perfume and cosmetic use) and medicinal aromatherapy. When aromatherapy is used for the treatment or prevention of disease, a precise knowledge of the bioactivity and synergy of the essential oils used, knowledge of the dosage and duration of application, as well as a medical diagnosis are required. At the scent level, the oils activate the limbic system and trigger emotions. When applied to the skin (commonly in form of "massage oils," i.e., 1%–10% solutions of essential oils in carrier oil), they activate thermal receptors and kill microbes and fungi. Internal application of essential oil preparations (mainly in pharmacological drugs; generally not recommended for home use) may stimulate the immune system, urine secretion, may have antiseptic activity, and so on.

Brief Relaxation Massages. A brief upper body massage is done for relaxation.

Guided Imagery for Healing. It is the art of creating mental images of reality or fantasy by using one's imagination and all five senses. The practice is widely used for relaxation, stress management, and reduction of pain and side effects from cancer treatment. This method is akin to creative visualization and led meditation. It is designed is to promote physical healing or attitudinal or behavioral changes. Practitioners act as prompters and orally outline scenes and/or give instructions on using imagery for self-help.

Relaxation Exercise. It teaches how self-hypnosis and progressive relaxation can help alleviate anxiety, sleep disturbances, fear, stress, pain, and tension. The exercises are geared to teach participants how to control these physiological "side effects" of cancer treatment.

Fatigue and Self-Hypnosis. Participants are taught how relaxation and self-hypnosis are used to manage the effects of fatigue.

Self-Hypnosis for Relaxation. Individuals with cancer often suffer from tremendous stress, which makes it difficult to cope and enjoy life. Through self-hypnosis techniques, they can get back the ability to relax, to reduce adverse symptoms from treatment, and to enhance their overall quality of life.

Stress Management Techniques. This program teaches relaxation procedures, diaphragmatic breathing, progressive muscle relaxation, and guided imagery.

Support groups

Professionally-led support groups at The Place of Wellness provide education, group discussion, guest speaker presentations, and supportive sharing for patients, family, and friends. These include the American Cancer Society's Man to Man Prostate Cancer Patient and Family Group, a group for caregivers, a bereavement group, a brain tumor networking group, a lung cancer network, ovarian cancer support group, sarcoma discussion group, and smoking cessation group.

Acupuncture

M. D. Anderson inpatients and outpatients can receive acupuncture services with a written physician order. There is a fee for service. Acupuncture involves placing metal needles in the skin to stimulate specific areas of the body. Research has shown that acupuncture can stimulate the natural healing process to restore health and well-being. Some cancer patients find that it relieves fatigue, pain, and nausea, and clear evidence supports the effectiveness of acupuncture to control chemotherapy-related nausea and vomiting.

Massage is also offered for a fee at The Place of Wellness. This service is for patients and their family members, and outpatients can self-refer for a brief relaxation massage but must obtain physician releases before scheduling a full-body massage. Inpatients may self-refer to receive bedside brief relaxation massage services in their rooms. Caregivers/family members may self-refer for chair massages or full-body massages. Full-body massage is fee for service, but chair massages are free. Certain criteria may prohibit patients from receiving massage therapy. Patients with certain medical conditions must consult with their physician and the massage therapist prior to any massage session. Some patients are not eligible for massage therapy, but others may be eligible with appropriate restrictions on pressure, site, and position.

Massage involves the stroking, kneading, or stretching of muscle groups. Evidence shows that massage can benefit many cancer patients and caregivers, physically and emotionally. Research suggests that stress-reduction programs tailored to the cancer setting, such as massage, may help patients cope with the side effects of treatment and improve quality of life after treatment. The use of massage therapy for cancer patients has become more common in recent years as a way to reduce pain, anxiety, and nausea.

Music therapy is an established healthcare profession that uses music to address the physical, emotional, cognitive, and social needs of individuals of all ages. The idea that music can improve health dates back to ancient Egypt, and current research indicates its positive effect on quality of life for children and adults with disabilities or illnesses such as cancer. Music therapy can be designed to promote wellness, manage stress, alleviate pain, express feelings, enhance memory, improve communication, and promote physical rehabilitation.

M. D. Anderson's Place of Wellness provides music therapy for children and adult inpatients, outpatients, and their families. A board-certified music therapist provides individual and group sessions, using passive listening or actively playing various musical instruments. No previous musical experience is required.

Music therapy is offered at no cost.

SELECTED RESOURCES

The *NIH Office of Dietary Supplements* supports research and disseminates results in the area of dietary supplements. It maintains a database of several hundred thousand references, the *International Bibliographic Information on Dietary Supplements (IBIDS).*

ConsumerLab.com ConsumerLab ("CL") provides independent test results and information to help consumers and healthcare professionals evaluate health, wellness, and nutrition products. It publishes results of its tests online, including listings of brands that have passed testing.

▶ Herbal supplements

American Botanical Council This nonprofit education and research organization disseminates science-based information promoting the safe and effective use of medicinal plants and phytomedicines.

Botanical.com This Web site contains an online version of "A Modern Herbal," by Mrs. Maud Grieve, originally published in 1931. Although written with the conventional wisdom of the early 1900s, it continues to be a leading authority on herbal harvesting and usage. An extensive index of common names for plants is accessible via the Web site's search engine.

ConsumerLab.com See information above.

Herb Research Foundation This member-supported nonprofit organization provides comprehensive scientific information on medicinal plants from a botanical library containing more than 300,000 scientific papers plus multiple online sources.

National Agricultural Library As part of the Agricultural Research Service of the U.S. Department of Agriculture (USDA), the National Agricultural Library (NAL), is one of four national libraries in the United States and a major international source for agriculture and related information.

Phytochemical and Ethnobotanical Databases Several searchable databases compiled by Jim Duke and Stephen Beckstrom-Sternberg, ethnobotanists of the USDA, include chemical constituents of plants.

Food and Drug Administration (FDA) Center for Food Safety and Applied Nutrition This center within the FDA is responsible for monitoring safety (voluntary adverse event reporting, labeling, claims, package inserts, and accompanying literature) and for taking action against any unsafe dietary supplement product after it reaches the market.

NAPRALERT is an acronym for NAtural PRoducts ALERT, the NIH Center for Botanical Dietary Supplements Research, located at the University of Illinois at Chicago. It is the largest relational database of world literature describing the ethnomedical or traditional uses, chemistry and pharmacology of plant, microbial and animal (primarily marine) extracts. This is a subscription/fee-based database.

▶ Complementary therapies, general

The *Alternative Medicine Homepage* Under the direction of a medical librarian of the Health Sciences Library System of the University of Pittsburgh, this Web site provides references to major bibliographic databases containing CAM resources.

Ask NOAH This New York Online Access to Help Web site provides key information in English and Spanish about numerous health topics including CAM therapies.

Operation Cure.All The Federal Trade Commission (FTC) is targeting false and unsubstantiated health claims on the Internet through Operation Cure.All—a law enforcement and consumer education campaign. This Web site offers information for consumers on how to recognize health fraud, guidance for businesses on how to market health products and services truthfully, and information about the FTC's initiatives.

National Center of Complementary and Alternative Medicine This center within the U.S. National Institutes of Health (NIH) supports rigorous research on CAM, trains researchers in CAM and disseminates information to the public and professionals on which CAM modalities work, which do not, and why.

American Association of Naturopathic Physicians (AANP) is the national professional society representing naturopathic physicians who are licensed or eligible for licensing as primary care providers.

American College for Advancement in Medicine This medical society is dedicated to educating physicians on the latest findings and emerging procedures in complementary/alternative medicine, with special emphasis on preventive/nutritional medicine for various diseases. (A prime interest for this organization is the use of chelation therapy.)

Center for Mind-Body Medicine offers experiences, perspectives, and tools for healing.

Duke University Medical Center *Cancer Patient Education Program: Complementary/Alternative Care* A Cancer Patient's Guide to Complementary and Alternative Medicine, 2nd ed. Editors: Kerry Harwood, RN, MSN, Director, and Christine Pickett, MS, RD, Cancer Center of Santa Barbara.

QuackWatch A member of Consumer Federation of America, Quackwatch is a nonprofit corporation whose purpose is to combat health-related frauds, myths, fads, and fallacies.

▶ Complementary therapies, cancer

American Cancer Society The cancer information, treatment options, and resources on this Web site include an extensive discussion of *Complementary and Alternative Therapies.*

Cancer Information Service of the National Cancer Institute (NCI) As the Federal Government's principal agency for cancer research and training, the National Cancer Institute conducts and supports research, training, health information dissemination, and other programs concerning cancer.

Commonweal Cancer Help Program Supportive programs for health professionals and people with cancer. Programs for patients emphasize informed choices for patients in integrating conventional cancer treatment with complementary treatment. Programs for physicians include CME credit workshops on relationship-centered care to find deeper satisfaction and meaning in the day-to-day practice of medicine.

The *National Cancer Institute Office of Cancer Complementary & Alternative Medicine* This office within the NCI provides reviews of some complementary therapies for cancer. It also reviews sets of *best cases* submitted by clinics providing complementary therapies.

Rosenthal Center for Alternative/Complementary Medicine, Columbia University Specializing in women's health, this center provides evidence-based reviews in addition to notices of current and proposed clinical trials.

Steve Dunn's Cancer Information Page This knowledgeable cancer survivor provides patients with tools for learning about the fundamentals of cancer, comprehending survival assessments, assessing both conventional and complementary research, and reading about other cancer survivors.

Recommended by the Cancer Patient Education Network (CPEN) of the National Cancer Institute (revised October 2000).

▶ Complementary therapies, legal issues

The Complementary and Alternative Medicine Law Blog provides general information on current legal developments pertaining to CAM, such as licensure and credentialing, dietary supplements, malpractice, and professional liability and ethical issues.

Texas State Board of Medical Examiners Standards for Physicians Practicing Integrative and Complementary Medicine.

▶ Complementary therapies, clinical trials

National Cancer Institute (NCI) clinical trials in complementary alternative/integrative therapies are listed at the Web site of the NCI's information service, *CancerNet*, (Step 1, choose all trials; Step 2, narrow search to Modality, complementary and alternative medicine.)

▶ Understanding cancer, the immune system, angiogenesis, and estrogen receptors

Recently developed concepts in cancer and its treatment are described by the National Cancer Institute series, *Science Behind the News*.

The resources listed above were taken from the Complementary/Integrative Web site found on M. D. Anderson (http://www.mdanderson.org/).

REFERENCES

1. Tasaki K, Maskarinec G, Shumay DM, et al. Communication between physicians and cancer patients about complementary and alternative medicine: exploring patients' perspectives. *Psychooncology.* 2002; 11:212.
2. Lafferty W, Bellas A, Baden A, et al. The use of complementary and alternative medical providers by insured cancer patients in Washington State. *Cancer,* 2004;100:1522.
3. Richardson MA, Sanders T, Palmer JL, et al. Complementary/alternative medicine use in a comprehensive cancer center and the implications for oncology. *J Clin Oncol.* 2000;18:2505.
4. Mind-Body Medicine: An Overview. http://nccam.nih.gov/health/backgrounds/mindbody.htm. [Cited December 27, 2005].
5. Kaplan G. Acupuncture. In: Leskowitz E, ed. *Complementary and Alternative Medicine in Rehabilitation.* St. Louis: Churchill Livingstone; 2003.
6. Kanakura Y, Niwa K, Kometani K, et al. Effectiveness of acupuncture and moxibustion treatment for lymphedema following intrapelvic lymph node dissection: a preliminary report. *Am J Chin Med.* 2002;30:37.
7. Vas J, Perea-Milla E, Mendez C. Acupuncture and moxibustion as an adjunctive treatment for osteoarthritis of the knee-a large case series. *Acupunct Med.* 2004;22:23.
8. Wang S, Wei H. Clinical application of moxibustion. *J Tradit Chin Med.* 2004;24:24–25.
9. Acupuncture. *JAMA.* 1998;280:1518.
10. Ernst E. Complementary therapies in palliative cancer care. *Cancer.* 2001;91:2181.
11. Lee H, Schmidt K, Ernst E. Acupuncture for the relief of cancer-related pain—a systematic review. *Eur J Pain.* 2005;9:437.
12. Paterson C, Britten N. Acupuncture as a complex intervention: a holistic model. *J Altern Complement Med.* 2004;10:791.
13. Hankey A. The scientific value of Ayurveda. *J Altern Complement Med.* 2005;11:221.
14. Padma TV. Ayurveda. *Nature.* 2005;436:486.
15. Patwardhan B, Warude D, Pushpangadan P, et al. Ayurveda and traditional Chinese medicine: a comparative overview. *Evid Based Complement Alternat Med.* 2005;2:465.
16. Boon HS, Cherkin DC, Erro J, et al. Practice patterns of naturopathic physicians: results from a random survey of licensed practitioners in two US States. *BMC Complement Altern Med.* 2004;4:14.
17. Girgis A, Adams J, Sibbritt D. The use of complementary and alternative therapies by patients with cancer. *Oncol Res.* 2005;15:281.
18. Novak KL, Chapman GE. Oncologists' and naturopaths' nutrition beliefs and practices. *Cancer Pract.* 2001;9:141.
19. Pizzorno JE. Naturopathic medicine—a 10-year perspective (from a 35-year view). *Altern Ther Health Med.* 2005;11:24.
20. Smith MJ, Logan AC. Naturopathy. *Med Clin North Am.* 2002;86:173.
21. Caulfield T, DeBow S. A systematic review of how homeopathy is represented in conventional and CAM peer reviewed journals. *BMC Complement Altern Med.* 2005;5:12.
22. Endrizzi C, Rossi E, Crudeli L, et al. Harm in homeopathy: aggravations, adverse drug events or medication errors? *Homeopathy.* 2005;94:233.
23. Ernst E. Is homeopathy a clinically valuable approach? *Trends Pharmacol Sci.* 2005;26:547.
24. Sato DY, Wal R, de Oliveira CC, et al. Histopathological and immunophenotyping studies on normal and sarcoma 180-bearing mice treated with a complex homeopathic medication. *Homeopathy.* 2005;94:26.
25. Gordon JS, Edwards DM. MindBodySpirit Medicine. *Semin Oncol Nurs.* 2005;21:154.
26. Astin JA. Why patients use alternative medicine: results of a national study. *JAMA.* 1998;279:1548.
27. Astin JA, Shapiro SL, Eisenberg DM, et al. Mind-body medicine: state of the science, implications for practice. *J Am Board Fam Pract.* 2003;16:131.
28. Wolsko PM, Eisenberg DM, Davis RB, et al. Use of mind-body medical therapies. *J Gen Intern Med.* 2004;19:43.
29. Energy Medicine: An Overview. http://nccam.nih.gov/health/backgrounds/energymed.htm. [Cited December 27, 2005].
30. DiNucci EM. Energy healing: a complementary treatment for orthopaedic and other conditions. *Orthop Nurs.* 2005;24:259.
31. Johnson M, Waite L, Nindl G. Noninvasive treatment of inflammation using electromagnetic fields: current and emerging therapeutic potential. *Biomed Sci Instrum.* 2004;40:469.
32. Mackay N, Hansen S, McFarlane O. Autonomic nervous system changes during Reiki treatment: a preliminary study. *J Altern Complement Med.* 2004;10:1077.
33. Olalde Rangel J. The systemic theory of living systems. Part IV: Systemic Medicine—The Praxis. *Evid Based Complement Alternat Med.* 2005;2:429.
34. Olalde Rangel J. The systemic theory of living systems and relevance to CAM: the theory (Part III). *Evid Based Complement Alternat Med.* 2005;2:267.
35. Olalde Rangel J. The systemic theory of living systems and relevance to CAM: the theory (Part II). *Evid Based Complement Alternat Med.* 2005;2:129.
36. Olalde Rangel J. The systemic theory of living systems and relevance to CAM: Part I: the theory. *Evid Based Complement Alternat Med.* 2005;2:13.
37. Burden B, Herron-Marx S, Clifford C. The increasing use of reiki as a complementary therapy in specialist palliative care. *Int J Palliat Nurs.* 2005;11:248.
38. Cook CA, Guerrerio JF, Slater VE. Healing touch and quality of life in women receiving radiation treatment for cancer: a randomized controlled trial. *Altern Ther Health Med.* 2004;10:34.
39. Kelly AE, Sullivan P, Fawcett J, et al. Therapeutic touch, quiet time, and dialogue: perceptions of women with breast cancer. *Oncol Nurs Forum.* 2004;31:625.
40. Weze C, Leathard HL, Grange J, et al. Evaluation of healing by gentle touch in 35 clients with cancer. *Eur J Oncol Nurs.* 2004;8:40.
41. Palmer RF, Katerndahl D, Morgan-Kidd J. A randomized trial of the effects of remote intercessory prayer: interactions with personal beliefs on problem-specific outcomes and functional status. *J Altern Complement Med.* 204;10:438.

42. Reece K, Schwartz GE, Brooks AJ, et al. Positive well-being changes associated with giving and receiving Johrei healing. *J Altern Complement Med.* 2005;11:455.

43. Dennis J. Alexander technique for chronic asthma. *Cochrane Database Syst Rev 2*: CD000995, 2000.

44. Jain S, Janssen K, DeCelle S. Alexander technique and Feldenkrais method: a critical overview. *Phys Med Rehabil Clin N Am.* 2004;15:811.

45. Stallibrass C, Sissons P, Chalmers C. Randomized controlled trial of the Alexander technique for idiopathic Parkinson's disease. *Clin Rehabil.* 2002;16:695.

46. Carter B. Clients' experiences of frozen shoulder and its treatment with Bowen technique. *Complement Ther Nurs Midwifery.* 2002;8:204.

47. Evans RCRosner AL. Alternatives in cancer pain treatment: the application of chiropractic care. *Semin Oncol Nurs.* 2005;21:184.

48. Corbin L. Safety and efficacy of massage therapy for patients with cancer. *Cancer Control.* 2005;12:158.

49. Field T, Hernandez-Reif M, Diego M, et al. Cortisol decreases and serotonin and dopamine increase following massage therapy. *Int J Neurosci.* 2005;115:1397.

50. Post-White J, Kinney ME, Savik K, et al. Therapeutic massage and healing touch improve symptoms in cancer. *Integr Cancer Ther.* 2003; 2:332.

51. Wilkie DJ, Kampbell J, Cutshall S, et al. Effects of massage on pain intensity, analgesics and quality of life in patients with cancer pain: a pilot study of a randomized clinical trial conducted within hospice care delivery. *Hosp J.* 2000;15:31.

52. Kohara H, Miyauchi T, Suehiro Y, et al. Combined modality treatment of aromatherapy, footsoak, and reflexology relieves fatigue in patients with cancer. *J Palliat Med.* 2004;7:791.

53. Milligan M, Fanning M, Hunter S, et al. Reflexology audit: patient satisfaction, impact on quality of life and availability in Scottish hospices. *Int J Palliat Nurs.* 2002;8:489.

54. Stephenson NL, Weinrich SP, Tavakoli AS. The effects of foot reflexology on anxiety and pain in patients with breast and lung cancer. *Oncol Nurs Forum.* 2000;27:67.

55. Mehling WE, DiBlasi Z, Hecht F. Bias control in trials of bodywork: a review of methodological issues. *J Altern Complement Med.* 2005;11:333.

56. Esteve Torres A. [Tui-Na, an oriental massage]. *Rev Enferm.* 2005;28:33.

57. . Biologically Based Practices: An Overview. http://nccam.nih.gov/health/backgrounds/biobasedprac.htm. [Cited December 27, 2005].

58. http://www.naturalstandard.com/. [Cited December 28, 2005].

59. Jonas W. Advising patients on the use of complementary and alternative medicine. *Appl Psychophysiol Biofeedback.* 2001;26:205.

60. Cartwright T, Torr R. Making sense of illness: the experiences of users of complementary medicine. *J Health Psychol.* 2005;10:559.

61. Burstein HJ. Discussing complementary therapies with cancer patients: what should we be talking about? *J Clin Oncol.* 2000;18:2501.

62. Ben-Arye E, Frenkel MMargalit RS. Approaching complementary and alternative medicine use in patients with cancer: questions and challenges. *J Ambul Care Manage.* 2004;27:53.

63. Fallowfield L, Jenkins V. Effective communication skills are the key to good cancer care. *Eur J Cancer.* 1999;35:1592.

64. Maguire P. Improving communication with cancer patients. *Eur J Cancer.* 1999;35:1415.

65. Frenkel M, Ben-Arye E, Baldwin CD, et al. Approach to communicating with patients about the use of nutritional supplements in cancer care. *South Med J.* 2005;98:289.

66. Cleeland CS, Gonin R, Hatfield AK, et al. Pain and its treatment in outpatients with metastatic cancer. *N Engl J Med.* 1994;330:592–596.

67. Cohen L, Serlin RC, Mendoza TR, et al. When is cancer pain mild, moderate or severe? Grading pain severity by its interference with function. *Pain.* 1995;61:277–284.

68. Zech DF, Grond S, Lynch J, et al. Validation of World Health Organization Guidelines for cancer pain relief: a 10-year prospective study. *Pain.* 1995; 63:65.

69. http://www.painfoundation.org/. [Cited December 28, 2005].

70. Jensen MP, Turner JA, Romano JM, et al. Coping with chronic pain: a critical review of the literature. *Pain.* 1991;47:249.

71. Keefe FJ, Salley AN, Jr, Lefebvre JC. Coping with pain: conceptual concerns and future directions. *Pain.* 1992;51:131.

72. Cohen L, Meyer TJ, Mark MM. Effects of psychosocial interventions with adult cancer patients: A meta-analysis of randomized experiments. *Health Psychol.* 1995;14:101.

73. Arathuzik D. Effects of cognitive-behavioral strategies on pain in cancer patients. *Cancer Nurs.* 1994;17:207.

74. Cohen L, Syrjala KL, Cummings C, et al. Hypnosis or cognitive behavioral training for the reduction of pain and nausea during cancer treatment: A controlled clinical trial. *Pain.* 1992;48:137–146.

75. Gaston-Johansson F, Fall-Dickson JM, Nanda J, et al. The effectiveness of the comprehensive coping strategy program on clinical outcomes in breast cancer autologous bone marrow transplantation. *Cancer Nurs.* 2000;23:277.

76. Graffam S, Johnson A. A comparison of two relaxation strategies for the relief of pain and its distress. *J Pain Symptom Manage.* 1987;2:229.

77. Sloman R. Relaxation and the relief of cancer pain. *Nurs Clin North Am.* 1995;30:697.

78. Syrjala KL, Donaldson GW, Davis MW, et al. Relaxation and imagery and cognitive-behavioral training reduce pain during cancer treatment: a controlled clinical trial. *Pain.* 1995;63:189.

79. Deng G, Cassileth BR. Integrative oncology: complementary therapies for pain, anxiety, and mood disturbance. *CA Cancer J Clin.* 2005; 55:109.

80. Cassileth BR, Vickers AJ. Massage therapy for symptom control: outcome study at a major cancer center. *J Pain Symptom Manage.* 2004; 28:244.

81. Alimi D, Rubino C, Pichard-Leandri E, et al. Analgesic effect of auricular acupuncture for cancer pain: a randomized, blinded, controlled trial. *J Clin Oncol.* 2003;21:4120.

82. Stephenson N, Dalton JA, Carlson J. The effect of foot reflexology on pain in patients with metastatic cancer. *Appl Nurs Res.* 2003;16:284.

83. Ward S, Donovan HS, Owen B, et al. An individualized intervention to overcome patient-related barriers to pain management in women with gynecologic cancers. *Res Nurs Health.* 2000;23:393.

84. Rimer B, Levy MH, Keintz MK, et al. Enhancing cancer pain control regimens through patient education. *Patient Educ Couns.* 1987;10:267.

85. Oliver JW, Kravitz RL, Kaplan SH, et al. Individualized patient education and coaching to improve pain control among cancer outpatients. *J Clin Oncol.* 2001;19:2206.

86. de Wit R, van Dam F, Zandbelt L, et al. A pain education program for chronic cancer pain patients: follow-up results from a randomized controlled trial. *Pain.* 1997;73:55.

87. Clotfelter CE. The effect of an educational intervention on decreasing pain intensity in elderly people with cancer. *Oncol Nurs Forum.* 1999;26:27.

88. Benor DE, Delbar V, Krulik T. Measuring impact of nursing intervention on cancer patients' ability to control symptoms. *Cancer Nurs.* 1998;21:320.

89. Spiegel D, Bloom JR. Group therapy and hypnosis reduce metastatic breast carcinoma pain. *Psychosom Med.* 1983;45:333.

90. Goodwin PJ, Leszcz M, Ennis M, et al. The effect of group psychosocial support on survival in metastatic breast cancer. *N Engl J Med.* 2001;345:1719.

91. http://www.mdanderson.org/departments/wellness/. [Cited December 29, 2005].

92. http://en.wikipedia.org/wiki/Reiki. [Cited January 6, 2006].

93. Leskowitz E. *Complimentary and Alternative Medicine in Rehabilitation.* St. Louis, Missouri: Churchill Livingstone; 2003.

94. Sharma RA, McLelland HR, Hill KA, et al. Pharmacodynamic and pharmacokinetic study of oral Curcuma extract in patients with colorectal cancer. *Clin Cancer Res.* 2001;7:1894.

Cancer Rehabilitation

Albert Hwang
Ki Shin

As previously stated in this text, the causes of cancer pain are numerous, with treatments directed at specific causes. Rehabilitation interventions for cancer pain are no exception, and can be useful in treating cancer-related musculoskeletal pain and neuropathic pain. The most prevalent problems seen in patients with cancer that can be addressed by appropriate rehabilitation care are functional impairments, pain, and psychological disturbances.[1]

Equally important to cancer patients as treating pain, cancer rehabilitation works to correct or minimize the disability associated with cancer and its treatments. In patients with advanced cancer, inpatient cancer rehabilitation can maximize quality of life by decreasing the burden of providing assistance for the cancer patient. The more patients can do for themselves, the more personal dignity they are able to maintain and the less help they require from those around them. For patients receiving active treatment, rehabilitation can address asthenia, impaired mobility, impaired self-care, and safe discharge issues. Examples of outpatient rehabilitation interventions include treatment of shoulder pain, lymphedema, and fatigue. Return-to-work and disability evaluations are important survivorship issues, which can also be addressed by the rehabilitation team.

CANCER REHABILITATION, GENERAL CONCEPTS

Physical rehabilitation is the process of returning a person to a higher level of function following illness, injury, or another debilitating event. The field of cancer rehabilitation continues to grow as advances in treatment increase cancer survivorship. For many, cancer is a chronic disease process leading to progressive disability. Cancer treatments, including chemotherapy, radiation therapy, and surgery, can contribute to functional deficits. Healthcare professionals should be aware of the benefits of rehabilitation for cancer patients. Early referrals can minimize disability early in the disease and throughout its course.

In 1978, Lehman identified functional problems in the cancer patient that could be improved with rehabilitation.[2] These include psychological impairments, generalized weakness, impairments in activities of daily living (ADLs), pain, impaired gait/ambulation, disposition issues, neurologic impairments, vocational assessments, impaired nutrition, lymphedema management, musculoskeletal difficulties, swallowing dysfunction, impaired communication, and skin management. According to Lehman, barriers to rehabilitation in the cancer patient include lack of identification of rehabilitation problems, lack of appropriate referral, patient too ill, prognosis too limited, and unavailable cancer rehabilitation services.

Patients with many different types of cancer can have impairments and functional deficits that are amenable to rehabilitation measures. In 2002, 403 patients were admitted to the University of Texas M. D. Anderson Cancer Center's inpatient rehabilitation unit. Primary tumors included brain and spine (28%), hematologic (14%), genitourinary (14%), lung (10%), orthopedic (8%), gastrointestinal (GI) (6%), breast (5%), head and neck (4%), and other (11%). Brain and spine tumor patients commonly had the rehabilitation diagnoses of hemiparesis or spinal cord injury. Hematologic patients' rehabilitation diagnoses were more frequently asthenia and dyspnea on exertion. Most of the patients admitted to the M. D. Anderson rehabilitation unit had the rehabilitation diagnosis of gait abnormality.

Many cancer patients have concurrent medical, physical, social, financial, and psychological issues. These contribute to disability and loss of function. Addressing these multiple problems is best accomplished with a comprehensive interdisciplinary team. Effective teamwork and communication are necessary for successful rehabilitation outcomes. Team members can include a physical therapist, occupational therapist, orthotist/prosthotist, speech therapist, case manager, social worker, rehabilitation nursing, nutritionist, and physiatrist. Implied in this approach is an understanding of each team member's role, reinforcing patient skills, and assisting in problem solving to achieve patient-defined goals. The active participation of oncologists, surgeons, pain specialists, and other medical specialists who can assist in managing the complex medical issues with which these patients present is also important for rehabilitation success.

Dietz classified four stages of rehabilitation needs specific to cancer patients: (1) preventive rehabilitation with the focus on limiting impairments or disabilities resulting from anticipated or continuing conditions or procedures, including deconditioning due to extended bed rest or isolation. Preventive therapies are initiated before or immediately after a treatment to prevent loss of function or disability; (2) restorative rehabilitation in a cured or controlled patient with disability has the goal of returning the patient to his or her previous level of function, such as before being given corticosteroid therapy; (3) supportive rehabilitation efforts are directed toward increasing self-care and mobility in patients with progressive cancer and disability; (4) palliative rehabilitation attempts to maintain comfort, function, and support, and to decrease the dependence of patients with advanced or end-stage cancer.[3]

Cancer rehabilitation can successfully occur in different settings depending on the extent of the cancer, the extent of the disability, and the resources available. For ambulatory patients with focal weakness, outpatient physical and occupational therapy can improve mobility and self-care issues. For patients requiring hospitalization after chemotherapy, surgery, or complications of treatment, inpatient physical and occupational therapies can address deficits in mobility and self-care to ensure a safe discharge. For patients with multiple rehabilitation issues, acute inpatient rehabilitation using a comprehensive interdisciplinary team may be necessary to coordinate mobility, self-care, cognitive, nutritional, and home care issues for discharge.

Experienced primary care physicians, oncologists, and surgeons can coordinate appropriate rehabilitation care for many of their cancer patients. However, the time and resources necessary to put together the appropriate cancer rehabilitation team are often not available. Rehabilitation for inpatient cancer patients with complicated problems and those with advanced disease may need the assistance of a cancer rehabilitation physician and the efforts of the interdisciplinary team in a tertiary cancer center to adequately address the rehabilitation issues. Due to the acute medical and surgical problems of advanced cancer patients, it is important to have ready access to oncologists, oncologic surgeons, and medical consultants for urgent evaluation and treatment. End-stage cancer rehabilitation can occur in a rehabilitation unit, palliative care unit, or hospice where symptom control and caregiver education needs can be addressed. With its emphasis on quality of life at any stage of disease, cancer rehabilitation can be arranged at home if safety issues are appropriately dealt with.

A challenge in cancer rehabilitation is the need to balance the benefits of therapy with the physiologic effects of tumor progression and aggressive cancer treatments. In patients with advanced disease, further rehabilitation therapies may not make appreciable differences in function, and can prevent patients from doing things by using limited patient time and energy resources. Similar to other treatments for advanced cancer patients, it is important to recognize when "enough is enough."

Rehabilitation is routine after common orthopedic procedures, including fracture repair, joint replacement, and amputation. Similar procedures are performed for treatment of primary bone tumors and metastatic bone disease. The rehabilitation treatments are similar, with specific restrictions depending upon the site, procedure, and extent of disease. Unlike tumor-specific or pathology-specific treatment, rehabilitation treatment can be site-specific, geared to functional deficits that are unique to the site of tumor involvement, surgical repair, or resection. With surgical advances, including limb salvage and partial resection with modular prostheses, rehabilitation is tailored to focus on intact and unstable structures, preventing further complications, and maximizing recovery of function. In addition, surgery can be preceded or followed by radiation treatment, which can delay wound healing, promote fibrosis, and contribute to joint contractures. Dedicated stretching and range of motion exercises, combined with modalities such as heat or ultrasound, can lessen these effects.

Some specific concerns unique to cancer rehabilitation that may not be present in traditional rehabilitation patients include precautions with thrombocytopenic patients, neutropenic patients, and patients with impending pathologic fractures. Cancer patients with neutropenia are more susceptible to opportunistic infection. Interactions with healthcare providers and other patients must be taken with special care directed toward hygiene and/or contact isolation. Similarly, patients with thrombocytopenia must be more cautious with fall precautions and trauma avoidance. Patients with cancers that have a propensity toward bone involvement (prostate, lung, renal, breast, multiple myeloma, thyroid, and so on) must be monitored closely for pain symptoms that could indicate the presence of an occult fracture. The presence of therapists and nurses experienced in these issues is important for successful outcomes in the rehabilitation of patients with advanced cancer.

A comprehensive rehabilitation patient evaluation begins with a traditional history and physical. Attention is paid to the cardiac, pulmonary, neurologic, and musculoskeletal systems to assess tolerance for activity and exercise. The patient's functional status is evaluated for mobility, self-care, and cognition. Accessibility of the patient's home, car, and work is determined. The patient's social situation is reviewed and specifically, attention is paid to who will be providing physical assistance for the patient at discharge. Frequently, a review of the patient's medical coverage and financial resources is necessary because equipment and services must be obtained after the patient is discharged. After this specialized evaluation, the patient's rehabilitation goals are determined, with the primary outcome measure being a safe discharge.

Improving patient function is primarily accomplished in therapy. Intact cognition, a willingness to participate, and patient motivation are each required for productive therapy. Therapy time is frequently used to educate the family and other caregivers in hygiene, transfer, and mobility techniques to help facilitate safe care. According to Mackey in 2000, family members as caregivers need to be assured that they will be taught how to safely care for and move their loved one.[4] They also need to be assured that they will not be asked to do more than they are physically or emotionally capable of doing. Proper education can decrease caregiver stress associated with providing care and the patient's concern about being a burden. Unfortunately for some patients, progressive disease leads to increasing disability, which requires rising levels of assistance from caregivers and family members. Ongoing rehabilitation and family education may be required during this transition.

Frequently, patients are bone marrow-suppressed after chemotherapy or radiation treatments, with depressed white blood cell counts, hemoglobin, and platelet counts. Adequate oxygenation to peripheral muscle is necessary to increase strength and endurance and recover from major surgery. Although relatively rare, spontaneous hemorrhage from thrombocytopenia has been documented.[5] The increased risk of falls in a hospitalized surgical or postchemotherapy patient can also increase the chance of significant bleeding. Hence, transfusions of red blood cells and platelets are frequently used to maximize oxygenation and reduce bleeding risk. Immunosuppression from chemotherapy, radiation treatments, steroids, and the cancer itself may increase the risk of infection in the cancer rehabilitation patient. This may be life-threatening and require systemic support and antibiotics or be relatively limited, causing only general fatigue and weakness. Diligent clinical awareness on the rehabilitation floor, a low threshold for laboratory and radiographic evaluations, and early initiation of antibiotic treatment can help minimize this risk.

Rehabilitation is an anabolic process. It strengthens muscle groups and increases endurance. Cancer is a catabolic process. It increases energy and nutritional requirements with increasing tumor burden. In addition, patients who have undergone major surgery have increased metabolic needs. If adequate nutrition is not maintained, efficient rehabilitation is impossible. Hence, nutritional supplementation either orally or enterally is often necessary in this patient population. Cancer patients frequently have symptoms of anorexia, nausea, or early satiety. Medications can be used to improve GI symptoms, improve GI motility, and stimulate the appetite.

Constipation is a frequent side effect of opiates and can be exacerbated by inactivity, neurologic dysfunction, decreased mood, fatigue, and pain. It can also contribute to anorexia, nausea, and satiety. A comprehensive bowel program may include stool softeners, suppositories, and enemas, and is necessary to maintain adequate bowel function. However, it is important to remember that rectal medications are contraindicated in the profoundly neutropenic or thrombocytopenic patient.

TRANSFER TRAINING

One of the most simple and practical rehabilitation techniques is the transfer. A transfer is a change in station or position; for example, to change from sitting in bed to standing. A person must transfer to get into a wheelchair or into a car. Patients cannot effectively mobilize until this can be accomplished. Depending on the patient's level of ability, a transfer may be sit to stand, stand and pivot, with a sliding board, or with a lift. After basic transfers are mastered, ambulation is frequently the next goal to increase mobility.

SHOULDER PAIN IN THE HEMIPARETIC PATIENT

Shoulder subluxation is often seen in hemiparetic patients and can cause significant shoulder pain. The humeral head is frequently subluxed inferiorly. Subluxation can be caused by weakness in the shoulder stabilizer muscles, including the supraspinatus muscle. A differential diagnosis for shoulder pain in a hemiparetic patient can also include complex regional pain syndrome, traction injury of the brachial plexus, rotator cuff tendonitis or tear, subacromial or subdeltoid bursitis, adhesive capsulitis, and heterotopic ossification. Diagnosis is made through physical examination and radiographic evaluation. Radiographic evaluation can also be used to quantify the amount of subluxation. The acromiohumeral interval is compared on each side with the arms in an unsupported position. Treatment of hemiparetic shoulder subluxation can include arm positioning, physical modalities such as ultrasound, and range of motion exercises. An arm sling can be useful for proper positioning and posture during ambulation. Use of a sling is discouraged when the patient is seated due to possible contribution to shoulder joint contracture. Additional interventions include biofeedback and functional electrical stimulation.

LYMPHEDEMA

Lymphedema occurs when lymph nodes or lymphatic vessels are resected or traumatized. Protein-laden lymph fluid accumulates in the subcutaneous tissues. The staging of lymphedema is based on a three-stage scale. In stage I, there is early accumulation of a lymph fluid that subsides with limb elevation. Pitting of the extremity may be present. In stage II, limb elevation alone rarely reduces tissue swelling and pitting is present. In late stage II, fibrosis is present and there may or may not be pitting of the extremity. Stage III is characterized by lymphostatic elephantiasis. Pitting is absent and the trophic skin is characteristically acanthotic with warty overgrowth. Tension and heaviness in the affected extremity is often reported followed by pain and reduced mobility. Numbness and a subjective reporting of decreased strength are also common. In addition, peripheral nerves can be compressed from swelling, causing neuropathic pain in the extremity. Recurrent erysipelas is another problem in the lymphedema patient, which is the result of a streptococcal cellulitis. This condition is characterized by localized erythema,

enhanced skin warmth, and, potentially, fever, nausea, and chills. Prompt evaluation is crucial and subsequent treatment with antibiotic therapy is warranted to prevent systemic illness. Treatment for lymphedema includes manual lymphatic drainage, compressive bandaging, fitting with compression sleeves, gloves or other garments, and specific exercises. It also involves a dedicated stretching and range of motion program for the affected joints and muscles. Assessment of limb volume is made before, during, and after treatment. This can be accomplished via water displacement, circumferential measurement using the truncated cone formulation, or perometer. Finally, it is important to educate the lymphedema patient in preventative measures. These should include a program of routine skin inspection, avoiding extremes in heat and cold, avoiding venipuncture, acupuncture, or injections on the affected side, and limiting excessive resistance exercise to the involved extremity.

SPASTICITY

Spasticity is defined as velocity-dependent resistance to passive movement across a joint. It is caused by increased muscle tone and is one of the positive findings of the upper motor neuron syndrome and can result from injury or tumor involvement of the brain or spinal cord. Spasticity affects gait and activities of daily living, can cause pain, and can contribute to joint contractures. However, spasticity can, at times, be beneficial to the rehabilitation patient. For example, a patient with hemiparesis may use knee extensor spasticity as muscle tone for weight bearing to assist in transfers.

Treatments for spasticity include physical and medical interventions. Proper positioning, passive range of motion exercises, serial casting, splints, and braces are commonly used physical interventions. Pharmacologic therapy includes medications such as tizanidine, dantrolene sodium, and baclofen. Tizanidine or dantrolene are often recommended for treating spasticity from primary brain pathology. The use of baclofen in patients with spasticity secondary to brain pathology is limited by its potential side effect of drowsiness. Spinal cord injury-associated spasticity is treated with baclofen and sometimes tizanidine. For severe spasticity associated with either brain or spinal cord injury, chemical neurolysis, botulinum toxin, and intrathecal baclofen are widely used.

BREAKTHROUGH PAIN IN REHABILITATION

Rehabilitation therapies and exercise can contribute to pain in cancer patients by causing activity-associated *breakthrough* pain. This is especially true in postoperative cancer patients or patients with extensive tumor burden. Short-acting oral, transmucosal, intravenous, and intrathecal preparations of narcotics are used to help patients tolerate rehabilitation therapies. These may be administered in addition to the regular dosing of *patient-controlled analgesia* or long-acting oral or transdermal preparations. Adequate pain control during intensive rehabilitation efforts in patients with significant tumor burden can become a balance between the detrimental effects of inactivity and the side effects of the pain medications.

CANCER-RELATED FATIGUE

In cancer patients, symptom burden is common, with as many as 80% of patients complaining of pain during the course of their disease,

90% with fatigue, 80% unintended weight loss, 90% nausea and vomiting, 80% confusion/agitation, 50% dyspnea, and 25% anxiety. Interestingly, these symptoms are also contributing causes for each other; for example, fatigue is worsened by pain, weight loss, nausea, and so on, and pain is exacerbated by fatigue, confusion, and agitation. Research has shown that tumor necrosis factor and other cytokines contribute to the expression of these common symptoms. A comprehensive rehabilitation treatment program for cancer pain should involve treatment for cancer-related fatigue.

The causes of cancer-related fatigue include metabolic issues related to the cancer itself, preexisting comorbid conditions (diabetes, cardiac, renal, or pulmonary disease), side effects from treatment (anemia, infection, fever, pain, anorexia, nausea, diarrhea, dehydration, electrolyte imbalances, malnutrition), effects from surgery, chemotherapy, radiation therapy, bone marrow transplant, and effects from medications. Other psychological and situational factors contributing to cancer fatigue include depression, anxiety, sleep disorders, personality disorders, adjustment issues, and vocational, financial, and family stressors.

The treatment of cancer-related fatigue is directed at its various causes. On the rehabilitation service this includes management of cancer-related anemia, correction of electrolyte imbalances, and correction of hypoxia via breathing treatments and supplemental oxygen. Psychological issues can be addressed with counseling as well as medications like antidepressants and neurostimulants. Alternative treatments such as biofeedback, acupuncture, muscle relaxation, and guided imagery techniques are sometimes used. Finally, traditional rehabilitation interventions for fatigue include promotion of good sleep hygiene, therapeutic exercise, and the use of energy conservation techniques.

For many hospitalized patients, especially those with prolonged intensive care unit (ICU) stays and longer hospitalizations, sleep-wake cycles may be severely altered. Sleep is often interrupted for nursing assessments, tests, and procedures. These patients also frequently take multiple medications, which can be sedating or, alternatively, cause agitation. A sleep hygiene program begins with recommendations to promote sleep by minimizing nighttime sleep interruptions, avoiding excessive activities in the evening, and avoiding daytime naps. Vigorous activities such as physical therapy are done during the day to promote the need for sleep at night. The patient's medication list should be reviewed, and unnecessary medications that can alter the central nervous system (CNS) should be discontinued. Sleep aids such as zolpidem or trazodone can help to regulate the sleep-wake cycle.

A common occupational therapy recommendation for managing cancer-related fatigue is the use of energy conservation techniques. This approach is based on the theory that an individual has a finite amount of energy for activity in a given day, and budgeting this amount of energy allows the patient to attain his or her most important goals. Essential activities should be prioritized and unnecessary tasks eliminated. Some activities should be delegated to those who can provide assistance. Labor-saving devices such as reachers and sock-aids are also helpful.

Therapeutic exercise can help in treating cancer-related fatigue. Exercise improves aerobic efficiency at the cellular level. Research in cancer patients has shown increased hemoglobin levels and decreased lactic acid levels after a conditioning program.[6] Exercise has also been shown to improve mood, immune response, appetite, and performance status. Therapeutic exercise requires patient motivation and consistent participation to achieve maximum benefit. A patient's comorbid conditions such as coronary artery disease or chronic obstructive pulmonary disease must be accounted for before initiating a therapeutic exercise program. Contraindications to exercise can include bone or joint pain and muscle weakness of recent origin, severe nausea with activity, fever, significant cachexia, profound thrombocytopenia, or anemia. A common exercise prescription will include mode, intensity, frequency, duration, and rate of progression. Mode is usually walking or a recumbent stationary bicycle. Intensity is 50% of cardiac capacity with a target heart rate of $0.5 \times (220 -$ patient's age). Initially, frequency can be three times a week. Duration can vary, but starting at 5–10 minutes a session is recommended. Rate of progression can also vary but should be gradual, that is, increasing sessions by 2 minutes per session per week. Patients may be at risk for falls, hence fall precautions and supervision from another individual are strongly recommended.

A combination of energy conservation techniques and therapeutic exercise is used to maximize activity and quality of life when treating cancer-related fatigue. It is important to recognize when a therapeutic exercise program is not practical; when a patient is using limited energy resources on exercise instead of necessary or more enjoyable activities.

NEUROGENIC BLADDER

Neurogenic bladder and bowel problems typically occur in patients with tumors of the brain, spinal cord, and lumbosacral plexus. Neurogenic bowel and bladder management is frequently addressed by the cancer rehabilitation team. In patients with spinal cord involvement, suprasacral neurogenic bladder problems can occur, which typically result in a hyperreflexic bladder with low urinary volumes, high bladder pressures, and diminished bladder compliance. In patients with an incomplete spinal cord lesion, adequate emptying with a sense of urgency can occur. Some patients with complete spinal cord lesions can have reflex incontinence and incomplete voiding due to detrusor-sphincter dyssynergia and bladder hyperreflexia. Some patients can have hypocontractility or areflexia with urinary retention and associated overflow incontinence if the lesion is at the sacral level. At times, there can be a mixed picture of upper motor neuron, hyperreflexic bladder and lower motor neuron, and areflexic bladder.

Management of lower motor neuron bladder compromise often involves the use of a condom catheter for men or indwelling catheter for females. When the sphincter tone is competent but the bladder tone diminished, an intermittent catheterization program is instituted.

Upper motor neuron bladder management involves the use of an intermittent catheterization program, which is usually combined with an anticholinergic medication such as oxybutynin to decrease detrusor tone and allow for greater bladder capacity.

An intermittent catheterization program initially requires daily measurements of postvoid residuals, the volume of urine left in the bladder after a void. This assessment can be performed noninvasively by an ultrasound bladder scanner or more accurately by straight catheterization and measurement. If the postvoid volumes are 100–150 cc or greater, an intermittent catheterization program is warranted. The patient is catheterized initially every 4 hours. The goal is to have catheter volumes not exceed 400–500 cc. If the volumes remain consistently below those numbers, the frequency of catheterizations can be decreased.

It is important to note that in the cancer population, life expectancy is a factor in rehabilitation management. Intermittent catheterization is the preferred method of management for patients who are unable to effectively void; however, an indwelling Foley catheter is also an option for patients with a limited life span, limited physical capabilities, or limited available assistance.

NEUROGENIC BOWEL

In patients with CNS lesions above the conus medullaris, an upper motor neuron bowel can occur with a spastic external anal sphincter and pelvic floor muscles. The tracts between the spinal cord and colon remain intact, so stool can still be propelled by reflex activity. With lesions below the conus medullaris, an areflexic lower motor neuron bowel dysfunction occurs with the myenteric plexus intrinsically moving stool slowly.

A complicating matter with cancer patients is opioid-induced constipation. Often a plain radiograph of the abdomen can help assess for obstipation before beginning a bowel program. If present, an enema is given to clean out the bowels and evacuate the rectal vault.

The goal of a bowel management program is to prevent fecal impaction. It begins with a proper diet, which should contain adequate amounts of fluid and fiber to create soft bulky stools, which can decrease bowel transit time. Medication usually involves a stool softener such as docusate sodium and a stimulant such as senna. Bisacodyl suppositories are also frequently used. To take advantage of the gastrocolic reflex, the patient can be placed on the commode 30 minutes after a meal.

DELIRIUM (ENCEPHALOPATHY)

Delirium is frequently underrecognized and is inappropriately managed in advanced cancer patients. An altered level of consciousness, abnormal attention, perception, memory, motor behavior, and a disrupted sleep-wake cycle are characteristics of delirium. A disorder of generalized CNS dysfunction, delirium is a common problem in all gravely ill patients, occurs in 26%–44% of cancer patients admitted to a hospital or hospice,[7] and it affects as many as 80% of patients with advanced cancer.[7,8] Delirium has an acute onset and follows a fluctuating course.[7,9] Patients with delirium have a variable level of arousal, ranging from stupor to hyperalertness and hypervigilance, with motor activity ranging from profound psychomotor retardation to severe hyperactivity. Short-term memory and other cognitive functions are generally impaired and delirious patients are frequently disoriented.[8] Metabolic perturbations are the most common cause of cancer-related delirium and include severe electrolyte disturbances, hypoxia, and hypercalcemia.[8] However, delirium typically involves multiple medical etiologies in addition to metabolic disturbances. These include infection, organ failure, adverse effects from medication, and, rarely, paraneoplastic syndromes.[10] The pharmacologic agents used in supportive care are more likely to cause altered sensorium than antineoplastics. Opioid treatment is a factor in approximately 60% of patients with delirium, and excluding terminal delirium, it may be reversible in 50% of the cases.[7] Managing delirium is, when possible, focused on correcting its etiology. For patients with end-stage disease, however, palliation is the goal.[11] Recommendations include (1) stabilizing the environment, including conversing with patients to help reorient them; (2) a well-lit room during the day with simple interventions such as providing the patient who normally wears them, glasses and hearing aids; (3) a dimmed but lit room at night to maintain optimal orientation and ward off fear and perceptual dysregulations; (4) limited sleep deprivation and noise reduction strategies.[11] Other therapeutic strategies that have demonstrated efficacy include reducing or withdrawing the psychoactive medication, opioid rotation, and hydration. Haloperidol is the most frequently used drug for delirium, but new neuroleptics such as risperidone and olanzapine are being assessed, thus far with benefit.[7] Medications can be eliminated and others substituted for them such as opioid rotation. Hydration and correction of electrolyte abnormalities should be ongoing. Neuroleptics can be used to address symptoms such as hallucinations and delusions.[11]

REHABILITATION OF PATIENTS WITH BRAIN TUMORS

Even small, low-grade malignant tumors can cause significant functional deficits when they reside in eloquent locations. The most common complications of brain tumors and their treatments include weakness, sensory loss, visuospatial deficits, hemineglect or bilateral visual deficits, ataxia, cognitive deficits, speech deficits, dysphagia, bowel and bladder dysfunction, psychological sequelae, endocrine imbalances, skin involvement, and fatigue.[12] Cranial nerve function should be assessed in patients with brain tumors because intervention can greatly ameliorate functional status. Visual and hearing deficits are often seen in patients with meningiomas, acoustic neuromas, and pituitary adenomas. Suprasellar lesions can cause bitemporal hemianopsia, but can also cause diminished visual acuity, scotomata, quadrantic deficits, and blindness of one or both eyes. When treating patients with visual deficits, rehabilitation should include an ophthalmology consultation. The patients can be trained to use compensationary techniques such as scanning, which can improve visuospatial awareness. Driving recommendations should be given before discharge, with plans for further evaluations as vision improves.[12] Balance abnormalities should also be addressed and can include dizziness, unsteadiness, vertigo, muscle weakness, and proprioceptive sensory loss. Many cancer-related problems and treatments can contribute to imbalance, including poor nutrition, anemia, anxiety, postural hypotension, and dehydration. Additionally, most brain tumor patients at M. D. Anderson have cognitive difficulties, which are often accompanied by confusion and frustration. A neuropsychological assessment can be helpful in defining a patient's cognitive strengths and weaknesses and can also help patients understand their own illness-related cognitive limitations.[13]

INTRODUCTION TO THE MODALITIES

Modalities[14] use physical energy to achieve a desired therapeutic effect. Most of the modalities used by physical and occupational therapists in a general rehabilitation setting can also be applied to cancer patients; however, some specific precautions must be taken. The modalities used in cancer rehabilitation include heat, cold, light therapy, electrostimulation, and massage.

▶ The physical agents: heat and cold

Physical agents use energy to speed healing and lessen pain. Any energy form, including pressure, heat, electricity, sound, or light can be used.

Heat is generally used to treat chronic processes. It decreases muscle spasms, pain, and joint stiffness. Physiologically, heat causes hyperemia, analgesia, hyperthermia, decreased muscle tone, and increased collagen elasticity. Heat is useful in treating muscle spasms, myofascial pain, joint stiffness, contractures, arthritis, collagen vascular diseases, and superficial thrombophlebitis. Contraindications to heat include ischemia, bleeding disorders, impaired sensation, acute trauma or inflammation, scar tissue, edema, atrophic skin, and poor thermal regulation. Heat should be avoided over areas of malignancy, since it may promote tumor growth.

There are three methods of applying heat: convection, conduction, and conversive heating. Convection requires contact between two surfaces at different temperatures with the resultant flow of one past the other. Examples include hydrotherapy, fluidotherapy, and contrast baths. Conduction involves transference of heat between two bodies at different temperatures, without movement of the conducting body. Examples include hot water, paraffin, and hot packs. Conversive heating uses nonthermal energy to heat tissues. Examples include heat lamps, shortwave diathermy, ultrasound, and microwave.

Heat can be superficial or deep. Superficial heat is used to maximize tissue temperature in the skin and subcutaneous fat. It can be used to heat joints with little soft tissue covering. Examples of superficial heating modalities are fluidotherapy, hydrotherapy, contrast baths, heating pads, and radiant heat, such as infrared lamps.

Deep heat is used to maximize tissue temperature at 3–5 cm below the skin surface. It is best used for deep structures such as ligaments, bones, muscles, and joint capsules. Examples of deep heat modalities include ultrasound, shortwave diathermy, and microwave diathermy. Ultrasound is often used to treat bursitis and tendinitis and can be used to treat degenerative arthritis or adhesive capsulitis. Ultrasound should be avoided over areas of malignancy. It is also contraindicated in patients with pacemakers and cemented hip arthroplasties. Shortwave diathermy is used to treat chronic prostatitis, pelvic inflammatory disease, myalgia, and back spasms. Microwave heat is used to speed the resolution of hematomas and to provide local hyperthermia in cancer patients where diffuse heat modalities may be contraindicated.

Cold is generally used to treat acute processes. It provides localized vasoconstriction, decreases acute inflammatory response, slows nerve conduction velocity, and decreases spasticity. Cold is useful in treating acute traumatic conditions, arthritis or bursitis flares, minor burns, and muscle spasticity. Contraindications to cold include arterial insufficiency, impaired sensation, and cryopathies such as cryoglobulinemia.

Cold is also transferred by three mechanisms: conduction, convection, and evaporation. Examples of cold conduction include ice packs and ice massage. Examples of cold convection include cold baths. The third form of cold transfer, evaporation, occurs when liquid molecules gain sufficient energy to enter the gaseous state. An example of an evaporation modality is the vapocoolant spray, which is generally used to treat myofascial pain in a "spray-and-stretch" technique, or for local anesthesia.

▶ Light therapy

Ultraviolet light therapy operates in the 2000–4000 Ångstrom range. It produces a nonthermal photochemical reaction with resultant alteration of DNA and cell proteins.

Physiologically, ultraviolet light is bactericidal and increases vascularization of wound margins. It increases vitamin D production and causes exfoliation of the skin. Ultraviolet light can typically be used to treat nonhealing wounds, psoriatic lesions, and folliculitis. Precautions should be used in patients with scars, acute renal or hepatic failure, severe diabetes, or hyperthyroidism. Ultraviolet light is contraindicated in pellagra, porphyria, sarcoidosis, lupus, and eczema.

▶ Electrotherapy

Electrotherapy uses electricity via surface electrodes or acupuncture needles to stimulate nerve or muscle. Physiologically, it has been shown to improve joint range of motion, increase muscle group contraction, increase circulation, decrease spasticity, promote wound healing, and inhibit pain fibers. It is used to treat musculoskeletal pain, neurogenic pain, and general systemic pain. It is also used to treat muscle disuse atrophy, wounds, circulatory disorders, and postherpetic neuralgia. Contraindications to treatment with electrotherapy include pregnancy, seizure disorder, recent fracture, active hemorrhage, or decreased sensation. Electrotherapy should also be avoided over areas of malignancy.

The primary device used in electrotherapy is called a transcutaneous electrical nerve stimulation (TENS) unit. The device applies an electrical signal through wires and electrodes, which are attached to the patient's skin. The electrodes are typically placed over a peripheral nerve distribution and pulsed signals are emitted. The frequency and intensity of the stimulation can be adjusted based on the type of treatment the practitioner is hoping to achieve. For example, a high-frequency, low-intensity stimulation is most effective in treating neuropathic pain. Alternately, a low-frequency, high-intensity stimulation delivered through acupuncture needles is most effective for treating acute musculoskeletal conditions. Treatment sessions with TENS units last between 30 minutes and 1 hour. Patients should not exceed more than 8 hours of TENS treatments a day.

The physiologic mechanism behind pain relief in TENS units remains controversial. It is based primarily on the gate control theory by Melzack and Wall,[15] which states that pain signals can be blocked at the spinal cord before they are transmitted to the brain. The TENS unit stimulates large Ia afferent nerve fibers that in turn stimulate the substantia gelatinosa in the spinal cord, which closes the gate on pain transmission to the thalamus. TENS has also been shown to release endogenous opioids into the bloodstream. Still, placebo effect accounts for 30%–35% of symptom relief.

Functional electrical stimulation (FES) is a more powerful form of electrical stimulation used in cancer rehabilitation. It uses electrical stimulation to provide functional utilization of paretic muscles. Multiple muscles can be activated in a coordinated fashion through FES to attain functional goals. FES can be employed to maintain muscle mass after an immobilizing injury, such as a spinal cord injury. It can also prevent complications from immobilization, such as deep venous thrombosis. FES has also been shown to slow the rate of bone loss in patients who have sustained a spinal cord injury. Functionally, FES can be used for muscle reeducation by providing feedback to enhance voluntary muscle control.

▶ Massage

Massage uses pressure and stretching in a rhythmic fashion on the soft tissues. It provides reflex vasodilatation with improvement in circulation. In addition, it increases lymphatic drainage, decreases muscle tightness, and can soften scars. Precautions must be taken not to massage over malignant tumors and open wounds or areas of nerve entrapment. Massage should also be avoided in acute inflammatory conditions and deep venous thrombosis.

RADIATION-INDUCED BRACHIAL PLEXOPATHY

Radiation is commonly used in the treatment of various cancers. Although effective, it has toxic effects on several organs and systems that are exposed during treatment. Radiation-induced neurotoxicity can involve both the CNS and the peripheral nervous system. One of the most common types of radiation nerve injuries is radiation-induced brachial plexopathy,[16] which occurs when radiotherapy is directed at the chest, axillary region, thoracic organs, and neck.

The radiation dose, treatment technique, and concomitant use of chemotherapy are all associated with the development of radiation injury to the brachial plexus. The mechanism is believed to be a combination of localized ischemia and failure of cellular proliferation. The result is fibrosis of the perineural soft tissues secondary to microvascular insufficiency.

The time interval from last dose of radiation to the first symptom of plexus disorder can vary from 7.5 months to 6 years. Sensory symptoms, such as numbness, paresthesia, and dysesthesia, along with swelling and weakness are the most common presenting symptoms. Only 18% of patients present with any significant pain, and pain is a major symptom in only 35% of patients.

On physical examination, the C5-C6 myotomes and dermatomes are most frequently involved. There may be weakness with shoulder abduction and elbow flexion on muscle strength testing, and light-touch sensation may be decreased along the C5 and C6 dermatomes. The C7 myotome and dermatome can also be involved. Also, there can be concomitant lymphedema in the axilla and upper extremity with or without cyanosis. Decreased range of motion along the scapulothoracic or glenohumeral joint may also be encountered if there is postsurgical fibrosis in these regions.

Electromyography is the test of choice in distinguishing between radiation-induced brachial plexopathy and other causes of nerve injury. Affected muscles will exhibit myokymia, which are spontaneous discharges accompanied by wavelike quivering. Also, paroxysmal motor unit action potentials may be present. Magnetic resonance imaging (MRI) of the brachial plexus often reveals low signal intensity on T2-weighted images, and computed tomography (CT) of the brachial plexus can reveal diffuse infiltration of the tissue planes. A tissue biopsy will show fibrosis of the neural elements and surrounding soft tissues, along with chronic perineural microvascular ischemia.

Treatment of radiation-induced brachial plexopathy involves physical therapy, occupational therapy, and medications. Surgery, such as glenohumeral joint arthrodesis or lymphatic bypass surgery is rarely indicated. Physical therapy should address weakness, pain, and lymphedema. Therapeutic exercise should be used to enhance flexibility, range of motion, and strength of the shoulder girdle muscles. A sling may be required to prevent shoulder subluxation. Transcutaneous electrical nerve stimulation may be used for pain control. Lymphedema can be treated with manual lymphatic drainage and graded pressure garments. Occupational therapy should address fine motor skills training and motor reeducation techniques. Hand or wrist orthoses may be useful in improving function. Pharmacologic management of neuropathic pain should involve anticonvulsants, such as gabapentin or pregabalin. Tricyclic antidepressants such as nortriptyline can also be used.

Complications of radiation-induced brachial plexopathy include lymphangitis, cellulitis, complex regional pain syndrome type II, shoulder subluxation, and contractures. Clinicians treating patients with radiation-induced brachial plexopathy should be aware of these complications and watch for their symptoms.

SEXUAL FUNCTION AFTER CANCER TREATMENT

The issues surrounding sexuality and fertility after treatment for cancer[17–20] are complex and are not familiar to most physicians and other health professionals who see cancer patients. Additionally, as various treatment modalities improve and expand, a greater number of patients survive longer, making reproductive health an increasingly important issue for cancer patients and their partners. Although cancer treatments often cause sexual dysfunction that remains following therapy and is more refractory to amelioration than other treatment sequelae, sexual counseling is not routinely provided in most oncology settings.[17] Among others, these issues are the impact of cancer treatment on sexual function, including erectile dysfunction, hormonal deficits, decreased sexual desire, resuming sex comfortably, optimizing sexual communication, advice on mitigating the effects of physical handicaps such as having an ostomy, dyspareunia, compromised fertility, and cancer recurrence due to hormone treatments.[18–20] Sexual dysfunction has, in fact, been documented in at least 50% of patients treated for breast, prostate, colorectal, or gynecological cancer.[18] For a detailed discussion of the various issues surrounding cancer and sexuality, the reader is referred to an excellent article by Leslie Schover[18] as well as books that can be obtained at no charge from the American Cancer Society.[19,20]

Management of sexual dysfunction in cancer patients should include a thorough history taking and frank discussion of the sexual goals the patient and his/her partner wish to achieve.

In women, treatment of breast cancer is often followed by premature menopause, and ovarian damage is a significant long-term sequela of adjuvant chemotherapy in premenopausal breast cancer survivors. Hormone replacement therapy is contraindicated in breast cancer patients who have undergone premature menopause because of the fear of tumor recurrence. Female breast cancer patients who have undergone mastectomy often avoid sexual intercourse due to negative emotional effects, changes in the female body image, and fear of partner rejection. Furthermore, use of antiestrogen treatment may cause soreness, dryness, vaginal atrophy, hot flashes, and decreased libido.

Women with cervical or ovarian cancer who have undergone pelvic surgery often share the same impairments and infertility as breast cancer patients. Cervical cancer patients often have vaginal fibrosis, pain with penetration due to stenosis, and decreased lubrication. Sexual rehabilitation in these patients should include discussion of vaginal dilators to prevent stenosis, artificial lubricants, and changes from customary sexual positions to minimize discomfort.

Testicular and prostate cancer patients also show signs of long-term sexual dysfunction, including hormonal changes and infertility. Sexual counseling in these patients should include the discussion of sperm banking if the patient wishes to reproduce following cancer treatment. Radiation to the pelvic area following surgical tumor resection can cause fatigue, diarrhea, bowel and bladder incontinence, and skin changes, all of which can lead to sexual dysfunction. Erectile dysfunction, painful and/or retrograde ejaculation, and changes in the male body image can also contribute to sexual dysfunction. Counseling patients with erectile dysfunction should include discussion of topical intraurethral medications, oral medications, intracavernosal injection therapy, and the possibility of a penile prosthesis.[21,22]

REFERENCES

1. Tunkel RS, Lachmann E, Ho ML. In: Grabois M, Garrison SJ, Hart KA, Lehmkuhl LD, eds. *Physical Medicine & Rehabilitation*. Massachusetts: Blackwell Science, Inc.; 2000:1697–1723.
2. Lehmann JF, DeLisa JA, Warren CG, et al. *Cancer rehabilitation: assessment of need, development and evaluation of a model of care. Arch Phys Med Rehabil.* 1978:410–419.
3. Dietz JH. Adaptive rehabilitation of the cancer patient. *Curr Probl Cancer.* 1980:1–56.

4. Mackey KM, Sparling JW. Experiences of older women with cancer receiving hospice care: significance for physical therapy. *Phys Ther.* 2000;80:459–468.

5. Quinones-Hinojosa A, Gulati M, Singh V, et al. Spontaneous intracerebral hemorrhage due to coagulation disorders. *Neurosurg Focus.* 2003;15(4):E3.

6. Dimeo F, Bertz H, Finke J, et al. An aerobic exercise program for patients with haematological malignancies after bone marrow transplantation. *Bone Marrow Transplant.* 1996;18(6):1157–1160.

7. Centeno C, Sanz A, Bruera E. Delirium in advanced cancer patients. *Palliat Med.* 2004;18:184–194.

8. Valentine AD, Passik SD, Massie MJ. Psychiatric and psychosocial issues. In: Levin VA, ed. *Cancer in the Nervous System*, 2nd ed. New York: Oxford University Press; 2002:572–589.

9. Michaud L, Burnand B, Stiefel F. Taking care of the terminally ill cancer patient: delirium as a symptom of terminal disease. *Ann Oncol.* 2004;15:iv199–iv203.

10. Friedlander MM, Brayman Y, Breitbart WS. Delirium in palliative care. *Oncology (Williston Park).* 2004;18:1541–1550.

11. Morrison C. Identification and management of delirium in the critically ill patient with cancer. *AACN Clin Issues.* 2003;14:92–111.

12. Gillis TA, Yadav R, Guo Y. Rehabilitation of patients with neurologic tumors and cancer-related central nervous system disabilities. In: Levin VA, ed. *Cancer in the Nervous System*, 2nd ed. New York: Oxford University Press; 2002:470–492.

13. Meyers CA, Kayl AE. Neurocognitive function. In: Levin VA, ed. *Cancer in the Nervous System*, 2nd ed. New York: Oxford University Press; 2002:557–571.

14. Strax TE, Cuccurullo S. Physical modalities, therapeutic exercise, extended bed rest, and aging effects. In: Cuccurullo SJ, ed. *Physical Medicine and Rehabilitation Board Review*, vol. 1. New York: Demos Medical Publishing; 2004:553–570.

15. Melzack R, Wall PD. Pain mechanisms: a new theory. *Science.* 1965;150:971–979.

16. Kaplan R. *Radiation-Induced Brachial Plexopathy.* emedicine.com, 2005.

17. Shover LR. Counseling cancer patients about changes in sexual function. *Oncology (Williston Park).* 13:1585–1591.

18. Shover LR. Sexuality and fertility after cancer. *Hematology Am Soc Hematol Educ Program.* 2005:523–527.

19. Sexuality and cancer for the woman who has cancer and her partner. American Cancer Society, 2004; www.cancer.org; 1–800.ACS.2345.

20. Sexuality and cancer for the man who has cancer and his partner. American Cancer Society, 2004; www.cancer.org; 1–800.ACS.2345.

21. Body JJ, Lossignol D, Ronson A. The concept of rehabilitation of cancer patients. *Curr Opin Oncol.* 1997;9(4):332–340.

22. Fialka-Moser V, Crevenna R, Korpan M, et al. Cancer rehabilitation: particularly with aspects on physical impairments. *J Rehabil Med.* 2003;35(4):153–162.

Practical Aspects of Cancer Pain and Symptom Management and Pediatric Palliative Care

Kathleen Larkin

"Freedom from pain should be regarded as a human rights issue."

INTRODUCTION

Over the last 40 years, the prognosis for the majority of children with malignancies has improved dramatically. It is estimated that one in 900 American adults is a survivor of childhood cancer.[1] National Institutes of Health data from 2001 are that 78.6% of children diagnosed with cancer have long-term survival or cure.[2] Survival from the most common childhood cancer, acute lymphoblastic leukemia (ALL), increased from 40% in the early 1970s to about 70% in the mid-1990s without a single new frontline therapeutic agent. This decrease in mortality is due to the development of multimodal treatment, including new chemotherapeutic agents, improved surgical and radiotherapy techniques, and enhanced support services. Improvements are also due to trial and error adjustments of therapeutic dosages and schedules resulting from the large number of children in clinical trials. The American Cancer Society found that 80%–90% of children 0–21 years old with ALL participated in clinical trials in 1992. In contrast, the study involvement rate in adults with cancer is only 2%–3%.

Multimodality treatment in children versus adults is often aimed at cure and can require multiple cycles of chemotherapy and procedures. Even when the chance of survival is low, the families of children commonly continue to pursue aggressive treatment. The improved prognosis resulting from this treatment has been accompanied by a significant increase in morbidity secondary to cancer therapy. The increased intensity and invasiveness of cancer treatment demands equally aggressive pain management.

Ninety percent of the children in the world live in developing countries, and despite pediatric cancers being highly treatable, worldwide 80% of children with malignancies die because of inaccessibility to medical care. Additionally, the prohibitive cost of care leads to geographic variations in survival. This has led to the development of standard guidelines for treating children by the World Health Organization (WHO), United Nations Children's Emergency Fund (UNICEF), International Union Against Cancer (UICC), and the International Society of Pediatric Oncology (SIOP). The goal is to make chemotherapy, supportive care drugs, and opioids for palliation uniformly available.[3] Even in the United States, access to care, race, and various other socioeconomic factors may impact survival rates.[4]

Each child with cancer will experience pain during the diagnosis and treatment of his or her disease. In comparison to adults, treatment-related pain is a relatively more prevalent problem than tumor-related pain. Other symptoms, including nausea and vomiting, sedation, and fatigue, are also primary sources of distress and

impaired quality of life among children with cancer, both during the phase of aggressive cancer-directed treatment and in palliative care.[5,6] Pain management must be regarded in the context of broad-based approaches to the alleviation of other symptoms and of non-painful sources of suffering and distress.

PAIN ASSESSMENT IN CHILDREN

An accurate pain assessment is an important first step in caring for a child's pain. Pain assessment in children can be a challenge for many reasons. Clinicians must be familiar with the varying anatomic, physiologic, pharmacologic, and psychological considerations in infants and children. Babies, children too young to speak, or cognitively impaired children are unable to communicate effectively when they are in pain. Often the parent is the best judge of the degree of pain experienced by the child. Many scales have been developed to aid the assessment of pain by healthcare providers. These serve to guide the appropriate level of pain intervention.

A complete assessment of pain will include a full medical history as well as characteristics of the pain: timing, location, quality, radiation, and exacerbating and alleviating factors. Previous medications and interventions for the pain and response to each are important to document (Table 16-1).

▶ Self-report measure of pain

This technique is most useful for verbal and cognitively aware children, usually children 6 years and older. The visual analog scales (VAS) are commonly used for adolescents and adults. Children must be able to understand numbers and proportions to properly assign a number to their perceived pain. Pictures of facial expressions are helpful in younger children between the ages of 4 and 8. These pictures show children exhibiting increasing levels of distress. Color analog scales have also been developed and used successfully in this age group. These scales do not, however, differentiate well between pain and anxiety in children.

▶ Behavioral observation

Children who are too young to self-report pain or who are cognitively impaired require observations of behavior to assess pain. Facial expressions, limb movement, and crying should be rated by the observer. These assessments can be misleading, however. Some children will lay immobile in bed due to severe movement-related pain.

Table 16-1

Types of Pain Measurement Tools in Children

Self-report, e.g., visual, numerical or color analog, Faces (Bieri or Wong-Baker), Oucher

Behavioral, e.g., FLACC, OSBD, PBCL, PPP

Physiologic measures, e.g., heart rate, "vagal tone," skin conductance

---

Table 16-3

Types of Pain due to Malignancy

Somatic pain, e.g., osteosarcoma, bony metastases

Visceral pain, e.g., hepatoblastoma

Neuropathic pain, e.g., neuroblastoma

Two scales commonly used to assess children with cancer are the Observational Scale of Behavioral Distress and the Procedure Behavior Checklist (PBCL). These behavioral scales measure fear and anxiety along with pain (Table 16-2). Validity data have shown that anxiety is rated more frequently than pain. Interrater reliability is always a potential problem.

A scale developed in the United Kingdom can help parents and healthcare providers assess the pain of nonverbal children. The Pediatric Pain Profile (PPP) evaluates 20 different types of pain cues including vocal cues, changes in posture, different movements, changes in facial expression and mood, and changes in sleeping and eating behaviors. The scale has been made into a record that parents can use to track pain at home (www.ppprofile.org.uk).[7]

▶ Physiologic measures

Measuring physiologic changes as a response to pain can be problematic. Heart rate, blood pressure, and respiratory rate can increase with pain but also as a result of myriad other reasons, including hypovolemia, fever, medications, and anxiety. Physiologic responses to pain can habituate in chronic pain. However, in certain situations these could be the observer's only available variables for assessing pain, for example, an intubated deeply sedated child in the intensive care unit.

CANCER CAUSING PAIN

All children with cancer will experience pain, whether due to their tumor or to cancer treatment. The WHO, recognizing the magnitude of the problem of pediatric cancer pain, produced a manual dedicated to the principles of pediatric cancer pain management and palliative care. Children reported pain prior to diagnosis in 62% of non-central nervous system (CNS) malignancies. Tumor-related pain resolves quickly in most children within 2 weeks of the initiation of cancer therapy. This time is shorter for hematologic malignancies compared to solid tumors. Studies show pain is present on average 74 days prior to beginning cancer therapy and lasts a median of 10 days after initiation of treatment in most patients.

Table 16-2

Pain Behaviors Measured in Children

Crying

Grimacing

Pulling away

Limited movement or splinting

Withdrawal from environment

Patients with metastatic disease did not have preceding pain longer than those without metastases.

In children admitted to the hospital with a diagnosis of cancer, pain is rated as the most prevalent symptom (84.4%).[8] Its incidence is high in the outpatient setting as well (35%). Breakdown of pain severity found 87% of inpatients rating their pain as moderate to severe and 53% rating it as being highly distressing. Reports of pain can vary by type of malignancy. In bone cancer, pain is the most common early symptom in children. Cancer-related bone pain is only partially correlated with the type and location of the tumor and with the number and size of malignant lesions.[9]

In pediatric tumors of the brain, commonly presenting symptoms are related to an increase in intracranial pressure rather than pain. However, in spinal cord tumors, most children present with pain before neurologic deficits appear. Metastatic spinal cord lesions are rare at the time of diagnosis. The most common cause of back and neck pain in pediatric oncology patients is metastatic disease. Back pain is caused by metastases in 63% of patients with solid tumors. Other less common causes in this population include infection, avascular necrosis of the femur causing low back pain, and development of a meningioma of the cervical spine after radiotherapy. Bone marrow expansion due to colony-stimulating factor or a recurrence in leukemia can be a cause of severe back pain.[10]

Tumor pain can be characterized as somatic, visceral, or neuropathic depending on the tissue being invaded (Table 16-3). Somatic pain often arises from bone and is well localized. Visceral pain is harder to localize and occurs when the thoracic or abdominal viscera are invaded, stretched, or compressed by tumor. It is described as deep, squeezing pressure with associated nausea and diaphoresis. Neuropathic pain arises when a tumor infiltrates or compresses nervous system tissue, whether peripherally or in the spinal cord. This pain can also be due to chemotherapy or radiation and is characterized by burning, electrical shooting pain associated with allodynia and hyperalgesia.

Tumor-related pain can recur at the time of relapse or metastatic spread, or in the terminal phase of the disease. A Finnish study found that 89% of children required scheduled pain medication during the terminal phase of their cancer care. Breakthrough pain, or pain requiring more than the scheduled pain medication, can occur in 50%–75% of cancer patients.[11] Severe cancer-related pain at the end of life occurs more commonly with solid tumors that have metastasized to the CNS or peripheral nervous system, resulting in neuropathic pain that is difficult to treat.

TREATMENT CAUSING PAIN

Once the child initiates cancer therapy, pain from treatment becomes more common than tumor-related pain, and two-thirds of the pain experienced by children with cancer has an iatrogenic origin. This is

Table 16-4

Treatment-Related Pain

Mucositis

Graft-versus-host disease

Phantom limb pain and other forms of postsurgical neuropathic pain

Infection

Chemotherapy-related pain

Postoperative pain

Procedure-related pain

    Needle puncture

    Lumbar puncture

    Bone marrow aspirate

    Nasogastric tube

    Central venous line placement/removal

true even more in pediatrics than in adults due to children living longer, having more relapses, and receiving aggressive multimodal treatment. Younger children and children with short disease duration are more concerned about procedural pain (Table 16-4).[12]

Mucositis

Microfloral invasion and colonization of mucosal tissues contribute to the pathophysiology of ulcerative oral mucositis. Mucositis is among the most frequent and severe complications of chemotherapy in children with cancer. Studies have shown that mucositis develops in about 40% of chemotherapy patients, 80% of bone marrow transplant (BMT) patients, and 100% of patients treated with radiotherapy to the head and neck.[13] Almost one-third of patients receiving chemotherapy for solid tumors experienced one or more episodes of mild to more severe oral mucositis. Chemotherapeutic agents such as paclitaxel, doxorubicin, or etoposide are independent risk factors. Low body mass is also associated with a slightly increased risk for the development of mucositis.[14] The average duration of mucositis is 7.9 days (range 3–23 days), and the mean duration of the most severe stage of mucositis is 4.81 days (range 2–13 days).[15]

There is a wide variation in the management of mucositis, despite publication of guidelines by the NIH. Treatments range from topical therapies to systemic antifungals and opioids. Topical therapies include saline, sodium bicarbonate, hydrogen peroxide, nystatin, viscous lidocaine, and dyclonine. Studies establishing a safe dose of oral lidocaine recommend 5 mL of 2% viscous lidocaine to swish only (not swallow) three times a day (2.5 mL for less than 6 years old).[16] Topical anesthetics carry the risk of anesthetizing the supraglottic and glottic aperture, thus predisposing children to aspiration. If oral mucositis pain cannot be controlled with topical solutions, second-line therapy includes opioids.

Multiple studies have found *chlorhexidine* mouth rinse to be more effective at reducing ulcerative lesions and the severity of mucositis in children than benzydamine.[17] The pain and severity of oral mucositis are significantly reduced by tooth brushing, 0.2% chlorhexidine mouth rinse, and 0.9% saline rinse.[18] Topical honey has been used successfully for mucositis pain in patients receiving radiation to the head and neck, with high compliance and advantageous weight gain in 55% of patients.[19] Three-drug combination

mouthwash (lidocaine, diphenhydramine, and sodium bicarbonate in normal saline) is effectively used when children develop mucositis of any severity.[20]

Sucralfate given preventively is effective in diminishing severe oral and intestinal mucositis in patients on high-dose chemotherapy alone or combined with total body irradiation before BMT. Patients receiving sucralfate also showed a significant reduction in the occurrence of diarrhea.[21] *Iseganan* is an analog of protegrin-1, a naturally occurring peptide with broad-spectrum microbicidal activity. It has been shown to be effective in preventing oral mucositis after chemotherapy.[22]

Several studies examined the therapeutic effect of *laser* therapy in the treatment of mucositis. Some studies suggest that low-level laser therapy can enhance natural wound healing and reduce pain in children suffering from oral mucositis.[23,24]

BMT mucositis

Autologous and allogeneic BMT require high-dose chemotherapy and sometimes irradiation. Mucositis is the leading side effect in these patients. The mouth pain after conditioning for BMT is more intense and lasts longer than chemotherapy-associated mucositis. Transplant mucositis tends to be continuous, requiring opioid infusion. Many studies tout the advantages of using patient-controlled analgesia (PCA) for this type of pain because children experienced greater comfort using less opioid compared to continuous infusion or nurse-administered pain medications. Comparing morphine, hydromorphone, and sufentanil in PCAs for mucositis pain in this population found morphine to have the fewest side effects. The sufentanil group developed tolerance and had inadequate pain control more than the patients in the other two groups. Remarkably, despite the common belief that fentanyl-series opioids should produce less itching than morphine and hydromorphone, sufentanil produced no less itching than the other two opioids in this study.

Palifermin is a version of keratinocyte growth factor and has been shown to markedly reduce the incidence of severe oral mucositis. Palifermin recipients used less opioid analgesics for mucositis, had a lower incidence of febrile neutropenia, and had significantly higher scores for functional well-being.[25] *Clarithromycin* has also been used for oral mucositis in BMT recipients.[26]

Surgery-related pain

Because children with cancer often have to undergo multiple surgeries during their treatment, postoperative pain control requires special attention. Often these children are undermedicated during and after their surgery. If the child has been receiving opioids preoperatively, it is important to reinstate their daily opioid requirement as their *baseline* to which additional opioids should be added for postoperative pain control. Opioid requirements in this population can be surprisingly high postoperatively. Extensive surgery for tumor resection cuts through tissue planes rather than dividing them anatomically and, therefore, may be more painful than analogous noncancer surgeries involving similar incisions and similar access to body compartments (Table 16-5).

A study of pediatric oncology patients found that this subpopulation of children suffered from more *breakthrough pain* after major surgery than other patients, despite their morphine consumption being twice as high as the other patients. When breakthrough pain occurs in these opioid-tolerant children, it is important to increase the baseline opioid infusion as well as the bolus dose available to avoid future breakthrough episodes. Interestingly, the study found that the use of laxatives correlated with fewer breakthrough pain events.[27]

Table 16-5

Oncologic Surgeries

Primary excision

Biopsy

Central venous line insertion and removal

Gastrostomy feeding

Surgical excision post-therapy

Table 16-6

Risk Factors for PHN

Older age

Greater rash severity

Prodrome

Severity of acute pain

Source: From Refs. 33 and 34.

Children with malignancies on opioids may be at higher risk of *awareness* during surgery. In adults, awareness under anesthesia is a rare event (0.1%–0.2%) but can be associated with significant psychological effects. In a large pediatric study, in which children were interviewed postoperatively to assess awareness, the incidence of true awareness was found to be 0.8%. Compared with adults, children require a larger concentration of anesthetic to achieve anesthesia. Minimum alveolar concentration (MAC) for awakening increases as age decreases but there have been very few MAC-awake studies conducted in children. Awareness happened more commonly when using nitrous, narcotic, and muscle relaxant where the increased need for opioids is not appreciated. Additional agents, such as volatile anesthetics or intravenous (IV) sedatives-hypnotics, should be added to minimize the risk of recall (unless contraindicated by hemodynamic instability). Dreaming was more frequent in children who were aware. No aware child reported distress, and no substantial difference was detected in behavior disturbance between aware and nonaware children. Children have different expectations, fears, and ways of managing stressful events than adults, which could account for the differences in sequelae secondary to awareness.[28]

▶ Infection

In immunocompromised children, infection can often be a source of pain. The most common sites of painful infections include perioral, perirectal, abdominal (e.g., Typhlitis—inflammation of the cecum), and skin infections at sites of IV access. This is due to the immunosuppressive effect of the therapy, particularly to neutropenia. Primary therapy should be aimed at treating the infection and usually the pain resolves.[29]

Acute and chronic pain due to herpes zoster

Varicella-zoster virus (VZV) is a significant cause of painful morbidity and occasional mortality in immunocompromised children. Patients can occasionally develop encephalitis.[30] Fortunately, children are less likely than adults to develop postherpetic neuralgia (PHN). The incidence of VZV infection in children following stem cell transplant varies from 23% to 67%, and is higher in children with leukemia or lymphoma than other types of cancer. Herpes zoster, caused by VZV reactivation affects 16.5% of children with ALL.[31] Zoster lesions most frequently affect the thoracic dermatomes in children.[32] Pain is a frequent feature associated with the rash in acute HZ. This pain is thought to be due to inflammatory changes induced by the virus in the skin, peripheral nerve, and spinal cord, as well as due to neuronal injury and dorsal root ganglion and dorsal horn cell loss. Pain usually attenuates over a period of weeks in children, but can occasionally persist longer.

PHN is considered to have developed after HZ if pain is still present after 3 months. Both HZ and PHN are associated with reduced sensitivity of the skin as well as allodynia in the affected dermatome (Table 16-6). Allodynia is frequently severe enough to be the dominant clinical feature of PHN. Among children with cancer or immunologic disorders, early antiviral treatment is highly recommended for prevention of PHN. Oral *famciclovir* is an effective and well-tolerated regimen for immunocompromised patients with HZ.[35] VZV can cause acute abdominal pain without skin manifestations in BMT recipients.[36]

Children who do suffer from established PHN are often treated similarly to adults, with tricyclic antidepressants, anticonvulsants, local anesthetics (topical, regional, systemic), opioids, and occasionally epidurals with local anesthetics and corticosteroids; there are no controlled trials regarding efficacy of any of these treatments in childhood. One study in adults recommends intrathecal corticosteroids.[37] In one case series, treatments for zoster-associated pain in children include standard analgesics in 68% of patients (nonsteroidal anti-inflammatory drugs [NSAIDs], acetaminophen, or mild opioids), tricyclic antidepressants in 44%, antiepileptic drugs in 21%, and topical local anesthetics in 12%. No patient was prescribed steroids. Several patients received nerve blocks for pain relief.[38]

▶ Graft-versus-host disease

Graft-versus-host disease (GvHD) is the second most common complication in children receiving BMT, with mucositis being the most common complication. The risk of *acute GvHD* has been considerably reduced over the past three decades by the use of prophylactic agents. It commonly affects the skin, liver, and gastrointestinal tract. Children can develop a maculopapular rash that often desquamates. The disease then leads to hepatomegaly with jaundice and ascites. Dysphagia and odynophagia result from desquamation, web and stricture formation, and reflux esophagitis due to inflammation of the gastrointestinal tract. Many patients have anorexia, nausea, lower abdominal pain, cramping, and diarrhea. Abdominal pain is most often treated with opioids. Muscle cramps are a common complaint. Rarely, myositis, with tender muscles and elevated muscle enzymes, may occur. Fasciitis often affects forearms and legs, causing significant limitations in range of motion and joint contractures. Patients may benefit from physical therapy and massage. Steroids and other immunomodulatory drugs may be used to treat GvHD once the disease is apparent.[29]

Chronic GvHD is the most common nonrelapse problem affecting long-term survivors of BMT. The incidence of chronic GvHD is lower in children but remains significant. A recent evaluation reported a chronic GvHD rate of 21.2% despite uniform GvHD prophylaxis with *methotrexate*.[39] Unfortunately, chronic GvHD is becoming more frequent due to the increasing use of non-HLA-matched donors, increasing age limits of transplantation, and the use of peripheral blood stem cells instead of bone marrow as the source of the graft. Children and adults frequently have very similar presentations of chronic GvHD.[40]

▶ Chemotherapy-related pain

Intravenous (IV) chemotherapy can cause significant pain on injection with particular agents such as leucovorin or thiotepa, even when the vein is intact. Thrombophlebitis can also occur after injection into a peripheral vein. However, central lines are used more commonly in children for delivering chemotherapy. This has decreased the risk of extravasation into the surrounding soft tissue when peripheral IVs are used. Extravasation of chemotherapeutic vesicant agents can result in significant tissue damage, alteration in limb function, and pain. Known chemotherapeutic vesicants include mechlorethamine, mitomycin-C, doxorubicin, daunomycin, vincristine, and vinblastine.[41] Other agents are more irritants than vesicants and can cause a burning sensation. Extravasation can involve a nerve, creating neuropathic pain. Children are more likely to develop nerve pain after the use of specific agents such as vincristine. Neuropathic pain can also develop after radiation therapy to the spine or peripheral nervous system. This can be treated with a decreased dose of vincristine, tricyclic antidepressants, or gabapentin.[42] Paclitaxel (Taxol), an effective antineoplastic agent for the treatment of solid tumors, produces a dose-limiting painful peripheral neuropathy.[43] Granulocyte colony-stimulating factor (GCSF) given to children to increase neutrophil production can cause bony pain.[44,45]

Delivery of cytotoxic agents *intrathecally* has possible complications as well, including arachnoiditis or meningeal irritation syndrome. Patients may complain of headache, nuchal rigidity, fever, nausea, and vomiting. There are reports of anterior lumbosacral radiculopathy after intrathecal methotrexate.[46]

Varieties of drugs commonly used in pediatric oncology are listed in Table 16-7 with their side effects. All the drugs cause nausea, vomiting, mucosal inflammation, and bone marrow toxicity.

Newer agents can produce pain by novel mechanisms. An antibody-based therapy *3F8* for stage-4 neuroblastoma binds to epitopes on small peripheral fibers, causing severe neuropathic abdominal and limb pain.

Thalidomide has been used for treating cancers and inflammatory disorders. Side effects associated with thalidomide include teratogenicity, peripheral neuropathy, and deep vein thrombosis. Somnolence, rash, and abdominal pain can occur with its use.[47] Thalidomide has a direct analgesic action on some forms of established neuropathic pain as well.[48]

▶ Procedural-related pain

During the course of a child's cancer therapy, they will be "stuck" with hundreds of needles. There is a great need for frequent blood sampling, as well as the delivery of IV medications, which make needles the biggest source of fear for pediatric oncology patients. Having an implanted port still requires a "poke" to access it. It is best to prepare children with an age-appropriate explanation before the procedure. Enlist the parents' cooperation prior to the needle puncture and assess the child's coping style. This should include an age-appropriate explanation of why the procedure is being done and what to expect.

Topical anesthesia can be utilized to diminish needle pain. Techniques include injection of local anesthetic at the procedure

Table 16-7

Commonly Used Drugs in Pediatric Malignancy

Class	Drug	Side effects
Vinca alkaloids	Vincristine	Neuropathy, constipation
	Vinblastine	Myositis
Antimetabolites	Methotrexate	Nephrotoxicity, lung fibrosis, hepatic fibrosis, CNS
	6-Mercaptopurine	Hepatic fibrosis
Alkylating agents	Cyclophosphamide	Hemorrhagic cystitis, sterility
	Ifosfamide	Nephrotoxicity, sterility
	Melphalan	Cardiomyopathy
	CCNU	Sterility, lung fibrosis, cardiomyopathy, late bone marrow toxicity
Antibiotics	Doxorubicin	Cardiomyopathy
	Daunorubicin	Cardiomyopathy
	Actinomycin-D	Hepatic fibrosis
	Bleomycin	Lung fibrosis
Platinum compounds	Cisplatinum	Nephrotoxicity, neurotoxicity
	Carboplatinum	Nephrotoxicity
Epipodophyllotoxins	Etoposide	CNS, secondary leukemia
Miscellaneous	Procarbazine	Hepatic fibrosis
	L-asparginase	Hepatic fibrosis, CNS
Steroids	Prednisolone	Bone, skeletal maturity

Source: From Ref. 29.

site, application of topical anesthetic creams, iontophoresis, and ultrasound. Local anesthetics pose a somewhat increased risk of systemic toxicity in infants due to decreased plasma protein concentration, higher free fraction, slower hepatic metabolism, slightly reduced plasma pseudocholinesterase activity, and decreased methemoglobin-reductase activity.[49]

The most commonly applied topical cream is EMLA cream (eutectic mixture of 2.5% lidocaine and 2.5% prilocaine). EMLA cream can be effective in reducing pain associated with venipuncture, assessing ports, or lumbar puncture. It is effective for anesthetizing the dermis only. There is a theoretical risk of methemoglobinemia secondary to the prilocaine component of EMLA but this is rare. EMLA can cause the unwanted side effect of vasoconstriction. The benefit of decreasing a child's distress usually outweighs the disadvantage of vasoconstriction. It is recommended to apply EMLA cream a minimum of 45 minutes prior to needle insertion, but the longer it is on, the better the anesthesia. Because of this time constraint, EMLA may be underutilized. Some advocate giving parents a tube for application at home before bringing the child in. There are reports of vasodilation after the cream has been on for 3 hours.

The prolonged onset of maximum analgesia is a significant handicap of EMLA cream. This has led to numerous drugs and techniques being developed to enhance the rate of onset of analgesia, such as

ELA-Max, ultrasound pretreatment, and amethocaine (tetracaine) microemulsion. ELA-Max (4% liposomal lidocaine) is a rapidly acting topical agent for intact skin that works by way of a liposomal delivery system. Studies demonstrate that a 30-minute application of ELA-Max is as safe and as effective as a 60-minute application of EMLA.[50] Additionally, ELA-Max is reported to cause less blanching of the skin, which may increase the success rate of IV insertion, and it has no prilocaine, eliminating the risk of methemoglobinemia.[51]

A topical formulation of the ester-type local anesthetic *amethocaine* is available abroad for reducing pain from cutaneous procedures such as venipuncture. Amethocaine gel (4%) is known to be more powerful with a shorter onset than EMLA; however, it produces greater systemic toxicity. It produces anesthesia within 30–45 minutes of application; its duration of action ranges from 4 to 6 hours. In the neonatal population, amethocaine was found to be ineffective at reducing the pain of heel prick and peripherally inserted central catheters.[52] A newer mixture called AMLI (2.5% amethocaine and 2.5% lidocaine) has been shown effective in relieving venous puncture pain in children. AMLI exhibits a shorter latency period than EMLA, while inducing fewer adverse effects than 4% amethocaine and EMLA.[53] Amethocaine 4% microemulsion has been developed in an attempt to achieve faster drug permeation, thus reducing the time to analgesic effect.[54]

Ultrasound pretreatment of skin increases permeation rates of hydrophobic topical medications like lidocaine. Applying an ultrasound device to the skin for 15 seconds followed by 5 minutes of 4% liposomal lidocaine cream has been shown to significantly reduce the pain of venipuncture.[55] A low-dose lidocaine *iontophoresis* system has been developed that provides topical anesthesia in children for venipuncture within 10 minutes.[56]

Another technique for reducing pain and anxiety during IV insertion is using subcutaneous *buffered lidocaine*. Buffered lidocaine is composed of 1 part sodium bicarbonate with 10 parts of 1% lidocaine. Buffering the pH from 7.0 to 7.4 reduces the pain associated with local anesthetic infiltration. This has been shown to be as effective as topical ELA-Max applied 30 minutes before IV insertion.[57]

A newer alternative is J-Tip, a needleless injection system that can be used for delivery of local anesthetic before IV cannulation. Eighty-four percent of pediatric patients reported no pain at the time of J-Tip lidocaine application compared to 61% in the EMLA group at the time of dressing removal.[58]

▶ Lumbar puncture

Lumbar puncture (LP) is a frequently performed procedure for diagnosis and treatment in pediatric oncology patients. The physical pain and psychological distress associated with this procedure can be great for a child. The most painful parts of this procedure are penetrating skin and contacting periosteum. Cutaneous analgesics, like EMLA, can help with the former and can ameliorate pain from deeper infiltration with injected local anesthetics. The dura is rarely a pain generator when doing an LP.

Positioning is often a distressing part of the LP, as well as the requirement for the patient to remain still for a prolonged period of time. Sometimes it is necessary to provide conscious sedation or a general anesthetic if a patient cannot voluntarily comply with these demands. Neck flexion is irrelevant to opening up the lumbar intervertebral spaces and is unnecessary. A thin, spinal needle with a noncutting tip should be considered for patients who complain of headaches from previous LPs.

In pediatrics, complications from LP are typically mild and short lasting. The frequency of positional and nonpositional headaches

after LP is lower in children than in adults, but not as rare as commonly taught. A study in the general pediatric population showed that 27% of the patients experienced headaches (positional headache in 9%), and 40% developed backache after LP. Frequency of complaints increased with patients' ages. It may be underestimated among preschool children due to their difficulty in expressing complaints.[59] Of children aged 10–12 years, 12% developed a headache, whereas in children aged 13–18 years, 50% developed a headache. With puberty, the incidence of headache increases in girls. Patients with higher cell counts in their cerebrospinal fluid had more frequent headaches than did patients without pleocytosis. Cannula gauge or bevel orientation of Quinkes did not influence outcome, which differs from the adult literature.[60]

A postdural puncture headache (PDPH) or spinal headache can be a debilitating complication after a LP. The classic PDPH usually presents within 24–48 hours after a LP. The headache is postural (i.e., is worsened with the upright position and relieved with supine positioning) and is frequently associated with nausea and vomiting. It is located most commonly over the occipital or frontal areas, and it has associated clinical manifestations such as blurred vision, neck and low back pain, and occasionally abducens nerve palsy and diplopia.[61] Conservative treatment of PDPH with hydration, caffeine, supine position, and mild analgesics will lead to resolution of symptoms in most children within several days. Pharmacologic treatments proposed for treating PDPH include sumatriptan, intravenous caffeine, theophylline, and adrenocorticotropic hormone (ACTH). Acupuncture has been proposed as well.[62] If the symptoms are severe and are not relieved within a few days, an autologous epidural blood patch may be necessary. The appropriate volume of autologous blood for a patch in children is 0.2–0.3 mL·kg^{-1}. In some cases, smaller amounts of blood may sufficiently relieve symptoms, but larger volumes, up to 0.64 mL·kg^{-1}, have also been used. Blood injection should be stopped if resistance is felt.[59] It is contraindicated to perform an autologous epidural blood patch in infected, leukemic, or other immunocompromised patients because of the risk of seeding the epidural or subarachnoid space either with infectious organisms or cancer cells.[61,63] The epidural placement of various nonblood materials, including dextran, albumin, fibrin glue, and gelatin, have been reported.

▶ Bone marrow biopsy

Bone marrow aspiration is more painful than LP. This can be due to factors, which include using a larger needle, intentionally contacting the sensitive periosteum, and suctioning the marrow. Local anesthetic does not adequately treat the discomfort of aspirating bone marrow. The best approach to alleviating a child's distress is by tailoring treatment to the individual patient. This can range from general anesthesia for an uncooperative 4-year-old, to guided imagery and hypnosis for a willing teenager. Other anesthetic options include propofol for brief anesthetics in patients with indwelling IV access, nitrous oxide with some volatile agent, or oral midazolam and ketamine.[64] Some literature has advocated the use of oral transmucosal fentanyl citrate (OTFC) for this population. At many centers, propofol is administered in combination with short-acting opioids, including alfentanil, remifentanil, or fentanyl for these procedures.[65]

An interesting study evaluated periosteal infiltration with bupivacaine for pain relief. Patients undergoing bilateral hip marrow aspirates had only one side infiltrated, thus serving as their own controls. Lower pain scores were recorded on the bupivacaine side for 3 days after the procedure.[66] One risk associated with this practice is an inadvertent intraosseous (marrow space) injection. Rapid systemic uptake of bupivacaine could lead to cardiac depression, arrhythmia, or seizures.

Central line

Central venous catheters are now more commonly used in children with cancer. Most are placed under a general anesthetic. For their removal, a brief general anesthetic is often called for. The indwelling line can be used to induce anesthesia with a sedative-hypnotic, like propofol. Then, anesthesia can be maintained with volatile agents while the line is being removed.

NONMALIGNANT/CHRONIC PAIN IN SURVIVORS

It is easy to overlook more common pain-producing states in a complex pediatric oncology setting. It must be remembered that these patients can suffer from acute appendicitis, nonspecific abdominal pain, benign headaches or migraines, as well as cancer-associated discomfort. In fact, acute appendicitis has a high diagnostic error rate in patients with leukemia.

Chronic pain in cancer survivors

Almost 70% of children diagnosed with cancer now live 5 or more years after diagnosis, and so the number of pediatric cancer patients who develop chronic pain related or unrelated to their disease or treatment has markedly increased. A conference on the long-term complications of treatment of children and adolescents with cancer assessed general health, mental health, functional status, activity limitations, cancer-related pain, and cancer-related anxiety/fears. Those at substantial risk for long-term complications were females, those with less education, and those with low household incomes.[67,68] Posttraumatic stress symptoms, particularly intrusive thoughts, avoidance, and arousal, are among the most common psychological after effects of childhood cancer for survivors and their parents.

Types of pain most commonly seen in cancer survivors are phantom limb pain, causalgia, complex regional pain syndrome, other forms of neuropathic pain in the limbs,[70] avascular necrosis of joints, unspecified abdominal pain (often associated with chronic GvHD), and headaches. These cases can prove difficult to manage because pain is often mentally associated with tumor recurrence, thus producing elevated anxiety in the patient and family. New forms of pain in a patient with a history of cancer should be considered as a potential recurrence until proven otherwise with diagnostic testing.

Pain after amputation

Chronic pain after a limb removal for treatment of malignancy can be due to stump pain or phantom pain. Stump pain may be due to neuroma formation, a poorly fitted prosthetic, recurrent tumor, or infection. Phantom limb is a neuropathic condition that is common in children and may appear even more frequently than in adults.[69] Krane and Heller reported that 100% (24/24) of young amputees had phantom sensations and 83% had phantom limb pain. Children's pain tends to decrease with time spontaneously, but a significant number will experience stump pain or phantom limb pain 1 year after loss of the limb. Preoperative limb pain or preoperative

chemotherapy may increase the incidence of phantom limb pain. Many analgesic modalities have been tried, with limited success. These include sympathetic blockade, tricyclic antidepressants, calcitonin, trigger point injections, psychotherapy, massage, biofeedback, and even dorsal rhizotomy or partial lobectomy. Preemptive analgesia has a role in minimizing the risk of phantom limb pain with preoperative regional anesthesia and gabapentin.[71] Applying a TENS unit to the contralateral extremity has been shown to effectively decrease the intensity of phantom sensations.[71] Recent brain imaging studies have demonstrated rapidly occurring plastic changes in cortical somatosensory organization following amputation. They have also shown regression of these patterns of abnormal cortical organization with effective therapies, including mirror-image physical therapy, early use of myoelectric prosthesis, and, in selected cases, opioids.[72,73]

Avascular necrosis

Survivors of childhood cancer are at risk of corticosteroid-induced osteonecrosis later in life. This can frequently be a cause of pain in this population, usually with extended weight bearing. A study reviewing magnetic resonance imaging (MRI) ankle scans in patients who survived childhood cancer showed that 67% of ankles had osteonecrosis. Older children had the highest incidence of the disease.[74] In selected cases, joint replacements can dramatically improve pain and reduce disability.

NONPHARMACOLOGIC TREATMENTS

Emerging evidence from randomized trials supports the value of nonpharmacologic approaches for alleviating distress and pain in pediatric oncology patients. When used as complementary techniques, these interventions can reduce the amount of pharmacologic treatment needed and minimize undesirable side effects. Studies have shown the effectiveness of combining several nonpharmacologic techniques. Deciding on whether to use pharmacologic versus nonpharmacologic approach requires an understanding of available techniques, consideration of the pain and anxiety associated with a given procedure, the child's age, behavior, coping skills, fear/anxiety, and past pain experience. Children who learn these skills can apply them to any new situation that causes distress or pain throughout their course of treatment and throughout their life.

Communication and preparatory information

One of the simplest adjuncts to pain management in children is verbally preparing them for procedures. Parents and clinicians can dramatically influence a child's experience of pain by discussing the specific sensations that the child will encounter. Giving children choices about how to reduce the pain gives them greater control and this alone can improve the perception of pain. Procedures should be done away from the child's room or "safe zone." Enlisting the parents' support can serve to decrease parental anxiety and the child's as well.

Physical techniques include massage, heat and cold stimulation, TENS units, and acupuncture. *Massage* is increasingly utilized for patients with cancer to treat pain, fatigue, stress/anxiety, nausea, and depression. Stress has been linked to increased tumor development by decreasing natural killer (NK) cell activity. The long-term effects of massage include reduced depression and hostility and increased urinary dopamine, serotonin values, NK cell number, and lymphocytes.[75]

Symptom scores have been reduced by approximately 50% after massage.[76] For a more extensive discussion of massage therapy, see Chap. 14.

Acupuncture has been shown to reduce pain intensity, fatigue, and nausea in cancer patients.[77–79] Zeltzer reported on acupuncture and hypnosis as techniques for reducing chronic pediatric pain and found that pain was significantly improved after six weekly sessions.[80] A more extensive discussion of acupuncture can be found in Chap. 14.

Behavioral techniques include exercise, relaxation, biofeedback, modeling, desensitization, and art and play therapy. These techniques have demonstrated efficacy in managing side effects in children on chemotherapy. *Exercise* has been shown to be beneficial in combating the fatigue associated with chemotherapy.[81] Behavioral interventions can effectively control anticipatory nausea and vomiting in pediatric cancer patients undergoing chemotherapy as well as reducing anxiety and distress accompanying invasive treatments.[82]

Cognitive therapy includes meditation, distraction, attention, imagery, thought stopping, hypnosis, music therapy, and psychotherapy. Cognitive-behavioral techniques (CBT) are commonly used to help a child mitigate anxiety and distress. These techniques vary based on the child's age and coping ability, level of fear and anxiety surrounding the procedure, and the pain expected to be generated by the procedure. Many studies show that CBT is effective for controlling nausea and vomiting secondary to chemotherapy. In younger children, *distraction* has been found to be useful. In children from the ages of 10 to 17, a computer-simulated technique of *virtual reality* has been effective as a distraction during outpatient chemotherapy.[83] *Hypnosis* can effectively reduce pain and anxiety in children undergoing bone marrow aspiration.[84,85]

Herbal supplements are gaining popularity but their use can be problematic due to an incomplete understanding of how they interact with cancer drugs. Concurrent use of herbal products with mainstream oncologic treatment should be undertaken cautiously until further research delineates the synergistic effects of these supplements.[86]

ANALGESIC MEDICATIONS

Pediatric research on the use of analgesics in cancer is limited. Approximately 50%–75% of the drugs used in pediatric medicine have not been studied adequately to provide appropriate labeling about dosing and side effects. In 1997, Congress passed the Food and Drug Administration Modernization Act (FDAMA), which encouraged pediatric drug development by providing incentives to manufacturers. This led to improved understanding of the pharmacokinetics of drugs in pediatric medicine, important dose changes, and improved drug safety for children (Table 16-8).[87]

Pain due to malignancy should be treated early by applying the WHO ladder (Table 16-9). Care should be taken to not overlook the problem of neuropathic pain that may not respond well to standard dosing of acetaminophen, NSAIDs, and opioids.

▶ Nonopioids

Acetaminophen is the most commonly used analgesic in the pediatric population. It inhibits prostaglandin synthesis primarily in the CNS. It avoids the sedation seen with opioids and the gastritis/platelet inhibition seen with NSAIDs. The safety and efficacy of

---

Table 16-8
Pain Management Basics
Preempt the development of pain
Provide a baseline of analgesia at rest
Adjust analgesics to the situation (e.g., procedure or mouth care)
Assess the level of pain by asking or examining patient
The correct dose of opioids is the one that adequately relieves pain

---

acetaminophen in children are well established.[88] However, it can cause hepatic and renal injury at high doses. Studies suggest oral dosing of 15 mg/kg every 4 hours. Rectal absorption is less, and an elevated dose of 30–40 mg/kg can be given once to attain equivalent blood levels. Due to the risk of bacteremia, rectal medication administration is usually avoided in the oncology population. The risk of developing toxic reactions to acetaminophen is lower in children than in adults. However, concerns about pediatric acetaminophen toxicity remain high because this drug is so widely used. Reports of liver toxicity in pediatric patients have associated a single acetaminophen dose of 120–150 mg/kg of body weight with hepatotoxicity. Fasting is linked to increased acetaminophen hepatotoxicity. Acetaminophen is contraindicated in neutropenic patients for whom monitoring fever is critical.

Aspirin (ASA) is a common analgesic that is avoided due to the increased risk of bleeding in the pediatric oncology population. Aspirin irreversibly inhibits platelet function, which adds significant risk to a cancer patient who might become thrombocytopenic during the course of treatment.

NSAIDs also are often contraindicated in this population because of the risks of bleeding. NSAIDs reversibly inhibit platelets, but the effect wears off sooner than aspirin when the drug is cleared. NSAIDs, if used carefully, are very effective analgesics, especially in combination with opioids. Care should be taken in giving antipyretics to neutropenic patients. NSAIDs cause platelet thromboxane inhibition. Therefore, NSAIDs are contraindicated in pediatric oncology patients at risk of thrombocytopenia. Conversely, in patients with advanced cancer who have adequate coagulation parameters, there is a role for NSAIDs as components of a multimodal analgesic regimen. There is ample research on the pediatric pharmacokinetics of NSAIDs but few studies have compared different types of NSAIDs in children. A meta-analysis evaluating NSAIDs for bone pain versus visceral pain found them equally effective. The pharmacokinetic characteristics of *ibuprofen* in children are similar to those in adults, and clinical experience suggests that ibuprofen is better tolerated by children than adults. Clinical trials of ibuprofen have shown the effective dose range to be 7.5–10 mg/kg.[89]

Table 16-9
WHO Ladder for Pediatric Cancer Pain
Step 1: Acetaminophen + NSAIDs
Step 2: Mild opioids
Step 3: Opioids (for severe pain, start at this step)

Cyclooxygenase-2 (COX-2) inhibitors[90–92] were developed to be more selective inhibitors of inducible prostanoid synthesis in leukocytes and in the nervous system, and to have diminished actions on platelets and on gastric mucosal integrity compared with traditional NSAIDs. Clinical trials in adults raised the concern that selective COX-2 inhibition may predispose patients to cardiac and vascular complications.[93] The relevance of these risks for healthy children or children with cancer is unknown. Renal effects, edema, and hypertension appear to be similar for conventional NSAIDs and COX-2-selective inhibitors.[94] Most available studies on COX-2 inhibitors in children are either small pharmacokinetic studies, small studies in children with arthritis, or studies in postoperative patients, especially those undergoing tonsillectomy.[95–97] Of the currently available COX-2s, the risk profile of *celecoxib* is most favorable. Celecoxib in children is cleared faster than in adults, is well-tolerated, and without significant side effects.[98] A safer alternative to COX-2s may be naproxen along with a proton pump inhibitor.

Combining adjuvants can provide additive analgesia and, with some drug combinations, less-than-additive toxicities. Ibuprofen can be dosed every 6–8 hours and acetaminophen every 4 hours up to 5 doses per day. The two drugs should not be administered in the same schedule (every 4 hours). On the basis of pharmacokinetics, alternating doses might be used every 6 hours so that one drug or the other is administered every 3 hours.[99]

▶ Opioids

Morphine

Morphine is the most commonly used mu-opioid agonist. There is flexibility in the routes by which it may be delivered (IV, PO, PR, SC, epidural, intrathecal). Morphine is converted to morphine-6-glucuronide (M6G), which is primarily responsible for the analgesic effect as well as side effects.[100] M6G is renally cleared and accumulates in patients with renal insufficiency. Age is the most important factor affecting morphine requirements and plasma morphine concentrations. Because morphine clearance is decreased in the first 3 months of life, the dose should be reduced by 50% for these young infants. Morphine has a half-life of 10–20 hours in preterm babies, whereas the half-life in young children can be as low as 2 hours. In full-term neonates, the volume of distribution is linear with age and weight. In vitro studies of fetuses up to 27 weeks indicated that morphine glucuronidation was approximately 10%–20% of that seen in adults, and it can be seen in premature infants as young as 24 weeks. Given IV, the pediatric dose of morphine is 0.1 mg/kg per dose (less for infants) (Table 16-10). Infusion dosing is 0.02–0.03 mg/kg/h; if less than 4 months old, decrease the dose to 0.015 mg/kg/h.[101]

Oral morphine is often the first choice for cancer patients with moderate to severe pain. The first-pass effect is considerable, so oral dosing should be three times greater than IV dosing. It has been demonstrated that children younger than 11 years had significantly higher morphine clearance than older children and also had a larger volume of distribution than adults. Hepatic blood flow and liver-to-body-weight ratio is greater in younger children. Studies suggest that a dose of at least 1.5 mg/kg/d is necessary to attain the minimum effective blood concentration (higher than adults dose of 1.0). Recommendations for starting most opioid-naïve patients on immediate-release oral morphine are 0.3 mg/kg every 4 hours.[102] Sustained-release (SR) oral morphine is available for use in pediatric oncology patients requiring long-acting opioids. Fluctuations in blood level are more marked in children than in adults due to the

shorter elimination half-life. Many centers now give SR morphine every 8 hours to provide steady-state analgesia.[102]

Once-a-day dosed morphine is called *Kadian*. It is constructed with time-release pellets that can be mixed with food. There is much more risk for under- or overdosing with a once-daily drug. Caution should be taken before using once-a-day dosing in children without sufficient research and adequate pain assessment.

Hydromorphone (Dilaudid)

Hydromorphone is often used when there are dose-limiting side effects associated with morphine. It is also available PO, IV, subcutaneously (SC), epidurally, or intrathecally. Studies of IV hydromorphone versus morphine in children demonstrate a potency ratio of 5:1. It is a preferred agent for SC infusion due to its high potency, high concentration, and hydrophilic nature. It can be specially prepared to a concentration of 50 mg/mL if needed. Hydromorphone is safe to use in patients with renal disease. There are no studies on its pharmacokinetics in infants. There is an oral immediate-release form of hydromorphone (Dilaudid IR) that has been studied in young subjects.[103] The new once-daily oral hydromorphone is called *Palladone*. To date, there has been no research on its use in children.

Methadone

Methadone is a long-acting opioid that has a growing role in pediatric palliative care. It has a variable half-life ranging from 6 to 24 hours after a single parenteral dose in opioid-naïve subjects. The parenteral to oral ratio is approximately 1:1.5 to 1:2. Converting the dose of other opioids to methadone has been problematic for some physicians. Delayed somnolence has occurred as a result. Methadone has therapeutic effects that extend beyond its opioid effect. It is a racemic mix, with the *l*-isomer working at the mu-receptor and the *d*-isomer working as an antagonist at the *N*-methyl-*D*-aspartate (NMDA) receptor.[104] This antagonism has been shown to prevent and possibly reverse opioid tolerance. Methadone's NMDA receptor antagonism makes it appropriate for consideration in cancer patients with neuropathic pain who do not respond to dose increases of other opioids. Methadone, if given to opioid-tolerant patients, acts more potently than in opioid-naïve patients. Therefore, converting to methadone in tolerant patients should be less than the guidelines suggest for naïve patients.

Care should be taken with dosing methadone. Many opioid conversion charts underestimate the potency of methadone, which can result in toxicity. Evaluate the patient's response to the first doses. If the patient becomes comfortable, extend the intervals or decrease the dose to minimize risk of oversedation. If the patient becomes sedated with dosing, hold subsequent doses until the patient shows signs of less sedation. Early in dosing, methadone as needed (prn) is appropriate until a schedule is established. Cancer patients should then be placed on a scheduled dose to avoid windows in pain coverage. With the long half-life, there is a risk of delayed sedation or possible overdose several days into treatment.

The efficacy of methadone is well known in adults, but there is limited clinical information on children or neonates. It can be taken orally, as a liquid, crushed, or IV. One study of methadone pharmacokinetics in children aged 1–18 years found a prolonged elimination half-life (19.2 hours) with a range of 3.8–62 hours. The great variability in half-life suggests that some pediatric patients may metabolize methadone as adults do, whereas others may have low plasma clearance rates. Methadone can be especially valuable in pediatric cancer patients with neuropathic pain that is poorly responsive to opioids

Table 16-10

Opioid Analgesic Initial Dosage Guidelines

Drug	Equianalgesic doses		Usual starting IV or SC doses and intervals		Parenteral oral dose ratio	Usual starting oral doses and intervals	
	Parenteral	Oral	Child <50 kg	Child >50 kg		Child <50 kg	Child >50 kg
Codeine	120 mg	200 mg	NR	NR	1:2	0.5–1.0 mg/kg q3–4h	30–60 mg q3–4h
Morphine	10 mg	30 mg (chronic)	Bolus: 0.1 mg/kg q2–4h	Bolus: 5–8 mg q2–4h	1:3 (chronic)	Immediate release: 0.3 mg/kg q3–4h	Immediate release: 15–20 mg q3–4h
		60 mg (single dose)	Infusion: 0.03 mg/kg/h	Infusion: 1.5 mg/h	1.6 (single dose)	Sustained release: 20–35 kg: 10–15 mg q8–12h	Sustained release: 30–45 mg q8–12h
Oxycodone	NA	15–20 mg	NA	NA	NA	0.1–0.2 mg/kg q3–4h	5–10 mg q3–4h
Methadone*	10 mg	10–20 mg	0.1 mg/kg q4–8h	1:2	1:1.5–1:2	0.15–0.2 mg/kg q4–8h	7–10 mg q4–8h
Fentanyl	100 µg (0.1 mg)	NA	Bolus: 0.5–1.0 µg/kg q1–2h	Bolus: 25–50 µg q1–2h	NA	NA	NA
			Infusion: 0.5–2.0 µg/kg/h	Infusion: 25–100 µg/h			
Hydromorphone	1.5–2.0 mg	6–8 mg	Bolus: 0.02 mg q2–4h	Bolus: 1 mg q2–4h	1:4	0.04–0.08 mg/kg q3–4h	2–4 mg q3–4h
			Infusion: 0.006 mg/kg/h	Infusion: 0.3 mg/h			
Meperidine† (pethidine)	75–100 mg	300 mg	Bolus: 0.8–1.0 mg/kg q2–3h	Bolus: 50–75 mg q2–3h	1:4	2–3 mg/kg q3–4h	100–150 mg q3–4h

NA = not available: NR = not recommended.

*Methadone requires additional vigilance, because it can accumulate and produce delayed sedation. If sedation occurs, doses should be withheld until sedation resolves. Thereafter, doses should be substantially reduced or the dosing interval should be extended to 8 to 12 hours (or both).

†Meperidine should generally be avoided if other opioids are available, especially with chronic use, because its metabolite can cause seizures. Note: Doses refer to patients older than 6 months. In infants younger than 6 months, initial doses per kg should begin at roughly 25% of the doses per kg recommended here. All doses are approximate and should be adjusted according to clinical circumstances,

Source: From Berde CB, Sethna NF. Analgesics in the treatment of pain in children. *N Engl J Med.* 2002;347:1094–1103.

or when opioid side effects are intolerable. It has been used successfully in a PCA for children with refractory cancer pain.[105]

Oxycodone

Oxycodone is a semisynthetic oral opioid used for moderate to severe pain relief that has no ceiling effect. It is available in the United States in short-acting oral form as tablets or as a liquid, and in the form of controlled-release tablets (marketed as OxyContin). It has a higher bioavailability and a slightly longer half-life than oral morphine in adults.[106,107] However, in children 2–20 years old, oxycodone has a higher clearance and a shorter half-life than morphine.

OxyContin is a long-acting form of oxycodone. It has a more rapid onset compared to MS Contin when swallowed whole. This preparation should not be given to children who cannot swallow pills, as chewing or crushing converts it to immediate release, which could be dangerous. The conversion from parenteral morphine equivalents to long-acting oxycodone should be done via short-acting oxycodone.[108] In recent years, abuse of OxyContin has emerged as a major public health issue. While occasional patients may sometimes have a favorable side-effect profile with OxyContin, in view of OxyContin's greater cost and drug diversion concerns, we do not believe that this formulation offers any unique advantages for most patients compared with less expensive alternatives for long-acting oral analgesia, such as sustained-release morphine or methadone.

Fentanyl

Fentanyl is a synthetic opioid that is 50–100 times more potent than morphine, and its potency varies depending on its mode of administration, that is, bolus versus infusion. Its advantage of rapid onset and rapid elimination is due to its lipophilic nature, which allows it to enter the brain more quickly than morphine or hydromorphone. This property makes it the ideal drug for short, painful procedures such as needle punctures or dressing changes.

In a preterm baby, the half-life of fentanyl has been shown to be prolonged in cardiac surgery. Clearance approaches adult levels by the first month and is even higher than adults in infants and children. When bolused, fentanyl can cause chest wall rigidity and make ventilation extremely difficult.[109] It can be infused, but its elimination half-life increases after prolonged infusion and it loses the benefit of rapid elimination. Some studies suggest that there may be less histamine released from fentanyl versus morphine, but pruritis is equal.

Due to the lipophilicity of fentanyl, it can be delivered through the mouth or skin. Transdermal use is ideal for pediatric patients who have constant severe pain and who cannot take oral medications.[110] It should not be used for opioid-naïve patients or patients whose pain is fluctuating rapidly, as it cannot be rapidly titrated. Once placed, the patch takes 18–24 hours to reach a steady state in the blood. There are reports of using fentanyl patches on children as young as 3 years. The equipotency ratio of transdermal fentanyl to oral morphine is a 25 mcg patch to 45 mg per day.

Transmucosal fentanyl (oral transmucosal fentanyl citrate [OTFC]) via a "lollipop" is an alternative way to provide painless opioid administration. Although data in children are limited, it can be used for those older than 2 years who weigh more than 10 kg. Initially OTFC seemed like a great breakthrough for pediatric pain relief, as it is less threatening and is readily acceptable to children. Absorption via the oral mucosa would bypass the first-pass effect to which oral fentanyl is subject. However, the reality is that there are numerous disadvantages to the fentanyl lollipop. Children cannot be prevented from chewing the lollipop and getting a larger release of fentanyl than intended. Children have also been known to refuse the lollipop before or midway through consumption, receiving only a partial dose. Time to complete the Oralet can be very variable, ranging from 5 to 45 minutes. Children also need to be constantly watched while consuming the lollipop. The increased incidence of nausea (12%), vomiting (31%), and postoperative respiratory events may also serve to limit clinical usefulness,[111–113] although it has been proven effective for bone marrow aspiration and lumbar puncture.

Oral delivery of the IV formulation of fentanyl is being reexamined and some distinct advantages are apparent: ease of administration, rapid single-swallow consumption, and rare partial dosing due to refusal. Oral delivery of the IV formulation of fentanyl bypasses buccal absorption but still results in similar plasma concentrations as an equivalent dose of OTFC. Oral liquid fentanyl has an acceptable taste, costs less, is commonly available, and facilitates a flexible dosing schedule.[114]

Meperidine

Meperidine is a synthetic opioid that has similar uses to morphine, with a shorter duration of action. Its most frequent use, in low-dose, is for the treatment of rigors due to postoperative anesthesia, blood transfusion, or amphotericin administration. However, its drawback is that its major metabolite, normeperidine, can accumulate and cause dysphoria, excitation, and seizures, especially in patients with renal dysfunction. For these reasons it is not recommended for use in chronic pain patients. It may be used instead of fentanyl for short procedures, as the duration of action is shorter than morphine. Neonates eliminate meperidine more slowly and, therefore, the drug should be avoided in this population.

Codeine

Codeine is historically the most commonly used weak opioid in the pediatric population for mild to moderate pain, and it is often regarded as the second step of the WHO ladder. Nevertheless, we discourage its use in most settings. At recommended doses (0.5–1 mg/kg), it is a very weak analgesic, and at higher doses, the frequency of side effects is quite high. Codeine is a prodrug that is effective only with conversion to morphine, and a remarkably high percentage of children

(46%) produced essentially no detectable morphine in a recent pediatric study.[115,116]

Hydrocodone

Hydrocodone, the opioid in Vicodin, is also considered a weak opioid. Knowledge of the weak opioids will allow the practitioner to phone in a prescription to a pharmacy when the patient needs immediate relief but may be far away from the provider. Tylenol with codeine as well as hydrocodone may be called in to a pharmacy in most locations in the United States.

Buprenorphine

In developing countries, mixed agonist-antagonists are used more frequently than in the United States for pain control due to tighter governmental regulation of mu-opioid agonists abroad. Morphine may be available only on a limited basis. Kappa agonists, for example, *buprenorphine*, are sometimes used to treat pediatric pain.[117] Using kappa or mixed agonists-antagonists is less than ideal, as somnolence or dysphoric reactions are more common and the antagonist could precipitate withdrawal in a patient taking mu agonists. The buprenorphine transdermal delivery system was introduced in 2001 for the treatment of chronic cancer pain, but there are no studies of its use in children to date.[118,119]

Tramadol

Tramadol is a synthetic analog of codeine that is used for the treatment of moderate pain. Tramadol is not primarily an opioid; rather it is a mixed 5HT-NE drug whose metabolite is probably a weak opioid. Its analgesic properties can be partially reversed by naloxone. It is known to produce less respiratory depression than the opioids. Centrally, tramadol exerts its action on monoaminergic systems, which contributes to its analgesic effect. Tramadol mainly inhibits noradrenaline uptake and promotes serotonin and noradrenaline release. Tramadol enhances the inhibitory activity of the descending pain pathways, resulting in a suppression of nociceptive transmission at the spinal level. Several clinical studies have shown that tramadol has peripheral local anesthetic properties (by an unknown mechanism) similar to lidocaine.[120] Tramadol has been given SC for postoperative analgesia.[121]

Peripheral acting opioids

The use of peripheral acting opiates could avoid the deleterious side effects of centrally acting opioids in pediatric cancer patients. *Loperamide* is an opioid agonist whose analgesic effects are mediated by the mu-opioid receptor peripherally. It does not cross the blood-brain barrier and can be antagonized by naloxone. Loperamide inhibits hyperalgesia when subcutaneously injected locally over a tumor.[122]

Diamorphine is an opioid gel that works particularly well on pain due to pressure sores occurring in palliative care. This type of pain does not respond well to oral analgesics. It is hypothesized that diamorphine gel binds to peripheral opioid receptors that are activated once inflammation is present.[123]

REFRACTORY CANCER PAIN

The majority of children can be kept adequately comfortable with dose escalation, adjuvants, and treatment of side effects. In 10% of

Table 16-11

Factors that May Influence Opioid Responsiveness

Type of pain (neuropathic)

Temporal pattern of pain (incident pain)

Tolerance – Progression of Disease

Individual factors

Drug specificity

Opioid metabolites

Route of administration

Source: From Ref. 124.

Table 16-12

Neuropathic Treatment Options

Neuroactive oral medications

   Tricyclic antidepressants

   Anticonvulsants (gabapentin, carbamazepine)

   Oral local anesthetics (mexiletine)

Nerve blockade (Local anesthetics, chemical or surgical neurolysis)

   Somatic or sympathetic

Spinal cord stimulation

Alpha-2 adrenergic agonists (clonidine, dexmedetomidine)

   Subarachnoid, epidural, IV, PO, Transdermal

children, however, more extensive management is required, as they are poorly responsive to opioids. This can be explained by many factors, such as changing nociception, receptor modulation, and production of inactive morphine metabolites (Table 16-11).[125]

When parents are surveyed after the death of their child with cancer, a high percentage report that the child experienced delays or incomplete effectiveness in achieving relief of pain and other symptoms.[6] In the adult oncology population, tumor spread, rather than tolerance, is the most common cause of rapid dose escalation. In children, predictors of intractable pain were identified as solid tumors metastatic to the spine, CNS, or major nerve plexus.

In 1995, the opioid requirements in children dying of cancer at Boston Children's Hospital and the Dana-Farber Cancer Institute were examined. One hundred and ninety-nine children were enrolled, and their opioid dose escalations were recorded. Twelve of these patients (6%) required greater than a hundredfold escalation over starting values or greater than 3 mg/kg/h, usually in the final weeks of life. Ranges of opioid dosing at the end of life were from 3.8 to 518 mg/kg/h of IV morphine equivalents. The highest infusion (518 mg/kg/h) occurred in an 18-month-old with a rhabdomyosarcoma with isolated metastases to the periaqueductal gray (PAG) matter. It was hypothesized that because the PAG is the site in the brainstem involved with mediating analgesia and defense reactions, metastases to this area made the patient extremely resistant to the analgesic effects of opioids.

Of the 12 children who required high-dose analgesia, two-thirds remained uncomfortable and required management beyond opioids, including epidural, spinal, or sedation. Those children who received sedation could not have their pain adequately controlled by other means. High-dose opioids should be continued along with sedatives to avoid having a patient who is in pain but too sedate to report it. The ethical issues of terminal sedation for the child with cancer are discussed elsewhere.[126]

Neuropathic pain is frequently resistant to opioids, so other classes of medication, such as tricyclic antidepressants, anticonvulsants, and local anesthetics, are often used (Table 16-12). The occurrence of central sensitization may perpetuate chronic neuropathic pain even when ongoing peripheral sensory input is absent. This sensitization, or windup, is thought to cause allodynia, hyperalgesia, and hyperpathia.

Adjuvant medications

While caring for a child in pain, a provider can increase opioid efficacy or reduce adverse effects by combining other drugs that are synergistic. Adjuvant analgesic is defined as *a heterogeneous group of drugs that have a primary indication other than pain but are analgesic in some painful conditions* (Table 16-13).

Clonidine

Clonidine, an alpha-2-adrenoceptor agonist commonly used in the treatment of hypertension, may reduce neuropathic pain. It has been administered spinally or epidurally for pain management, or orally as an anxiolytic/analgesic in pediatric palliative care. It directly acts on alpha-2 receptors to inhibit pain transmission along adrenergic pathways at the spinal cord. Studies show it decreases opioid requirements and/or improves pain relief in palliative cancer care. Clonidine is available as a patch and has been used in chronic neuropathic pain conditions.[128]

Anticonvulsants

The overlap between the pathophysiologic mechanisms of epilepsy models and neuropathic pain models supports the rationale for trying antiepileptic drugs (AEDs) in the treatment of neuropathic pain.[129]

Table 16-13

Analgesic Adjuvants

Alpha-2 agonist

NSAID

NMDA receptor antagonist

Anticonvulsant

Antidepressant

Corticosteroid

Stimulant

Skeletal muscle relaxant

CCK antagonist

Gabapentinoids

NK-1 receptor antagonist

Source: From Ref. 127.

This class of drugs was originally applied to lancinating or paroxysmal neuropathic pain, but is now also applied to cases with burning pain or allodynia.[130,131]

Gabapentin is the most commonly used anticonvulsant for pain. It compares favorably with others in its class with respect to side effects and complications, as there is a reduced risk of hematologic, hepatic, or autoimmune complications with gabapentin. Dose response and maximum dose tolerated have been known to vary widely. Oral clearance is directly related to creatinine clearance, with the slope of the relationship greater in African American patients. Children younger than 5 years have demonstrated higher and more variable clearance values than older children.

In children, one should start administering gabapentin conservatively with a twice-a-day dosing. The larger dose should be in the evening to time the sedative side effect with sleep onset. It is recommended to start adolescents on 50 mg in the morning and 100 mg in the evening. Younger children should start at 25 mg in the morning and 50 mg in the evening. Currently, the smallest capsule made is 100 mg. It can be dissolved in juice and fractionated to the appropriate dose. After several days, if this starting dose is tolerated, one can increase to three-times-a-day dosing. The evening dose should remain the largest. Doses should be increased by 50% until one of three events occur: (1) analgesia is reached; (2) dose-limiting side effects of sedation, headache, or change in memory; (3) dosing reaches 50–60 mg/kg/day.

Older anticonvulsants have also been used to relieve lancinating neuropathic cancer pain, including carbamazepine, phenytoin, clonazepam, and valproic acid (Table 16-14). These drugs work by reducing paroxysmal discharges of central and peripheral neurons as in epilepsy. Dizziness, fatigue, and somnolence occurred more frequently among patients on carbamazepine than those taking gabapentin. More patients on carbamazepine (19%) discontinue treatment because of rash.[132]

Oxcarbazepine is a second-generation AED. There is increasing evidence that oxcarbazepine may be effective in treating neuropathic pain refractory to other AEDs, such as carbamazepine and gabapentin. It has an improved safety and tolerability profile compared with other standard AEDs.[133]

Table 16-14

Anticonvulsants in Pain Management

Valproic acid

Carbamazepine

Phenobarbital

Lamotrigine

Phenytoin

Levetiracetam

Oxcarbazepine

Topiramate

Zonisamide

Gabapentin

Pregabalin

Ethosuximide

Lamotrigine and *topiramate* are two newer AEDs that have been used to treat neuropathic pain. Unfortunately, their risk of side effects is high. Side effects appear in about one-half of the children receiving topiramate, and in about one-third of those treated with lamotrigine. Most side effects were considered mild to moderate, but caused the drug to be discontinued in about 10% of the patients due to them. The most common side effects of topiramate were poor appetite, drowsiness, speech difficulties, nervousness, and weight loss. Physicians should avoid giving topiramate to children with eating disorders or low weight. Topiramate has been found to cause a nonanion gap metabolic acidosis, which occurs more commonly in children than in adults.[134] Rash, headache, and sleep disturbances were seen with lamotrigine. Physicians should avoid giving lamotrigine to children with sleeping disorders.[135]

Pregabalin is a new anticonvulsant for peripheral neuropathic pain approved by the U.S. Food and Drug Administration (FDA) in December 2004. Pregabalin and gabapentin have structures similar to gamma-aminobutyric acid (GABA) and have similar mechanisms of action, modulating calcium influx in calcium channels. The primary difference between the two drugs is that pregabalin is more potent than gabapentin, so smaller doses are required and dose-related side effects are less. Trials show adults treated with pregabalin titrated up to 600 mg/day given in two or three doses had a significant reduction in their pain score.[136–138]

▶ Antidepressants

The analgesic efficacy of the tricyclic antidepressants for many painful disorders has been well established, and they are frequently used in cancer pain patients. The analgesic effect of the tricyclic antidepressants in this population is not directly related to antidepressant activity but rather to enhance morphine analgesia. Neuropathic tumor pain characterized by continuous dysesthesias is believed to be the most favorable indication for antidepressant therapy.[139] The analgesic response is usually observed within 5 days of attaining an adequate dose. Antidepressants can improve depression, enhance sleep, and decrease perception of pain. *Amitriptyline* has been shown to increase the plasma concentration of morphine.

Common side effects of tricyclic compounds include antimuscarinic effects, such as dry mouth, impaired visual accommodation, urinary retention, and constipation; antihistaminic effects (sedation); and sympatholytic effects (orthostatic hypotension). *Nortriptyline* tends to have fewer anticholinergic side effects compared to amitriptyline. The choice of antidepressant should be based on the side-effect profiles of the different agents and the greatest benefit to the patient, for example, using the side effect of somnolence for patients with difficulty sleeping. An electrocardiogram (ECG) should be obtained prior to initiating therapy to rule out QT prolongation.

The pharmacokinetics of these agents in children can be different than in adults. The increased rate of metabolism in children may suggest the appropriateness of twice-a-day dosing. Dosing should be started at night, and a second smaller dose may be added in the morning as needed. It can be helpful to check blood levels before discontinuing the drug due to ineffectiveness. The ECG should be repeated if dosing exceeds the standard dose, as QT changes can be asymptomatic.

Selective serotonin reuptake inhibitors (SSRIs) have less side effects, but appear less effective than tricyclic antidepressants as analgesics.[140] Onloxetine, an SNRI, has some evidence for pain relief in adults.

Neuroleptics

There has been significant controversy about whether the conventional neuroleptics have analgesic properties. A review of older neuroleptics concluded that the evidence for effectiveness was sparse, except for methotrimeprazine. It has been used as an analgesic in adults with cancer. *Methotrimeprazine* is a phenothiazine antipsychotic also used in palliative care for the management of terminal agitation and nausea/vomiting. As an antiemetic, 62% showed some improvement in nausea or vomiting.[141] Neuroleptics may sedate patients, diminishing their ability to express pain, and should never be substituted for opioid analgesia. Some older neuroleptics may have a limited role as antiemetics, such as phenothiazines and butyrophenones. However, a review of the newer atypical neuroleptics (olazapine, risperidone, quetiapine) concluded that the atypicals do have analgesic effects.[142]

Bisphosphonates

The treatment of bone pain that responds poorly to opioids can be improved by administering bisphosphonates. These agents exert an inhibitory effect on bone resorption and may prevent pathological fractures. *Pamidronate*, a potent bisphosphate, can significantly reduce pain and pathological fractures caused by bone metastases.[140]

Steroids

A number of studies document the beneficial effects of corticosteroids on many cancer-related symptoms, including pain, appetite, energy level, general well-being, and depression. They have been proven useful for their antiinflammatory qualities and reduction of edema associated with tumors. Short-term use of high doses has been recommended for epidural cord compression (Table 16-15). High doses are usually analgesic and are sometimes used empirically for other pain crises.[140]

Corticosteroids also may attenuate spontaneous discharges from injured nerves. They may be used alone or as adjuvants in combination with other palliative or antineoplastic treatments. Steroids may help prevent nausea, vomiting, and hypersensitivity reactions to treatment with chemotherapy or radiation. They are also commonly used as appetite stimulants in patients with advanced cancer.[143] *Dexamethasone* is the most frequently used steroid due to its high potency, longer duration of action, and minimal mineralocorticoid effects.

Radionucleotides

Radionucleotides have been used to treat painful osseous metastasis in adults. In children, ^{131}I-meta-iodobenzylguanidine is used for the treatment of bone pain in disseminated neuroblastoma. In one study, patients no longer required opioids after three treatments. Side effects include thrombocytopenia and cystitis.[144]

Table 16-15

Steroid Use in Pediatric Cancer Pain Management

Bone pain due to metastatic disease

Cerebral edema due to primary or metastatic disease

Epidural spinal cord compression

Possibly neuropathic pain

Antihistamines

Clinical trials have demonstrated that antihistamines have direct and adjuvant analgesic activity, although the exact mechanism of action is unknown. There are reports of patients with advanced cancer pain refractory to oral, IV, and epidural opioids who obtained sustained pain relief after the repeated administration of *diphenhydramine*.[145]

Stimulants

Psychostimulants have a unique role as adjunctive medication for pain management. Amphetamines have an analgesic effect, which is thought to be mediated by central and descending spinal inhibitory pathways. *Dextroamphetamine* has been shown to potentiate the effects of opioids in adult postoperative patients. Daytime sedation is a common and potentially dose-limiting side effect of the opiate analgesics in palliative care. Psychostimulants counteract opioid-induced sedation and can allow dose escalation of opioids in cancer patients who were previously limited in dosing by somnolence. The use of psychostimulants may be limited by side effects, such as weight loss, anxiety, insomnia, or tolerance to their antisedative effects.

Methylphenidate is a psychostimulant that is used most commonly to treat attention deficit hyperactivity disorder and has been shown to reverse cognitive dysfunction in adult cancer patients. Methylphenidate is used to ameliorate opioid-induced somnolence, to augment the analgesic effects of opioids, to treat depression, and to improve cognitive function in patients with cancer.[146] Methylphenidate is thought to act on dopamine transport descending noradrenergic and serotoninergic spinal inhibitory pathways. The use of dextroamphetamine and methylphenidate was reviewed in 11 children receiving opioids for cancer and other chronic pain. Somnolence was reduced, and safety, efficacy, and tolerability were high.

Preliminary studies of *donepezil*, an acetylcholinesterase inhibitor used in Alzheimer's, show possible benefit in treating opioid-related sedation.[147]

Ketamine

Ketamine has been used for neuropathic pain secondary to its activity at the NMDA receptor. It is also useful for refractory pain or opioid-induced hyperalgesia (0.1–0.2 mg/kg/hr IV or 1–2 mg/kg every 4–6 hours orally). It can be applied as a topical gel for the treatment of neuropathic pain. The analgesic effects of the gel are thought to be due to ketamine's peripheral action at opioid and Na+−K+ channels. A small study of five patients reported a pain score decrease from 8.8 to 1.6 at initial application of topical ketamine, with no significant side effects.[148]

Topical delivery systems differ from transdermal delivery systems in that they target a site immediately adjacent to the site of delivery rather than using the skin as an alternate systemic delivery system. There are currently only a limited number of topical therapies available for the relief of somatic pain (NSAIDs, capsaicin, lidocaine).

SIDE EFFECTS IN CHILDREN

Any evaluation of analgesic response to an opioid must include an assessment of side effects. In children, the common side effects of opioids may not be volunteered and must be asked about. Each child can have varying side effects to the same dose of drug. If any of the side effects are intolerable (e.g., dreams that are frightening), the opioid should be switched. Within the first week of treatment with opioids, tolerance to sedation, nausea and vomiting, and pruritus occur. However, tolerance does not develop to the constipating effects of opioids, so children must be placed on laxatives when they begin treatment with opioids (Table 16-16).

Nausea and vomiting

With the development of stronger methods of fighting cancer through chemotherapy and radiation therapy, the incidence of nausea and vomiting has increased in pediatric oncology. Nausea and vomiting affect between 20% and 70% of patients with advanced cancer. They are ranked first and third as the most distressing side effects of chemotherapy in adults. They can be severe enough to require hospitalization for dehydration or the cessation of treatment due to the severity of the nausea. Early and aggressive treatment is the best way to manage this symptom.

More than 50% of children experience anticipatory nausea before chemotherapy, which is a conditioned response associated with anxiety. Children under the age of 6 years have been shown to

Table 16-16

Management of Opioid Side Effects

Side effect	Treatment
Constipation	1. Prescribe regular use of stimulant and stool-softener laxatives (fiber, fruit juices often are insufficient).
	2. Ensure adequate water intake.
Sedation	1. If analgesia is adequate, try dose reduction.
	2. Unless contraindicated, add nonsedating analgesics, such as acetaminophen or NSAIDs, and reduce opioid dosing as tolerated.
	3. If sedation persists, try methylphenidate or dextroamphetamine, 0.05–0.2 mg/kg PO BID in early morning and midday.
	4. Consider an opioid switch.
Nausea	1. Exclude disease processes (e.g., bowel obstruction, increased intracranial pressure).
	2. Antiemetics (ondansetron, hydroxyzine)
	3. Consider an opioid switch.
Urinary retention	1. Exclude disease processes (e.g., bladder neck obstruction by tumor, impending cord compression, hypovolemia, renal failure).
	2. Avoid other drugs with anticholinergic effects (e.g., tricyclic antidepressants, antihistamines).
	3. Consider short-term use of bethanechol or Tamsulosin (Flomax).
	4. Consider short-term catheterization.
	5. Consider opioid dose reduction if analgesia is adequate or an opioid switch if analgesia is inadequate.
Pruritus	1. Exclude other causes (e.g., drug allergy, cholestasis).
	2. Prescribe antihistamines, micro dose naloxone, low dose nalbuphine.
	3. Consider an opioid dose reduction if analgesia is adequate or consider an opioid switch.
Respiratory depression mild to moderate	1. Awaken and encourage to breathe.
	2. Apply oxygen.
	3. Withhold opioid dosing until breathing improves; reduce subsequent dosing by at least 25%.
Severe	1. Awaken if possible, apply oxygen, and assist respiration by bag and mask as needed.
	2. Titrate small doses of naloxone (0.02 mg/kg increments as needed): stop when respiratory rate increases to 8–10/min in older children or 12–16/min in infants: do not try to awaken fully with naloxone.*
	3. Consider a low-dose naloxone infusion or repeated incremental dosing.
	4. Consider short-term intubation in occasional cases if risk of aspiration is high.
Dysphoria, confusion, hallucinations	1. Exclude other pathology as a cause for these symptoms before attributing them to opioids (e.g., hypoxia, sepsis, metabolic disturbance).
	2. When other causes have been excluded, change to another opioid.
	3. Consider adding a neuroleptic such as haloperidol (0.01–0.1 mg/kg PO OR IV every 8 h to a maximum dose of 20 mg/d).
Myoclonus	1. This usually is seen in the setting of high-dose opioids or, alternatively, rapid dose escalation.
	2. No treatment may be warranted if this is infrequent and not distressing to the child.
	3. Consider an opioid switch or treat with clonazepam (0.01 mg/kg PO every 12 h to a maximum dose of 0.5 mg/dose) or a parenteral benzodiazepine (e.g., diazepam) if the oral route is not tolerated.

NSAIDs = Nonsteroidal antiinflammatory drugs.
*Do not give a bolus dose of naloxone, because severe pain and symptoms of opioid withdrawal may ensue.

have fewer symptoms.[149] In the adult literature, severity can be predicted by being female or by having a history of motion sickness, anxiety, and prior chemotherapy.

Our knowledge of the mechanisms controlling nausea and emesis has improved but is still incomplete. Serotonin receptors are known to play a role in the mediation of chemotherapy-induced nausea, and selective antagonists to subgroup 3 of the serotonin receptors have been very effective in treating nausea and vomiting. Metoclopramide, which is known to act on dopaminergic receptors, also acts on serotonin receptors. Substance P may play a role in nausea and vomiting. Studies show that antagonism of the neurokinin-1 receptor can reduce the incidence of vomiting from radiation and chemotherapy and can be especially helpful in treating delayed emesis.[150]

Antiemetic treatment should begin prior to therapy and should be maintained until the stimulus is gone. Doses of antiemetics should be scheduled, and any change in the patient's symptoms should warrant investigation as to other causes of nausea and vomiting (e.g., increased intracranial pressure [ICP]). Other factors shown to play a role in nausea and vomiting are the effect of a roommate who is vomiting, pretreatment anxiety, and the taste of the drug.

Chemotherapeutic agents have known emetogenicity that can vary slightly between adults and children.[151] Treatment factors that increase the severity of nausea and vomiting are an increased dose and decreased infusion time. Chemotherapy combinations containing *platinum* compounds have been found to be highly emetogenic despite double antiemetic therapy. Complete antiemetic coverage for the combination of *vincristine*, *cyclophosphamide*, and *dactinomycin* is poor. For most of the severely emetogenic chemotherapy protocols, patients experienced good prevention of nausea and vomiting less than 60% of the time, despite the use of two antiemetic agents.[152]

Most of the randomized control studies on antiemetics have been done in adults and must be extrapolated to the pediatric population. However, this extrapolation is not always reliable, as there may be differences in pediatric half-life or side effects. With children, drug choice may be limited by route of administration or the minimal dose available of a pill or patch may be too high for a small patient.[151]

▶ Radiation-induced nausea and vomiting

As many as 40%–80% of patients undergoing radiotherapy experience nausea and vomiting, depending on the site of irradiation. Radiation-induced nausea and vomiting (RINV) is mediated through both chemoreceptor trigger zone and peripheral mechanisms. The most emetogenic treatments are whole-body, cranial, and abdomen, with abdominal irradiation clearly the worst offender (Table 16-17). Radiotherapy may be delivered over a 6–8-week

period, and prolonged symptoms of nausea and vomiting affect quality of life. Uncontrolled nausea and vomiting may result in children delaying or refusing further radiotherapy. The incidence and severity of nausea and vomiting depend on radiotherapy-related factors (single and total dose, fractionation, irradiated volume, radiotherapy techniques) and patient-related factors (gender, age, general health, concurrent or recent chemotherapy, psychological state, tumor stage). Current antiemetic guidelines recommend the use of 5-HT$_3$ antagonists with or without a steroid for prophylaxis.[153,154]

▶ 5-HT$_3$ antagonists

The development of serotonin 5-HT$_3$-receptor antagonists dramatically improved the treatment of chemotherapy-induced nausea and vomiting (Table 16-18).

Ondansetron, a selective serotonin 5-HT$_3$-receptor antagonist, is widely used to treat chemotherapy- and radiation-induced nausea and vomiting in children. This treatment regimen is effective against acute nausea and vomiting, but it fails to control delayed nausea and vomiting. There seem to be fewer side effects (headache, constipation) with ondansetron in the pediatric population than in adults. In comparative trials, ondansetron was significantly more effective at reducing nausea and vomiting than metoclopramide or chlorpromazine. When used in children undergoing conditioning therapy (including total body irradiation) prior to bone marrow transplantation, ondansetron was significantly better at controlling nausea and vomiting than combined perphenazine and diphenhydramine therapy.[155] Intravenous and oral ondansetron have been shown to be equally effective in the prevention of nausea and emesis in pediatric patients receiving moderately/highly emetogenic chemotherapy.[156] Dosing in children varies in the literature. Most studies dose intravenously at 0.15 mg/kg/dose three times a day or 5 mg/m^2/dose.

Granisetron is a potent and highly selective 5-HT$_3$-receptor antagonist. Its selectivity may help to explain why granisetron has less adverse side effects than ondansetron. Its efficacy and tolerability in children on chemotherapy has been proven.[157] The pharmacokinetics can vary greatly, and a shorter dosing interval should be considered because in some children the half-life is shorter than in adults.[158] *Dolasetron* is another 5-HT$_3$-receptor antagonist. Pediatric studies found efficacy with a dose of 1.8 mg/kg IV or PO.[159,160] There was a trend toward a shorter half-life in younger children. *Tropisetron*, another selective 5-HT$_3$-receptor antagonist, has been assessed in the prevention of acute vomiting in children receiving chemotherapy for solid tumors. It was found to be very effective in controlling acute, and to a lesser extent delayed, nausea and vomiting in children.[161] *Ramosetron* is a selective serotonin 5-HT$_3$-receptor antagonist with an affinity higher than that of the previously available drugs, ondansetron, granisetron, and tropisetron. It is well tolerated in children. Ramosetron is as effective as the others in this class but seemed exceptionally efficacious for longer periods (up to 48 hours) after treatment.[162]

The 5-HT$_3$ antagonists have been extensively compared. Tropisetron (0.2 mg/kg/24 h) and granisetron (40 mcg/kg/24 h) were compared in the prevention of nausea and vomiting in children receiving highly emetogenic chemotherapy for various malignancies. Granisetron was found to be more effective than tropisetron, especially in patients heavier than 25 kg.[163] Other studies concluded that granisetron, ondansetron, dolasetron, and tropisetron had the same antiemetic efficacy, which declined with treatment time.[164,165]

A single dose of the 5-HT$_3$ antagonists is as effective as multiple doses or a continuous infusion. The oral route has been shown to be

Table 16-17

Disease-Induced Vomiting

Tumor exudates or sloughed tissue from metastasis causing toxic effects

High or low ICP

Stretching an organ capsule

Inflammation of the GI tract

GI obstruction

Treatment with opioid

Table 16-18

Antiemetic Agents*

Agent	Antiemetic efficacy		Routes of administration	Frequency	Dose-limiting side effects
	Acute	Delayed			
5-HT₃ receptor antagonists: ondansetron, granisetron, dolsertron	Marked	Minimal	PO, IV	Daily	Headache, constipation with prolonged administration
Dexamethasone	Moderate as a single agent	Moderate	PO, IV	Daily, BID	Hyperglycemia
Tetrahydrocannabinol	Moderate	?	PO	q4h	Drowsiness, dysphoria, "high"
Scopolamine	Moderate	?	Transdermal	q72h	Dry mouth
Metoclopramide	Marked	Moderate	IV, PO	2–3 h	EPS,† sedation
Thiethylperazine	Marked	?	PO, PR, IV, IM	4 h	EPS, agitation
Perphenazine	Marked	?	PO, PR, IV, IM	4 h	EPS, agitation
Prochlorperazine	Moderate	?	PO, PR, IV, IM	4 h	EPS, agitation
Chlorpromazine	Moderate	?	PO, PR, IV, IM	4–6 h	EPS, orthostatic hypotension, sedation
Droperidol	Moderate	?	IV, IM	Infusion	Somnolence, agitation, prolong QT

EPS = extrapyramidal symptoms; 5-HT₃ = 5-hydroxytryptamine subtype 3; PR = per rectum; IM = intramuscular.
*See text for dosage recommendations.
†More frequent in children than in adults.

as efficacious as the IV route of administration, even with chemotherapy of high emetic risk.[166] There is, however, a paucity of data about the effectiveness of 5-HT₃ antagonists in the infant population.

A new class of agents, the substance P antagonists, has been developed for the control of emesis. *Aprepitant*, the first of this class, is a potent and selective NK₁ RA antagonist with a long duration of action. It was approved by the FDA for the prevention of both acute and delayed chemotherapy-induced nausea and vomiting, with particular efficacy in the delayed phase. Clinical trials demonstrate that triple therapy (NK₁ receptor antagonist, ondansetron, and dexamethasone) is superior to standard therapy (ondansetron and dexamethasone) or an NK₁ receptor antagonist alone, in controlling acute as well as delayed nausea and vomiting.[167,168]

▶ Other antiemetic agents

Steroids are very useful for potentiating the effects of other antiemetics (Table 16-19). They do have an immunosuppressive effect that must be considered. They may directly affect lymphoid malignancies and laboratory data. There are no clear dosing recommendations for children. *Dexamethasone* can be started at a dose of 10 mg/m² to a maximum of 10 mg once a day, a dose that can be doubled in refractory cases.

Scopolamine (hyoscine) is an anticholinergic agent that is effective for motion sickness. It can be used to prevent nausea and vomiting with chemotherapy. Because it comes in a single patch form, it cannot be used in small children.

Antihistamines have some antiemetic properties. Dimenhydrinate (Dramamine) and diphenhydramine have been used for motion sickness and are useful in combination with other antiemetics.

Phenothiazines were commonly used before the 5-HT class was available. The piperazine class is more effective than antiemetics. Prochlorperazine (Compazine), thiethylperazine (Torecan), and perphenazine (Trilafon) are in this class. This class of drugs is limited by the incidence of extrapyramidal side effects, which can be eliminated by giving the drugs very slowly (over an hour) with an antihistamine.

Metoclopramide, which has also been used to treat delayed nausea and vomiting, acts centrally and peripherally as an antiemetic. Children are at a higher risk of extrapyramidal side effects than adults, and the risk increases greatly above a dose of 1.5 mg/kg. Therefore, prophylaxis with diphenhydramine is recommended.

Lorazepam has been successfully used in combination with other antiemetics for treatment of nausea and vomiting in children. Its amnestic and anxiolytic effects are thought to be helpful for preventing anticipatory nausea.

Droperidol has been linked to cases of QT prolongation, torsade de pointes (TdP), and sudden death, leading the U.S. FDA to issue a warning about its use. A report on 20 infants and children undergoing cardiac surgery showed that droperidol significantly prolonged the QTc time to abnormal values. The prolongation was prompt and resolved within 30 minutes, and no clinically relevant cardiac arrhythmias were observed.[169]

The antiemetic studies of *haloperidol* were reviewed. In the postoperative setting, it was found to be antiemetic above a dose of 0.25 mg. For chemotherapy and radiation therapy, however, no conclusions about its efficacy could be drawn. Side effects include extrapyramidal symptoms and sedation seen at doses above 3 mg. For children, valid data are unavailable.[170]

Olanzapine, an atypical antipsychotic, possesses a unique neurotransmitter binding profile that is similar to methotrimeprazine.

Table 16-19

Antiemetic Algorithm for Initial Cycle of Chemotherapy or Radiotherapy*

Goal	Emetogenicity of the chemotherapy or radiotherapy	Treatment
Prophylaxis to prevent acute symptoms	High	5-HT$_3$ receptor antagnist, steroid
	Moderate	5-HT$_3$ receptor antagonist
	Mild	5-HT$_3$ receptor antagonist
Rescue (treatment of breakthrough acute symptoms): advance up ladder, starting after agents already given for prophylaxis	Any	1. 5-HT$_3$ receptor antagonist 2. Steroid 3. Lorazepam 4. Scopolamine (if >40 kg) 5. Dronabinol (if >6year old) 6. Metoclopramide (with diphenhydramine)
Prophylaxis to prevent delayed symptoms	High	Steroid (consider metoclopramide or 5-HT$_3$ receptor antagonist if breakthrough emesis in the first 24 h)
	Moderate	None (consider metoclopramide or 5-HT$_3$ receptor antagonist if breakthrough emesis in the first 24 h)
	Mild	None
Rescue (treatment of breakthrough delayed symptoms); advance up ladder, starting after agents already given for prophylaxis	Any	1. Dexamethasone 2. Metoclopramide 3. 5-HT$_3$ receptor antagonist 4. Lorazepam, dronabinol, scopolamine

5-HT$_3$ = 5-hydroxytryptamine subtype 3.
*Data from the Dana-Farber Cancer Institute and Children's Hospital, Boston.

It has been shown to improve symptoms in patients who suffered nausea resistant to initial treatment with traditional antiemetics.[171]

▶ Cannabis

The discovery of the *endocannabinoid system* led to a renewed interest in the use of cannabinoids for the management of nausea, vomiting, and weight loss arising either from cancer or from cancer treatment. The endocannabinoid system has been found to be a key modulator in pain perception, emesis, and reward pathways.[172] One of the proven indications for the use of the synthetic cannabinoid (dronabinol) is chemotherapy-induced nausea and vomiting. Other possible effects that may prove beneficial include appetite stimulation, analgesia, antitumor effect, mood elevation, muscle relaxation, and relief of insomnia.[173]

The effect of delta-9-tetrahydrocannabinol (THC) appears to be mediated by cannabinoid receptors in the nucleus tractus solitarius. To date, clinical trials have not compared the antiemetic effects of cannabinoids with the newer agents. Moreover, all studies have involved oral use of cannabinoids, which may be less effective than sublingual or inhaled cannabinoids. While not recommended as first-line treatment, cannabinoids may be used as adjuvant treatment to enhance the effects of existing antiemetic agents, because the mechanisms of cannabinoid-induced antiemesis differ from other agents.[174]

A review of 1366 chemotherapy patients revealed that cannabinoids were more effective than prochlorperazine, metoclopramide, chlorpromazine, thiethylperazine, haloperidol, domperidone, or alizapride. In crossover trials, patients preferred cannabinoids for future chemotherapy cycles. Some potentially beneficial side effects occurred more often with cannabinoids: euphoria, attaining a "high," or drowsiness. Harmful side effects also occurred more often with cannabinoids: dizziness, dysphoria or depression, hallucinations, paranoia, and arterial hypotension. Patients given cannabinoids were more likely to withdraw due to side effects. Negative side effects are likely to limit their use in pediatric cancer care.[175]

Studies in animals have found cannabinoid receptors widely distributed in the central and peripheral nervous systems, similar to morphine. Several animal studies have shown that THC enhances pain relief from morphine. Pain studies in humans have had mixed results. There have been positive analgesic effects in cancer patients with severe pain that is resistant to conventional analgesics. Studies have shown THC to be an equivalent analgesic to codeine. It has shown to be morphine sparing in adults with nociceptive pain, and its role in neuropathic pain is promising.[176]

The acute and long-term risks of therapeutic cannabinoids may limit their widespread use in the pediatric population. Short-term immunosuppressive effects are not well established. Cannabis smoke is a probable risk factor for cancer and lung damage. There is a risk of developing dependence on THC, which is highest in adolescents (especially those with conduct disorders) and in children with psychiatric disorders. Families of children with terminal cancer may regard cannabinoid dependence as an acceptable risk for gain of therapeutic effects.[177,178]

Complementary antiemetics

Ginger, which has been used traditionally for controlling emesis, showed good activity against chemotherapy-induced nausea and vomiting in one trial.[179] Nonpharmacological methods such as acupressure and acustimulation are good adjunct methods for treating nausea and vomiting. *Acupuncture* has demonstrated equal efficacy to metoclopramide in preventing postoperative nausea and vomiting in children.[180] Hypnosis has been shown to be effective for nausea as well. Sleep has also been shown to be an antiemetic. Since many mediators are involved in emesis induced by chemotherapy, combinatorial treatment is more efficacious than a single drug.[181]

▶ Itch

Pruritus is one of the more common side effects of opioid treatment in children with cancer. Diphenhydramine can be used to treat opioid-induced itching. Nalbuphine can be used if diphenhydramine is ineffective. In children and adolescents, a small-dose naloxone infusion (0.25 mcg/kg/h) has been shown to significantly reduce the incidence and severity of opioid-induced side effects, such as itching and nausea, without affecting opioid-induced analgesia.[182]

DRUG ROUTES

Analgesics should be administered by the route that is least painful and most effective. Oral administration of medications is the first choice for most pediatric patients. It is simple, reliable, and inexpensive. It is less invasive and more comfortable than many of the alternatives. This route is potentially unfeasible if a patient is experiencing extreme nausea and vomiting or ileus. Some children refuse to cooperate with oral medication due to fear or delirium.

Intramuscular is a painful route of administration and is avoided in the pediatric oncology population. Per rectum (PR) is also undesirable. It has variable absorption and carries a risk of infection in children with neutropenia that is often associated with cancer treatment.

IV dosing of medications is ideal if an indwelling catheter is in place. This route allows quick effect and rapid titration of drug levels. First-pass effect is bypassed so bioavailability is complete. Infusions can produce a relatively constant level of relief. Placing an IV line in a patient without venous access is the only drawback. Small pumps can be used for home infusions in the palliative care setting.

Subcutaneous delivery of medication has a role for the child who cannot tolerate oral medication and who has poor IV access. A small (27 g) angiocath can be placed under the skin and opioid can be infused at a low rate. Sites most preferable for infusion include the abdomen, thorax, and thigh. The site should be changed every 3–5 days. Drugs should be concentrated so that the volume infused subcutaneously can be small (less than 3 mL/h). This route has been used for PCA bolusing as well. Morphine and hydromorphone are the most commonly used opioids subcutaneously. This technique is appropriate for small home-infusion pumps as well. Techniques to make this route less painful include placing EMLA cream on the site of infiltration prior to administration or mixing lidocaine into the opioid to be infused. Only 1% lidocaine in a 1:9 ratio with the opioid solution should be used. Lidocaine infusion should not exceed 1.5 mg/kg/h.

▶ Patient-controlled analgesia

PCA has a large role in pediatric oncologic pain relief (Table 16-20). A computer-controlled device allows patients to bolus themselves alone or on top of a continuous infusion of opioid. The use of background infusions is more frequent in children than adults and may improve analgesia, but at the risk of increased adverse events such as respiratory depression. Careful consideration must go into the

Table 16-20

Advantages of Patient-Controlled Analgesia in Children

Permits individual titration of medication to pain intensity and pharmacokinetics/pharmacodynamics

Permits child to have control and decrease anxiety

Permits child to balance analgesia against side effects

Diminished sedation

ordering of opioid bolus size, lockout, and continuous infusion. The child should be monitored (respiratory rate, oxygen saturation, and level of sedation) and the PCA doses adjusted as needed.[183]

For mucositis, studies have shown PCA to be more effective than nurse-administered opioids in the pediatric population. Children on PCAs required less morphine, had less sedation, and experienced equivalent analgesia to the group with continuous-infusion morphine controlled by healthcare providers.

Children older than 6 years often benefit from the control of a PCA. There are instances of children between 4 and 6 years old benefiting from a PCA as well, who likely represent a population of young children who have become "medically sophisticated" over the course of cancer treatment. However, the younger the child, the higher the risk of poor pain control due to failure of the child to associate pushing the PCA button with pain relief. Putting the button in the hands of understanding children allows them to control their level of analgesia. By using the bolus, they can also determine their own balance between analgesia and side effects. In children with mucositis who require IV boluses more frequently, a PCA with a basal infusion is appropriate. With a PCA, the patient can time the boluses with mouth care and at other times of increased discomfort.

▶ Nurse/parent-controlled analgesia

PCA is safe because when patients become sedated, they will not press the button. Having others press the PCA button could lead to an overdose. However, the medical literature supports nurses controlling the PCA button with few adverse outcomes. In the home palliative care population, parents are instructed to use the PCA with good effect. Parents of chronically ill or dying children are often quite astute at gauging their child's level of pain. Children in the home care setting are often opioid-tolerant, and the risk of hypoventilation with a PCA is less. In the acute postoperative setting, parental use of PCA has lead to oversedation and death in opioid-naïve patients. In a study of parent-controlled PCA, 1.7% of children required naloxone for treatment of apnea or desaturation.[184] Often in these cases, parental education regarding the PCA was less than optimal, or risk factors for hypoventilation were underappreciated. Before parents are allowed to control the PCA they should be instructed on pain assessment, the effects of opioids, and dosing guidelines. If children have been sent home for palliative care, parents should be able to immediately contact a clinician who can advise them about dose adjustments and side effects. They should be reassured before, during, and after their child's death that it was the cancer, not the drug delivery for comfort, causing the death.

▶ Patient-controlled epidural analgesia

Many studies support the use of IV PCA in pediatrics. In contrast, little has been reported about the ability of children to use patient-controlled epidural analgesia (PCEA). A study evaluating the use of PCEA in children postoperatively found satisfactory analgesia in 90%.[185] The volume required in PCEA has been found to be 50% less than a continuous epidural with no demand bolus.[186] Careful attention should be paid to the total hourly local anesthetic dose to avoid exceeding the recommended limits.

▶ Peripheral nerve catheters

There has been an increase in the use of peripheral nerve catheters for pain control, which are also available in a patient-controlled delivery system. Children who had perineural catheters (popliteal and fascia iliaca compartment block) inserted and infused with ropivacaine obtained satisfactory analgesia to localized limb pain.[187]

▶ Transdermal PCA

A patient-controlled iontophoretic transdermal system using fentanyl has been developed for use in adults. A study comparing it with an IV morphine PCA resulted in similar opioid-related side effects and equivalent analgesia between the groups.[188] There are no studies of its use in children.

There are case reports on the use of intracerebroventricular drug delivery for analgesia in palliative patients.[189]

DRUG DOSING INTERVALS

Analgesics for a child should be scheduled to facilitate maximum pain relief with minimum side effects. If the painful stimulus is constant, for example, mucositis, analgesics should be given around the clock or continuously. If pain is intermittent or there are episodes of increased pain (e.g., mouth care), analgesics should be prescribed PRN. PRN doses can best be estimated as 5%–10% of the 24-hour analgesic requirement. Another technique is to estimate a PRN bolus equal to a patient's hourly infusion rate. One must be prepared to escalate analgesics rapidly after they are started (Table 16-21). A rule of thumb for daily adjustment is to increase the daily basal dose to the previous day's 24-hour total (basal + PRN).

Tolerance refers to "the progressive decline in the potency of an opioid with continued use, such that increasingly higher doses are required to achieve the same analgesic effect." Tolerance to a particular opioid does not completely transfer over to another opioid. Cross-tolerance is not complete. This should be recalled when switching from one drug to another. *Physical dependence* is a "physiologic state characterized by withdrawal after discontinuation of the opioid" (Table 16-22).

Addiction is a "psychological and behavioral syndrome characterized by drug craving and aberrant drug use."

Table 16-21

Analgesic Dosing and Drug Metabolism in Children Cancer Pain Report, WHO

Children metabolize drugs faster than adults (larger liver per kg of body weight)

Because drugs clear more rapidly in children, more frequent drug dosing is required. For example, oral SR-morphine used twice daily in adults is required 3-times-daily in children

Table 16-22

Withdrawal Symptoms

Anxiety, insomnia, restlessness

Yawning

Diaphoresis, mydriasis

Lacrimation, rhinorrhea

Stomach cramps, vomiting, diarrhea

Fever, chills

Muscle spasm, tremors

Tachycardia, hypertension

Seizure

These terms should all be explained to parents and older children because there is often a hesitation caused by fear of addiction to take opioids appropriately. Reassure them that addiction without a history of prior abuse is extremely rare. A study evaluating 12,000 adult patients receiving opioids reported that only four cases of addiction developed in patients without a history of previous drug addiction.

OPIOID ROTATION

If pediatric oncology patients experience inadequate pain relief or intolerable side effects from one opioid, then changing to another opioid can sometimes improve symptoms. Because of incomplete cross-tolerance, analgesia can improve by rotating drugs. Each opioid affects a different subset of receptors in the CNS; therefore, changing medication may improve side effects.[140] However, clinical evidence for opioid rotation in children is observational and uncontrolled.[190]

A retrospective study was done to determine the therapeutic value of opioid rotation in a large pediatric oncology center. Mucositis was the most common cause of pain (70%). Other causes of pain were bony, postoperative, or neuropathic pain. The opioid was rotated either for excessive side effects, with or without adequate analgesia, or tolerance. Adverse opioid effects were resolved in 90% of cases and there was no significant loss of pain control. All failures occurred when morphine was rotated to fentanyl.[191]

There is incomplete cross-tolerance when converting opioids, so it is recommended to reduce the dose to 50% of the equianalgesic dose when switching from one opioid to another. If converting to long-acting methadone, less than half of the equianalgesic dose is often required (see appendix D). Careful assessment for pain control and opioid side effects is prudent after opioid rotation, particularly in the first 5 days after the switch.

INTERVENTIONAL PAIN MANAGEMENT

For the majority of children with cancer pain, the WHO's three-step analgesic ladder provides adequate management with oral, transdermal, or IV options. However, this is not sufficient for some children. Interventional treatment of cancer pain should be considered the fourth step in the WHO analgesic ladder. This would include visceral and peripheral nerve blocks, spinal/epidural administration of local anesthetics, opioids, alpha-2 agonists, spinal cord stimulation, and surgical interventions.[192]

Spinal/epidural catheters

Spinal (subarachnoid) or epidural drug delivery has been successfully to control pain in terminal pediatric malignancies. A small dose of opioid administered intrathecally provides increased analgesia with fewer opioid side effects than with IV administration. An intrathecal or epidural catheter can be tunneled to port implanted subcutaneously. Pediatric patients in whom this approach should be considered are those with dose-limiting side effects from opioid infusions and those whose pain is poorly responsive to massive opioid infusion. Combined mixtures of opioid, local anesthetic, and alpha-2 adrenergic agonists have shown the most efficacy in intraspinal infusions. Dosing should be based on preprocedural opioid use converted to a parenteral equivalent dose of morphine. Incomplete cross-tolerance should be accounted for if opioids other than morphine are being used. The initial epidural morphine dose is equal to 10% of the 24-hour parenteral equivalent morphine dose. The initial subarachnoid morphine dose is 10% of the epidural dose. This should fall within the range of 0.1–20 mg of morphine a day.[193]

Timing a procedure for pain palliation can be challenging. These children are quite ill; thus, the procedures should optimally be carried out in the operating room. An anesthetic delivered to a child who is close to death could be detrimental. The procedure should be done in a sterile setting. An implantable catheter placed too early could lead to infection if it remains implanted for months. The risk:benefit ratio can change daily, and pain relief from the interventional procedure must be critically weighed against the risk of placing the port, catheter, and so on. This population of patients also carries the risk of thrombocytopenia secondary to chemotherapy and may require platelet transfusion prior to the procedure. A 2–3-day trial catheter should ideally be tested prior to implantation, which will determine clinical efficacy and drug dosing criteria.

There are many case reports of successful pain control in pediatric palliative care using interventional techniques. For example, an intrathecal catheter in a 15-year-old girl with high-grade osteogenic sarcoma of the right femur diminished her somnolence and improved her pain control for 2 months until death. Morphine and clonidine at doses of 0.7 mg and 340 mcg per day were started based on her previous epidural dose requirements.[193] The intrathecal catheters have been kept in place for as long as 18 months.[194]

A subcutaneous intrathecal port can allow more mobility and ease of care for a child with cancer. However, it requires another "poke" into the port chamber.

A comparison of intraspinal drug administration with aggressive comprehensive medical management for refractory cancer pain revealed better pain relief in patients given intraspinal drug treatment (over a 50% reduction in VAS scores), with less opioid side effects. Quality of life was significantly improved by reduced fatigue and depressed level of consciousness. Survival was improved in patients with an intraspinal infusion (though it was not statistically significant), but there is anecdotal evidence that patients with better pain control live longer. These patients may eat better, be more active, and have more "will to live." Immune system function may even improve due to the lessened stress response.[195]

Risks associated with placement of a neuraxial catheter include bleeding, infection, headache, backache, and nerve injury. The incidence of infection in long-term epidural catheters in children is reported to be 2.4%. This can be minimized by careful monitoring of the site. Bleeding may occur during catheter placement or removal, and coagulation should be optimal around these events (Table 16-23).

Table 16-23

Advantages of Spinal over Epidural Drug Delivers

Small dose/volume of medication

Lower infusion rates

Limited tachyphylaxis and systemic toxicity

Surveillance for infection simpler (draw off CSF)

Less fibrosis at catheter tip

Children have been discharged to hospice care or home with both systems, with visiting nurse follow up.[193] Studies that look at the cost-effectiveness of implantable devices in adults found that after 3 months, the implantable pump was more economical than a tunneled epidural catheter.

Some considerations for catheter placement in the pediatric population are:

1. Catheters should be placed under effective sedation or general anesthesia to avoid undue stress in the child.

2. Catherter tip should be verified intraoperatively by fluoroscopy and contrast injection to ensure proper level and to ensure that the catheter is not obstructed by spinal or epidural metastases.

3. Catheter should be tunneled at time of placement to increase longevity.

4. Opioid alone is often insufficient in the pediatric population. The addition of local anesthetic is often necessary to obtain analgesia.

5. Catheter tip needs to be at or above the appropriate dermatomal level of the child's pain, as local anesthetic has a limited spread in the epidural space.

   (a) Pain above the umbilicus calls for a thoracic epidural.

   (b) Pain below the umbilicus calls for a lumbar spinal catheter. This allows the greatest flexibility in escalating the local anesthetic without unwanted leg weakness.

6. Care must be taken with systemic opioids after the spinal or epidural catheter has been placed. Deafferentation of the painful input might lead to sedation in the patient, in which case systemic opioids will need to be reduced. A rapid reduction in systemic opioids, however, might lead to signs and symptoms of withdrawal. Therefore, dosing after a catheter placement must be tailored to the patient, and frequent clinical assessments are recommended.

7. The IV route must be maintained for rescue medications or other needed medications for itch, anxiety, sleep, or terminal air hunger.

Spinal cord stimulator

The use of spinal cord stimulators in pediatric cancer patients is limited but they can be helpful in neuropathic states. Settings that may be amenable to this therapy include postthoracotomy pain and radicular lower extremity pain after tumor resection.

Cryoanalgesia and radiofrequency ablation

Cryoanalgesia, freezing the offending nerves down to −75°C, is safe with no dysesthesias due to preservation of the neurolemma to allow regeneration. This technique is short-lived. Radiofrequency lesioning of a nerve may provide pain relief of a lasting nature. Both procedures are rarely performed in children.

Neurolytic blocks

Pain from visceral tumors in adults can be treated with neurolytic blocks, such as celiac plexus block or hypogastric plexus block, using phenol or alcohol. These modalities are underutilized and should be considered for children with pain due to upper abdominal malignancy. There are several case reports of treating refractory abdominal pain in children with neuroblastoma or hepatoblastoma with a neurolytic celiac plexus block. These blocks should be performed by experienced practitioners of pediatric regional anesthesia and pain management.

Surgery

Neurodestructive surgery had a larger role in cancer therapy in the past when opioids, adjuvants, and regional anesthesia were not being used as effectively. There is significant morbidity associated with these procedures, including paralysis, paresthesias, and urinary dysfunction. Pain returns within a year in 40% of the patients. Currently, the most common neurosurgical procedure performed for children at the end of life is decompressive laminectomies for pain due to acute spinal cord compression.

Percutaneous cordotomy is a procedure in which the spinothalamic tract, responsible for the transmission of nociception, is interrupted to relieve pain. It has demonstrated utility for patients with unilateral pain due to cancer. Occasionally, bilateral cordotomies may be required as mirror pain can develop on the contralateral side.[197]

PALLIATIVE CARE

Cancer is the most common cause of nontraumatic death in children. Approximately 25% of children diagnosed with cancer will die of their disease or its complications.[198] Orchestrating a peaceful transition into death for the patient and family requires skill, planning, and teamwork. The WHO has defined palliative care as the active total care of a patient whose disease is not responsive to curative treatment. Control of pain and other symptoms, and understanding associated psychological, social, and spiritual problems in dying children is paramount.

Pediatric patients have heterogeneous physiologic factors and developmental issues. The needs of the dying child are fundamentally different from those of an adult. Parents are more involved in caregiving and decision-making. Most pediatricians desire to maintain involvement.[199,200] Pediatric palliative care is an integrated and holistic approach to a child and his or her family facing a life-threatening illness. It seeks to meet the emotional, physical, psychological, and spiritual needs of the child and family. It allows the family to make plans calmly, with forethought, by bringing up difficult topics early in a supportive way.[201] Any child or family living with a life-threatening illness would benefit from the involvement of a palliative care team.

The pediatric palliative care team is a multidisciplinary team comprised of individuals who can address the physical, psychosocial, spiritual, and practical needs of the patient and family. It is important that members are team players, good communicators with the family, who can provide continuity of care and be a reassuring presence until the end. There should be a coordinator appointed to respond quickly to questions from the family. Team members should be skilled at assessing pain in young, nonverbal, cognitively impaired children and experienced with pharmacologic and nonpharmacologic pain management. It is also important that team members have knowledge of childhood development vis-à-vis the concepts of illness and death, and that they recognize that a child may mature or regress during the process of dying.

Many resources and models are available for establishing a palliative care service.[202] The American Academy of Pediatrics has an integrated model for providing care to terminal children.[203] *The Initiative for Pediatric Palliative Care*—a consortium of U.S. organizations that work to improve care of children and families—offers interdisciplinary and interactive educational resources for free at www.ippcweb.org.[7]

In 2003, legislation seeking to improve palliative and end-of-life care for children was introduced in both the U.S. House and Senate. The Children's Compassionate Care Act (S. 1629) and the Pediatric Palliative Care Act (H.R. 3127) called for creating pediatric palliative care projects and providing grants to expand services and research in this area. Such a program allows children to seek curative treatment while also receiving hospice and other palliative care services. It also expands hospice eligibility by waiving the Medicare requirement that a patient must have a life expectancy of 6 months or less to qualify for such care.

When palliative care begins is not an exact point, but rather represents a continuum from diagnosis and treatment to death. Studies show that the concept of palliative care should be introduced to the child and family early, preferably when the diagnosis of a life-threatening disease is first made. This timing avoids an abrupt transition to palliative care near the end of life, when the family may view the switch as "giving up."[204,205] The primary medical team can have conflicting goals of trying to cure and seeking quality of life for their patient. Therefore, it can be advantageous to involve the palliative care team whose main goal is to focus on comfort care and quality of life. The team will work to assure that the child and family receive excellent pain control and other comfort measures, get the information families want to participate in decisions about care, receive emotional and spiritual support and practical assistance, obtain expert help in planning for care outside the hospital, and continue getting good services in the community. A palliative care team tries to coordinate and tailor a package of services that best suits a family's values, beliefs, wishes, and needs in whichever setting the child is receiving care.[206]

There are multiple *psychosocial* dilemmas surrounding a family with a dying child.[207] There is the difficulty of living with uncertainty, varying coping styles among family members, and the need for control in choices around the child. Caregivers can help alleviate suffering by questioning, listening attentively, being present, and showing compassion.

Palliative care includes concern for a child and family's *spiritual* needs. Studies that have looked into spiritual issues in pediatric hospice and palliative care show that spirituality is important to dying children.[208] It may involve a particular religion the family practices, but spirituality encompasses much more than a practice of a particular faith tradition. Spiritual anguish can lead to suffering and worsened physical pain. A provider must be attuned to the often silent difficulties a child and family may be experiencing. A team member must be willing to explore existential questions with the child in an open, respectful way. Families stress the importance of conducting religious or cultural rituals at the end of life.[209]

Awareness of death in children

According to classical developmental theory, children do not fully comprehend the irreversibility of death until approximately ages 11 to 16 years. However, some have a surprising awareness of the fact that they are going to die. Even those as young as 4 years pick up cues from the physiologic changes in their bodies and the reactions of parents or hospital staff and can have an advanced understanding of disease and the concept of death.[210] Overwhelmingly, children want to know that they are dying (95% in a study of 50 children aged 8 to 17). Some advocate including children as young as 6 in end-of-life discussions. Others believe children younger than 11-years-old cannot grasp the concept of their mortality to the degree needed to make rational treatment decisions. Dying children often signal their awareness and distress about dying indirectly. These signals can be picked up as opportunities to discuss end-of-life issues with the child. A younger child might exhibit separation anxiety or generalized anxiety. Preadolescents may express their distress through drawings, or become tearful, agitated, lethargic, hostile, and refuse to eat or be treated. Adolescents may display the need to discuss end-of-life issues by expressions of rage, concerns about appearance, and a heightened awareness of time. As the end of life approaches, children might turn completely inward, a process called *decathexis*.

Few pediatric oncology training programs offer formal training on how to approach end-of-life communication with dying children and their families. Even experienced oncology providers can struggle to find a way to initiate these discussions. Various recommendations have been posited for discussing the transition to comfort care or introducing the terminal nature of a child's disease. Most recommend ensuring privacy and adequate time for discussion, presenting things simply and honestly, allowing for expressions of sympathy by the family, and being free to empathize with them. Remind all involved that there will be follow-up discussions as well as opportunities to address new concerns as they arise. Discussion about resuscitation status should be brought up in subsequent meetings but before parents are in the midst of a crisis. This discussion should be worded very carefully to correct erroneous thoughts parents might have about the meaning of "do not resuscitate (DNR)."

Issues surrounding how best to communicate with children who are dying of cancer are seminal because providing information and actively addressing their concerns can enhance the cooperation of the child, reduce anxiety, and lighten the burden of secrecy. Withholding information from them might lead to feelings of isolation and mistrust. Parents often pass on only hopeful information thinking that the truth may cause depression, when in actuality this divides a child from those who can best help them understand and deal with their experience. Sharing information with a child from the beginning of the illness can help establish trust. When discussing end-of-life issues with children, the caregiver should already have a trusting relationship and a rapport with the child. Time should be allotted for children to ask questions and for fears to be dispelled: "Is it going to hurt?," "Will I be able to breathe?" In seriously ill adults or children, uncertainties about the future often provoke a profound sense of loss of control. What a child needs to know may be age-dependent. Most will worry about the impact of the disease and medical treatments on their daily lives and on the family. Sometimes children will act out their concerns with disruptive behaviors. When these concerns are addressed, these disruptive behaviors often disappear.[210]

▶ Home vs. hospice vs. hospital

Data from the United States and Western Europe show that 52% of children and adolescents and 30% of young adults with progressive cancers die at home.[211] Many parents believe that their child will be happier at home because of the familiar surroundings, easier access to family and friends, fewer disruptions in family life, and the opportunity to eat their preferred foods.[207] There may be cultural variations in this belief. There is some evidence that parents grieve better if the child dies at home, possibly due to fewer feelings of helplessness and increased intimacy. Others believe that family relationships remain more stable when the child dies in the hospital.

The choice of home care has to take into account practical issues such as healthcare provider access and financial resources. Having a team always available can be a challenge. Because the overall number of children who die at home is small, there are few healthcare workers skilled in this field. Adult hospice workers may not have the skills to handle the different medical, social, and psychological needs of the family with a dying child.

Freestanding pediatric hospices are now growing in the United States and United Kingdom. These are tailored specifically to the pediatric palliative care patient, providing options such as pet visitation, long-term bereavement, and social services for the family.[212] Hospital-based palliative care rooms exist in only a few hospitals. These can provide access to quality care but in a less relaxing setting and with less continuity of care due to shift workers.

▶ Pain management in palliative care

Parents report that relieving suffering is their first priority and extending life is secondary. Reviews of adult patients dying with cancer reveal end-of-life priorities: pain and symptom management, strengthening relationships with loved ones, and avoiding inappropriate prolongation of death.[213] It can be assumed this is similar for children, though no studies show this.

A *pain plan* should be made with the input of the child and family. The team must anticipate and plan for pain crises and symptom management. The family should be prepared for premortem signs and symptoms (such as agonal breathing) and postmortem details. One should discuss all management options and their impact on quality of life with the goal of giving a sense of control to family. It is important to stress that medications are to relieve pain and not to hasten death.

A multimodal approach to pain should be used from the beginning.[214] A provider should clarify what the pain means to the patient and what pain is, as opposed to fear, sadness, or feelings of isolation. Cultural and religious beliefs may have an effect on the goals for pain treatment. It should be clarified that the goal of the medical team is to achieve pain relief with minimal sedation or side effects. It must be discussed with the family what acceptable side effects will be. Common misconceptions held by families about pain medications should be explored. These may include fear of addiction or hastening death if analgesics are given.

Pain assessment in the chronically or extremely ill child can be challenging. Standard tools assessing heart rate, sweating, and facial expression are less reliable in this stage. Parents as caregivers are often the best able to assess pain in their child (Table 16-24).

Table 16-24
Pain Management Basics in Pediatric Palliative Care
Keep it simple
Try oral first unless presence of nausea or rapidly escalating pain
Stick with one drug until reaching dose-limiting side effects
Treat round the clock rather than PRN

Near the end of life, pain experienced by terminal children tends to be due more to the progressing cancer than to the treatments used. The literature reveals that 80% of children with advanced cancer, regardless of tumor type, will experience pain.[6] Patients with a solid tumor or metastasis to the central or peripheral nervous systems will most likely have more pain for a longer duration.

It is appropriate to start with the WHO Analgesic Ladder[215] but the provider must be flexible and act quickly if pain starts to escalate. Consider an NSAID if there are bony metastases (avoid this in patients with a risk of bleeding). Oxycodone is the first-line opioid for moderate pain as there is no ceiling and, unlike codeine, it can be metabolized by all children. It also has a better side-effect profile than codeine. For severe pain that is constant, switch to immediate-release and sustained-release morphine. Avoid agonist-antagonist opioids because of the ceiling effect these drugs have. Demerol should be avoided because of its toxic metabolite. Opioid rotation should be considered when dose-limiting side effects have been reached.

Adjuvants should be utilized to minimize side effects and to work synergistically with opioids. These include steroids, bisphosphonates for bony metastasis, tricyclics, and antiepileptic drugs for neuropathic pain. If a sleep aid is desired, try amitriptyline. If sedation and dry mouth are bothersome, try nortriptyline. Interventions such as epidural, intrathecal, or neurolytic blocks should be considered early. Steroids can cause euphoria when given to treat pain due to visceral distention, bony destruction, or cerebral edema.

Many complementary nondrug therapies that have been used by pediatric oncology patients through treatments can be used at the end of life as well,[216] for example, hypnosis, acupuncture, guided imagery, and meditation.[217–219] Favorite pets can be brought in. At this stage, touch is very important for the parent-child relationship; parents can find it very beneficial to learn therapeutic touch techniques. Story telling about the child can be helpful to promote life memories before death.

Side effect management in palliative care

One must be vigilant about detecting side effects once pain management is achieved. Pediatric palliative caregivers should anticipate and aggressively treat the most common side effects. Sedation can occur, especially if the patient was sleep-deprived before the initiation of pain management. Allow the patient to "catch up," but if sedation persists, consider adding dextroamphetamine and methylphenidate. Treat histamine release with diphenhydramine. Treat nausea and vomiting early and aggressively to avoid aversion to opioid treatment. Treat constipation prophylactically with sodium docusate or senna. Increase these doses as you increase opioids. Myoclonus can develop at high doses of opioids, which can be treated by lowering the opioid or using benzodiazepines. If it persists, consider switching to another class of opioids. Respiratory distress due to narcotics is extremely rare in cancer patients on chronic opioids, but it remains a major fear for caregivers and family members. If a patient does seem to have a lowered respiratory rate or decreased responsiveness, do not give naloxone. Most likely it is due to disease progress, but one could lower the opioid dose briefly to see if there is improvement.

Medication route

The practitioner must be flexible and rapidly make changes, as a child may need all medications rapidly converted from oral to intravenous. Near the end of life, a transdermal patch might be too slow

to achieve analgesia and hard to titrate; plus, generalized anasarca may limit its uptake. Transmucosal fentanyl is not ideal as mental status starts to diminish. IV medications should be administered at the end of life when there is poor oral intake and decreased level of consciousness. The SC route can be used if there is no IV access. The IM route should never be used in palliative care, where comfort is paramount. If the goal is to get the child home to die, one must consider mobility and manageability of drug delivery systems. An intrathecal or epidural catheter, if placed early, can be the most effective way to control a pain crisis if the pain is localized.[214]

Medication dosing

At the end of life, analgesics should be dosed around the clock to prevent pain. Start with a short-acting opioid every 4 hours plus breakthrough doses as needed. Then, after a day or two, when opioid requirements are established, convert to long-acting opioids. Dosing should be scheduled to allow uninterrupted sleep, if possible. There should be a plan for PRN analgesics to gain rapid control of breakthrough pain, preferably the immediate-release form of the long-acting drug. The rescue dose of short-acting opioid should equal 5%–10% of the patient's 24-hour requirement. The provider should expect logarithmic escalation in pain and medication requirements when a patient is actively dying, and titrations should be in significant increments of both the short- and long-acting opioid. Remember that there is no maximum dose for opioids in the final stages of dying.

Palliative treatment of cancer

Many families want to continue treating their child even when it is known that there is no chance of survival. This might be because of a desire to extend the child's life, holding out for a miracle, or to treat symptoms of the disease.[220,221] Each treatment should be balanced with consideration for the child's quality of life.

Palliative chemotherapy or radiation

In the effort to minimize suffering, one must understand that continued chemotherapy will affect quality of life. There will be more time spent in the hospital setting and more potential side effects or adverse events. Despite this, there are studies that suggest quality of life is improved in teenagers undergoing palliative chemotherapy (Table 16-25). Providers must be very clear with parents about what their goal of continuing treatment is: to alleviate suffering or to prolong life. Providing treatment might serve mainly to extend hope in the family. Etoposide is an agent that has been helpful in pediatric

---

Table 16-25

Indications for Palliative Radiation for the Reduction of Symptoms

Pain relief from bony/pulmonary metastases

Pain relief from tumors infiltrating nerve root and soft tissue

Controlling bleeding, fungation, or ulceration

Avoiding impending obstruction of airway, ureter, and so on

Decreasing symptoms from brain metastasis

Source: From Ref. 222.

palliative chemotherapy for refractory neuroblastoma, germ cell tumors, brain tumors, and rhabdomyosarcoma.[223] Acute lymphoblastic leukemia that has relapsed may be temporarily controlled with vincristine, methotrexate, prednisone, and 6-mercaptopurine.

Children who most commonly receive radiotherapy for symptomatic metastases have diagnoses of neuroblastoma, Ewing's sarcoma, and osteosarcoma.[224] Radiation oncology emergencies include spinal cord compression or vena cava obstruction.

▶ Nonpain symptoms

Almost 90% of children who have a cancer-related death die while experiencing two to eight troubling symptoms. With improved symptom control and end-of-life care, these patients might suffer less before they die. It is during the last month of life that the terminal child experiences the majority of disease- and treatment-related symptoms.[6] On average, a child has 11 symptoms in the last week of life.[225] The most common distressing symptoms rated by parents after the death of their child include fatigue, poor appetite, pain, and dyspnea.[220] These symptoms were felt by parents to contribute significantly to their child's suffering. Thus, symptom management often becomes the first priority for parents. Common psychological symptoms include being worried, sad, irritable, or nervous.[226]

Fatigue

Fatigue is the most common symptom experienced by a child dying of cancer.[6,226] Because there are multiple causes, fatigue can be difficult to treat. Contributing to the feeling are the disease, treatment, pain, sleep-cycle disturbance, medication side effects, a hopeless feeling or depression, and respiratory compromise. To begin treating this symptom, a careful evaluation of underlying causes should be undertaken. Exercise has been suggested to relieve fatigue in cancer patients.

Respiratory symptoms

Respiratory symptoms in pediatric terminal care are common. Forty percent of children dying of cancer will have problems with secretions or dyspnea in the last 3 months of life. Many reports rate dyspnea or "an uncomfortable awareness of breathing" as a significant contributor to suffering. Respiratory symptoms are seen most commonly with solid tumors that have metastasized to the lungs and pleural spaces. Dyspnea may also result from extrapulmonary causes, including generalized cachexia and fatigue that affects the respiratory muscles.

Opioids are often effective in relieving feelings of suffocation due to impaired oxygen exchange, without inciting significant respiratory depression. A quarter of the 4-hour opioid dose has been shown to be effective in relieving dyspnea.[227] Others have studied nebulized opioids.[228] Supplemental oxygen has been shown to be helpful, even when oxygen saturation is normal. However, an oxygen delivery device may be more stressing than relieving for the child. A fan may be less invasive and still help with feelings of dyspnea. Occasional bronchoconstriction can respond to bronchodilators.

Alternatively, benzodiazepines can serve a role in managing the anxiety associated with dyspnea. So as not to create any confusion, assure the family that the medications are to help their child not mind the breathlessness. Pneumonia should be treated with an antibiotic. Dyspnea due to congestive heart failure in the setting of chemotherapy cardiomyopathy can be treated with an angiotensin-converting enzyme (ACE) inhibitor or diuretics. Draining a pleural effusion can be greatly helpful in alleviating shortness of breath, though the relief is often short-lived. Chest tubes or sclerosis may produce more discomfort than they are worth in the terminal child.[229]

Pruritus

Pruritus is quite common and can be distressing in pediatric palliative care patients. There are several possible etiologies causing pruritus, such as dry skin, opioids, and liver or renal failure. Scheduled diphenhydramine may be helpful.

Disturbed sensorium

Toward the end of life, agitation, sedation, and confusion can become prominent. A provider must investigate a differential diagnosis to look for reversible causes. Possible contributors include medications, electrolytes, and liver or kidney failure. Work-up should be pursued only if it is painless and could find a reversible cause. If a child is nonverbal and appears agitated, consider dyspnea or pruritus as possible causes. Treatment of disturbed sensorium could include opioid rotation or sedation.

Depression

Signs and symptoms of depression are prevalent among children who suffer from cancer.[6] Assessing only neurovegetative symptoms may miss some cases of depression that would be found by asking about feelings of hopelessness, helplessness, worthlessness, guilt, and suicidal ideation. One study found the question, "Are you depressed?" the best screening tool for adults. This might not apply to all children in palliative care. Caregivers should treat depression early in children with advanced cancer. Starting a selective serotonin reuptake inhibitor or a tricyclic antidepressant is the mainstay of treatment. A psychostimulant should be considered for treatment of depression in the palliative setting, as its effects are seen more rapidly.

Anxiety

Anxiety can play a large role in children with terminal cancer. Benzodiazepines can be used to enhance the analgesics and reduce the child's anxiety level. It is best to use these agents for the short term or intermittently due to a waning anxiolytic effect and possible psychomotor impairment.

Bleeding

Children dying of cancer quite commonly are coagulopathic. As platelet levels fall, a child may develop spontaneous bleeding from the nose or gastrointestinal tract. Palliative platelet transfusion should be discussed early with the family. This usually cannot be done in a home setting due to the short-lived nature of platelets.

Blood products should not be automatically given for children in palliative care. Antifibrinolytic agents like tranexamic acid (TXA) or aminocaproic acid (ACA) have been used. The family should be prepared if this is an anticipated symptom. Dark sheets can be helpful to minimize the frightening appearance of blood to the family.

Anemia

In children with malignancies that affect the bone marrow, anemia and thrombocytopenia can be quite common. If a child develops symptoms from anemia (dizziness, shortness of breath, tachycardia, fatigue), after discussion with the family, treatment can be appropriate in the palliative setting. Avoid blood draws to check labs;

transfusions should be guided by clinical examination and response to delivered blood products. Erythropoietin can be considered.

Seizures

Yet another distressing event for patients and families is when a child experiences seizures in the terminal phase of life. These should be anticipated in a child with a primary or metastatic brain lesion, and benzodiazepines should be readily available. They can also occur in the setting of hypocoagulability, leading to spontaneous intracranial hemorrhages. If the seizures are new in onset, imaging studies should be sought, as a new mass, if detected, could respond to palliative radiation therapy. Diazepam is used most frequently for rapid IV control of seizures. If seizures break through existing anti-seizure medications that the patient is taking, consider increasing the dose or adding short-acting benzodiazepines.

Increased intracranial pressure

In children with brain tumors, increased ICP may become problematic at the end of life. This may manifest as headache, nausea, vomiting, and lethargy. Palliative radiation therapy is the first-line treatment. But if maximum doses of radiation have been reached, then an increased dose of IV dexamethasone can be used. Shunting a child with advanced cancer may be considered, but the risks and benefits must be thoroughly discussed with the family.

Spinal cord compression

New onset back pain in pediatric cancer patients should be investigated, as new epidural metastasis could lead to spinal cord compression. The majority of spinal metastases present with back pain, before neurologic deficits are apparent. After a thorough physical examination, a MRI should be obtained to rule out compression. Early intervention minimizes long-term sequelae. Studies show that if patients with spinal cord compression are treated while they are still walking, 89%–94% of patients will remain ambulatory. Treatment consists of steroids and radiation therapy.[230]

Fever

How aggressively a caregiver works up and treats a fever can be problematic. Clarify goals of care with the family and assess the infection's impact on the patient's quality of life. Treatment can be empiric, without lab work. For example, treat for a urinary tract infection without sending urine off to the lab if the patient complains of dysuria. Most families, during the chemotherapy regimen, were taught to aggressively identify and treat infections, so this new approach may be hard to accept. It is important to discuss with the family the treatment options and expected course if treatment is withheld. The discomfort of a fever should be treated with acetaminophen and possibly ibuprofen.

Nutrition and hydration

Anorexia and cachexia are common in advanced cancer for multifactorial reasons. Studies suggest that terminal cancer patients can achieve adequate hydration with smaller volumes.[231] Some feel that thirst and hunger can contribute to a patient's suffering, while others believe that a decline in oral intake is natural in the disease course and not associated with hunger or thirst. The goal of nutrition and fluid management, therefore, should be aimed at alleviating hunger/thirst and preserving the social aspect of meals. An appetite stimulant such as megestrol acetate can be used. More invasive approaches such as feeding tubes or total parenteral nutrition should be carefully considered by the patient, family, and caregiver for effect on quality of life.

Nausea

Nausea is quite common in the end of life for a pediatric cancer patient and the cause should be investigated. It could be due to opioid therapy, abdominal tumor advancement, increased ICP, or severe constipation. Selective 5-HT antagonists have been effective against nausea. If nausea is refractory to the above, dexamethasone and lorazepam should be added. Phenothiazines can be administered with diphenhydramine to avoid extrapyramidal side effects. Other therapeutic options include acupuncture, rotating opioids, or changing the opioid dosing schedule to keep the child's blood levels within the therapeutic window. If a child suffers from anticipatory vomiting, benzodiazepines can help. If nausea is movement-induced, scopolamine should be tried.

Constipation

Constipation happens frequently in children with terminal cancer due to drugs, immobility, and poor oral intake. Other less common causes include gastrointestinal obstruction or neurologic deficit. A physical examination should be done and an abdominal x-ray obtained to evaluate the cause. A bowel regimen should be started any time a patient starts on opioids. Rectal laxatives should be the last line of treatment for severe constipation, as they can have a considerable negative effect on quality of life. Oral naloxone can be used for opioid-induced bowel obstruction. Intestinal obstruction normally is an indication for surgery, but cancer patients can be too infirm to tolerate surgery, so medical management may be best. Symptoms of gastrointestinal obstruction should be treated with morphine, scopolamine, and haloperidol or corticosteroids.[232]

Insomnia

In children with cancer, there can be several causes of insomnia, including pain, anxiety, and depression. Treatment of this condition is guided by cause. If there is difficulty initiating sleep or staying asleep due to pain, a larger dose of long-acting opioid should be given at night. If pain is not the primary cause, symptoms generally improve with a small dose of tricyclic antidepressant or with a tetracyclic antidepressant like trazodone. Benzodiazepines should not be used for long-term sleep disturbances. When used chronically, they can disrupt sleep cycles and produce tolerance and dependence.

Last moments

Symptoms that become visible in the last few days of life include increasing weakness, drowsiness, loss of interest in food or drink, and difficulty swallowing. In this phase, supporting the family and treating signs and symptoms of suffering are paramount. Often, conversion from oral to IV medications has to occur at this point. Open, ongoing, consistent communication between the provider and the family is important during this time.[6] Explaining that death is imminent but that the time course could be hours to days helps clarify the family's expectations. Even when the child is comfortable, the presence of a caregiver is valued. Someone should be available to pronounce the children if they are not in the hospital setting.

▶ Terminal sedation

When a patient's pain and agitation can no longer be managed despite the caregiver's best effort, terminal sedation should be considered. Initially, opioids are escalated, but due to tolerance or dose-limiting side effects, pain sometimes cannot be controlled. Sedation with opioids alone might not suffice. Benzodiazepines, barbiturates, or neuroleptics can be added to the continuous opioid infusion. Expect rapid progression of symptoms requiring rapid, aggressive titration of medications to obtain comfort in the final days and hours. Dose adjustments should be made in response to the child's suffering and not the suffering of the family. Medications should be given by continuous infusion, and doses should be escalated by 50% as needed. One should avoid giving medications by "IV push" so that if the death occurs rapidly after the last dose, a causal relationship is not assumed by the family.

The family should be prepared for the changes in respiration that precede death. The death rattle is most common in children with lung disease or brain tumors.[233] The child is often unconscious by this point, and so is not disturbed by this symptom. Drying secretions with scopolamine or *l*-hyoscyamine drops can reduce the rattle.

▶ Autopsy

This delicate topic is best brought up premortem to give the family time to consider the option. Most consenting families believe the autopsy will be helpful to other patients. It also can serve a role in the bereavement process when a family returns for a follow-up discussion after the autopsy.

▶ Barriers to palliative care

An inexperienced caregiver may fear that his or her management of pain and suffering may hasten the child's death. The principle of double effect,[234] arising from moral theology, justifies the possibility of an early death in the pursuit of alleviating suffering (Table 16-26).

Thus, the good effect of pain control in a child dying of cancer can justify the possible bad effect of hastening death. Yet overall, it is extremely unlikely for there to be a causal relationship between the two (Table 16-27). Other ethicists have cited logical and practical difficulties with these of the Principle of Double Effect in palliative care.

Table 16-26

Barriers to Optimal Pediatric Palliative Care

Education of providers: few teachers

Limited resources for research

No evidence-based practice guidelines, few prospective trials

Emotional impact of caring for a dying child

Difficulty of effectively dealing with children at different stages of development

Poor reimbursement for time-intensive services

Research challenges in the dying child

Source: From Refs. 235–237.

Table 16-27

Principle of Double Effect

An action that has both good and bad effects is not immoral if:

The action itself is morally good

The bad effect can be foreseen but not intended

The good effect cannot be achieved by way of the bad effect

The good effect must outweigh the bad effect

Quality assessments

Interviewing parents after the death of their child provides a degree of quality assessment in pediatric end-of-life care. The most common difficulty cited by parents is communication difficulties between parents and providers, especially regarding the shift to end-of-life care and adequate pain control.[238] Staff members similarly reported feeling inexperienced in communication with patients and families about end-of-life issues, transition to palliative care, and DNR status. Fifty-four percent of providers report that adequate support is not available for palliative care providers.[239]

Caregivers' role in bereavement process

This can be considered one of the most important roles the caregiver can play. There are several ways to support the parents and siblings after the loss of a child. Give ample time to review medical events surrounding the death and to answer questions. Dispel misconceptions siblings may have about dying.[240] There are copious educational materials and support groups for grieving parents and children. It is helpful to conduct a memorial service at the hospital or in the community to emphasize to the family how loved the child was by caregivers. A child's death is so shocking that the bereavement period is often longer than average, but be aware of signs of grief becoming pathological. Parents can feel cut off from close relationships they made with caregivers. If possible, plan cards or phone calls during the following year, especially around challenging times like birthdays, holidays, or anniversaries. This lets parents know that they and their child are not forgotten and may give them an opportunity to ask lingering questions.

Caring for the caregivers

Caring for a dying child is extremely rewarding but may engender powerful negative emotions in the caregiver. Some have described feelings of failure, helplessness, or sadness at the loss of a life cut short. These emotions must be acknowledged so as to not become a barrier to effective communication and decision-making.[210] Studies suggest a higher incident of alcoholism, marital discord, and suicide in caregivers. Several etiologies behind this include confronting death, which emphasizes our finite nature, the cumulative grief associated with repeated loss, and the inability to achieve idealistic goals. Prevention and management of stress includes recognizing stress in oneself and one's colleagues, setting limits, clarifying roles and goals, team support meetings, regular exercise, and clarifying unresolved personal issues around death and dying.

CONCLUSION

There is a critical lack of research into best practice for pediatric palliative care. Some cite the delicate nature of death and dying for the family as the reason for the paucity in data. Future research goals in pediatric palliative care should include the characteristics of cancer-related death, end-of-life decision-making, outcomes of symptom-directed interventions, a cost analysis of pediatric palliative care, and the profiles of survivors (family members and healthcare providers). More research should also be done in communication, suffering, and quality of life.[235]

Finally, "A kind word and a caring attitude are remembered for decades."[235]

ACKNOWLEDGMENTS

Many thanks to Charles Berde & Joanne Wolfe for all their work in this field & assistance with this chapter.

REFERENCES

1. Gunderman RB. Psychosocial issues in pediatric oncology: what the radiologist needs to know. *Pediatr Radiol.* 2000;30(1):7–13.
2. Surveillance, Epidemiology, and End Results (SEER), Cancer Statistics Review, 1975–2003, National Cancer Institute, NIH.
3. Usmani GN. Pediatric oncology in the third world. *Curr Opin Pediatr.* 2001;13(1):1–9.
4. Tammemagi CM, Nerenz D, Neslund-Dudas C, et al. Comorbidity and survival disparities among black and white patients with breast cancer. *JAMA.* 2005;294(14):1765–1772.
5. Drake R, Frost J, Collins JJ. The symptoms of dying children. *J Pain Symptom Manage.* 2003;26(1):594–603.
6. Wolfe J, Grier HE, Klar N, et al. Symptoms and suffering at the end of life in children with cancer. *N Engl J Med.* 2000;342:326–333.
7. New Tools to Improve Clinical Competency in Pediatric Pain Management. Understanding Pain in Children Who Cannot Speak. Cancer Pain Release, WHO, Vol. 16, Nos. 3 & 4, 2003.
8. Collins JJ, Byrnes ME, Dunkel IJ, et al. The measurement of symptoms in children with cancer. *J Pain Symptom Manage.* 2000;19:363–377.
9. Marec-Berard P. Cancer-related bone pain in children. *Arch Pediatr.* 2005;12(2):191–198.
10. Antunes NL. Back and neck pain in children with cancer. *Pediatr Neurol.* 2002;27(1):46–48.
11. Gomez-Batiste X. Breakthrough cancer pain: prevalence and characteristics in patients in Catalonia, Spain. *J Pain Symptom Manage.* 2002;24:45–52.
12. Ljungman G, Gordh T, Sorensen S, et al. Pain in pediatric oncology: interviews with children, adolescents and their parents. *Acta Pediatr.* 1999;88:623–630.
13. Sonis ST, Eilers JP, Epstein JB, et al. Validation of a new scoring system for the assessment of clinical trial research of oral mucositis induced by radiation or chemotherapy. Mucositis Study Group. *Cancer.* 1999;85(10):2103–2113.
14. Raber-Durlacher JE. Oral mucositis in patients treated with chemotherapy for solid tumors: a retrospective analysis of 150 cases. *Support Care Cancer.* 2000;8(5):366–371.
15. Turhal NS. Efficacy of treatment to relieve mucositis-induced discomfort. *Support Care Cancer.* 2000;8(1):55–58.
16. Elad S, Cohen G, Zylber-Katz E, et al. Systemic absorption of lidocaine after topical application for the treatment of oral mucositis in bone marrow transplantation patients. *J Oral Pathol Med.* 1999;28:170–172.
17. Cheng KK. Prevention of oral mucositis in paediatric patients treated with chemotherapy a randomized crossover trial comparing two protocols of oral care. *Eur J Cancer.* 2004;40(8):1208–1216.
18. Cheng KK. Evaluation of an oral care protocol intervention in the prevention of chemotherapy-induced oral mucositis in paediatric cancer patients. *Eur J Cancer.* 2001;37(16):2056–2063.
19. Biswal BM. Topical application of honey in the management of radiation mucositis: a preliminary study. *Support Care Cancer.* 2003;11(4): 242–248.
20. Turhal NS. Efficacy of treatment to relieve mucositis-induced discomfort. *Support Care Cancer.* 2000;8(1):55–58.
21. Castagna L. Prevention of mucositis in bone marrow transplantation: A double blind randomized controlled trial of sucralfate. *Ann Oncol.* 2001;12(7):953–955.
22. Bradford WZ. A Phase III, Randomized, Double-blind, Placebo-controlled, Multinational Trial of Iseganan for the Prevention of Oral Mucositis in Patients Receiving Stomatotoxic Chemotherapy *Leuk Lymphoma.* 2003;44(7):1165–1172.
23. Genot MT, Klastersky J. Low-level laser for prevention and therapy of oral mucositis induced by chemotherapy or radiotherapy. *Curr Opin Oncol.* 2005;17(3):236–240.
24. Wong SF, Wilder-Smith P. Pilot study of laser effects on oral mucositis in patients receiving chemotherapy. *Cancer J.* 2002;8(3):247–254.
25. Spielberger R. Palifermin for Oral Mucositis after Intensive Therapy for Hematologic Cancers. *N Engl J Med.* 2004;351(25):2590–2598.
26. Yuen KY. Effects of clarithromycin on oral mucositis in bone marrow transplant recipients. *Haematologica.* 2001;86(5):554–555.
27. Flogegard H. Characteristics and adequacy of intravenous morphine infusions in children in a paediatric oncology setting. *Med Pediatr Oncol.* 2003;40(4):233–238.
28. Davidson AJ. Awareness During Anesthesia in Children: A Prospective Cohort Study. *Anesth Analg.* 2005;100:653–661.
29. MacKenzie JR. Complications of treatment of paediatric malignancies. *Eur J Radiol.* 2001;37(2):109–119.
30. Koc Y, Miller KB, Schenkein DP, et al. Varicella zoster virus infections following allogeneic bone marrow transplantation: frequency, risk factors, and clinical outcome. *Biol Blood Marrow Transplant.* 2000;6:44–49.
31. Leung TF. Incidence, risk factors and outcome of varicella-zoster virus infection in children after haematopoietic stem cell transplantation. *Bone Marrow Transplant.* 2000;25(2):167–172.
32. Takayama N, Yamada H, Kaku H, Minamitani M. Herpes zoster in immunocompetent and immunocompromised Japanese children. *Pediatr Int.* 2000;42(3):275–279.
33. Nagasako EM. Rash severity in herpes zoster: correlates and relationship to postherpetic neuralgia. *J Am Acad Dermatol.* 2002;46(6):834.
34. Dworkin RH. Acute pain in herpes zoster: the famciclovir database project. *Pain.* 2001;94(1):113–119.
35. Tyring S. A randomized, double-blind trial of famciclovir versus acyclovir for the treatment of localized dermatomal herpes zoster in immunocompromised patients. *Cancer Invest.* 2001;19(1):13–22.
36. Itoh M, Tohoku KS. Acute abdominal pain preceding cutaneous manifestations of varicella zoster infection after allogeneic bone marrow transplantation. *J Exp Med.* 2001;195(1):61–63.
37. Kotani N, Kushikata T, Hashimoto H, et al. Intrathecal methylprednisolone for intractable postherpetic neuralgia. *N Engl J Med.* 2000;343:1514–1519.
38. Haanpaa M. Allodynia and pinprick hypesthesia in acute herpes zoster, and the development of postherpetic neuralgia. *J Pain Symptom Manage.* 2000;20(1):50–58.
39. Neudorf S, Sanders J, Kobrinsky N, et al. Allogeneic bone marrow transplantation for children with acute myelocytic leukemia in first remission demonstrates a role for graft versus leukemia in the maintenance of disease-free survival. *Blood.* 2004;103(10):3655–3661.
40. Higman MA, Vogelsang GB. Chronic graft versus host disease. *Br J Haematol.* 2004;125(4):435–454.
41. Kassner E. Evaluation and treatment of chemotherapy extravasation injuries. *J Pediatr Oncol Nurs.* 2000;17(3):135–148.
42. Uhm JH, Yung WK. Neurologic complications of cancer therapy. *Curr Treat Options Neurol.* 1999;1:428–437.
43. Polomano RC. A painful peripheral neuropathy in the rat produced by the chemotherapeutic drug, paclitaxel. *Pain.* 2001;94(3):293–304.
44. Fischmeister G, Kurz M, Haas OA, et al. G-CSF versus GM-CSF for stimulation of peripheral blood progenitor cells (PBPC) and leukocytes in healthy volunteers: comparison of efficacy and tolerability. *Ann Hematol.* 1999;78:117–123.
45. Milkovich G, Moleski RJ, Reitan JF, et al. Comparative safety of filgrastim versus sargramostim in patients receiving myelosuppressive chemotherapy. *Pharmacotherapy.* 2000;20:1432–1440.
46. Koh S. Anterior lumbosacral radiculopathy after intrathecal methotrexate treatment. *Pediatr Neurol.* 1999;21(2):576–578.

47. Laffitte E. Thalidomide: an old drug with new clinical applications. *Expert Opin Drug Saf.* 2004;3(1):47–56.

48. Schwartzman RJ. Thalidomide has activity in treating complex regional pain syndrome. *Arch Intern Med.* 2003;163(12):1487–1488; author reply 1488.

49. Carceles MD. Amethocaine-lidocaine cream, a new topical formulation for preventing venopuncture-induced pain in children. *Reg Anesth Pain Med.* 2002.

50. Eichenfield LF. A clinical study to evaluate the efficacy of ELA-Max (4% liposomal lidocaine) as compared with eutectic mixture of local anesthetics cream for pain reduction of venipuncture in children. *Pediatrics.* 2002;109(6):1093–1099.

51. Koh JL, Harrison D, Myers R, et al. A randomized, double-blind comparison study of EMLA and ELA-Max for topical anesthesia in children undergoing intravenous insertion. *Paediatr Anaesth.* 2004;14(12):977–982.

52. O'Brien L. A critical review of the topical local anesthetic amethocaine (Ametop) for pediatric pain. *Paediatr Drugs.* 2005;7(1):41–54.

53. Cárceles MD. Amethocaine-lidocaine cream, a new topical formulation for preventing venopuncture-induced pain in children. *Reg Anesth Pain Med.* 2002;27:289–295.

54. Arévalo MI. Rapid skin anesthesia using a new topical amethocaine formulation: a preclinical study. *Anesth Analg.* 2004;98:1407–1412.

55. Becker BM. Ultrasound with topical anesthetic rapidly decreases pain of intravenous cannulation. *Acad Emerg Med.* 2005;12(4):289–295.

56. Zempsky WT. Evaluation of a low-dose lidocaine iontophoresis system for topical anesthesia in adults and children: a randomized, controlled trial. *Clin Ther.* 2004;26(7):1110–1119.

57. Luhmann J. A comparison of buffered lidocaine versus ELA-Max before peripheral intravenous catheter insertions in children. *Pediatrics.* 2004;113(3):e217–e220.

58. Jimenez N. A comparison of a needle-free injection system for local anesthesia versus EMLA for intravenous catheter insertion in the pediatric patient. *Anesth Analg.* 2006;102(2):411–414.

59. Ylönen P. Management of postdural puncture headache with epidural blood patch in children. *Paediatr Anaesth.* 2002;12(6):526.

60. Ebinger F. Headache and backache after lumbar puncture in children and adolescents: a prospective study. *Pediatrics.* 2004;113(6):1588–1592.

61. Campanini R. Perioperative headaches in an adolescent: a most complex situation. *J Adolesc Health.* 2004;34(6):535–539.

62. Harrington BE. Postdural puncture headache and the development of the epidural blood patch. *Reg Anesth Pain Med.* 2004;29(2):136–163

63. Bucklin BA. Clinical Dilemma: A Patient with Postdural Puncture Headache and Acute Leukemia. *Anesth Analg.* 1999;88:166–167.

64. Annequin D, Carbajal R, Chauvin P, et al. Fixed 50% nitrous oxide oxygen mixture for painful procedures: a French survey. *Pediatrics.* 2000; 105:E47.

65. Barnes C, Downie P, Chalkiadis G, et al. Sedation practices for Australian and New Zealand paediatric oncology patients. *J Paediatr Child Health.* 2002;38(2):170–172.

66. Chern B, McCarthy N, Hutchins C, Durrant ST. Analgesic infiltration at the site of bone marrow harvest significantly reduces donor morbidity. *Bone Marrow Transplant.* 1999;23:947–949.

67. Crom DB, Chathaway DK, Tolley EA, et al. Health status and health-related quality of life in long-term adult survivors of pediatric solid tumors. *Int J Cancer Suppl.* 1999;12:25–31.

68. Hudson MM. Health Status of Adult Long-term Survivors of Childhood Cancer. *JAMA.* 2003;290(12):1583–1592.

69. Krane EJ, Heller LB. The Prevalence of Phantom Sensation and Pain in Pediatric Amputees. *J Pain Symptom Manage.* 1995;10:21–29.

70. Mekhail N. Complex regional pain syndrome type I in cancer patients. *Curr Rev Pain.* 2000;4(3):227–233.

71. Rusy LM, Troshynski TJ, Weisman SJ. Gabapentin in phantom limb pain management in children and young adults: report of seven cases. *J Pain Symptom Manage.* 2001;21:78–82.

72. Flor H. Neuroelectric source imaging of steady-state movement-related cortical potentials in human upper extremity amputees with and without phantom limb pain. *Pain.* 2004;110(1-2):90–102.

73. Birbaumer N. Reorganization of motor and somatosensory cortex in upper extremity amputees with phantom limb pain. *J Neurosci.* 2001;21(10):3609–3618.

74. Chollet CT. Childhood cancer survivors: an at-risk cohort for ankle osteonecrosis. *Clin Orthop Relat Res.* 2005;(430):149–155.

75. Hernandez-Reif M. Breast cancer patients have improved immune and neuroendocrine functions following massage therapy. *J Psychosom Res.* 2004;57(1):45–52.

76. Cassileth BR. Massage therapy for symptom control: outcome study at a major cancer center. *J Pain Symptom Manage.* 2004;28(3):244–249.

77. Shen J. Acupuncture: evidence and implications for cancer supportive care. *Cancer Pract.* 2001;9(3):147–150.

78. Alimi D. Analgesic effect of auricular acupuncture for cancer pain: a randomized, blinded, controlled trial. *J Clin Oncol.* 2003;21(22): 4120–4126.

79. Vickers AJ. Acupuncture for postchemotherapy fatigue: a phase II study. *J Clin Oncol.* 2004;22(9):1731–1735.

80. Zeltzer LK. A phase I study on the feasibility and acceptability of an acupuncture/hypnosis intervention for chronic pediatric pain. *J Pain Symptom Manage.* 2002;24(4):437–446.

81. Adamsen L., Midtgaard J., Roerth M., Andersen C., Quist M. & Moeller T. Transforming the nature of fatigue through exercise: qualitative findings from a multidimensional exercise programme in cancer patients undergoing chemotherapy. *Eur J Cancer Care.* 2004;13:362–370.

82. Redd WH, Montgomery GH, DuHamel KN, Behavioral intervention for cancer treatment side effects. *J Natl Cancer Inst.* 2001;93(11):810–823.

83. Schneider SM. Virtual reality as a distraction intervention for older children receiving chemotherapy. *Pediatr Nurs.* 2000;26(6):593–597.

84. Wild MR. The efficacy of hypnosis in the reduction of procedural pain and distress in pediatric oncology: a systematic review. *J Dev Behav Pediatr.* 2004;25(3):207–213.

85. Liossi C. Clinical hypnosis in the alleviation of procedure-related pain in pediatric oncology patients. *Int J Clin Exp Hypn.* 2003;51(1):4–28.

86. Deng G. Complementary therapies for cancer-related symptoms. *J Support Oncol.* 2004;2(5):419–426; discussion 427–429.

87. Roberts R. Pediatric drug labeling: improving the safety and efficacy of pediatric therapies. *JAMA.* 2003;290(7):905–911.

88. Lesko SM, Mitchell AA. The safety of acetaminophen and ibuprofen among children younger than two years old. *Pediatrics.* 1999;104:E39.

89. Autret-Leca E. A general overview of the use of ibuprofen in paediatrics. *Int J Clin Pract* 2003;135(suppl):9–12.

90. Goldstein JL, Silverstein FE, Agrawal NM, et al. Reduced risk of upper gastrointestinal ulcer complications with celecoxib, a novel COX-2 inhibitor. *Am J Gastroenterol.* 2000;95:1681–1690.

91. Leese PT, Hubbard RC, Karim A, et al. Effects of celecoxib, a novel cyclooxygenase-2 inhibitor, on platelet function in healthy adults: a randomized, controlled trial. *J Clin Pharmacol.* 2000;40:124–132.

92. Laine L, Harper S, Simon T, et al. A randomized trial comparing the effect of rofecoxib, a cyclooxygenase 2-specific inhibitor, with that of ibuprofen on the gastroduodenal mucosa of patients with osteoarthritis. Rofecoxib Osteoarthritis Endoscopy Study Group. *Gastroenterology.* 1999;117: 776–783.

93. Kuehn BM. FDA panel: keep COX-2 drugs on market: black box for COX-2 labels, caution urged for all NSAIDs. *JAMA.* 2005;293(13): 1571–1573.

94. Fowles RE. Potential cardiovascular effects of COX-2 selective nonsteroidal antiinflammatory drugs. *J Pain Palliat Care Pharmacother.* 2003;17(2):27–50.

95. Stempak D, Gammon J, Klein J, et al. Single-dose and steady-state pharmacokinetics of celecoxib in children.[see comment]. *Clin Pharmacol Ther.* 2002;72(5):490–497.

96. Foeldvari I, Burgos-Vargas R, Thon A, Tuerck D. High response rate in the phase I/II study of meloxicam in juvenile rheumatoid arthritis. *J Rheumatol.* 2002;29(5):1079–1083.

97. Pickering AE, Bridge HS, Nolan J, Stoddart PA. Double-blind, placebo-controlled analgesic study of ibuprofen or rofecoxib in combination with paracetamol for tonsillectomy in children. *Br J Anaesth.* 2002;88(1):72–77.

98. Fahey SM. Use of NSAIDs and COX-2 inhibitors in children with musculoskeletal disorders. *J Pediatr Orthop.* 2003;23(6):794–799.

99. American Academy of Pediatrics. Committee on Drugs. Acetaminophen toxicity in children. *Pediatrics.* 2001;108(4):1020–1024.

100. Klepstad P, Kaasa S, Borchgrevink PC. Start of oral morphine to cancer patients: effective serum morphine concentrations and contribution from morphine-6-glucuronide to the analgesia produced by morphine. *Eur J Clin Pharmacol.* 2000;55:713–719.

101. Bouwmeester NJ. Developmental pharmacokinetics of morphine and its metabolites in neonates, infants and young children. *Br J Anaesth.* 2004;92(2):208–217.

102. Hunt A. Population pharmacokinetics of oral morphine and its glucuronides in children receiving morphine as immediate-release liquid or sustained-release tablets for cancer pain. *J Pediatr.* 1999;135(1):47–55.

103. Durnin C. Pharmacokinetics of oral immediate-release hydromorphone (Dilaudid IR) in young and elderly subjects. *Proc West Pharmacol Soc.* 2001;44:79–80.

104. Davis AM, Inturrisi CE. D-Methadone blocks morphine tolerance and N-methyl-D-aspartate-induced hyperalgesia. *J Pharmacol Exp Ther.* 1999;289:1048–1053.

105. Sabatowski R. Patient-controlled analgesia with intravenous L-methadone in a child with cancer pain refractory to high-dose morphine. *J Pain Symptom Manage.* 2002;23(1):3–5.

106. Lugo RA. The pharmacokinetics of oxycodone. *J Pain Palliat Care Pharmacother.* 2004;18(4):17–30.

107. Kokki H. Pharmacokinetics of oxycodone after intravenous, buccal, intramuscular and gastric administration in children. *Clin Pharmacokinet.* 2004;43(9): 613–622.

108. Czarnecki ML. Controlled-release oxycodone for the management of pediatric postoperative pain. *J Pain Symptom Manage.* 2004; 27(4):379–386.

109. Muller P, Vogtmann C. Three cases with different presentation of fentanyl-induced muscle rigidity—a rare problem in intensive care of neonates. *Am J Perinatol.* 2000;17:23–26.

110. Collins JJ, Dunkel IJ, Gupta SK, et al. Transdermal fentanyl in children with cancer pain: feasibility, tolerability, and pharmacokinetic correlates. *J Pediatr.* 1999;134:319–323.

111. Wheeler M. Uptake pharmacokinetics of the Fentanyl Oralet in children scheduled for central venous access removal: implications for the timing of initiating painful procedures. *Paediatr Anaesth.* 2002;12(7): 594–599.

112. Binstock W. The effect of premedication with OTFC, with or without ondansetron, on postoperative agitation, and nausea and vomiting in pediatric ambulatory patients. *Pediatr Anesth.* 2004;14(9):759.

113. Klein EJ. A randomized, clinical trial of oral midazolam plus placebo versus oral midazolam plus oral transmucosal fentanyl for sedation during laceration repair. *Pediatrics.* 2002;109(5):894–897.

114. Wheeler M. The pharmacokinetics of the intravenous formulation of fentanyl citrate administered orally in children undergoing general anesthesia. *Anesth Analg.* 2004;99(5):1347–1351.

115. Williams. Codeine phosphate in paediatric medicine. *Br J Anaesth.* 2001;86(3):413–421.

116. Williams DG. Pharmacogenetics of codeine metabolism in an urban population of children and its implications for analgesic reliability. *Br J Anaesth.* 2002;89(6):839–845.

117. Cowan A. Buprenorphine: new pharmacological aspects. *Int J Clin Pract Suppl.* 2003;133:3–8, 23–24.

118. Sorge J. Transdermal buprenorphine in the treatment of chronic pain: results of a phase III, multicenter, randomized, double-blind, placebo-controlled study. *Clin Ther.* 2004;26(11):1808–1820.

119. Sittl R. Equipotent doses of transdermal fentanyl and transdermal buprenorphine in patients with cancer and noncancer pain: results of a retrospective cohort study. *Clin Ther.* 2005;27(2): 225–237

120. Robaux S. Tramadol added to 1.5% mepivacaine for axillary brachial plexus block improves postoperative analgesia dose-dependently. *Anesth Analg.* 2004; 98(4):1172–1177.

121. Altunkaya H. The postoperative analgesic effect of tramadol when used as subcutaneous local anesthetic. *Anesth Analg.* 2004; 99(5):1461–1464.

122. Menendez L. Analgesic effects of loperamide in bone cancer pain in mice. *Pharmacol Biochem Behav.* 2005;81(1):114–121.

123. Flock P. Pilot study to determine the effectiveness of diamorphine gel to control pressure ulcer pain. *J Pain Symptom Manage.* 2003;25(6): 547–554

124. Arcuri E. Opioid nonresponsiveness in cancer pain can be reversible. A serendipitous conclusion of a refrospective analysis. *J Pain Symptom Manage.* 2000; 20(6):393–394.

125. Mercadante S. Opioid poorly-responsive cancer pain. Part 1: clinical considerations. *J Pain Symptom Manage.* 2001;21(2):144–150.

126. Truog RD. Barbiturates in the care of the terminally ill. *N Engl J Med.* 1992;327(23):1678–1682.

127. Sawynok J. Topical and peripherally acting analgesics. *Pharmacol Rev.* 2003;55(1):1–20.

128. Kalso E. Improving opioid effectiveness: from ideas to evidence. *Eur J Pain.* 2005;9(2):131–135.

129. Pan HL, Eisenach JC, Chen SR. Gabapentin suppresses ectopic nerve discharges and reverses allodynia in neuropathic rats. *J Pharmacol Exp Ther.* 1999;288:1026–1030.

130. Tremont-Lukats IW, Megeff C, Backonja MM. Anticonvulsants for neuropathic pain syndromes: mechanisms of action and place in therapy. *Drugs.* 2000;60:1029–1052.

131. Backonja MM. Anticonvulsants (antineuropathics) for neuropathic pain syndromes. *Clin J Pain.* 2000;16:S67–S72.

132. Ecevit C. Effect of carbamazepine and valproate on bone mineral density. *Pediatr Neurol.* 2004;31(4):279–82

133. Carrazana E. Rationale and evidence for the use of oxcarbazepine in neuropathic pain. *J Pain Symptom Manage.* 2003; 25(5 Suppl): S31-5.

134. Groeper K. Topiramate and metabolic acidosis: a case series and review of the literature. *Paediatr Anaesth.* 2005;15(2):167–170.

135. Schechter T. Adverse reactions of Topiramate and Lamotrigine in children. *Pharmacoepidemiol Drug Saf.* 2005;14(3):187–192.

136. Guay DR. Pregabalin in neuropathic pain: a more "pharmaceutically elegant" gabapentin? *Am J Geriatr Pharmacother.* 2005;3(4):274–287.

137. Freynhagen R, Strojek K, Griesing T, et al. Efficacy of pregabalin in neuropathic pain evaluated in a 12-week, randomized, double-blind, multicentre, placebo-controlled trial of flexible- and fixed-dose regimens. *Pain.* 2005;115(3):254–263.

138. Neafsey PJ. Lyrica (pregabalin): neurontin replacement? *Home Healthc Nurse.* 2005;23(9):563–564.

139. Sindrup SH, Jensen TS. Efficacy of pharmacological treatments of neuropathic pain: an update and effect related to mechanism of drug action. *Pain.* 1999;83:389–400.

140. Mercadante S. Opioid poorly-responsive cancer pain. Part 3. Clinical strategies to improve opioid responsiveness. *J Pain Symptom Manage.* 2001;21(4):338–354.

141. Kennett A. An open study of methotrimeprazine in the management of nausea and vomiting in patients with advanced cancer. *Support Care Cancer.* 2005; 13(9): 715–21.

142. Fishbain DA. Do The Second-Generation "Atypical Neuroleptics" Have Analgesic Properties? A Structured Evidence-Based Review. *Pain Med.* 2004;5(4):359–365.

143. Wooldridge JE. Corticosteroids in advanced cancer. Oncology (Williston Park). 2001;15(2): 225–234; discussion 234–236.

144. Gaze MN. Feasibility of dosimetry-based high-dose 131I-meta-iodobenzylguanidine with topotecan as a radiosensitizer in children with metastatic neuroblastoma. *Cancer Biother Radiopharm.* 2005;20(2): 195–199.

145. Santiago-Palma J, Fischberg D, Kornick C, et al. Diphenhydramine as an analgesic adjuvant in refractory cancer pain. *J Pain Symptom Manage.* 2001;22:699–703.

146. Rozans M. Palliative uses of methylphenidate in patients with cancer: a review. *J Clin Oncol.* 2002;20(1):335–339.

147. Slatkin NE. Treatment of opiate-related sedation: utility of the cholinesterase inhibitors. *J Support Oncol.* 2003;1(1):53–63.

148. Gammaitoni A. Topical Ketamine Gel: Possible Role in Treating Neuropathic Pain. *Pain Med.* 2000;1(1):97–100.

149. Komada Y, Matsuyama T, Takao A, et al. A randomized dose-comparison trial of granisetron in preventing emesis in children with leukemia receiving emetogenic chemotherapy. *Eur J Cancel.* 1999;35:1095–1101.

150. Hesketh PJ, Gralla RJ, Webb RT, et al. Randomized phase 11 study of the neurokinin 1 receptor antagonist CJ- 11,974 in the control of cisplatin-induced emesis [see comments]. *J Clin Oncol.* 1999;17:338–343.

151. Gralla RJ, Osoba D, Kris MG, et al. Recommendations for the use of antiemetics: evidence-based, clinical practice guidelines. American Society of Clinical Oncology [published erratum appears in *J Clin Oncol* 1999; 17:38601.] *J Clin Oncol.* 1999;17:2971–2994.

152. Small BE. Survey ranking of emetogenic control in children receiving chemotherapy. *J Pediatr Hematol Oncol.* 2000;22(2):125–1232.

153. Goldsmith B. First choice for radiation-induced nausea and vomiting—the efficacy and safety of granisetron. *Acta Oncol.* 2004;43(Suppl. 15): 19–22.

154. Feyer PC. Radiotherapy-induced nausea and vomiting (RINV): antiemetic guidelines. *Support Care Cancer.* 2005;13(2):122–128.

155. Culy CR. Ondansetron: a review of its use as an antiemetic in children. *Paediatr Drugs.* 2001;3(6):441–479.

156. White L. A comparison of oral ondansetron syrup or intravenous ondansetron loading dose regimens given in combination with dexamethasone for the prevention of nausea and emesis in pediatric and adolescent patients receiving moderately/highly emetogenic chemotherapy. *Pediatr Hematol Oncol.* 2000;17(6):445–455.

157. Aapro M. Granisetron: an update on its clinical use in the management of nausea and vomiting. *Oncologist.* 2004;9(6):673–686.

158. Wada I. Pharmacokinetics of granisetron in adults and children with malignant diseases. *Biol Pharm Bull.* 2001;24(4):432–435.

159. Coppes MJ, Lau R, Ingram LC, et al. Open-label comparison of the antiemetic efficacy of single intravenous doses of dolasetron mesylate in pediatric cancer patients receiving moderately to highly emetogenic chemotherapy. *Med Pediatr Oncol.* 1999;33:99–105.

160. Coppes MJ, Yanofsky R, Pritchard S, et al. Safety, tolerability, antiemetic efficacy, and pharmacokinetics of oral dolasetron mesylate in pediatric cancer patients receiving moderately to highly emetogenic chemotherapy. *J Pediatr Hematol Oncol.* 1999;21:274–283.

161. Cappelli C. Tropisetron: optimal dosage for children in prevention of chemotherapy-induced vomiting. *Pediatr Blood Cancer.* 2005;45(1):48–53.

162. Rabasseda X. Ramosetron, a 5-HT3 receptor antagonist for the control of nausea and vomiting. *Drugs Today (Barc).* 2002;38(2):75–89.

163. Aksoylar S. Comparison of tropisetron and granisetron in the control of nausea and vomiting in children receiving combined cancer chemotherapy. *Pediatr Hematol Oncol.* 2001;18(6):397–406.

164. Forni C. Granisetron, tropisetron, and ondansetron in the prevention of acute emesis induced by a combination of cisplatin-Adriamycin and by high-dose ifosfamide delivered in multiple-day continuous infusions. *Support Care Cancer.* 2000;8(2):131–133.

165. Karamanlioglu B. Comparison of oral dolasetron and ondansetron in the prophylaxis of postoperative nausea and vomiting in children. *Eur J Anaesthesiol.* 2003;20(10):831–835.

166. Kris MG. Consensus proposals for the prevention of acute and delayed vomiting and nausea following high-emetic-risk chemotherapy. *Support Care Cancer.* 2005;13(2):85–96.

167. de Wit R. Addition of the oral NK1 antagonist aprepitant to standard antiemetics provides protection against nausea and vomiting during multiple cycles of cisplatin-based chemotherapy. *J Clin Oncol.* 2003;21(22):4105–4111.

168. Chawla SP. Establishing the dose of the oral NK1 antagonist aprepitant for the prevention of chemotherapy-induced nausea and vomiting. *Cancer.* 2003;97(9):2290–2300.

169. Stuth EA. Droperidol for perioperative sedation causes a transient prolongation of the QTc time in children under volatile anesthesia. *Paediatr Anaesth.* 2004;14(10):831–837.

170. Buttner M. Is low-dose haloperidol a useful antiemetic?: A meta-analysis of published and unpublished randomized trials. *Anesthesiology.* 2004;101(6):1454–1463.

171. Jackson WC. Olanzapine for intractable nausea in palliative care patients. *J Palliat Med.* 2003;6(2):251–255.

172. Martin BR. Mechanism of action of cannabinoids: how it may lead to treatment of cachexia, emesis, and pain. *J Support Oncol.* 2004;2(4):305–314; discussion 314–316.

173. Walsh D. Established and potential therapeutic applications of cannabinoids in oncology. *Support Care Cancer.* 2003;11(3):137–143.

174. Radbruch L. Review of cannabinoids in the treatment of nausea and vomiting. *Schmerz.* 2004;18(4):306–310.

175. Tramer MR. Cannabinoids for control of chemotherapy induced nausea and vomiting: quantitative systematic review. *Br Med J.* 2001;323(7303):16–21.

176. Naef M. The analgesic effect of oral delta-9-tetrahydrocannabinol (THC), morphine, and a THC-morphine combination in healthy subjects under experimental pain conditions. *Pain.* 2003;105(1-2):79–88.

177. Hall W. Cannabinoids and cancer: causation, remediation, and palliation. *Lancet Oncol.* 2005;6(1):35–42.

178. Bagshaw SM. Medical efficacy of cannabinoids and marijuana: a comprehensive review of the literature. *J Palliat Care.* 2002;18(2):111–122.

179. Ernst E, Pittler MH. Efficacy of ginger for nausea and vomiting: a systematic review of randomized clinical trials. *Br J Anaesth.* 2000;84(3):367–371.

180. Butkovic D. Comparison of laser acupuncture and metoclopramide in PONV prevention in children. *Paediatr Anaesth.* 2005;15(1):37–40.

181. Mahesh R. Cancer chemotherapy-induced nausea and vomiting: role of mediators, development of drugs and treatment methods. *Pharmazie.* 2005;60(2):83–96.

182. Maxwell LG. The Effects of a Small-Dose Naloxone Infusion on Opioid-Induced Side Effects and Analgesia in Children and Adolescents Treated with Intravenous Patient-Controlled Analgesia. *Anesth Analg.* 2005;100(4):953–958.

183. McDonald AJ. Patient-Controlled Analgesia: An Appropriate Method of Pain Control in Children *Paediatr Drugs.* 2001;3(4):273–284.

184. Monitto CL. The Safety and Efficacy of Parent-/Nurse-Controlled Analgesia in Patients Less than Six Years of Age *Anesth Analg.* 2000;91(3):573–579.

185. Birmingham PK. Patient-Controlled Epidural Analgesia in Children: Can They Do It? *Anesth Analg.* 2003;96(3):686–691.

186. Antok E. Patient-Controlled Epidural Analgesia Versus Continuous Epidural Infusion with Ropivacaine for Postoperative Analgesia in Children *Anesth Analg.* 2003;97(6):1608–1611.

187. Duflo F. Patient-controlled regional analgesia is effective in children: a preliminary report. *Can J Anaesth.* 2004;51(9):928–930.

188. Viscusi ER. Patient-Controlled Transdermal Fentanyl Hydrochloride vs Intravenous Morphine Pump for Postoperative Pain *JAMA.* 2004;291(11):1333–1341.

189. Vojkovic SJ. Case study report of two palliative care patients receiving intracerebroventricular (ICV) analgesia. *J Palliat Care.* 2003;19(4):280–283.

190. Quigley C. Opioid switching to improve pain relief and drug tolerability. *Cochrane Database Syst Rev.* 2004;(3):CD004847.

191. Drake R, Longworth J, Collins JJ. Opioid rotation in children with cancer. *J Palliat Med.* 2004;7(3):419–422.

192. Miguel R. Interventional treatment of cancer pain: the fourth step in the World Health Organization analgesic ladder? *Cancer Control.* 2000;7(2):149–156.

193. Saroyan JM, Schechter WS, Tresgallo ME, Granowetter L. Role of intraspinal analgesia in terminal pediatric malignancy. *J Clin Oncol.* 2005;23(6):1318–1321.

194. Baker L. Evolving spinal analgesia practice in palliative care. *Palliat Med.* 2004;18(6):507–515.

195. Smith TJ. Randomized Clinical Trial of an Implantable Drug Delivery System Compared With Comprehensive Medical Management for Refractory Cancer Pain. *J Clin Oncol.* 2002;20(19):4040–4049.

196. Shimazaki M. Intrathecal phenol block in a child with cancer pain—a case report. *Masui.* 2003;52(7):756–758.

197. Yegul I. Bilateral CT-guided percutaneous cordotomy for cancer pain relief. *Clin Radiol.* 2003;58(11):886–889.

198. Wolfe J. Caring for the Child With Cancer at the Close of Life. *JAMA.* 2004;292:2141–2149.

199. Hynson JL, Sawyer SM, Paediatric palliative care: Distinctive needs and emerging issues *J Pediatr Child Health.* 2001;37:323.

200. Sumner LH. Lighting the way: improving the way children die in America. *Caring.* 2003; 22(5):14–28

201. Weinstein SM. Integrating palliative care in pediatrics. *Curr Pain Headache Rep.* 2004;8(4):281–283.

202. Kane JR. Alleviating the suffering of seriously ill children. *Am J Hosp Palliat Care.* 2001;18(3):161–169.

203. Committee on Bioethics and Committee on Hospital Care, American Academy of Pediatrics. Palliative Care for Children *Pediatrics.* 2000;106(2):351–357.

204. Wolfe J, Mar N, Grier H, et al. Understanding of prognosis among parents of children who died of cancer: impact on treatment goals and integration of palliative care. *JAMA.* 2000;284(19):2469–2475.

205. Schmidt LM. Pediatric end-of-life care: coming of age? *Caring.* 2003; 22(5):20–22.

206. Curtis JR. Studying communication about end-of-life care during the ICU family conference: development of a framework. *J Crit Care.* 2002; 17(3):147–160.

207. Vickers JL, Carlisle C Choices and controls: parental experiences of pediatric terminal home care. *J Pediatr Oncol Nurs.* 2000;17:12–21.

208. Davies B, Brenner P, Orloff S, Sumner L, Worden W. Addressing spirituality in pediatric hospice and palliative care. *J Palliat Care.* 2002;18(1):59–67.

209. Barnes LJ, Plotnikoff GA, Fox K, et al. Spirituality, religion, and pediatrics: intersecting worlds of healing. *Pediatrics.* 2000;104(6):899–908.

210. Beale EA. Silence is not golden: communicating with children dying from cancer. *J Clin Oncol.* 2005;23(15):3629–3631.

211. Higginson IJ, Thompson M. Children and young people who die from cancer. *Br Med J.* 2003;327:478–479.

212. Zwerdling T. Unique aspects of caring for dying children and their families. *Am J Hosp Palliat Care.* 2000;17(5):305–311.

213. Singer PA, Martin DK, Kelner M. Quality end-of-life care: patients' perspectives. *JAMA.* 1999;281(2):163–168.

214. Galloway KS, Yaster M. Pain and symptom control in terminally ill children. *Pediatr Clin North Am.* 2000;47(3):711–746.

215. Garro LC. Culture, pain and cancer. World Health Organization Ladder. Cancer pain relief and palliative care. Technical report series 804. Geneva: World Health Organization, 1990. *J Palliat Care.* 1990;6(3):34–44.

216. Scrace J. Complementary therapies in palliative care of children with cancer: a literature review. *Paediatr Nurs.* 2003;15(3):36–39.

217. Daveson BA. Music therapy in palliative care for hospitalized children and adolescents. *J Palliat Care.* 2000 Spring;16(1):35–38.

218. Driessnack M. Remember me: mask making with chronically and terminally ill children. *Holist Nurs Pract.* 2004;18(4):211–214.

219. Rollins JA. New initiatives in end-of-life care. *Pediatr Nurs.* 2002;28(3):292–293.

220. Wolfe J, Mar N, Grier H, et al. Understanding of prognosis among parents of children who died of cancer: impact on treatment goals and integration of palliative care. *JAMA.* 2000;284(19):2469–2475.

221. Goldman A, Heller KS. Integrating palliative and curative approaches in the care of children with life-threatening illnesses. *J Palliat Med.* 2000;3(3):353–359.

222. Paulino AC, Palliative radiotherapy in children with neuroblastoma. *Pediatr Hematol Oncol.* 2003;20(2):111–117.

223. Porcu P, Bhatia S, Sharma M, et al. Results of treatment after relapse from high-dose chemotherapy in germ cell tumors. *J Clin Oncol.* 2000;18(6):1181–1186.

224. Deutsch M. Radiotherapy for symptomatic metastases to bone in children. *Am J Clin Oncol.* 2004;27(2):128–131.

225. Drake R. The symptoms of dying children. *J Pain Symptom Manage.* 2003;26(1): 594–603.

226. Collins JJ, Byrnes ME, Dunkel IJ, et al. The measurement of symptoms in children with cancer. *J Pain Symptom Manage.* 2000;19(5):363–377.

227. Allard P, Lamontagne C, Bernard P, et al. How effective are supplementary doses of opioids for dyspnea in terminally ill cancer patients? A randomized continuous sequential clinical trial. *J Pain Symptom Manage.* 1999;17(4):256–265.

228. Gavin R. Nebulized Fentanyl for Palliation of Dyspnea in a Cystic Fibrosis Patient *Respiration.* 2004;71(6):646–649.

229. Ripamonti C. Management of dyspnea in advanced cancer patients. *Support Care Cancer.* 1999;7(4):233–243.

230. Abrahm JL. Management of pain and spinal cord compression in patients with advanced cancer. ACP-ASIM End-of-life Care Consensus Panel. American College of Physicians-American Society of Internal Medicine. *Ann Intern Med.* 1999;131(1):37–46.

231. Morita T, Tsunoda J, Inoue S, et al. Perceptions and decision-making on rehydration of terminally ill cancer patients and family members. *Am J Hosp Palliat Care.* 1999;16(3):509–516.

232. Laval G, Girardier J, Lassauniere JM, et al. The use of steroids in the management of inoperable intestinal obstruction in terminal cancer patients: do they remove the obstruction? *Palliat Med.* 2000;14(1):3–10.

233. Morita T, Tsunoda J, Inoue S, et al. Risk factors for death rattle in terminally ill cancer patients: a prospective exploratory study. *Palliat Med.* 2000;14(1):19–23.

234. Sulmasy DP, Pellegrino ED. The rule of double effect: clearing up the double talk. *Arch Intern Med.* 1999;159(6):545–550.

235. Wolfe J, Friebert S, Hilden J. Caring for children with advanced cancer integrating palliative care. *Pediatr Clin North Am.* 2002;49(5):1043–1062.

236. Quill TE. The rule of double effect—a critique of its role in end-of-life decision making. *N Engl J Med.* 1997;337(24):1768–1771.

237. Collins JJ. Palliative care and the child with cancer. *Hematol Oncol Clin North Am.* 2002;16(3):657–670.

238. Hilden JM. Attitudes and Practices Among Pediatric Oncologists Regarding End-of-Life Care: Results of the 1998 American Society of Clinical Oncology Survey. *J Clin Oncol.* 2000;19(1):205–212.

239. Contro NA. Hospital Staff and Family Perspectives Regarding Quality of Pediatric Palliative Care, *Pediatrics.* 2004;114(5)1248–1252.

240. American Academy of Pediatrics. Committee on Psychosocial Aspects of Child and Family Health. The pediatrician and childhood bereavement. *Pediatrics.* 2000;105(2):445–447.

INTERVENTIONAL TECHNIQUES AND OTHER SPECIALIZED APPROACHES

Neuraxial Infusions

CHAPTER
17

Phillip Phan
Madhuri Are
Allen W. Burton

INTRODUCTION

According to the World Health Organization (WHO), an estimated 6.6 million people die from cancer every year.[1] With cancer progression, 65%–85% of patients with advanced cancer will experience pain.[2] As many as 80% of cancer patients describe their pain as having moderate to severe intensity.[2] The WHO has established an algorithm for a three-step analgesic ladder that can be used to treat cancer pain.[1] However, approximately 10%–20% of cancer patients fail to achieve pain relief from using the three-step analgesic ladder.[3,4] This failure arises either from pain that is refractory to opioids or the inability of the patients to tolerate the side effects of the opioids at higher doses.

It has been suggested that a fourth, "interventional" step should be added to the three-step WHO analgesic ladder[3–5] (Fig. 17-1), which would encompass the vast armamentarium of interventional procedures to help alleviate pain that is not controlled with pharmacologic treatment. Neuraxial therapy is a major class of interventions and involves the administration of epidural and intrathecal analgesics at the level of the spinal cord.

Administration of neuraxial or spinal analgesics offers some advantages over irreversible neurodestructive procedures to control pain, that is, neurolytic blockade. It can be very effective in patients with multiple pain sites, such as those who have advanced cancer with multiple sites of metastases. An indwelling neuraxial catheter allows the opioid dosage to be titrated and rotation of analgesic agents, if necessary. The use of intraspinal opioids is selective for the pain transmission pathway at the spinal level, without any discernable effect on the motor, sensory, or sympathetic system.

MECHANISM

Intraspinally administered opioids modulate pain transmission by acting on receptors in the dorsal horn of the spinal cord. Morphine was the first intraspinal opioid administered, and it is the standard of comparison for other intraspinally active analgesics.[6,7] Afferent noxious stimuli converge in the dorsal horn of the spinal cord where the primary nociceptive neuron synapses with the wide dynamic range interneurons and the second-order nociceptive neuron in the spinothalamic tract. Opioid receptors are concentrated in the dorsal horn in the laminae I, II, V, and X of the spinal cord. Agonism of these opioid receptors helps to suppress afferent nociceptive input from pain sites.[8,9] Specifically, opioids are believed to modulate

nociceptive inputs by decreasing release of pain pathway-associated peptides, such as substance P, from small diameter afferent fibers.[10] In addition, opioids also act on pain-transmission pathways by suppressing postsynaptic excitability of second-order neurons at the level of the spinal cord.[10] The goal of intraspinal analgesics, including opioids, is local inhibition of nociceptive transmission at the spinal cord level.

INTRASPINAL ANALGESICS

Many medications have been investigated as intraspinal analgesics, but data from controlled clinical studies are very limited. Opioids as a class of intraspinal analgesics have been the most extensively studied.[11,12] Morphine is the only opioid approved for spinal administration by the U.S. Food and Drug Administration (FDA), although there is a growing body of literature supporting the use of others. Other opioids that have been used intraspinally as reported in the literature include hydromorphone, fentanyl, sufentanil, meperidine, and methadone.[13–15] Caution must be exercised with meperidine and methadone as limited safety data are available.

Efficacy of intraspinal analgesics is affected by three major factors. The patient's characteristics, such as age, weight, and height, can affect the distribution of medication within the spinal column.[16] The route of administration, epidural versus intrathecal, also plays an important role in determining the onset as well as the duration of the intraspinally administered drug.[11] Most importantly, the physical and chemical properties of the drug itself will determine its overall efficacy.[11]

The target of intraspinal analgesics is the receptor system within the spinal cord. Specifically for opioids, the target is the opioid mu receptors located within the dorsal horn. Many of the pharmacokinetic and pharmacodynamic properties of intraspinal opioids are related to their lipid solubility, specifically their ability to diffuse across the dura, spread within the cerebrospinal fluid, and diffuse into the dorsal horn. The oil-water coefficient of an analgesic agent is a good indicator of the hydrophilicity or hydrophobicity of that agent. Morphine, with an oil-water coefficient of 1.40, is a hydrophilic opioid. Thus, morphine will take longer to diffuse across the dura, and to diffuse into the spinal cord. Correspondingly, this hydrophilicity will result in slow receptor saturation, longer onset to peak action, and longer time to clearance from the spinal cord.[17,18] Slow clearance of hydrophilic morphine from spinal cerebrospinal fluid accounts for delayed respiratory depression sometimes seen

Treatment of cancer pain

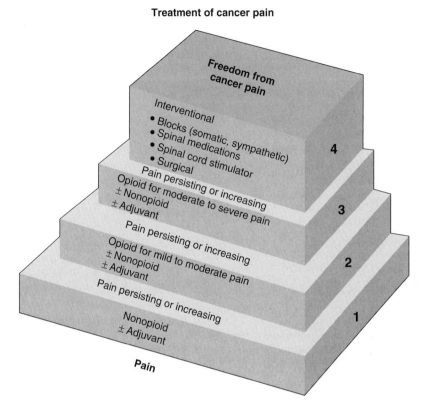

Freedom from cancer pain

Interventional
- Blocks (somatic, sympathetic)
- Spinal medications
- Spinal cord stimulator
- Surgical

4

Pain persisting or increasing
Opioid for moderate to severe pain
± Nonopioid
± Adjuvant

3

Pain persisting or increasing
Opioid for mild to moderate pain
± Nonopioid
± Adjuvant

2

Pain persisting or increasing
Nonopioid
± Adjuvant

1

Pain

FIGURE 17-1 WHO ladder with step 4 "Interventional Pain Management" added. *(Adapted from Miguel R. Interventional treatment of cancer pain: the fourth step in the WHO analgesic ladder? Cancer Control. 2000;7:149–156; Krames ES. Interventional pain management: appropriate when less invasive therapies fail to provide adequate analgesia. Med Clin North Am. 1999;83:787–808.)*

with intraspinally administered morphine. This is due to the rostral spread of morphine remaining within cerebrospinal fluid and morphine's action on the respiratory centers in the brainstem.[19] This delayed effect is, however, rarely seen in opioid-tolerant patients.

Sufentanil, with an oil-water coefficient of about 1800, is the prototypical hydrophobic opioid.[20] Once administered either via epidural or the intrathecal route, this hydrophobic agent quickly diffuses across the dura and is taken up into the spinal cord and vascular system. Receptor saturation of the spinal cord level corresponding to the catheter tip location is expected to be relatively rapid. Sufentanil is rapidly cleared from the intraspinal space.[20]

OTHER INTRASPINAL AGENTS

Clonidine is a well-studied analgesic that is considered to be useful as an adjuvant agent for treating neuropathic pain states.[21] Clonidine acts on central alpha-2 adrenergic receptors, thereby modulating the spinal pain pathway. Clonidine binds to postsynaptic alpha-2 receptors within the dorsal horn and activates the descending noradrenergic inhibitory systems.[22,23] This spinal mechanism explains why clonidine is a poor analgesic when administered systemically.[24] Clonidine is hydrophobic, with an oil-water coefficient that is similar to fentanyl. It is quickly taken up from the cerebrospinal fluid and has a pronounced local effect at the spinal level.[25,26] Use of spinal clonidine has been investigated for postoperative pain control and cancer pain management.[27,28] When clonidine is combined with an opioid, the intraspinal opioid requirement is

less and tolerance takes longer to develop.[29] The main side effect of intraspinally administered clonidine is postural hypotension.[30]

Spinally administered local anesthetics have a synergistic effect when combined with opioids. Bupivacaine, an amide local anesthetic, is commonly used in postoperative epidural infusions, but is also widely used via the intrathecal route in combination with opioids for cancer pain. Like clonidine, bupivacaine is more effective when used in combination with opioids than opioids alone for the treatment of neuropathic pain; however, bupivacaine is also used to treat nociceptive pain.[31,32] The mechanism of local anesthetics involves blockade of voltage-sensitive sodium channels and preventing the generation and conduction of nerve impulses across pain transmission pathways.[32] As with other local anesthetics, bupivacaine dosing is limited by the occurrence of motor blockade at higher local anesthetic concentrations. Intrathecally administered, bupivacaine can cause a motor block at doses as low as 10 mg/day. However, with slow dose titration, bupivacaine doses up to 25–30 mg/day can be used without producing a motor blockade. At lower doses, with an intrathecal patient-controlled demand dose, an interesting case report showed promising efficacy for its use in treating patients with refractory pain.[33]

Ziconotide, a calcium channel blocker, produces its analgesic effect by selectively blocking neuronal N-type voltage-sensitive calcium channels.[34] Calcium channel blockade prevents calcium ion influx and neurotransmitter release. This selectively inhibits transmission of primary afferents located in the dorsal horn of the spinal cord. Ziconotide is currently being evaluated in clinical studies for the treatment of severe chronic pain that is refractory to systemic opioid therapy.[34] Its approval for intrathecal use by the U.S. FDA was obtained in December 2004. This will become the first agent developed specifically for intraspinal administration against chronic pain states. It may be useful as a sole agent or as a coanalgesic with intraspinal opioids.

Neostigmine is another interesting nonopioid that may have a role as an intraspinal analgesic.[35,36] Cholinergic mechanisms are involved in the transmission of pain pathways within the spinal cord.[37] Neostigmine is a water-soluble anticholinergic, which does not cross the blood-brain barrier. Thus, when it is injected intrathecally, neostigmine has a long-acting central effect. The drug has efficacy and minimal toxicity, but initial trials have demonstrated troublesome systemic side effects,[38] which are commonly dose-related. They include nausea, vomiting, and somnolence.

A number of other alpha-2 adrenergic agonists, local anesthetics, calcium-channel blockers, and drugs from other classes (gamma-aminobutyric acid [GABA] agonists, N-methyl-D-aspartate [NMDA] antagonists) have been delivered via the intraspinal route to treat intractable cancer pain, with varying degrees of success. According to a 2002 review, satisfactory analgesia has been reported with the use of such agents delivered intraspinally;[32] however, most are currently considered to be investigational vis-à-vis intraspinal therapy. Clinical guidelines were published in 2000 but were recently revised in 2003. These guidelines function as a basis for decision-making in the form of a treatment algorithm that can be used to direct intraspinal therapy (Fig. 17-2).[15,39] A specific set of algorithms were released for treating cancer pain.[40]

Indications

As discussed earlier, intraspinal analgesics are effective in modulating pain pathways at the spinal level. The significant side effects from systemic high-dose opioid administration (including nausea, constipation, confusion, increased somnolence, or lethargy) can be minimized with intraspinal delivery of opioids. Deposition of opioids into close proximity of spinal cord receptors disseminates potent analgesia with potential sparing of side effects. If the opioid is delivered into the epidural space, only 20%–40% of the systemic dose is required to achieve equianalgesia with systemic opioids. The intrathecal route is even more potent, requiring only 10% of the systemic dose for equianalgesia.[15,18–20,32,40] This therapy is effective for two broad groups of patients: those with refractory pain syndromes and those with intolerable opioid-related side effects.[41,42] The ability to treat pain effectively while minimizing these side effects has a significant impact on quality of life.[43]

Patient selection

When a comprehensive trial of pharmacologic therapy fails to provide adequate analgesia or leads to unacceptable side effects, consideration may be given to alternative modalities. These modalities include parenteral opioid infusions, neuraxial medication infusion, neurolytic blockade, and other procedures such as vertebroplasty. Consultation with a pain specialist may help select patients most likely to benefit from one or another of these interventions. One advantage of intraspinal analgesia is that a trial of therapy can be undertaken with minimal risk to the patient. If no benefit is seen with a trial of intraspinal therapy, a more permanent catheter or pump system need not be implanted. The trial is described in more detail later. With the placement of a permanent system, that is, intrathecal pump, deciding on which cancer patients will benefit from such implantation is complex and involves multiple factors.

The role of interventional therapies must be placed in the proper context. In most cases, they cannot be employed as the sole treatment for cancer pain. Spinal analgesia should be used as part of a multimodality approach in treatment of cancer pain.[44–46] As discussed previously, the etiologies of cancer pain are diverse, and nociception is one portion of the constellation of symptoms experienced

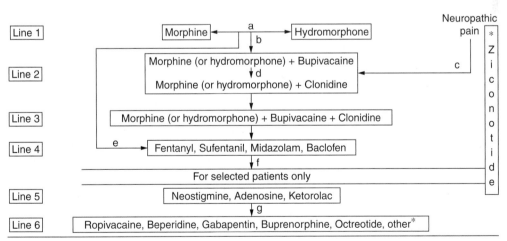

*The specific line to be determined after FDA review.
**Potential spinal analgesics: Methadone, Oxymorphone, NMDA antagonists.
a. If side effects occur, switch to other opioid.
b. If maximum dosage is reached without adequate analgesia, add adjuvant medication (Line 2).
c. If patient has neuropathic pain, consider starting with opioid monotherapy (morphine or hydromorphone) or, in selected patients with pure or predominant neuropathic pain, consider opioid plus adjuvant medication (bupivacaine or clonidine), (Line 2).
d. Some of the panel advocated the use of bupivacaine first because of concern about clonidine-induced hypotension.
e. If side effects or lack of analgesis on second first-line opioid, may switch to fentanyl (Line 4).
f. There are limited preclinical data and limited clinical experience; therefore, caution in the use of these agents should be considered.
g. There are insufficient preclinical data and limited clinical experience; therefore, extreme caution in the use of these agents should be considered.

Figure 17-2 Intrathecal analgesia algorithm. (*From Hassenbusch SJ, Portenoy RK, et al. Polyanalgesic Consensus Conference 2003: an update on the management of pain by intraspinal drug delivery—report of an expert panel. J Pain Symptom Manage. 2004;27(6):540–563.*)

by the cancer patient. Consequently, a comprehensive multidisciplinary approach to treatment of cancer pain is optimal. It includes the appropriate palliative antineoplastic therapy, management of systemic analgesics and adjuvant pain medications, behavioral and psychiatric support and, finally, interventional therapies. In general, interventional pain procedures are not expected to completely eliminate the need for pain medications; rather, the intent is to significantly help alleviate cancer pain, reduce the overall analgesic need, and thereby minimize associated opioid-related side effects.

Communication

Effective communication with the patient's treatment team, including oncologists, primary care providers, and consultants, is important for achieving an optimal outcome. The interventional procedure selected should be coordinated with the overall cancer treatment. For example, the cancer patient may undergo chemotherapy with resultant thrombocytopenia. In such situations, the interventional procedure must be carried out prior to chemoinduction or afterward when the patient's platelet count has normalized. Typically, other members of the patient's healthcare team are informed about the planned interventional procedure and given a chance to participate in the decision and to express any concerns they may have.

Detailed history and physical examination

Taking a thorough patient history and conducting a physical examination, including a complete neurologic evaluation prior to the procedure, is critical. Interventional procedures for pain control generally involve placing needles and/or catheters near tissues, including nerves and eloquent central nervous system structures. The objective of the intervention is to disrupt or modulate nociceptive pathways. Intrathecal infusion of opioids and local anesthetics will not only block pain transmission but at higher doses may also reversibly block sensory and motor function. Consequently, it is important to have a thorough understanding of the patient's neurologic and functional status before and after the procedure. Changes such as sensory and motor blockade are closely monitored after procedures, especially when high doses of local anesthetics are being utilized. The use of high-dose local anesthetics needs to be carefully explained to patients who may otherwise fear that they have become paralyzed if a motor block is induced.

Another important aspect of the preprocedure evaluation is to assess the patient's overall symptom burden and level of psychological distress. If these are very high, the effect of the intervention to decrease nociception may be disappointing in its seeming lack of overall effectiveness.

Delivery of intraspinal analgesics

Intraspinal delivery of opioids and other agents can be achieved by different approaches, including epidural bolus, intermittent intrathecal injection, and continuous epidural and intrathecal infusions. Continuous infusion via either the epidural or intrathecal route requires the use of a catheter system and either external or implantable infusion pumps to deliver the analgesic medications. There is little consensus on when to use the intrathecal versus the epidural route of administration and when to use an implantable versus external pump (Fig. 17-3). With prolonged epidural infusions of greater than 6–9 months, complications with catheter obstruction, fibrosis, and loss of analgesic efficacy have been observed, leading

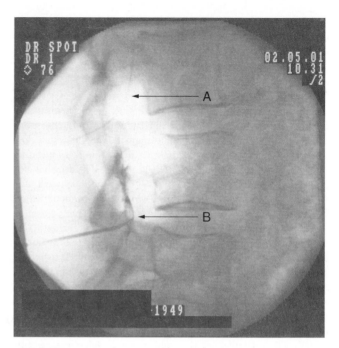

FIGURE 17-3 Intrathecal (A) versus epidural (B) catheter placement. *(Courtesy of A. Burton, M. D. Anderson Cancer Center).*

most clinicians to favor the intrathecal route for long-term intraspinal analgesic infusions.[46,47]

Many factors are considered in the decision to use an external pump system versus an implantable pump. The factors supporting an external system include a short life expectancy (<3 months), the need for frequent patient-controlled doses (such as with severe incident pain), the need for an epidural infusion (which generally requires infusion volumes too great for the implanted pump), the lack of reprogramming/refilling capabilities near the patient's home, payer constraints, as well as the ability of the patient and family to take care of an externalized catheter system.[48–50] We use various catheters for our external systems, including a tunneled Arrow Flex-Tip catheter (Arrow, Inc., Reading, PA), the Du Pen's epidural catheter (Bard Access Systems, Inc., Salt Lake City, UT) , and the Sims epidural portacath (Sims-Deltech, St. Paul, MN) (Fig. 17-3).

Factors supporting the use of an implantable intrathecal pump include a longer life expectancy (>3 months), access to pump refill/reprogramming capabilities, diffuse pain (e.g., widespread metastasis), and a favorable response to an intrathecal trial.[50] The cost of an implanted intrathecal pump has a role in the decision to use it for cancer patients. We recently published our decision-making algorithm (Fig. 17-4). An economic analysis of an implantable versus externalized pumps demonstrated that a 3-month life expectancy is the approximate "break-even" point for the implanted pump to become more cost-effective than the externalized pump system.[51,52]

Implanted infusion pump systems utilize either a fixed (factory preset at 0.5 or 1.0 cc/day) or programmable flow rate. All implantable pumps come with a refillable drug reservoir. In addition, they all have an access port and a side port system that allows for direct injection of a drug into the implanted catheter system. FDA-approved fixed infusion pump systems include Codman's model 400 (Raynham, MA), Medtronic's IsoMed (Minneapolis, MN), and Arrow's M-3000 (Walpole, MA). Changing the dose in a fixed-rate pump requires that the medication concentration be changed, mandating a pump refill each time the dose is adjusted.

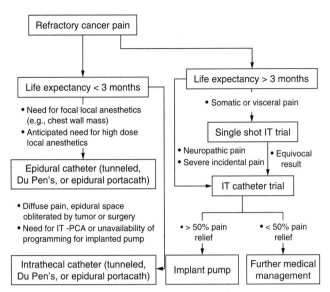

FIGURE 17-4 Decision algorithm for intraspinal therapy. *(Modified from Burton AW, Rajagopal A, Shah HN, et al. Epidural and intrathecal analgesia is effective in treating refractory cancer pain. Pain Med. 2004;5:239.)*

These implantable pumps come with a variety of reservoir volumes (up to 60 cc), which can be selected based on the patient's needs and body habitus.

Medtronic Inc. (Minneapolis, MN) produces Synchromed I and II programmable pumps that can hold up to 20 cc and 40 cc of medication, respectively. They can be programmed to deliver a single bolus, time-specific boluses, or a complex regimen of continuously infused intrathecal analgesic. A function exists for a patient-controlled "demand dose" via a remote control, but this application has not yet been approved for use in the United States. While these fixed rate and programmable pumps can be used to deliver either epidural or intrathecal medications, these pumps are more suited to intrathecal delivery. Epidural infusions usually require a significantly higher daily volume, and thus are typically managed with an external pump system.[50]

▶ Intraspinal analgesic trial

To properly explore the potential value of intraspinal analgesia for a given patient, an intrathecal therapeutic trial must first be undertaken. This trial is instituted to demonstrate the efficacy of intraspinal medication in improving pain control, the patient's level of functioning, and overall quality of life. There is no standard for neuraxial trials, although numerous approaches have been advocated.[40,50,53,54] Patients undergoing catheter-external pump systems do not require a therapeutic trial, as the trial procedure and catheter "implant" procedure are virtually identical. For consideration of intrathecal catheter-pump implantation, our preference is to pursue a single shot (one subarachnoid opioid or opioid/local anesthetic injection) trial in most cases. If the analgesia is equivocal or the patient has a severe incidental pain syndrome, a tunneled intrathecal catheter trial is performed, usually with opioid/local anesthetic or opioid/clonidine in combination. Also, in some cases when we anticipate the need for local anesthetic combination therapy, an intrathecal catheter trial is helpful in adjusting and achieving the right opioid and local anesthetic mix prior to pump implantation. Criteria for a successful intraspinal opioid trial are variable, with

some effective indicators being reduction in pain scores, improvement in function, decreased opioid requirement, as well as a reduction in opioid-related side effects.[50]

▶ Pump implantation surgery

Prior to surgery, the patient is again evaluated for any change in medical as well as neurologic status since the last clinic preoperative visit. Consent must be obtained with all the patient's questions answered. The position of the pump pocket, usually in the subcutaneous tissues of the lower abdominal wall on the right or left side, should also be discussed with the patient and marked prior to the operation. The pump should not be positioned close to prior surgical sites such as colostomy, polyethylene glycol (PEG) tube, or externalized drains.

The patient is then taken back into the operating room. The procedure may be done under general anesthesia or monitored anesthetic care (sedation plus local anesthesia). The entire surgery must be performed under usual surgical aseptic precautions with the use of preoperative prophylactic antibiotics to minimize the chance of perioperative infection. Using fluoroscopic guidance, a spinal catheter is placed up to a specific level for optimal analgesia. Our preference is to place a purse-string of nonabsorbable suture around the catheter in addition to the anchoring device. Next, the pump is implanted in the lower quadrant of the abdomen via an 8-cm incision (Fig. 17-5). A malleable tunneling rod is used to bring a catheter around the flank to connect it to the abdominal pump. The pump is then filled with the appropriate intrathecal medication solution and programmed to prime with the agent to be infused. Once the pump is secure within the pump pocket, both wounds in the back and anterior abdominal sites are copiously irrigated with antibiotic solution. Both incisions are closed using interrupted 3-0 Vicryl sutures to close the subcutaneous fascia. Once the wound edges are approximated, we use either a running 3-0 polydioxanone (PDS) absorbable suture or skin staples for skin closure. This wound is further reinforced with adhesive and Steri-strips. A final dressing is placed over both wound incisions. The patient is observed overnight and released home the next morning. Instructions are given to the patient upon discharge regarding follow-up care, pump refill date, safety precautions, and routine postoperative wound care, including 10 days of oral antibiotics per our preference. The patient

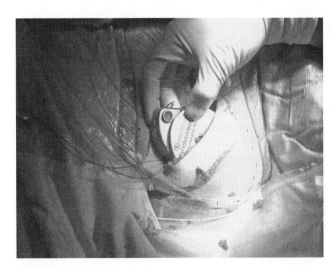

FIGURE 17-5 Surgical placement of the intraspinal infusion pump into the left lower quadrant of the abdomen. *(Courtesy Burton A, M. D. Anderson Cancer Center)*

should be instructed to keep in touch with the clinic in the coming week as we titrate the pump medication regimen for optimal pain control as needed.

▶ Efficacy of intraspinal opioids in cancer pain

Intrathecal delivery of opioids has been shown to reduce pain levels in patients with intractable cancer pain.[47,50,55–59] A review of the literature from 1999 found that intrathecal delivery of morphine by an implanted infusion pump provided "good to excellent" pain relief, accompanied by increased activity and improved quality of life of patients with intractable pain.[59] Furthermore, the results of three recent studies of intrathecal therapy demonstrate the effectiveness of this therapy for managing severe cancer pain.[50,55,56] Two of the studies examined the effectiveness of intrathecal drug delivery systems for managing continuous severe cancer pain.[50,55] The third study examined the effectiveness of intrathecal therapy for episodic or breakthrough pain.[56]

Our group at M. D. Anderson reported our results utilizing intraspinal analgesia in 87 of 4107 evaluated patients using a previously mentioned algorithm.[50] Retrospective evaluation of 8-week follow up revealed improved pain control, decreased oral opioid intake, and decreased drowsiness and mental clouding. This study analyzed the effectiveness of intraspinal analgesia on pain reduction by comparing pain scores, oral opioid intake, and self-reported symptoms before and after the intraspinal intervention. After administration of intraspinal analgesia, either via the epidural or intrathecal route, there was a significant reduction in the proportion of patients in severe pain (with pain score 7–10, Numerical Rating System) from 86% to 17% ($p < 0.001$). The patient numerical pain scores decreased significantly from 7.9 +/− 1.6 to 4.1 +/− 2.3 ($p < 0.001$). Oral opioid intake decreased from a 588 mg/day morphine-equivalent daily dose (MEDD) to 294 mg/day ($p < 0.001$). Self-reported drowsiness and mental clouding (0–10) also significantly decreased from 6.2 +/− 3.0 and 5.4 +/− 3.4 to 3.2 +/− 3.0 and 3.1 +/− 3.0, respectively ($p < 0.001$).

In a prospective, randomized, multicenter clinical trial, an implanted intrathecal drug delivery system was shown to improve pain control, reduce toxicities, and improve survival in cancer patients with refractory pain.[55] At study entry, all patients ($n = 202$) had unrelieved cancer pain, as indicated by their visual analog pain scores of ≥5 on a 0–10 scale. Patients were randomized to receive either morphine via intrathecal delivery and comprehensive medical management per the 1994 AHCPR Cancer Pain Relief guidelines, or comprehensive medical management alone. At week 4 of follow up, 60 (84.5%) of the 71 patients in the intrathecal delivery arm achieved clinical success, as indicated by a ≥20% reduction in visual analog scale pain scores or a ≥20% reduction in toxicity. By contrast, in the comprehensive medical management arm, only 51 (70.8%) of 72 patients achieved clinical success. Mean toxicity scores declined in the intrathecal delivery and comprehensive medical management-only arm by 50% and 17%, respectively ($p = 0.004$). Further, the intrathecal delivery group had significant reduction in fatigue and depressed level of consciousness ($p < 0.05$). A slightly greater improvement in 6-month survival was seen in the intrathecal delivery group compared to medical management-only group (53.9% vs. 37.2%, $p = 0.06$). It is, however, worth nothing that new medical management techniques such as opioid rotation have not yet been compared to the use of implantable drug delivery systems.

In a third study, Rauck et al. evaluated intrathecal drug delivery systems for the management of episodic or breakthrough pain in a prospective, open-label study.[56] In this study of 119 cancer patients

with refractory cancer pain and/or uncontrollable side effects, the best analgesia was achieved when the patients managed their pain with an implantable, patient-controlled intrathecal drug delivery system. Such a system allowed patients to self-administer a bolus dose of morphine sulfate on demand. Results of the study showed that the mean numerical analog pain score significantly decreased from 6.1 to 4.2 at month 1 ($p < 0.01$, $n = 99$), and was maintained through month 7 ($p < 0.01$, $n = 14$) and month 13 ($p < 0.05$, $n = 10$). In addition, the MEDD was significantly reduced throughout the study ($p < 0.01$). Overall success (≥50% reduction in numeric analog pain score, system opioid use, or severity of opioid side effects) was reported in 83% of patients at month 1 and in 91% of patients at month 4.

Clearly, intraspinal analgesic therapy is one effective option for pain control in cancer patients with difficult to control refractory pain or with refractory opioid side effects.

▶ Complications

Complications of intraspinal analgesia fall into two broad categories: device-related or drug-related. Device-related complications include wound infection, catheter breakage/migration, and catheter tip granuloma. There is a growing body of literature about sterile granuloma formation at the catheter tip, which is being increasingly reported. The consensus is that this is related to highly concentrated medications, especially morphine, and the index of suspicion should be high in patients with a new pain in their back, prompting magnetic resonance imaging (MRI) evaluation and appropriate management.[60]

Drug-related complications include dosing/programming errors, misfiring, and the spectrum of opioid-related side effects, including nausea, sedation, urinary retention, pruritus, and respiratory depression. These side effects are minimized through patient monitoring and careful dose adjustments, and double-checking device programming prior to the patient's departure from the clinic. In general, in a stable patient who begins to have side effects shortly after pump refill, the programming should be promptly double-checked and drug changed if needed.

In cases of suspected pump malfunction, a plain radiograph should be ordered to check catheter patency. Next, a dye study with injection of contrast via the side port may reveal catheter malposition or disruption. Pump battery life is approximately 5 years, with the more recent devices lasting longer than older devices. Algorithms for device assessment have been published and if the practitioner is in doubt, the pump manufacturer should be consulted.[61] Implanted pumps have a wound infection rate of less than 5%, although an infection may lead to pump explant and local treatment. Leaving the pump in place has been advocated in some cases.[62] Rare, but serious infections reinforce the need for strict asepsis both at implant and with pump refill.

CONCLUSION

Cancer pain management is a complicated challenge. It requires a thorough understanding of the cancer disease process, the pain diagnosis, and the treatment modalities available to treat the painful condition. In addition to pain, the patient often presents with a constellation of symptoms arising from his or her cancer and the oncologic treatment. Full utilization of all available treatment modalities should help to optimize the patient's pain control and quality of life. In selected cases, neuraxial intervention via an epidural or intrathecal delivery system can help the physician and patient achieve effective control of cancer pain, minimize opioid-related side effects, and thereby optimize quality of life. In the modern era, palliative care can and should utilize these modalities to become both "high-touch" and "high-tech," which need not be mutually exclusive concepts in the care of the cancer patient.

REFERENCES

1. World Health Organization. *Cancer Pain Relief and Palliative Care.* 2nd ed. Geneva: World Health Organization; 1996:12–15.
2. Lesage P, Portenoy RK. Trends in cancer pain management. *Cancer Control.* 1999;6:136–145.
3. Miguel R. Interventional treatment of cancer pain: the fourth step in the WHO analgesic ladder? *Cancer Control.* 2000;7:149–156.
4. Krames ES. Interventional pain management: appropriate when less invasive therapies fail to provide adequate analgesia. *Med Clin North Am.* 1999;83:787–808.
5. Waldman SD. The role of spinal opioids in the management of cancer pain. *J Pain Symptom Manage.* 1990;5:163.
6. Ventafridda V, Spoldi E, Caraceni A, et al. Intrathecal morphine for cancer pain. *Acta Anaesthesiol Scand Suppl.* 1987;85:47–53.
7. Chaney MA. Side effects of intraspinal and epidural opioids. *Can J Anaesth.* 1995;42:891–903.
8. Saeki S, Yaksh TL. Suppression of nociceptive responses by spinal mu agonists: effects of stimulus intensity and agonist efficacy. *Anesth Analg.* 1993;77:265.
9. Yaksh TL. Spinal opiates: a review of their effect on spinal function with an emphasis on pain processing. *Acta Anaesthesiol Scand.* 1987;31:25.
10. Sosnowski M, Yaksh TL. Spinal administration of receptor-selective drugs as analgesics: new horizons. *J Pain Symptom Manage.* 1990;5:204.
11. Yaksh TL, Noueihed R. The physiology and pharmacology of spinal opiates. *Annu Rev Pharmacol Toxicol.* 1985;25:433.
12. Zieglgansberger W. Opiate actions on mammalian spinal neurons. *Int Rev Neurobiol.* 1984;25:243.
13. Coda BA, Brown MC, Schaffer R, et al. Pharmacology of epidural fentanyl, alfentanil, and sufentanil in volunteers. *Anesthesiology.* 1994;81:1149–1161.
14. Jacobson L, Chabal C, Brody MC, et al. Intrathecal methadone: a dose-response study and comparison with intrathecal morphine 0.5 mg. *Pain.* 1990;43:141–148.
15. Hassenbusch SJ, Portenoy RK, Cousins M, et al. Polyanalgesic Consensus Conference 2003: an update on the management of pain by intraspinal drug delivery—report of an expert panel. *J Pain Symptom Manage.* 2004;27:540–563.
16. Payne RM. CSF distribution of opioids in animals and man. *Acta Anaesthesiol Scand Suppl.* 1987;31:38.
17. Cousins MJ, Mather LE. Intrathecal and epidural administration of opioids. *Anesthesiology.* 1984;6:276.
18. Max MB, Inturrisi CE, Kaiko RF, et al. Epidural and intrathecal opiates: CSF and plasma profiles in patients with chronic cancer pain. *Clin Pharmacol Ther.* 1985;38:631.
19. Gourlay CK, Cherry DA, Cousins MJ. Cephalad migration of morphine in CSF following lumbar epidural administration in patients with cancer pain. *Pain.* 1985;23:317.
20. Miguel R, Barlow I, Morrell M, et al. A prospective, randomized double-blind comparison of epidural and intravenous sufentanil infusions. *Anesthesiology.* 1994;81:346–352.
21. Sullivan AF, Dashwood MR, Dickenson AH. Alpha-2 adrenoreceptor modulation of nociceptor in rat spinal cord: location, effects, and interactions with morphine. *Eur J Pharmacol.* 1987;138:169–177.
22. Yaksh TL. Pharmacology of spinal adrenergic systems which modulate spinal nociceptive processing. *Pharmacol Biochem Behav.* 1985;22:845–858.
23. Ono H, Mishima A, Ono S, et al. Inhibitory effects of clonidine and tizanidine on release of substance P from slices of rat spinal cord and antagonism by alpha-adrenergic receptor antagonists. *Neuropharmacology.* 1991;30:585–589.
24. Segal IS, Jarvis DJ, Duncan SR, et al. Clinical efficacy of oral-transdermal clonidine combinations during the perioperative period. *Anesthesiology.* 1991;74:220–225.
25. Jarrott B, Conway EL, Maccarrone C, et al. Clonidine: understanding its disposition, sites, and mechanism of action. *Clin Exp Pharmacol Physiol* 1987;14:471–479.
26. Filos KS, Goudas LC, Patroni O, et al. Hemodynamic and analgesic profile after intrathecal clonidine in humans. A dose-response study. *Anesthesiology.* 1994;81:591–601.
27. Eisenach JC, DuPen S, Dubois M, et al. Epidural clonidine analgesia for intractable cancer pain. The Epidural Clonidine Study Group. *Pain.* 1995;61:391–399.
28. Hassenbusch SJ, Gunes S, Wachsman S, et al. Intrathecal clonidine in the treatment of intractable pain: a phase I/II study. *Pain Med.* 2002;3:85–91.
29. Coombs DW, Saunders RL, Fratkin JD, et al. Continuous intrathecal hydromorphone and clonidine for intractable cancer pain. *J Neurosurg.* 1986;64:890–894.
30. Eisenach JC, Tong CY. Site of hemodynamic effects of intrathecal alpha 2-adrenergic agonists. *Anesthesiology.* 1991;74:766–771.
31. Deer TR, Caraway DL, Kim CK, et al. Clinical experience with intrathecal bupivacaine in combination with opioid for the treatment of chronic pain related to failed back surgery syndrome and metastatic cancer pain of the spine. *Spine J.* 2002;2:274–278.
32. Walker SM, Goudas LC, Cousins MJ, et al. Combination spinal analgesic chemotherapy: a systematic review. *Anesth Analg.* 2002;95:674–715.
33. Buchser E, Durrer A, Chedel D, et al. Efficacy of intrathecal bupivacaine: how important is the flow rate? *Pain Med.* 2004;5:248–252.
34. Staats PS, Yearwood T, Charapata SG, et al. Intrathecal ziconotide in treatment of refractory pain in patients with cancer or AIDS: a randomized controlled trial. *JAMA.* 2004;291:63–70.
35. Almeida RA, Lauretti GR, Mattos AL. Antinociceptive effect of low-dose intrathecal neostigmine combined with intrathecal morphine following gynecologic surgery. *Anesthesiology.* 2003;98:495–498.
36. Grant GJ, Piskoun B, Bansinath M. Intrathecal administration of liposomal neostigmine prolongs analgesia in mice. *Acta Anaesthesiol Scand.* 2002;46:90–94.
37. Naguib M, Yaksh TL. Antinociceptive effects of spinal cholinesterase inhibition and isobolographic analysis of the interaction with mu and alpha 2 receptor systems. *Anesthesiology.* 1994;80:1338–1348.
38. Hood DD, Eisenach JC, Tuttle R. Phase I safety assessment of intrathecal neostigmine methylsulfate in humans. *Anesthesiology.* 1995;82:331–345.
39. Bennett G, Burchiel K, Buchser E, et al. Clinical guidelines for intraspinal infusion: report of an expert panel. PolyAnalgesic Consensus Conference 2000. *J Pain Symptom Manage.* 2000;20:S37–S43.
40. Smith TJ, Coyne PJ. How to use implantable intrathecal drug delivery systems for refractory chronic cancer pain. *J Support Oncol.* 2003;1:73–76.
41. Kedlaya D, Reynolds L, Waldman S. Epidural and intrathecal analgesia for cancer pain. *Best Pract Res Clin Anaesthesiol.* 2002;16:651–655.
42. Krames E. Implantable devices for pain control: spinal cord stimulation and intrathecal therapies. *Best Pract Res Clin Anaesthesiol.* 2002;16:619–649.
43. Gallagher RM. Epidural and intrathecal cancer pain management: prescriptive care for quality of life. *Pain Med.* 2004;5:235.
44. Lubenow TR, Ivankovich AD. Intraspinal narcotics for treatment of cancer pain. *Semin Surg Oncol.* 1990;6:173.
45. Practice guidelines for cancer pain management. A report by the American Society of Anesthesiologists Task Force on Pain Management, Cancer Pain Section. *Anesthesiology.* 1996;84:1243–1257.
46. Patt RB, Jain S. Therapeutic decision-making for invasive procedures. In: Patt RB, ed. *Cancer Pain.* Philadelphia: Lippincott; 1993:275–283.
47. Crul BJ, Delhaas EM. Technical complications during long-term subarachnoid or epidural administration of morphine in terminally ill cancer patients: a review of 140 cases. *Reg Anesth.* 1991;16:209–213.
48. Exner HJ, Peters J, Eikermann M. Epidural analgesia at the end of life: facing empirical contraindications. *Anesth Analg.* 2003;97:1740–1742.
49. Mercadante S. Epidural treatment in advanced cancer patients (letter). *Anesth Analg.* 2004;98:1503.
50. Burton AW, Rajagopal A, Shah HN, et al. Epidural and intrathecal analgesia is effective in treating refractory cancer pain. *Pain Med.* 2004;5:239.
51. Bedder MD, Burchiel K, Larson A. Cost analysis of two narcotic delivery systems. *J Pain Symptom Manage.* 1991;6:368.
52. Hassenbusch SJ. Cost modeling for alternative routes of administration of opioids for cancer pain. *Oncology.* 1999;13:63–67.

53. Burton AW, Hassenbusch SJ. The double catheter technique for intrathecal medication trial: a brief clinical note and report of five cases. *Pain Med.* 2001;2:352–354.

54. Krames ES. Intraspinal opioid therapy for chronic nonmalignant pain: current practice and clinical guidelines. *J Pain Symptom Manage.* 1996; 11:333–352.

55. Smith TJ, Staats P, Deer T, et al. Randomized clinical trial of an implantable drug delivery system compared with comprehensive medical management for refractory cancer pain: impact on pain, drug-related toxicity, and survival. *J Clin Oncol.* 2002;20:4040–4049.

56. Rauck RL, Cherry D, Boyer MF, et al. Long-term intrathecal opioid therapy with a patient-activated, implanted delivery system for the treatment of refractory cancer pain. *J Pain.* 2003;4:441–447.

57. Hassenbusch SJ, Pillay PK, Magdinec M, et al. Constant infusion of morphine for intractable cancer pain using implanted pump. *J Neurosurg.* 1990;73:405–409.

58. Krames ES, Gershow J, Glassberg A, et al. Continuous infusion of spinally administered narcotics for the relief of pain due to malignant disorders. *Cancer.* 1985;56:696–702.

59. Gilmer-Hill HS, Boggan JE, Smith KA, et al. Intrathecal morphine delivered via subcutaneous pump for intractable cancer pain: a review of the literature. *Surg Neurol.* 1999;51:12–15.

60. Follett KA. Intrathecal analgesia and catheter-tip inflammatory masses. *Anesthesiology.* 2003;99:5–6.

61. Burton AW, Conroy B, Garcia E, et al. Illicit substance abuse via an implanted intrathecal pump. *Anesthesiology.* 1998;89:1264–1267.

62. Boviatsis EJ, Kouyialis AT, Boutsikakis I, et al. Infected CNS infusion pumps. Is there a chance for treatment without removal? *Acta Neurochir (Wien).* 2004;146:463–467.

Nerve Blocks and Related Procedural Pain Management Techniques

CHAPTER 18

Fayez Kotob
Óscar A. de Leon-Casasola

BACKGROUND

Pain produced by cancer growth may be somatic, visceral, or neuropathic in origin. History, physical examination, and dedicated radiologic studies have proven to be successful in determining the origin of the pain and helpful in determining the type of pain component(s) that the patient is experiencing. Therefore, oral, transdermal, or transmucosal pharmacologic therapy with opioids, and adjuvant therapy, including anticonvulsants, oral local anesthetics, tricyclic antidepressants, steroids, and others can be tailored to the types of pain the patient is experiencing. Adequate pain control is experienced by 80%–90% of patients treated with these regimens.[1] To be effective, this therapy is conducted by applying aggressive guidelines over time.[1] However, for the remaining 10%–20% of patients, an alternative approach is needed, which is usually invasive.[2] Patients who experience severe side effects from opioid and/or adjuvant medications are also candidates for invasive therapy. Longterm epidural or subarachnoid techniques have been used with success in these patients.[2] Various modes of administration and drug combinations are available. Although controlled trials of these interventions have been scarce, anecdotal experience from around the world along with recent consensus relating to treatment approaches serve to guide pain clinicians toward potentially successful approaches that may be followed to obtain adequate pain relief.[3]

At the other end of the spectrum are patients with early stage abdominal cancer who experience considerable visceral pain. These include patients with pancreatic cancer without evidence of metastasis outside the pancreas, and those with cervical or endometrial cancer without invasion of the parametrium. Neurolysis of the sympathetic axis in the form of celiac plexus blocks, splanchnic nerve blocks, or superior hypogastric plexus blocks has proven efficacy for managing visceral pain in this patient population.

Another invasive technique that may be useful for patients with cancer-related pain is epidural steroid injections for neuropathic pain. Neuraxial steroid injections can assist in decreasing the severity of neuropathic pain, giving the practitioner a window in which adjuvant analgesics can be titrated over a period of 4–6 weeks without compromising the quality of analgesia and exacerbating psychosocial issues in these patients.

Approximately 10% of patients with cancer also experience pain that is unrelated to tumor growth.[4] In addition to pharmacologic therapy and counseling if needed, procedural approaches can be useful in treating the pain condition, with the same indications as in the general population. These approaches include trigger point injections, peripheral nerve blocks, interlaminar/transforaminal epidural steroid injections, sympathetic chain blocks, and others.

This chapter discusses the indications, applications, success rate, and complications associated with some of these procedures (Table 18-1).

NEUROLYSIS OF THE SYMPATHETIC AXIS

Stretching, compressing, invading, or distending visceral structures can result in poorly localized noxious, visceral pain. Such pain is often described as vague, deep, squeezing, crampy, or colicky. Other indicators include referred pain (e.g., shoulder pain that appears when the diaphragm is invaded with tumor) and nausea/vomiting due to vagal irritation.

Visceral pain associated with cancer may be relieved with oral pharmacologic therapy that includes combinations of nonsteroidal anti-inflammatory drugs (NSAIDs), including nonspecific and COX-2 inhibitors, opioids, and adjuvant medications. Neurolytic blocks of the sympathetic axis are also effective in controlling visceral cancer pain and should be considered as important adjuncts to pharmacologic therapy to relieve severe cancer pain. However, these blocks rarely eliminate cancer pain because patients frequently experience coexisting somatic and neuropathic pain. Therefore, oral pharmacologic therapy must be continued, albeit at lower doses. The goals of performing a neurolytic block of the sympathetic axis are to maximize the analgesic effects of opioid or nonopioid analgesics and to reduce the dosage of these agents to alleviate side effects.

Because neurolysis techniques have a narrow risk-benefit ratio, undesirable effects due to neurolytic blocks can be minimized by using sound clinical judgment and assessing the probable effect of the technique on each patient. A detailed description of the techniques used for these blocks is beyond the scope of this review but is available elsewhere.[5] This chapter describes several different approaches that can be used to achieve neurolysis, including the celiac plexus block, superior hypogastric block, and ganglion impar block.

▶ Celiac plexus block

The celiac plexus is situated retroperitoneally in the upper abdomen at the level of the T_{12} and L_1 vertebrae, anterior to the crura of the diaphragm. The celiac plexus surrounds the abdominal aorta and the celiac and superior mesenteric arteries. The plexus is composed of a network of nerve fibers, from both the sympathetic and the parasympathetic systems. It contains two large ganglia that receive

Table 18-1

Clinical Application of Interventional Blocks for Cancer Pain Management

Indications and Contraindications of Interventional Procedures for the Treatment of Cancer Pain

Indications	Contraindications
Intractable pain	Irreversible coagulopathy
Refractory pain to optimized conventional therapy	Generalized infection
	Local infection at the block site
Beyond reasonable adverse effects. Caused by pharmacologic treatment	Reduced mental status
	Patient refusal
Fast pain relief is desired	
Block as a mean to treat opioid side effect (celiac block to resolve constipation)	
Rib lesion and rib pathologic fracture	
Perioperative analgesia (including preemptive)	

used with significant success in patients with acute or chronic pancreatitis.[6] Likewise, patients with cancer in the upper abdomen who have a significant visceral pain component have responded well to this block.[7]

Three approaches used to block nociceptive impulses from the upper abdominal viscera include the retrocrural (or classic) approach, the anterocrural approach, and neurolysis of the splanchnic nerves. For all of these approaches, the needles are inserted at the level of the first lumbar vertebra, 5–7 cm from the midline. The tip of the needle is then directed toward the body of L_1 for the retrocrural and anterocrural approaches and to the body of T_{12} for neurolysis of the splanchnic nerves. More recently, computed tomography (CT) and endoscopic ultrasound (EUS) guidance techniques have allowed pain specialists to perform neurolysis of the celiac plexus via a transabdominal approach. This approach is frequently used when patients are unable to tolerate either the prone or lateral decubitus position or when their liver is so enlarged that a posterior approach is not feasible. There is accumulating evidence that EUS-guided celiac neurolytic blockade has a superior analgesic outcome compared to CT-guided celiac block, with less of an incidence of adverse effects.[8,9]

Drugs and dosing

For neurolytic blocks, 50%–100% alcohol, 20 mL per side, is used. Injected by itself, alcohol can produce severe pain. Thus, it is recommended to first inject 5–10 mL of 0.25% bupivacaine 5 minutes prior to the injection of alcohol or to dilute 100% alcohol by 50% with local anesthetic (0.25% bupivacaine). Phenol in a 10% final concentration may also be used; this has the advantage of being painless on injection. Both agents seem to have the same efficacy.

sympathetic fibers from the three splanchnic nerves (greater, lesser, and least). The plexus also receives parasympathetic fibers from the vagus nerve. Autonomic nerves supplying the liver, pancreas, gallbladder, stomach, spleen, kidneys, intestines, and adrenal glands, as well as blood vessels, arise in the celiac plexus (Fig. 18-1).

Neurolytic blocks of the celiac plexus are used to treat malignant and chronic nonmalignant pain. The celiac plexus block has been

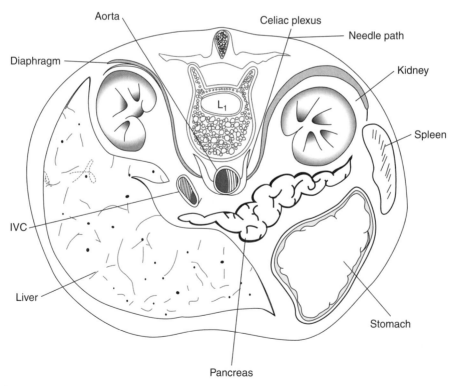

FIGURE 18-1 Topographic landmarks of celiac block.

Complications

Complications associated with celiac plexus blocks are related to the technique used: retrocrural,[6] transcrural,[7] or transaortic.[10] In a prospective, randomized study of 61 patients with cancer of the pancreas, Ischia et al. compared the efficacy and incidence of complications associated with these three approaches to celiac plexus neurolysis.[11] Orthostatic hypotension occurred more often with the retrocrural (50%) or splanchnic (52%) approach compared to the anterocrural approach (10%). In contrast, transient diarrhea was more frequent with the anterocrural approach (65%) than with the splanchnic nerve block technique (5%), but not the retrocrural approach (25%). The incidence of dysesthesia, interscapular back pain, reactive pleurisy, hiccups, or hematuria was not statistically different among the three groups.

The incidence of complications from neurolytic celiac plexus blocks was recently determined by Davis in 2730 patients having blocks performed from 1986 to 1990.[12] The overall incidence of major complications (e.g., paraplegia, bladder, and bowel dysfunction) was 1 in 683 procedures. However, the report does not describe which approach or approaches were used to perform the blocks.

The following are some of the essential aspects in the diagnosis and management of specific complications:

Malposition of the needle is avoided when radiologic imaging precedes the injection of a neurolytic agent, as the tip of the needle may be intravascular, in the peritoneal cavity, or in a viscus. Imaging techniques currently used include biplanar fluoroscopy, CT, or ultrasound guidance. However, no study has evaluated the superiority of one technique over the others. Wong and Brown suggest that the use of radiologic imaging does not alter the quality of the block or the incidence of complications. Their conclusions were drawn from a retrospective study of 136 patients with pancreatic cancer pain treated with a celiac plexus block with or without radiologic control of the needle tip location.[13] It is not, however, clear how many of those patients had radiologic imaging. Assuming that 50% of the patients did not, then the upper 95% confidence limit for complications is 5%.[14]

Orthostatic hypotension can occur up to 5 days after the block in 1%–3% of patients. Treatment includes resting in bed, avoiding sudden changes in position, and replacing fluids. Once compensatory vascular reflexes are fully activated, this side effect disappears. Wrapping the lower extremities from the toes to the upper thighs with elastic bandages has been successful in patients who developed orthostatic hypotension, and thus needed to walk during the first week after the block.

Backache may result from local trauma during needle placement resulting in a retroperitoneal hematoma, from alcohol irritation of the retroperitoneal structures, or from injury to the lumbar plexus. Patients with a backache should have at least two hematocrit measurements with a 1-hour interval. If there is a decrease in the hematocrit, radiologic imaging is indicated to rule out a retroperitoneal hematoma. A urine analysis positive for red blood cells suggests renal injury.

Retroperitoneal hemorrhage is rare; however, in patients who present with orthostatic hypotension, the possibility of hemorrhage must be ruled out before assuming that it is a physiologic response to the block. Patients who present with backache and orthostatic hypotension after a celiac plexus block should be admitted to the hospital for serial hematocrit monitoring. If the hematocrit level is low or decreasing, patients should undergo radiologic evaluation to rule out injury to the kidneys, aorta, or other vascular structures. A surgical consult should be obtained as soon as feasible.

Diarrhea may occur due to the sympathetic block of the bowel. Treatment includes hydration and antidiarrheal agents. Oral loperamide is a good choice, although any anticholinergic agent can be used. Matson and colleagues reported near-fatal dehydration from diarrhea following this block.[15] In debilitated patients, diarrhea must be treated aggressively.

Abdominal aortic dissection has also been reported.[16,17] The mechanism of aortic injury is direct damage with the needle while the block is being administered. As expected, the anterocrural approach is more frequently associated with this complication. This approach should be avoided if atherosclerotic disease of the abdominal aorta is present.

Paraplegia and *transient motor paralysis* have occurred after a celiac plexus block.[17–23] These neurologic complications may occur due to a spasm of the lumbar segmental arteries that perfuse the spinal cord.[24] In fact, canine lumbar arteries undergo contraction when exposed to low concentrations of alcohol.[25] Empirical data suggest that alcohol should not be used if there is evidence of significant atherosclerotic disease of the aorta, suggesting that the circulation to the spinal cord may also be impaired. However, a report of paraplegia after phenol use[18] suggests that factors such as direct vascular injury, neurologic injury, or retrograde spread to the spinal cord may come into play. These complications further support the use of radiologic imaging when the block is administered.

Efficacy

To date, three randomized,[11,26,27] controlled trials and one prospective study[28] have evaluated the efficacy of celiac plexus neurolysis for pain due to cancer of the upper abdomen. In a prospective, randomized study, Ischia et al. looked at the efficacy of three different approaches to celiac plexus neurolysis in pancreatic cancer.[11] Of 61 patients with pancreatic cancer pain, 29 (48%) experienced *complete* pain relief after the neurolytic block. The remaining 32 patients (52%) required further therapy for residual visceral pain due to technical failure in 15 patients and neuropathic/somatic pains in 17 patients. The second trial,[26] which compared the procedure with oral pharmacologic therapy in 20 patients, concluded that celiac plexus neurolysis resulted in an equal reduction in visual analog pain score (VAPS) as therapy with a combination of NSAIDs and opioids. However, opioid consumption was significantly lower in the group of patients who underwent neurolysis compared to the group receiving oral pharmacologic therapy during the 7 weeks of the study. Moreover, the incidence of side effects was greater in patients who received oral pharmacologic therapy compared to those who had a neurolysis block.

Wong and collaborators[29] recently published the results of their controlled, randomized study. Their results are welcome in light of a lack of sufficient, properly designed comparative studies between neurolytic techniques and comprehensive medical management (CMM). Their conclusions are encouraging. However, several issues need to be considered:

1. Patients enrolled in the study did not have severe pain at study entry. Mean pain scores at baseline were 4.4 ± 1.7 in the neurolytic celiac plexus block (NCPB) group and 4.1 ± 1.8 in the CMM group. This is a surprising finding in patients with this type

of malignancy, and may reflect ethnic and racial differences in pain perception and reporting by the population enrolled in the study.

2. Although the authors reported a significant reduction in pain scores 1 week after therapy when comparing the NCPB group to the CMM group, the difference between the two groups may not be clinically important. Patients assigned to the NCPB group reported mean pain scores of 2.1 ± 1.4, whereas those randomized to the CMM group reported pain scores of 2.7 ± 2.1 in the same time interval. Moreover, the statistical difference was found when the percentage of reduction from baseline for the NCPB and the CMM group was analyzed separately (53% reduction from baseline for the NCPB group, $p = 0.05$ versus the 27% reduction observed in the CMM group, $p = 0.01$). It is not clear whether the difference between the two groups is statistically significant.

3. In analyzing these results, I also believe that it is important to note that most patients (93%) used opiates during the first week of therapy with similar amounts of opiates being administered to the two treatment groups. In fact, opiate consumption increased with time during the study, with no differences between groups at the different time intervals. Moreover, the incidence of side effects was not different between the two treatment groups at any point in time.

4. Likewise, quality of life (QOL) measurements and the physical and functional well-being subscales of the FACT-PA did not differ between groups at any evaluation point.

Two important questions stem from these results: (1) Can the authors truly conclude that the major finding of the study was that NCPB significantly improves pain relief in patients with advanced pancreatic cancer compared with those who received optimized CMM? (2) Based on these results, are we justified to submit a patient with advanced pancreatic cancer to a NCPB considering the potential side effects and complications associated with this procedure?

As with every study, it is important to recognize that these results only apply to the population studied, under the conditions of a particular study protocol design. The critical issue here is that *all* patients had nonresectable disease due to extrapancreatic metastasis, which suggests that patients were likely to have other pain components, such as somatic and/or neuropathic, that are not responsive to a NCPB.[3] This is because neurolytic blocks of the sympathetic axis are effective in treating visceral pain only. Moreover, previous studies have suggested that when there is evidence of disease outside of the pancreas, such as celiac and/or portal adenopathy, the success rate of this block decreases significantly.[30] In the study by De Cicco and collaborators, long-lasting pain relief was described in 9/9 patients (95% confidence interval of 60–100) when contrast medium spread in the four quadrants and in 10/21 patients (95% confidence interval of 26–70) when contrast spread in three quadrants. None of the 75 patients with contrast spread in two or one quadrant experienced long-lasting pain relief.[30] Thus, the presence of adenopathy due to metastasis is a poor prognostic factor to success of the block. The results of the study by Wong and collaborators further support the notion that NCPB should *not be* performed in patients with advanced *unresectable* carcinomas of the pancreas or in those with evidence of disease in the locoregional lymph nodes. This block should be reserved for patients without evidence of extravisceral disease, in whom there is a guarantee that there is only a visceral pain component.

A prospective, nonrandomized study compared 41 patients treated according to the World Health Organization guidelines for cancer pain relief with 21 patients treated with a neurolytic celiac plexus block.[28] The authors concluded that this technique can play an important role in managing pancreatic cancer pain.

Since one of the three studies that used a randomized, controlled design compared different approaches to the celiac plexus one and had no control group,[11] and the other study compared the procedure with an analgesic drug,[26] it is not possible to estimate the success rate of this technique from the literature. In contrast, the results of a meta-analysis that evaluated the results of 21 *retrospective* studies in 1145 patients concluded that adequate to excellent pain relief can be achieved in 89% of patients during the first 2 weeks after the block.[31] Partial to complete pain relief continued in approximately 90% of the patients who were alive after 3 months and in 70%–90% of patients during the 3-month interval before death. Moreover, the efficacy was similar in patients with pancreatic cancer as in those with other intra-abdominal malignancies of the upper abdomen. However, these results are based on *retrospective* evaluations that may not yield reliable information or may be subject to publication bias. In addition, diverse statistical techniques used for the analysis must account for the heterogeneity produced by the patients' selection criteria, technical differences in the performance of the blocks, choice of neurolytic agents and doses, diversity in the tools for the evaluation of pain, and goals of therapy. Thus, the meta-analysis must be interpreted with caution as the reports may be overly enthusiastic.

New perspectives

As previously discussed, oral pharmacologic therapy with opioids, NSAIDs, and adjuvant analgesics is frequently used to treat cancer pain. However, evidence suggests that chronic use of high doses of opioids may have a negative effect on immunity.[32] Thus, analgesic techniques that lower opioid consumption may have a positive effect on patient outcomes. Lillemoe and colleagues showed in a prospective, randomized trial that patients with nonresectable cancer of the pancreas who received splanchnic neurolysis lived longer than patients who did not.[33] These findings may be the result of lower opioid use in the neurolysis patients who not only had better-preserved immune functions, but also experienced fewer side effects (e.g., nausea and vomiting), thus allowing them to eat better. Unfortunately, the study by Wong et al. contradicts these findings as patients randomized to the neurolytic block did not have a prolonged survival rate.[29] As noted, this may be because patients in both groups consumed the same amount of opiates, thus negating the potential beneficial effect of the block.

▶ Superior hypogastric plexus block

Cancer patients with tumor extension into the pelvis may experience severe pain that is unresponsive to oral or parenteral opioids. In addition, excessive sedation or other side effects may limit the acceptability and utility of oral opioid therapy. A more invasive approach is needed to control pain and improve the quality of life of these patients.

Pelvic pain associated with cancer and chronic nonmalignant conditions may be alleviated by blocking the superior hypogastric plexus.[34–36] Analgesia to the organs in the pelvis is possible because the afferent fibers innervating these structures travel in the sympathetic nerves, trunks, ganglia, and rami. Thus, a sympathectomy for visceral pain is analogous to a peripheral neurectomy or dorsal rhizotomy for somatic pain. In a study conducted at Roswell Park Cancer Institute in 1993, it was suggested that visceral pain is an important component of the cancer pain syndrome experienced by patients with cancer of the pelvis, even in advanced stages.[35] Therefore, percutaneous neurolytic blocks of the superior hypogastric plexus should be considered more frequently as an option for patients with advanced stages of pelvic cancer.

The superior hypogastric plexus is situated in the retroperitoneum, bilaterally extending from the lower third of the fifth lumbar vertebral body to the upper third of the first sacral vertebral body. The technique for the blockade has been described elsewhere.[34–36]

Complications

The combined experience of more than 200 cases at the Mexican Institute of Cancer, Roswell Park Cancer Institute, and M. D. Anderson Cancer Center indicates that neurologic complications do not occur as a result of this block.[36]

Efficacy

The effectiveness of the block was originally demonstrated by documenting a significant decrease in pain via VAPS. In this study, Plancarte et al. showed that this block was effective in reducing VAPS scores in 70% of patients suffering from cancer-related pelvic pain.[34] The majority of the enrolled patients had cervical cancer. In a subsequent study, 69% of the patients had decreased VAPS scores. Moreover, a mean daily opioid morphine reduction of 67% was seen in the success group (736 ± 633 reduced to 251 ± 191 mg/day), and 45% in the failure group (1443 ± 703 reduced to 800 ± 345 mg/day).[35] In a more recent multicentric study, 159 patients with pelvic pain associated with cancer were evaluated. Overall, 115 patients (72%) had satisfactory pain relief after one or two neurolytic procedures. Mean opioid use decreased by 40% from 58 ± 43 to 35 ± 18 equianalgesic mg/day of morphine 3 weeks after treatment in all patients studied. This decrease in opioid consumption was significant for both the success group (56 ± 32 reduced to 32 ± 16 mg/day) and the failure group (65 ± 28 reduced to 48 ± 21 mg/day.[36] Success was defined in these two studies as the ability to reduce opioid consumption by at least 50% in the 3 weeks following the block and a decrease in pain scores below 4/10 using a VAPS system.[35,36]

In a recent case report, Rosenberg and colleagues reported on the efficacy of this block in a patient with severe chronic nonmalignant penile pain after transurethral resection of the prostate.[37] Although the patient did not receive a neurolytic agent, a diagnostic block performed with 0.25% bupivacaine and 20 mg of methylprednisolone acetate was effective in relieving the patient's pain for more than 6 months. The usefulness of this block in chronic benign pain conditions has, however, not been adequately documented.

Ganglion impar block

The ganglion impar is a solitary retroperitoneal structure located at the level of the sacrococcygeal junction. This unpaired ganglion marks the end of two sympathetic chains. Visceral pain in the perineal area associated with malignancies may be effectively treated with neurolysis of the ganglion impar (Walther's).[38] Patients who will benefit from this block frequently present with a vague, poorly localized pain that is frequently accompanied by sensations of burning and urgency. However, the clinical value of this block is not clear as the published experienced with it is limited.

This block may be performed with the patient in the left lateral decubitus position with the knees flexed, in the lithotomy position, or in the prone position. The easiest approach is with the patient in the prone position, where a 20-g 1.5-inch needle is inserted through the sacrococcygeal ligament in the midline. The needle is then advanced until the tip is placed posterior to the rectum.

No complications have been reported with this block.

MORE PERIPHERAL BLOCKS

▶ Trigger point injections

Therapeutic injections of local anesthetics, with or without corticosteroid, into trigger points, which are subcutaneous foci of localized muscle spasm, may provide lasting relief of myofascial pain.[39] This bedside procedure is particularly useful when muscle spasms arise as a result of prolonged bed rest and for pain that follows thoracotomy, mastectomy, or radical neck dissection. Diffuse subcutaneous injection of corticosteroids and local anesthetics may be useful for treating acute herpes zoster or postherpetic neuralgia. Botulinum toxins are a reasonable alternative to local anesthetics for refractory or frequently recurrent trigger points.[40,41] Analgesia produced by botulinum toxins considerably supersedes that produced by corticosteroids. The higher cost of the drug compared to local anesthetics raises a clinician dilemma, although it seems to be justified in selected cases.[40,41]

▶ Epidural steroid injections

Epidural steroid local injection of anesthetics generally do not provide lasting relief for back pain due to progressive neoplastic lesions. However, they may be useful for the short-term control of neuropathic pain associated with tumor growth into nerve structures, allowing the slow titration of anticonvulsants and tricyclic antidepressants to therapeutic levels.

▶ Sympathetic chain local anesthetic blocks

Local anesthetic injections administered in a series of blocks may contribute to lasting pain relief in the setting of posttraumatic sympathetically maintained pain (e.g., complex regional pain syndrome [CRPS] types I and II).[42–44] Although infrequent, such symptoms may arise as a result of tumor invasion of nervous system structures (e.g., brachial or lumbosacral plexopathy), in which case either local anesthetic blockade of the stellate ganglion or lumbar sympathetic chain has been used with some success to relieve pain. Additionally, there is evidence that a perioperative stellate ganglion block in patients with a history of upper extremity CRPS can significantly reduce the recurrence rate of this disease process.[41]

Stellate ganglion block may provide persistent relief of sympathetically maintained pain affecting the head, neck, and arm. Stellate ganglion neurolysis is hazardous because of the close proximity of other important structures (brachial plexus, laryngeal nerves, epidural and subarachnoid space, vertebral artery) and the potential for injury because of inaccurate needle placement. Moreover, the patient has the risk of experiencing a Horner's syndrome that may be long-lasting. If local anesthetic injections have been documented to provide temporary relief of pain, surgical extirpation of the first thoracic ganglia may be considered, or neurolysis may be performed cautiously using radiological guidance and small volumes of injectate.[45]

Neurolytic lumbar sympathetic block is most applicable for pain in the lower extremities due to lymphedema or reflex sympathetic imbalance, although there are anecdotal reports of its use for rectal and pelvic pain.[46]

▶ Intrathecal and epidural neurolysis

Subarachnoid (intrathecal) injections of alcohol or phenol continue to play an important role in the management of intractable cancer pain in carefully selected patients, particularly in countries where neuromodulation has not been widely utilized. Neurolytic neuraxial block produces pain relief by chemical rhizotomy. Since alcohol and phenol destroy nervous tissue indiscriminately, careful attention to the selection of the injection site, volume and concentration of injectate, and selection and positioning of the patient are essential to avoid neurologic complications.[47,48] Most authorities agree that neither alcohol nor phenol offer a clear advantage except for variations in specific gravity properties that may facilitate positioning of patient.[49,50] With the exception of perineal pain, alcohol is usually preferred, since most patients are unable to lie on their painful side, as is required for intrathecal phenol neurolysis. In one of the analyses of 13 published series documenting treatment with intrathecal rhizolysis of more than 2500 patients, Swerdlow reported that 58% of patients obtained "good" relief; "fair" relief was observed in an additional 21%, and in 20% of patients "little or no relief" was noted.[49] Average duration of relief is estimated at 3–6 months, with a wide range of distribution. Reports of analgesia persisting from 1 to 2 years are fairly common.[51] In a representative series using alcohol ($n = 252$) and phenol ($n = 151$), a total of 407 and 313 blocks were performed, respectively.[52,53] In these two series, neither motor weakness nor fecal incontinence occurred, and out of eight patients with transient urinary dysfunction, incontinence persisted in just one.

Subarachnoid neurolysis can be performed at any level up to the midcervical region, above which the risk of drug spread to medullary centers and the potential for cardiorespiratory collapse increases.[54] Blocks in the region of the brachial outflow are best reserved for patients with preexisting compromise of upper limb function. Similarly, lumbar injections are avoided in ambulatory patients, as are sacral injections in patients with normal bowel and bladder function. Hyperbaric phenol saddle block is relatively simple and is particularly suitable for many patients with colostomy and urinary diversion. Until recently, epidural neurolysis was performed infrequently. Results were inferior to those obtained with subarachnoid blockade, presumably because the dura acts as a barrier to diffusion, resulting in limited contact between the drug and targeted nerves.[53,55]

PERIPHERAL NERVE BLOCKS

▶ Pathophysiology of malignant peripheral neuropathy

Peripheral nerves' involvement in generating cancer pain is usually a result of one of three major pathologies: tumor invasion of the nerve, cancer treatment-induced neuropathy, and a postsurgical complication (Table 18-2).

▶ The role of peripheral nerve blockade in cancer pain management

Although peripheral nerve blockade has a limited role in the management of cancer pain,[56] it has great value for particular cancer pain manifestations, including perioperative pain management, other types of acute cancer pain, such as pathologic rib fractures, and in chronic peripheral pain conditions where life expectancy is short or the patient is not a candidate for other palliative protocols or procedures. For example, neoplastic head and neck pain is frequently difficult to control because of rich sensory innervations of the structures. In selected patients, blockade of involved cranial and/or upper cervical nerves is very helpful. Blockade of the ganglia of the trigeminal nerve at the foramen ovale at the base of skull or its branches may be beneficial for facial pain.[57] As in other blocks,

Table 18-2

Pathophysiology of Peripheral Nerve Neuropathic Pain

Tumor invasion of the nerve	Cervical plexopathy
	Brachial plexopathy
	Chest wall pain
	Malignant lumbosacral plexopathy
	Tumor-related mononeuropathy
	Cranial neuralgias
	Paraneoplastic peripheral neuropathy
	Acute vascular occlusion (upper or lower extremity)
Posttherapeutic	
Following chemotherapy	Postchemotherapy peripheral neuropathy
	Femoral head avascular necrosis
	Post-intraarterial infusion plexopathy
Following radiation	Postimbolization
	Postirradiation plexopathy
	Chronic radiation myelopathy
	Radioosteonecrosis
	Raynaud's syndrome
Postsurgical	Postthoracotomy syndrome
	Postmastectomy syndrome
	Postradical neck dissection syndrome
	Postoperative frozen shoulder
	Phantom pain syndromes (extremities or breast)
	Stump pain

Note: This list covers only peripheral malignant neuropathy, not all cancer pain syndromes.

peripheral blockade is either performed for temporary purposes with local anesthetics, or ablative (neurolytic vs. radiofrequency).

▶ Classification of peripheral nerve blockade

Temporary peripheral blockade

This can be achieved by single or periodically repeated injections or by placement of a perineural catheter. In all cases, a local anesthetic, such as bupivacaine or mepivacaine is used. Other medication can be added to the local anesthetic to intensify the block (clonidine), prolong the block (epinephrine, clonidine), or enhance analgesia (corticosteroids, opioids).[58] Despite various case reports, clinical observation and mini-trials demonstrating varying levels of coanalgesic effects, to date; there is no credible evidence that steroids or opioids enhance peripheral blockade compared to their proven efficacy with neuraxial blocks.[59]

Minor diagnostic or therapeutic procedures (e.g., peripherally inserted central catheters or central venous line insertion, bone marrow biopsy, lumbar puncture, dental procedures) performed on patients with active cancer, patients undergoing aggressive cancer treatment, or debilitated patients at the end of life, can cause these patients overwhelming bouts of breakthrough pain, ordinarily not experienced by other patients.[60] This pain can be attenuated by intradermal, subcutaneous, or deeper tissue infiltration of a local anesthetic, traditionally lidocaine, provided that the procedure's duration is short. Radiation-induced or chemotherapy-induced mucositis can be alleviated by topical viscous lidocaine,[61] or topical dibucaine films, with analgesia lasting up to 6 hours.[62]

In the pediatric population suffering from cancer, various diagnostic or therapeutic procedures, like those mentioned above, can be distressing. Preplanning for the procedures is important for pain relief and stress reduction. Age-appropriate approaches and explanations to the children along with parental input are crucial for the management of pain and distress. Sedation is often required. However, even the pain of venipuncture can be excruciating for pediatric patients. Topical blockade with a eutectic mixture of the local anesthetics lidocaine and prilocaine (EMLA), tetracaine gel (amethocaine), and lidocaine iontophoresis can be used for cutaneous analgesia before any procedure. Adequate sedation or general anesthesia should be readily available for reducing procedure-related cancer pain in children.[63]

Diagnostic blocks are administered only with local anesthetic as their function is to elucidate the nature and site of pain and to test the benefit of hypoesthesia or anesthesia produced by the block versus the existing experience of pain. Some patients might prefer pain over feeling numbness or a lack of sensation.[64] When a diagnostic block produces satisfactory analgesia, treatment options are dictated by the illness, patient, and his/her enviroment. Such options include recurring periodic injections, insertion of a perineural catheter, or neurolytic (ablative) blocks. Single temporary blocks can be diagnostic and therapeutic. However, the latter effect does not become evident until some time after the block. It is not unusual for peripheral blocks administered with local anesthetics to reduce or eliminate the analgesic requirement in distinct localized cancer pain presentations.[65] This is particularly true following prolonged peripheral neural blocks that last for hours in the postoperative period, and therefore reduce postoperative opioid requirements and substantially assuage postoperative pain.

Therapeutic single peripheral blocks are performed perioperatively for several purposes. These can be used as adjuncts or they can be the primary anesthetic used. Preoperative peripheral blocks serve as preemptive analgesia and the literature supports their utility in this setting. Prolonged peripheral neural blockade that lasts hours in the postoperative period reduces acute postoperative pain.

Therapeutic reccuring injections are used when painless mobility of a limb is required for physical rehabilitation therapy, and are particularly suited to patients with lympedema or frozen shoulders. Intraarticular periodic injections are one application. Recurring blocks are also performed when intial or subsequent blocks provided an acceptable length of analgesia duration. The optimal intervals between these injections depend on various factors. However, the clinician's judgement guides the schedule. In a United States-like healthcare system, financial considerations are extremely important, and advanced communications with health insurance providers are necessary to avoid denial of reimbursement.

Peripheral blockade (single or recurring) with longer acting local anesthetics such as bupivacaine can provide hours of relief until a more permanent solution can be devised. This window of analgesia can also provide time to titrate systemic medications such as corticosteroids, antidepressants, and anticonvulsants.

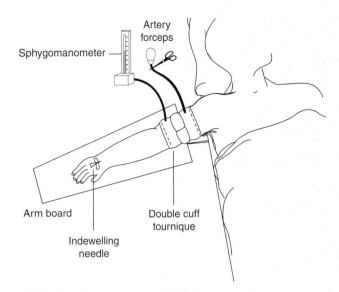

FIGURE 18-2 Diagram representing Bier block.

The *Bier block* is the oldest anesthetic regional technique, described in 1808 by Auguste Bier in Germany, and is an alternative approach to peripheral blocks (Fig. 18-2). Briefly, an intravenous bolus of a local anesthetic, customarily lidocaine 5%, sets off anesthesia on the arm below the elbow or the leg below the knee for up to 60 minutes.[66,67] Onset of anesthesia is rapid, and reasonable muscle relaxation can be obtained. As an anesthetic method, intraoperative Bier block application is limited to procedures lasting less than an hour and that is to circumvent increasing discomfort from the tourniquet.[66,67] Bier block is successfully employed to produce analgesia for patients with sympathetically-maintained pain (SMP) of the extremity. SMP of the extremities is a common occurrence among patients with cancer that invades neural plexi or following intraoperative iatrogenic nerve injuries. The use of an analgesic Bier block is based on the same concept underlying the use of therapeutic blocks. First an initial diagnostic session is scheduled. If satisfactory, recurring blocks are performed periodically. Frequency varies among patients, but the interval between the blocks is typically from 1 to 4 weeks. Adjuvants such as clonidine can be injected to follow or to be mixed with local anesthetic and it is thought to reduce tourniquet pressure pain.[68] Neostigmine greatly speeds the amount of time it takes for the effect of the block to be felt.[67] Clonidine, ketamine, ketorolac, and neostigmine all substantially reduce tourniquet pain.[67] A study from Greece showed that the addition of clonidine 1 μg/kg or ketamine 0.1 mg/kg to lidocaine given during Bier block delays the onset of unbearable tourniquet pain and decreases analgesic consumption for tourniquet pain relief, even though ketamine demonstrated greater analgesic potency.[69] Clonidine, ketorolac, and bretylium tosylate, in particular, provide prolonged postoperative analgesia.[67,70] Other medications have been used, including meperidine, fentanyl, tramadol, and labetalol with variable reports on efficacy.[71] Adding a steroidal agent to the local anesthetic did not provide any benefit.[72]

Perineural infusion catheters allow continuous infusion and/or repeated bolusing of local anesthetic. This resembles the concept of epidural patient-controlled analgesia (PCA), which prolongs the neural blockade and modulates breakthrough pain.[73] Catheters are inserted percutaneously, blindly or under ultrasonographic guidance, or surgically by direct vision. The latter is typically performed intra-operatively, commonly following amputative procedures. Catheter placement is often preceded by a diagnostic block or the block is applied at the time of the insertion. The condition of the patient and the patient's clinical situation dictate the timing of catheter placement. Catheters are usually tunneled subcutaneously so that they are secured in place. The length of treatment is usually a few days.[73] In most situations, catheters remain in place during the early postoperative phase. In certain circumstances, these catheters are left embedded longer if they provide sufficient analgesia, serve a purpose (improved quality of life or to facilitate a rehabilitative or medical treatment), and if proper care for their maintenance is available. Occasionally, patients can be discharged to their home or to a care facility with their peripheral catheter remaining in place. Portable pumps are used to control the infusion, but only after at-home follow-up by a trained healthcare professional has been arranged.[74,75] Agencies of the visiting nurse association are a good choice for finding people to provide this help. Convincing evidence suggests that continuous peripheral nerve blocks provided at home improve postoperative analgesia, sleep quality, and patient satisfaction while decreasing supplemental opioid requirements and opioid-related side effects.[74] Furthermore, a basal infusion after moderately painful surgery maximizes analgesic benefits, whereas PCA bolus doses decrease the basal rate and increase the duration of infusion.[75] These observations have not yet been made for perineural analgesic infusions in cancer pain patients. Although common sense would predict similar success, this cannot be assumed without valid data due to the variable and special needs of cancer patients. Our limited observation at Roswell Park Cancer Institute is promising and in accord with the reports of Ilfeld and Enneking.[74,75] Currently, there are two types of peripheral blockade catheters, stimulating and nonstimulating. Multiple reports of inaccurate catheter placement that occurred in a substantial number of cases,[76] led to the development of stimulating catheters. These were recently introduced to the world of anesthesiology and are thought to provide the possibility of improved catheter positioning adjacent to the nerve or plexus.[76] However, in hands that are not familiar with using the electric stimulator, blind placement might prove to be more accurate.[77] Some papers reported higher secondary block failure after placement of nonstimulating catheters, compared to stimulating catheters. This, besides the higher cost and usual skepticism that accompanies new procedures, has engendered controversy about which catheters are most appropriate.[76,77]

Neurolytic (ablative) peripheral blockade

In addition to neuraxial and sympathetic neurolytic blocks, peripheral neurolytic blocks can be effective as a conventional analgesic therapy.[78] However, they can cause unacceptable long-term or permanent motor loss along with pain blockade. This makes them an unfavorable choice which should be reserved for intractable, otherwise unmanageable, pain. They are most beneficial for patients who have a limited life expectancy. The effects from neurolytic blocks of somatic nerves usually last as long as 6 months. Recent advances in pharmacologic approaches and intraspinal techniques have narrowed the indications and need for neurolytic peripheral blocks. Yet in developing and poor parts of the world, neurolytic blocks in general are much more affordable than the newer alternatives. The use of neurolytic peripheral blocks is not limited to the management of pain. They are also useful for the treatment of spasticity in patients with central nervous system lesions or who have a spinal cord injury.

Modern minimally invasive neurolytic techniques can be divided into chemical, radiofrequency, cryoneurolysis, and surgical ablation.[79] *Chemical neurolysis* involves injecting a destructive chemical such as alcohol-glycerol or phenol, substances that affect neural tissue.[79] Radiofrequency neuroablation involves percutaneous introduction of insulated needles to localize nociceptive tracks followed by placement of a pinpoint heat lesion. The extent of the lesion can be controlled by the size of the probe, duration of application, and temperature at the tip of the needle.[79] Since a more precise controlled lesion can be created, radiofrequency neuroablation is more advantageous than chemical peripheral neurolysis and is undeniably preferred for cordotomy, rhizotomy, and ganglionotomy. Like radiofrequency neuroablation, contemporary cryoneurolysis has a similar advantage in the ability to produce a controlled lesion. *Cryoneurolysis* is based on the concept that freezing neural structures leads to axonal degeneration. It involves positioning cryoprobes on particular pain generators that are identified by electric stimulation using a radiofrequency technique. Following identification of these pain generators, they are frozen to −70°C. The main advantage of cryoneurolysis is that the neural injury is reversible and regeneration is more likely to occur without neuritis and dysesthesias than when other techniques are used.[79] The main disadvantage is that analgesia may be short-lived. In general, cryoneurolysis is preferred for noncancer patients who have a long life expectancy. Occasionally, *surgical interruption* of peripheral or cranial nerves can be done. Multiple level surgical rhizotomies of the dorsal root entry zone and ganglia are occasionally performed.[79]

▶ Clinical approach to peripheral nerve blockade

Preprocedure

This is perhaps the most important step of the block. Thorough knowledge of the anatomic region of the block, the characteristics of the blocking agent (including pharmacologic and nonpharmacologic), and good skills for conducting the procedure are essential. Appropriate patient selection and education adds to the success of the procedure. A full clinical evaluation should be instituted along with obtaining informed consent (Fig. 18-3).

The ideal patient for receiving therapeutic blocks is one with a localized source of pain that responded well to a diagnostic block, who is lacking coagulopathies, blood-borne infection, or infection at the proposed needle insertion site. The block must be performed in a sterile fashion and under monitored conditions that meet standards of care and safety.

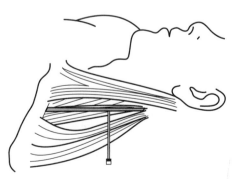

FIGURE 18-3 Diagram representing an example of peripheral plexus block: the interscalene approach to brachial plexus block.

Indications and techniques

The usefulness of peripheral therapeutic blocks is limited to areas of the body in which interruption of both motor and sensory function will not interfere with functional status.[80] Localized headaches, thoracic pain, and limb pain are the most common sites for such blocks.[80] Peripheral blocks could also be disadvantageous because each peripheral nerve sensorily innervates multiple levels, and, conversely, multiple nerves sensorily innervate common local areas of the body.[80]

Ultimately, peripheral blocks involve more than one nerve, which is why most are done at the level of the plexi. Somatic pain and mononeuropathies compared to multineuropathic pain respond more favorably to local anesthetic blockade.

Blocks with proven success rate in cancer pain include gasserian ganglion blocks for cranial and facial pain, intercostal blocks for chest wall metastasis and pathological rib lesions, and paravertebral blocks for radicular pain.[81] Patients whose pain is relieved by a local anesthetic peripheral block may benefit from a neurolytic (neuroablative) block. The paravertebral block is most common peripheral nerve neurolytic block.

A historic, but now uncommon, procedure involves instilling a local anesthetic (usually bupivacaine) or a neurolytic chemical (usually phenol) for the temporary or neuroablative relief of pain from metastatic disease to the neck, arms, chest, brachial plexus, thorax, or abdomen. This block is particularly effective for rapidly controlling acute exacerbations of cancer pain in terminally ill patients.[66,81,82]

Table 18-3 presents a list of the most encountered peripheral blocks in cancer pain management and their corresponding indication.

Medications

Choosing among short-acting and long-acting *local anesthetics* should be tailored to each individual patient. This is equally true for the purpose and anatomic location of the block. Local anesthetics can be variably diluted to suit the desired effect and minimize systemic toxicity, particularly if used for peripheral infusion through a catheter. Peripheral infusions of 3–8 mL/h of lidocaine 1%–2%, ropivacaine 0.2%–0.3%, or bupivacaine 0.125%–0.25% provide good analgesia in most cases.[73,81] Lidocaine is the most common local anesthetic used in the Bier block. Customarily, 50 mL lidocaine 5% for the arm and 100 mL lidocaine 5% for the leg is used.[66] Alternatively, equal volumes of bupivacaine 0.25% or ropivacaine 0.2% can be used,[66] although the block is not prolonged and there is a greater risk of side effects. In small or debilitated patients, dosing is lidocaine 3 mg/kg.[66] Common side effects of local anesthetics include pain at the injection site, lightheadedness, tremor, confusion, hypotension, blurred vision, tinnitus, dizziness, euphoria, lethargy, nausea, agitation, and hallucination. Serious but uncommon side effects include seizures, respiratory arrest, status asthmaticus, coma, and cardiac arrhythmias including extrasystole, bradycardia, and heart block. Management of these adverse reactions is by withdrawing the medication if the patient is undergoing infusion and supportive treatment targeting the specific reaction(s).

Clonidine, in doses of 0.5 μg/kg or greater, enhances and prolongs the effect of local anesthetics in peripheral blocks.[73,83] A similar effect is produced with 150 μg of clonidine administered in intraarticular blocks. Side effects of clonidine, namely bradycardia and hypotension, increase with doses higher than 1.5 μg/kg.[83] Clonidine's other common side effects include dry mouth and drowsiness. Serious side effects include sever hypotension and rebound hypertension. Intraarticular administration of neostigmine at 500 μg produces significant analgesia. However, several studies did not document any advantage of adding neostigmine to peripheral nerve blocks.[83] In the perineural continuous block of the lower extremities, fentanyl at 25 μg in 4 mL sterile water as a bolus injection improves analgesia when tachyphylaxis develops.[73] Subsequently, a dose of fentanyl 1 μg/mL can be added to the infused solution.[73] This effect of fentanyl has not been proven, yet, it might be worthwhile to test it in upper extremity

Table 18-3

The Most Encountered Peripheral Blocks in Cancer Pain Management and their Corresponding Indication

Region	Nerve/Structure	Indication
Head	Gasserian ganglion	Trigeminal neuralgia, postherpetic neuralgia of the face
	Supratrochlear, supraorbital, infraorbital	Facial neuralgia
	Maxillary, mandibular	Trigeminal neuralgia, postherpetic neuralgia of the face
	Greater occipital	Occipital neuralgia, postherpetic neuralgia of the head
	Glossopharyngeal	Jaw pain
Neck	Superficial cervical plexus	Postradical neck dissection syndrome
Upper Extremity	Brachial plexus	Brachial plexopathy, postmastectomy syndrome, UE-CRPS
Thorax	Intercostal	Intercostal neuralgias, metastatic rib pain, postthoracotomy syndrome
	Interpleural	Metastatic disease to the neck, arms, chest, brachial plexus, thorax, or abdomen
Groin	Iliohypogastric, ilioinguinal	Postherniorrhaphy syndrome
Lower Extremity	Sacroiliac joint	Sacroilitis
	Sciatic	Sciatic neuralgia
	Femoral	Femoral neuralgia
	Lateral femoral cutaneous	Meralgia paresthetica

continuous catheter infusions. Some anesthesiologists add *sodium bicarbonate* (alkalinizing agent) to lidocaine to speed up the onset of single injection blocks. A common practice is to add 1 mL of sodium bicarbonate (8.4%, 10 mEq/L) solution to 10 mL of lidocaine 1%–2%. This addition seems to reduce the feeling of burning that follows local cutaneous infiltration with lidocaine, perhaps by increasing the pH of the solution. Other adjuvants added to local anesthetics include ketamine, which demonstrated excellent analgesic effects in perineural continuous infusions,[73,84] tramadol, morphine, buprenorphine, which may enhance and prolong blocks[83] and vasoconstrictors (epinephrine, phenylephrine, ephedrine, norepinephrine). Caution must be exercised when adding vasoconstrictors, especially epinephrine, as they have the potential for causing ischemic neurotoxicity in peripheral nerves.[85]

Botulinum toxin is an evolving pharmacologic blocking agent. Several reports have shown its beneficial analgesic effects following muscle infiltration of the drug into the sites of surgical resection, such as for as mastectomy, placement of tissue expanders,[86] or hemorrhoidectomy.[87] Hemorrhoids are a common presentation in cancer of the rectum. The role of botulinum toxins in pain medicine in general, and in cancer pain and palliative care in particular, has yet to be clearly defined. However, botulinum toxin has demonstrated therapeutic value in patients with debilitating spastic syndromes, musculoskeletal pain syndromes (both malignant and nonmalignant), myofascial pain syndromes, and headaches.

For neuroablative procedures, the choice of medications is based on the desired onset of nerve destruction. Absolute alcohol diffuses faster than phenol. Phenol, at lower doses, acts as a local anesthetic rather than as a neurolytic. Phenol thus produces less pain at the injection site than absolute alcohol, although the quality of analgesia from the block is also reduced. Other agents used include glycerol and chlorocresol. Additives to phenol include glycerin, corticosteroids, and bupivacaine. Careful hemodynamic and neurologic monitoring is mandatory during administration of chemical neurolysis. Although these blocks can be performed using blind techniques by extremely skilled interventionalists, radiography-assisted positioning of the tip of the needle is preferred.

Complications

Serious side effects from regional anesthetic interventions with local anesthetics are rare.[88] The incidence of death during regional anesthesia is usually caused by cardiac arrest, most commonly reported from neuraxial approaches. Permanent disabling injuries are mostly seen in nerve blocks of the eye (retrobulbar > peribulbar) (23%) rather than from neuraxial opiates or neurolytic blocks (21%), and finally in neuraxial and peripheral blocks (20%).[89] For peripheral neural blockade, complications usually occur from poor procedural technique. Complications include local anesthetic systemic toxicity, infections, block failure, overblocking (spread to unintended neural structures or block prolongation), neuritis, transient neurologic symptoms, nerve damage and its sequelae (e.g., paraplegia), and death.[88] Advances in regional anesthetic instrumentation, development of newer local anesthetics with better safety profiles, and the introduction of ultrasonogram-guided techniques have significantly reduced these events.

There is the risk of block failure during neurolytic blockade. This failure is usually due to overlapping sensory innervation of the painful region, transient neurolysis, neuritis, and deafferentation pain as the effect of the block diminishes. Selecting the patients who are likely to succumb before the development of neuropathic pain (i.e., within 6 months) generally circumvents these complications.[88]

VERTEBROPLASTY

Many cancer patients with metastatic vertebral compression fractures (VCFs) or osteoporotic VCFs present with movement-related back pain. Percutaneous vertebroplasty (PV) is a minimally invasive procedure, which involves injecting an opacified bone cement (usually polymethymethacrylate or PMMA) into the fractured vertebral body to alleviate pain and possibly enhance structural stability (see Fig. 8a and b). This procedure is performed under fluoroscopic guidance by placing needles using a uni- or bipedicular approach. PMMA is injected in a carefully controlled manner to avoid unintentionally spreading cement into the spinal canal. The injection is stopped when the cement approaches the posterior third of the vertebral body. PV has shown efficacy in treating VCF-related pain in cancer patients.[90]

NEURODESTRUCTIVE PROCEDURES

Neurosurgical palliative techniques have fallen into less favor as more medications and reversible, titratable, lower risk techniques have largely replaced these procedures. Pituitary ablation entails destruction of the gland by means of the injection of a small quantity of alcohol through a needle positioned transnasally under light general anesthesia. This technique is effective in relieving pain originating from disseminated bony metastases, particularly secondary to hormone-dependent tumors (breast and prostate).[91] Commissural myelotomy has reported efficacy for treating cancer pain that is refractory to more conservative therapy.[91] Percutaneous cordotomy produces a thermal lesion within the substance of the spinal cord and reliably relieves unilateral truncal and lower limb pain.[91] As with pituitary ablation, this technique necessitates a high degree of skill and expertise, but using this technique often produces profound pain relief, while avoiding the risks of a major neurosurgical procedure.

CONCLUSION

The availability of different techniques for neuraxial drug delivery has presented an effective alternative for patients experiencing uncontrolled pain after optimal and aggressive oral/transdermal and adjuvant therapy. Drug compounding is necessary to meet the different drug requirements that patients may have.

Neurolysis of the sympathetic axis appears to be a safe, cost-effective approach to treating visceral pain associated with cancer. The benefits include improved analgesia, reduced opioid consumption, favorable economic implications, and superior clinical effects due to the deleterious properties of high-dose chronic opioid therapy. Current knowledge and techniques used to perform these blocks allow these procedures to be performed safely and expeditiously. Pain practitioners should consider the role of these blocks in adjuvant therapy for the optimal treatment of cancer pain.

REFERENCES

1. Jacox A, Carr DB, Payne R. New clinical-practice guidelines for the management of pain in patients with cancer. *N Engl J Med*. 1994;330(9): 651–655.
2. Portenoy RK. Managing pain in patients with advanced cancer: the role of neuraxial infusion. *Oncology (Williston Park)*. 1999;13(Suppl. 2):7–8.
3. Bennett G, Burchiel K, Buchser E, et al. Clinical guidelines for intraspinal infusion: report of an expert panel. PolyAnalgesic Consensus Conference 2000. *J Pain Symptom Manage*. 2000;20:S37–S43.

4. Foley KM. Advances in cancer pain. *Arch Neurol.* 1999;56:413–417.

5. Regional anesthetic techniques for the management of cancer pain. In: Urmey W, ed. *Techniques in Regional Anesthesia and Pain Management.* Vol. 1, No. 1. Philadelphia: WB Saunders; 1997.

6. Singler RC. An improved technique for alcohol neurolysis of the celiac plexus block. *Anesthesiology.* 1982;56:137–141.

7. Firdousi FH, Sharma D, Raina VK. Palliation by coeliac plexus block for upper abdominal visceral cancer pain. *Trop Doct.* 2002;32(4):224–226.

8. Gress F, Schmitt C, Sherman S, et al. A prospective randomized comparison of endoscopic ultrasound- and computed tomography-guided celiac plexus block for managing chronic pancreatitis pain. *Am J Gastroenterol.* 1999;94:900–905.

9. Gress F, Schmitt C, Sherman S, et al. Endoscopic ultrasound-guided celiac plexus block for managing abdominal pain associated with chronic pancreatitis: a prospective single center experience. *Am J Gastroenterol.* 2001;96(2):409–416.

10. Ischia S, Luzzani A, Ischia A, et al. A new approach to the neurolytic block of the coeliac plexus: the transaortic technique. *Pain.* 1983;16:333–341.

11. Ischia S, Ischia A, Polati E, et al. Three posterior percutaneous celiac plexus block techniques: a prospective randomized study in 61 patients with pancreatic cancer pain. *Anesthesiology.* 1992;76:534–540.

12. Davis DD. Incidence of major complications of neurolytic coeliac plexus block. *J Royal Soc Med.* 1993;86:264–266.

13. Wong GY, Brown DL. Celiac plexus block for cancer pain. In: Urmey W, ed. *Techniques in Regional Anesthesia and Pain Management.* Vol. 1, No. 1. Philadelphia: WB Saunders; 1997.

14. Hanley JA, Lippman-Hand A. If nothing goes wrong, is everything all right? Interpreting zero numerators. *JAMA.* 1983;249:1743–1745.

15. Matson JA, Ghia JN, Levy JH. A case report of a potentially fatal complications associated with Ischia's transaortic method of celiac plexus block. *Reg Anesth.* 1985;10:193–196.

16. Sett SS, Taylor DC. Aortic pseudoaneurysm secondary to celiac plexus block. *Ann Vasc Surg.* 1991;5:88–91.

17. Kaplan R, Schiff-Keren B, Alt E. Aortic dissection as a complication of celiac plexus block. *Anesthesiology.* 1995;83:632–635.

18. Galizia EJ, Lahiri SK. Paraplegia following coeliac plexus block with phenol. Case report. *Br J Anaesth.* 1974;46:539–540.

19. Lo JN, Buckley JJ. Spinal cord ischemia a complication of celiac plexus block. *Reg Anesth.* 1982;7:66–68.

20. Cherry DA, Lamberty J. Paraplegia following coeliac plexus block. *Anaesth Intensive Care.* 1984;12:59–61.

21. Woodham MJ, Hanna MH. Paraplegia after coeliac plexus block. *Anaesthesia.* 1989;44:487–489.

22. van Dongen RT, Crul BJ. Paraplegia following coeliac plexus block. *Anaesthesia.* 1991;46:862–863.

23. Jabbal SS, Hunton J. Reversible paraplegia following coeliac plexus block. *Anaesthesia.* 1992;47:857–858.

24. Wong GY, Brown DL. Transient paraplegia following alcohol celiac plexus block. *Reg Anesth.* 1995;20:352–355.

25. Brown DL, Rorie DK. Altered reactivity of isolated segmental lumbar arteries of dogs following exposure to ethanol and phenol. *Pain.* 1994;56:139–143.

26. Mercadante S. Celiac plexus block versus analgesics in pancreatic cancer pain. *Pain.* 1993;52:187–192.

27. Rathmell JP, Roland T, DuPen SL. Management of pain associated with metastatic epidural spinal cord compression: use of imaging studies in planning epidural therapy. *Reg Anesth Pain Med.* 2000;25:113–116.

28. Ventafridda GV, Caraceni AT, Sbanotto AM, et al. Pain treatment in cancer of the pancreas. *Eur J Surg Oncol.* 1990;16:1–6.

29. Wong GY, Schroeder DR, Carns PE, et al. Effect of neurolytic celiac plexus block on pain relief, quality of life, and survival in patients with unresectable pancreatic cancer: a randomized controlled trial. *JAMA.* 2004;291:1092–1099.

30. De Cicco M, Matovic M, Balestreri L, et al. Single-needle celiac plexus block: is needle tip position critical in patients with no regional anatomic distortions? *Anesthesiology.* 1997;87:1301–1308.

31. Eisenberg E, Carr DB, Chalmers TC. Neurolytic celiac plexus block for treatment of cancer pain: a meta-analysis. *Anesth Analg.* 1995;80:290–295.

32. Yeager MP. Morphine inhibits spontaneous and cytokine-enhanced natural killer cell cytotoxicity in volunteers. *Anesthesiology.* 1995;83:500–508.

33. Lillemoe KD, Cameron JL, Kaufman HS, et al. Chemical splanchnicectomy in patients with unresectable pancreatic cancer: a prospective randomized trial. *Ann Surg.* 1993;217:447–457.

34. Plancarte R, Amescua C, Patt RB, et al. Superior hypogastric plexus block for pelvic cancer pain. *Anesthesiology.* 1990;73:236–239.

35. de Leon-Casasola OA, Kent E, Lema MJ. Neurolytic superior hypogastric plexus block for chronic pelvic pain associated with cancer. *Pain.* 1993;54:145–151.

36. Plancarte R, de Leon-Casasola OA, El-Helaly M, et al. Neurolytic superior hypogastric plexus block for chronic pelvic pain associated with cancer. *Reg Anesth.* 1997;22:562–568.

37. Rosenberg SK, Tewari R, Boswell MV, et al. Superior hypogastric plexus block successfully treats severe penile pain after transurethral resection of the prostate. *Reg Anesth Pain Med.* 1998;23:618–620.

38. Plancarte R, Amescua C, Patt RB. Presacral blockade of the ganglion of Walther (ganglion impar). *Anesthesiology.* 1990;73:A751.

39. Travel JG, Simons DG. *Myofascial Pain and Dysfunction: The Trigger Point Manual.* Baltimore: Williams & Wilkins; 1983.

40. Kamanli A, Kaya A, Ardicoglu O, et al. Comparison of lidocaine injection, botulinum toxin injection, and dry needling to trigger points in myofascial pain syndrome. *Rheumatol Int.* 2004. [Epub ahead of print].

41. Swam RA, Karanikolas M, Cousins MJ. Anaesthetic techniques for pain control. In: Doyle D, Hanks G, Cherny NI, et al., eds. *Oxford Textbook of Palliative Medicine,* 3rd ed. New York: Oxford University Press; 2004:378–396.

42. Payne R. Neuropathic pain syndromes, with special reference to causalgia and reflex sympathetic dystrophy. *Clin J Pain.* 1986;2:59–73.

43. de Leon-Casasola OA. Interventional procedures for cancer pain management: when are they indicated? *Cancer Invest.* 2004;22:630–642.

44. Warfield CA, Crews DA. Use of stellate ganglion blocks in the treatment of intractable limb pain in lung cancer. *Clin J Pain.* 1987;3:13.

45. Racz GB, Holubec JT. Stellate ganglion phenol neurolysis. In: Racz GB, ed. *Techniques of Neurolysis.* Boston: Kluwer; 1989:133–143.

46. Cousins MJ. Anesthetic approaches in cancer pain. *Adv Pain Res Ther.* 1990;16:249–273.

47. Peyton Wt, Semansky EJ, Baker AB. Subarachnoid injection of alcohol for relief of intractable pain with discussion of cord changes found at autopsy. *Am J Cancer.* 1937;30:709.

48. Smith MC. Histological findings following intrathecal injections of phenol solutions for relief of pain. *Br J Anaesth.* 1963;36:387–406.

49. Swerdlow M. Intrathecal neurolysis. *Anaesthesia.* 1978;33:733–740.

50. Katz J. The current role of neurolytic agents. *Adv Neurol.* 1974;4:471–476.

51. Swerdlow M. Subarachnoid and extradural blocks. *Adv Pain Res Ther.* 1979;2:325–337.

52. Hay RC. Subarachnoid alcohol block in the control of intractable pain. *Anesth Analg.* 1962;41:12–16.

53. Stovner J, Endresen R. Intrathecal phenol for cancer pain. *Acta Anaesthesiol Scand.* 1972;16:17–21.

54. Holland AJC, Youssef M. A complication of subarachnoid phenol blockade. *Anaesthesia.* 1979;34:260–262.

55. Racz GB, Heavner J, Haynsworth R. Repeat epidural phenol injections in chronic pain and spasticity. In: Lipton S, Miles J, eds. *Persistent Pain,* vol. 5. Orlando: Grune & Stratton; 1985:157–179.

56. Doyle D. Nerve blocks in advanced cancer. *Practitioner.* 1982;226:539–544.

57. Madrid JL, Bonica JJ. Cranial nerve blocks. In: Bonica JJ, Ventafridda V, eds. *Advances in Pain Research & Therapy,* vol 2. New York: Raven Press; 1979;4638.

58. Eisenach JC. Local anesthetic adjuvants—neuraxial vs. peripheral blockade. In: *SYLLABUS, 29th Annual Spring Meeting.* American Society of Regional Anesthesia & Pain Medicine. Orlando, Florida. 2004:43–47.

59. Weller RS, Butterworth J. Opioids as local anesthetic adjuvants for peripheral nerve block. *Tech Reg Anesth Pain Mgmt.* 2004;8:123–128.

60. Cherny NI. Cancer pain syndromes. In: Melzack R, Wall PD, eds. *Handbook of Pain Management: A Clinical Companion to Wall and Melzack's Textbook of Pain.* Edinburgh: Churchill Livingstone; 2003: 603–639.

61. Knox JJ, Puodziunas AL, Feld R. Chemotherapy-induced oral mucositis. Prevention and management. *Drugs Aging.* 2000;17:257–267.

62. Yamamura K, Yotsuyanagi T, Okamoto T. Pain relief of oral ulcer by dibucaine-film. *Pain.* 1999;83:625–626.

63. Maxwell L, Yaster M. The myth of conscious sedation. *Arch Pediatr Adolesc Med.* 1996;150:665–667.

64. Loser JD. Neurosurgical approaches in palliative care. In: Doyle D, Hanks G, MacDonald N, eds. *Oxford Testbook of Paliative Medicine.* Oxford: Oxford Medical Publications; 1993:221–229.

65. Lynch M, Katz NP. Cancer pain management: I. *Hosp Physician.* 2000;1–12.

66. Mulroy MF. Intravenous regional anesthesia. In: Mulroy MF, ed. *Regional Anesthesia: An Illustrated Procedural Guide, 3rd ed.* Philadelphia: Lippincott Williams & Wilkins; 2002:183–189.

67. Viscomi C. Bier blocks: new tricks for an old dog. *ASRA News.* June;2–3.

68. Reuben SS, Rosenthal EA, Steinberg RB, et al. Surgery on the affected upper extremity of patients with a history of complex regional pain syndrome: the use of intravenous regional anesthesia with clonidine. *J Clin Anesth.* 2004;16:517–522.

69. Gorgias NK, Maidatsi PG, Kyriakidis AM, et al. Clonidine versus ketamine to prevent tourniquet pain during intravenous regional anesthesia with lidocaine. *Reg Anesth Pain Med.* 2001;26(6):512–517.

70. Hord AH, Rooks MD, Stephens BO, et al. Intravenous regional bretylium and lidocaine for treatment of reflex sympathetic dystrophy: a randomized, double-blind study. *Anesth Analg.* 1992;74:818–821.

71. Hord ED, Stojanovic MP, Vallejo R, et al. Multiple Bier blocks with labetalol for complex regional pain syndrome refractory to other treatments. *J Pain Symptom Manage.* 2003;25:299–302.

72. Taskaynatan MA, Ozgul A, Tan AK, et al. Bier block with methylprednisolone and lidocaine in CRPS type I: a randomized, double-blinded, placebo-controlled study. *Reg Anesth Pain Med.* 2004;29:408–412.

73. Evans H, Steele SM, Nielsen KC, et al. Peripheral nerve blocks and continuous catheter techniques. *Anesthesiol Clin North America.* 2005;23:141–162.

74. Ilfeld BM, Enneking FK. A portable mechanical pump providing over four days of patient-controlled analgesia by perineural infusion at home. *Reg Anesth Pain Med.* 2002;27:100–104.

75. Ilfeld BM, Enneking FK. Continuous peripheral nerve blocks at home: a review. *Anesth Analg.* 2005;100:1822–1833.

76. Boezaart AP. The stimulating catheter: is it useful? *ASRA News.* February 2005;8 (continued on 10-1).

77. Grant SA. Why I prefer a nonstimulating catheter. *ASRA News.* February 2005; 9 (continued on 16).

78. Lema MJ. Invasive procedures for cancer pain. Pain Clinical Updates. 1998;6:1–9.

79. Kim PS. Interventional cancer pain therapies. *Semin Oncol.* 2005;32: 194–199.

80. Tasker RR. Management of nociceptive, deafferentation and central pain by surgical intervention. In: Fields HL, ed. *Pain Syndromes in Neurology.* Boston: Butterworths; 1990:143.

81. Fischer HB. Peripheral nerve blocks for cancer pain. *Curr Anaesth Crit Care.* 2001;12:309–314.

82. Lema MJ, Myers DP, de Leon-Casasola OA. Pleural phenol therapy for the treatment of chronic esophageal cancer pain. *Reg Anesth.* 1992;17:166–170.

83. Habib AS, Gan TJ. Role of analgesic adjuncts in postoperative pain management. *Anesthesiol Clin North America.* 2005;23:85–107.

84. Carpenter KJ, Dickenson AH. NMDA receptors and pain—hopes for novel analgesics. *Reg Anesth Pain Med.* 1999;24:506–508.

85. Tsui BC, Wagner A, Finucane B. Regional anaesthesia in the elderly: a clinical guide. *Drugs Aging.* 2004;21:895–910.

86. Layeeque R, Hochberg J, Siegel E, et al. Botulinum toxin infiltration for pain control after mastectomy and expander reconstruction. *Ann Surg.* 2004;240:608–613.

87. Davies J, Duffy D, Boyt N, et al. Botulinum toxin (Botox) reduces pain after hemorrhoidectomy: results of a double-blind, randomized study. *Dis Colon Rectum.* 2003;46:1097–1102.

88. de Médicis É, de Leon-Casasola OA. Local anesthetic toxicity in the ambulatory setting. In: Stele SM, Nielsen KC, Klein SM, eds. *Ambulatory Anesthesia & Perioperative Analgesia.* New York: McGraw-Hill; 2005: 207–213.

89. Ben-David B. Complications of regional anesthesia: an overview. *Anesthesiol Clin North America.* 2002;20:665–667.

90. Fourney DR, Schomer DF, Nader R, et al. Percutaneous vertebroplasty and kyphoplasty for painful vertebral body fractures in cancer patients. *J Neurosurg Spine 1.* 2003;98:21–30.

91. Lahuerta J, Lipton S, Miles J, et al. Update on percutaneous cervical cordotomy and pituitary alcohol neuradenolysis: an audit of our recent results and complications. In: Lipton S, Miles J, eds. *Persistent Pain*, vol 5. New York: Grune & Stratton; 1985:197–223.

The Role of Palliative Surgery

Alexandra M. Easson
Peter W.T. Pisters

INTRODUCTION

Palliative surgery is an important part of the management of pain in patients with advanced cancer. Appropriate and timely surgical referral can alleviate or prevent the development of significant pain and other uncomfortable symptoms in the context of multidisciplinary palliative care. Palliation means "affording relief, not cure . . . to reduce the severity of."[1] Palliative surgery may therefore be characterized as "interventions where the major goal is the relief of symptoms and suffering, not the prolongation of life, for patients for whom there is no chance of cure."[2,3] Palliative procedures may be beneficial for terminally ill patients whose deaths are imminent, but such procedures may also be helpful for patients with indolent or recurrent disease whose deaths are months or years away.

Like conventional surgery, palliative surgery encompasses a wide spectrum of procedures, with differing levels of invasiveness, requirements for anesthesia, inherent technical difficulty, and attendant risks. Careful patient selection and preparation are required to determine which patients will experience improved quality of life and relief of symptoms with acceptable morbidity. In addition, because surgical interventions offer local tumor control only, the potential benefits of local treatment must be assessed in the context of the patient's disease process as a whole.

Pain has been described as "an unpleasant sensory and emotional experience associated with actual or potential tissue damage or described in terms of such damage,"[4] and is always a subjective experience. The conditions for which palliative surgical procedures are useful are often those in which pain is only one of many symptoms that cause distress and suffering for the patient. Pharmacological pain management must therefore remain an important adjunct before, during, and after surgical intervention.

This chapter outlines some of the conditions for which palliative surgery can and should be considered. It then discusses the decision-making approach that a surgeon should undertake before embarking on a palliative surgical procedure. Finally, this approach will be demonstrated with several clinical examples.

PALLIATIVE SURGICAL PROCEDURES

Locally advanced, recurrent, or metastatic tumors can cause pain by diverse mechanisms, including direct invasion of nerves by cancer cells, compression, stretching, or obstruction of surrounding soft tissues, organ capsules, nerves, or hollow organs. Surgical interventions that may be useful for palliation include resection, diversion, drainage procedures, stabilization via orthopedic techniques, and neurosurgical techniques.

▶ Resection

Biopsy

Increased or newly apparent pain may be the first sign that a tumor has recurred locally or has metastasized. New pain at follow-up should prompt a search for recurrence in a cancer patient, including radiologic imaging, tumor marker measurements, and physical examination. When recurrence is found, surgeons are occasionally called upon to perform incisional or excisional biopsies of newly discovered masses to help guide the palliative treatment of patients.

Complete resection

Complete resection of the primary tumor at the initial surgery plays a key role in the prevention of pain by reducing the risk of local recurrence. Increasingly, neoadjuvant chemotherapy and/or radiation are used before surgical resection for locally advanced tumors to improve local control rates. Incomplete resection will result in painful recurrences that may be impossible to treat surgically and difficult to manage by other means. Therefore, one of the most important roles of a surgical oncologist is to prevent pain by ensuring appropriate management of the primary tumor.

For the patient who presents with metastatic disease, surgery may be an important part of gaining control of the local disease even if cure is not possible. Once a tumor has infiltrated a nerve root, surgery is unlikely to be helpful, so earlier surgical intervention may be warranted to prevent this occurrence despite distant metastases. Palliative radical resections such as esophagectomy, pancreaticoduodenectomy, and pelvic exenteration have been described for the purposes of symptom control.[5] The results of surgery may be gratifying, and in select patients, improvements in quality of life can be dramatic even if survival is not lengthened.

Complete resection may also be appropriate to manage local recurrences or to manage the painful sequelae of metastases. Locally advanced, recurrent, or metastatic soft tissue tumors may result in difficult wound problems because of pain, ulceration, or fistula formation causing odor, discharge, or bleeding. Social interactions may be affected because the symptoms are often apparent to others. Examples include ulcerating breast tumors; eroding head and neck tumors; enterocutaneous or perineal fistulas draining bile, stool, or urine; and bulky axillary or inguinal nodal metastases causing progressive lymphedema and limited function. Surgical resection, if negative margins can be obtained, with or without radiation therapy may result in significantly improved quality of life. In this setting, the patient has often already had several attempts at local tumor control with surgery and/or radiation therapy. This previous therapy increases the complexity and potential morbidity of any planned local resection. For example, resection of a tumor through irradiated tissue may require the transfer of soft tissue and/or a muscle flap from an unirradiated area. A resection of a recurrent anal cancer after failed chemoradiation may require a two-team approach, where the surgical oncologist removes the tumor with an abdominal-perineal resection and a plastic surgeon fills the perineal defect by mobilizing a gracilis muscle or rectus abdominis soft tissue flap.

Debulking procedures

In general, surgical resection should not be performed unless a complete resection can be achieved, as the tumor will simply recur. For some tumors, however, incomplete or debulking resections are appropriate. These include slow-growing tumors (e.g., metastatic carcinoid or thyroid cancer), or when effective anticancer therapy can be given postoperatively to treat the residual tumor (e.g., ovarian cancer).

Amputation may be necessary for extremity lesions such as soft tissue sarcomas and melanomas. It is usually a secondary procedure after failed limb-conserving therapy. Unless it is absolutely necessary for palliation of pain or fungation or to prevent major hemorrhage, amputation should be avoided in the presence of metastatic disease.

▶ Relief of obstruction

Mechanical obstruction of an organ or viscus is common in patients with advanced cancer and can cause significant pain and distress. Extrinsic compression or intrinsic tumor growth can obstruct the respiratory, gastrointestinal, biliary, vascular, or urologic systems partially or completely, acutely, or chronically. Recognizing the symptoms of impending obstruction followed by early intervention can prevent a sudden life-threatening crisis. Relief from obstruction can facilitate many months of symptom-free survival and is most successful when there is a single site rather than multiple sites of obstruction.[6]

The symptoms resulting from obstruction depend on the site of obstruction and the organ(s) involved. Before acting to relieve the obstruction, it is important to confirm that symptoms are, in fact, due to obstruction. For example, bronchial obstruction is only one of many causes of shortness of breath. Treatment to relieve an obstruction should only be undertaken if the obstructive symptoms significantly contribute to the patient's overall distress and symptom burden. Modalities used to assess obstruction include radiologic imaging (angiography, fluoroscopy, ultrasonography, or computed tomography [CT]), and endoscopy.

Various procedures can relieve obstructive symptoms.[2] Local ablation using laser, electrocautery, cryotherapy, or photodynamic therapy can be effective in easily accessed areas such as the trachea and rectum. Percutaneously placed gastric, biliary, or bladder drains may effectively decompress obstructed viscera, but require an external drainage catheter. Endoscopic and/or fluoroscopic placement of stents through an obstructed lumen can also provide effective relief. Internal stents, long used in the biliary tree, esophagus, bronchus, and ureters, are now available for the small bowel, colorectum, and major blood vessels. More invasive techniques to manage obstruction include surgical bypass and/or tumor resection, using minimally invasive or open techniques. These often provide the best

long-term relief of obstruction but require a general anesthetic and are accompanied by a higher risk of morbidity and death.

▶ Drainage of effusions

An accumulation of fluid in the abdomen, pleural space, or pericardium is common in terminally ill cancer patients. In the palliative setting, surgical drainage is not necessary unless the effusion causes significant symptoms that would be relieved by draining the fluid. In addition to causing pain, the fluid can compress nearby organs contributing to shortness of breath, and, in the abdomen, early satiety, abdominal distension, and decreased mobility. Pericardial effusions can be life-threatening.

Percutaneous fluid drainage is the simplest intervention. It offers rapid but temporary relief of symptoms as the effusion will recur unless the underlying cause is treated. More definitive surgical procedures vary in their degrees of invasiveness. An external drainage catheter with or without a sclerosing agent is commonly used for pleural and pericardial effusions.[7] Thoracoscopic or open drainage of the pleural cavity with decortication, pericardiectomy, or creation of a pericardial window are treatments that may be effective but require general anesthesia. The degree of invasiveness chosen is determined by the severity of symptoms, the underlying disease, and the patient's condition.

In malignant ascites, the most commonly used treatment is therapeutic paracentesis. Up to 5 liters of fluid can be drained through a needle inserted through the abdominal wall with or without ultrasound guidance, resulting in significant but temporary symptom relief. A physician must do this, either at a house call or during a hospital visit. The fluid soon reaccumulates with a return of the associated symptoms; patients may require paracentesis two or three times per week, and usually become very symptomatic while waiting for their next drainage. Internal drainage shunts have been described, but are infrequently used in malignant ascites due to high complication rates.[8] Percutaneous catheters (without sclerosis) are increasingly being used for malignant ascites. Adam et al. reviewed 31 published series (680 patients) of percutaneously placed intra-abdominal drainage catheters for malignant ascites. Such catheters provided effective palliation in 70% of cases; the most common complications were catheter-related sepsis and occlusion.[9] Percutaneous catheters can be managed by nurses or caregivers at home, which is especially important as patients become less mobile near the end of their lives.

▶ Bone metastases

Pain is the most common presentation of skeletal metastases. Pain occurs in two-thirds of patients with radiologically evident metastases but may develop before the lesion is visible. Radiation therapy, systemic anticancer therapy, and pain medication are the usual first lines of management. Orthopedic surgery may be indicated when one of the following conditions arises: (1) impending fracture, (2) pathological fracture, (3) spinal instability, or (4) spinal cord or cauda equina compression.

Impending fracture

By the time a large, lytic bony metastasis is visible on an x-ray film, considerable involvement and destruction of the bony cortex has occurred, and the risk of fracture is high. Pain is usually present. Radiation therapy may not be the best choice for large lesions because it may temporarily weaken the bone and increase fracture risk. Primary surgical stabilization of the bone, followed by radiation, may be advantageous as internal fixation is easier when the bone is intact.

Orthopedic surgeons are attempting to define which patients with bone metastases would benefit from surgical treatment to prevent painful fractures.[10] Mirels proposed a scoring system for estimating the risk of fracture based on the site of a metastasis, severity of pain, radiographic appearance, and size of the lesion;[11] this system appears to be better than clinical judgment alone.[12] A recent randomized trial of radiation versus surgery for bony metastases of the femur recommended surgery if the axial cortical involvement was >30 mm; otherwise, radiation therapy was recommended.[13]

Pathological fracture

Breast cancer is the most common cancer-related cause of fracture, followed by myeloma, lung cancer, prostate cancer, and renal cell cancer. The most common site of pathological fracture is the long bone of the femur, but a fracture can occur in any bone. In one large series of breast cancer patients, surgical treatment of bone metastases decreased pain postoperatively in 77% of patients, and increased function in 65%.[14] Unlike in trauma patients, the vast majority of these fractures will not heal for a variety of reasons. This results in a high rate of fixation failure after surgical stabilization. In one series, the overall rate of failure of fixation was 11%, and it was 20%–24% in diaphyseal fractures and distal femur metastases, resulting in additional operations, complications, and loss of function.[15] Recognition of this fact has resulted in improvements in the surgical treatment of cancer-related pathological fractures. These include intermedullary fixation or bone prostheses rather than splinting to allow rapid return to function and hardware that provides permanent support rather than depending on the bone to heal for strength; such improvements have reduced failure rates to 2%.[10] Local irradiation 12–14 days postoperatively does not interfere with fracture healing, provided the fracture is adequately stabilized.

Spinal instability

Spinal instability may result from widespread vertebral metastases and cause pain so severe that the patient is unable to sit, stand, or walk. No discrete fracture of the vertebrae is seen, but there is destruction of bone with vertebral collapse. The pain is due to instability, and surgical stabilization is required for pain relief. The spine can be stabilized by either an anterior or posterior approach.

Spinal cord or cauda equina decompression

Spinal cord or cauda equina compression occurs in 5%–20% of patients with vertebral metastases.[16] It may occur with spinal instability or in isolation. Treatment depends on the duration, severity, and rapidity of the onset of symptoms. Pain is usually the first manifestation, and is frequently localized to the site of the disease, followed by motor dysfunction, weakness, paresthesia, and sensory loss. When spinal cord compression is suspected, urgent investigation with magnetic resonance imaging or CT myelography followed by surgical decompression is critical. Spinal decompression is indicated for a patient with a recent onset of symptoms, particularly paraplegia or urinary retention of less than 24 hours, spinal compression localized to no more than three segments, and a life expectancy of at least 3 months. The spine must be stabilized at the time of decompression; laminectomy alone is contraindicated, as it will cause spinal instability with increasing kyphosis, increasing pain, and neurologic deficit.

▶ Neurosurgical procedures

Neurosurgical procedures for pain relief are no longer commonly used because of the effectiveness of pharmacologic and less-invasive interventional techniques. However, neurosurgical procedures may be considered when all else has failed to control pain; the severity of the pain warrants surgery, and there are no medical contraindications to the procedure.

For cancer patients, neurosurgical pain relief procedures are usually ablative, involving division or destruction of the nerves responsible for the pain. A procedure should be undertaken only if disruption of the nerve is likely to help in pain control. The lowest or most peripheral point relative to the location of the pain is usually the most appropriate site for the procedure. Nociceptive pain is the most responsive to ablative techniques; however, the presence of pain other than nociceptive pain should not rule out the procedure, as the ablative techniques may provide enough pain control to enable effective pharmacological management of the remaining pain.[17] Because both motor and sensory fibers overlap in a single nerve, even select division of a nerve may result in significant motor and sensory disturbances.

Peripheral neurectomy

Destruction of the nerves may be accomplished by various modalities, including destruction by radiofrequency ablation, chemical neurolysis, or open techniques. Chest wall pain due to a paraspinal tumor involving a nerve at or distal to the neural foramen can be effectively relieved by peripheral neurectomy, as the resulting motor loss is relatively insignificant.[18] A body of evidence demonstrates benefit from ablation of the trigeminal or glossopharyngeal nerves in patients with head and neck cancers.[19]

Neurolytic celiac plexus blockade (NCPB) has been shown to prevent or significantly relieve severe pain in 70%–90% of patients with pancreatic cancer in several randomized trials and should be considered for all patients whose tumors are believed to be incurable.[20–22] In NCPB, neurolytic agents (50% ethanol, 6% phenol, or absolute alcohol) are injected on either side of the aorta at the level of the celiac plexus. In one randomized trial, pain relief was reported in 85% of patients postoperatively; although two-thirds of patients had return of pain before death, pain scores remained lower when compared to patients who did not receive NCPB.[21] NCPB also prevented the development of severe pancreatic pain in patients without pain at time of laparotomy. Interestingly, an increased survival time was also found for those who received NCPB.

Pain due to any tumor involving the celiac plexus will respond to this technique. For patients not undergoing surgery, NCPB can be done percutaneously.[23,24] In a meta-analysis of 989 patients who received NCPB percutaneously, pain was relieved in 89% of patients initially and in 70%–90% until death.[20] NCPB decreases narcotic requirements, adds little morbidity, and may increase survival.

Hypophysectomy

Hypophysectomy involves ablation or destruction of the pituitary gland through a stereotactic transsphenoidal approach and has been used to manage severe pain from diffuse bone metastases in cancer patients. The mechanism of this pain relief is not understood but may be stimulation of the hypothalamic pain-suppressing capability. Although hypophysectomy is not commonly performed, a recent study has demonstrated benefit in select patients.[25]

Cordotomy

Cordotomy involves division of the anterolateral quadrant of the spinal cord, which contains the spinothalamic tract. The procedure results in selective loss of temperature and pain perception on the contralateral side several segments below the level of the division. Cordotomy may be useful to treat well-localized, unilateral, lower extremity or perineal pain due to direct nerve plexus invasion by rectal or gynecological cancers. The procedure may be done percutaneously or with an open technique.[26]

SURGICAL DECISION-MAKING

▶ Selection of procedure

The surgeon may select from a wide spectrum of palliative surgical procedures, with differing levels of invasiveness, anesthetic requirements, technical complexity, and attendant risk. The decision of which option to recommend is dependent on the disease process, the anatomy of the region of interest (guided by imaging studies), the risk-benefit ratio for the procedure, and the available technical expertise. Developments in the fields of minimally invasive surgery and interventional radiology have been of particular importance as they may be associated with lower morbidity compared to open procedures. It should be noted that laparoscopy in the abdomen requires the use of a general and paralyzing anesthetic, which may be a major contributor to morbidity. Generally, the most minimally invasive effective procedure is chosen so as to result in the least discomfort, morbidity, and time in hospital. However, this should not result in withholding more invasive procedures in appropriately selected patients when these procedures will be more effective for the relief of symptoms.

An exploration of alternatives to surgery may avoid an operation. Examples include the use of photodynamic therapy to treat recurrent chest wall tumors,[27] laser therapy for recurrent head and neck cancers,[28] and stenting or laser ablation for intraluminal tumors causing obstruction.[2] Aggressive medical management of malignant bowel obstruction or the placement of a venting gastrostomy tube may allow patients with carcinomatosis to live without a nasogastric tube.[6]

▶ Selection of patients

An approach to the selection of patients who will benefit from palliative surgery considers the following: (1) disease factors, which require knowledge of the diagnosis, natural history of the cancer, and patient's prognosis; (2) physical factors, which include the patient's medical status, personality, expectations, and social supports; and (3) societal factors, which provide the cultural, ethical, legal, and economic context.

Disease factors

Determining the benefits and optimal timing of a palliative surgical intervention requires an understanding of the patient's underlying disease, particularly its natural history, treatment, and the symptoms it produces. An understanding of the prognosis of a particular patient, as well as the other options for palliative therapy, is essential. It may be reasonable to consider a palliative pelvic resection for pain in a patient with recurrent anal cancer, for example, if he or she has had a long disease-free interval, and lung and liver metastases that have responded to chemotherapy; in contrast, such a decision may not be reasonable for a patient who presents with pelvic pain from local recurrence and widespread metastases several months after the initial potentially curative treatment. While resection may be technically feasible, surgery is a local treatment only, and aggressive surgical therapy will not alter the systemic progression of disease. Knowledge of the natural history of the disease may also allow

the anticipation of complications, enabling earlier and potentially less morbid procedures. Operative morbidity and mortality rates are significantly higher after emergency rather than scheduled procedures.[29] Colonic resection in metastatic colorectal cancer, for example, is often offered to patients with obstructive symptoms to prevent acute obstruction, while recognizing that this will not alter the progression of metastatic disease.

An assessment of prognosis is essential to determine a risk/benefit ratio for the proposed surgical intervention. It is often helpful to discuss the anticipated disease course with the primary physician caring for the patient, especially the patient's response to and future eligibility for anticancer therapy. Studies of the ability of physicians to predict prognosis in advanced cancer patients have yielded mixed results. A prospective study found that clinicians estimated prognosis quite accurately when asked whether or not a patient with terminal cancer was expected to live 6 months.[30] In another study of terminal cancer patients, however, treating physicians tended to overestimate the survival of patients and, in particular, failed to predict who would die within 2 months.[31] Several clinical prognostic indices have been developed for terminal cancer patients; these combine objective clinical criteria such as weight loss and performance status (patient function) with clinician estimates.[32,33] Other less well-defined factors also impact on prognosis. In one study, extent of disease and quality of life together predicted survival better than each parameter alone in patients with breast cancer.[34] In another study, symptom distress alone predicted survival in lung cancer patients.[35]

Advances in medical therapy may significantly alter the natural history of disease. The dramatic improvement in survival for patients with gastrointestinal stromal tumor (GIST) with the use of imatinib is a recent example. Palliative surgical procedures may now also be contemplated, although it was not a rational option in the past. Surgeons must keep aware of such advances in therapy.

Physical factors

As with any operation, the patient's overall physical status is an important consideration when deciding on the magnitude of an intervention and the patient's operative risk. An assessment of the risk of operative morbidity and mortality is of major importance. This risk is a function of the degree to which the surgery disrupts normal physiologic function, the choice of anesthetic, the technical complexity of the procedure, and the general health status of the patient and his or her ability to withstand operative trauma. Factors known to increase operative risk include increased age, the presence of underlying cardiac, renal, hepatic, or respiratory disease; poor performance status; and concurrent illness, such as sepsis, anemia, and uncontrolled metabolic abnormalities. The preoperative assessment score using the American Society of Anesthesiologists Classification of Physical Status correlates well with postoperative mortality.[36]

Asthenia, anorexia, and cachexia are common interrelated systemic symptoms that occur in many terminally ill cancer patients, and all may contribute to the weakness and weight loss seen with advanced illness. Patients with these symptoms have significantly higher complication and mortality rates after surgical intervention.[37] Decreased mobility from asthenia results in increased postoperative pulmonary complications. Anorexia leads to decreased oral intake, and the resultant malnutrition affects healing and immune function. If cachexia is present, the anabolism required for healing and immune function is further impaired. The presence of these symptoms preoperatively should caution against aggressive surgical intervention.

Psychosocial factors

Since the goals of the procedure are the relief of suffering and improvement in quality of life, the patient's own perceptions and wishes are perhaps the most crucial determinants in procedure selection. A patient's decisions will be shaped by his or her personality, education, social situation, finances, religious beliefs, culture, employment, and personal relationships. Some time must be spent getting to know what is important to the patient. A few directed questions may be helpful, such as "Of all the symptoms that you have, which one bothers you the most?" and "If I were able to fix this symptom for you, would this significantly improve your life?" Since every procedure carries with it potential morbidity, only those procedures that will potentially improve symptoms important to the patient should be performed.

Patient treatment choices are also determined by what the patient and family understand about the disease and prognosis. Weeks et al. found that the patients' decisions about whether to undergo aggressive therapy were related to their perception of their own survival.[30] Cancer patients tended to overestimate their life expectancy; those who believed that there was at least a 10% chance that they would die within 6 months were more likely to favor less aggressive therapies. A patient's acceptance (or not) of his or her own mortality will shape the tone of the discussion. Psychiatric conditions must also be kept in mind; Chochinov et al. found that patients who did not acknowledge their prognosis (9.5% of 200 advanced cancer patients) were almost three times more likely to be clinically depressed than those who did.[38]

Societal factors

Treatment options are influenced by the economic, cultural, socioeconomic, ethical, and legal environment in which the patient, family, and physician reside. The choice of procedure will be affected by the available community and personal resources available. These factors include the location where the patient is cared for after the procedure (hospital, hospice, or home), the expertise of the caregivers (nurse, family, palliative care physicians, or home healthcare aids), and the equipment available (e.g., portable pain pumps or ostomy equipment). A procedure should make ongoing care as easy as possible for the patient and the caregivers. For example, an external drainage tube may be less invasive but will require management of a drainage bag; an internal stent placement may be more invasive but may require less care. Cost of the intervention may be a consideration for some families.

▶ Pharmacological Pain Management during Palliative Surgical Interventions

Cancer patients undergoing palliative procedures may already be receiving appropriate but high doses of narcotics and other pain medications. Patients who undergo an effective surgical intervention will require reassessment of their pain medications after the palliative procedure. The doses, especially of the long-acting medications, may need to be titrated down and provisions made to allow for appropriate doses of breakthrough medications until a new threshold is attained. This is especially important after interventions that offer rapid relief, such as paracentesis for malignant ascites or biliary decompression by endoscopic or percutaneous stent placement.

Another concern is that the high preoperative dosages of pain medication that patients require may complicate the postoperative course, especially in hospitals that also treat noncancer patients. The additional pain medications needed for postoperative pain may result in dosages that are so high that physicians used to managing routine postoperative pain may become uncomfortable. For this reason, in our institutions, it is routine to ask the palliative care pain service to manage both pre- and postoperative pain in advanced cancer patients.

CLINICAL EXAMPLES

▶ Soft tissue metastases from lung cancer

A 67-year-old woman with metastatic nonsmall cell lung cancer had just completed a course of palliative chemotherapy, and her lung lesions were stable. She had, however, developed a soft tissue metastasis on her anterior abdominal wall (Fig. 19-1), and the lesion continued to grow despite chemotherapy. Local irradiation was tried with no effect and she was referred for consideration of metastatectomy.

Her projected survival was at least 6 months, her performance status was good, and she had no other major medical problems. The tumor on her abdominal wall was the major source of her complaints. As the tumor grew, it became more painful, and she required increasing doses of narcotics, which affected her concentration and level of alertness. In addition, the tumor was beginning to produce increasing odor and discharge, which made her reluctant to participate in social events and to leave her house. After extensive discussion, it was decided to remove her abdominal wall tumor, recognizing that this would have no effect on the overall progress of her disease. The defect in the abdominal muscles was replaced with a plastic mesh and a large skin flap was mobilized to cover the skin defect (Fig. 19-2). She went home 7 days postoperatively and was able to stop taking pain medication. Five months later, she developed increasing weakness and shortness of breath due to disease progression and resumed palliative chemotherapy. She died 18 months later with no problematic soft tissue recurrence.

A 75-year-old man was referred for consideration of surgical resection of a painful soft tissue metastasis from lung cancer on his back (Fig. 19-3). He had finished chemotherapy and radiation, and his primary lung cancer was stable. Radiation therapy had been

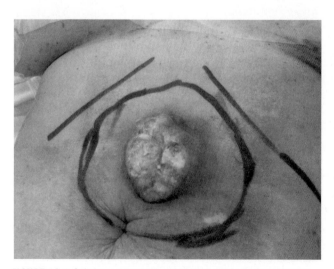

FIGURE 19-1 Soft tissue metastasis on abdominal wall from metastatic lung cancer. The patient had pain controlled by pain medication; equally distressing was the odor and discharge from the wound which is preventing her from leaving her house.

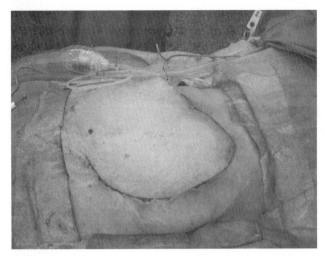

FIGURE 19-2 The tumor was resected, the abdominal wall defect replaced with prosthetic mesh, and skin and soft tissue of the remaining abdominal wall moved to cover the skin defect.

given to the soft tissue metastasis with no effect. However, he had just recovered from his second diagnosis of pneumonia; he was short of breath, and had a chronic cough. In addition, examination of his chest wall revealed multiple soft tissue metastases, including a large axillary metastasis. When the surgeon first saw the patient, the

mass on his back was the only one that was symptomatic. Technically, the mass could have been removed and the defect closed with a skin flap. However, over a short period of time, the other masses began to enlarge and became symptomatic. In addition, his anesthetic risk was believed to be high because of his poor respiratory status. Surgical resection was not offered and he underwent further palliative chemotherapy with some improvement in the pain from the metastasis.

▶ Resection of axillary and groin metastases

A 56-year-old woman with slowly growing lung cancer had a recurrence in the lung that was stable on chemotherapy. In addition, she had an axillary metastasis (Fig. 19-4) that was growing despite local radiation therapy, causing her pain and limiting her movement. Her performance status was excellent, and she was otherwise well. An axillary dissection was performed. Tumor was found close to but not involving the brachial plexus. Because the axilla had been previously irradiated, the soft tissue in the area was replaced with a latissimus dorsi musculocutaneous flap (Fig. 19-5). She did very well; 1 year later (Fig. 19-6), she had no pain in her arm and she was able to play golf. Her lung lesions were growing, however, and her chemotherapy regimen was changed.

A 70-year-old man with metastatic anal cancer had undergone an abdominal-perineal resection 1 year earlier to remove his primary cancer after it had not responded to chemotherapy. He had lung metastases that had not changed for 9 months and a lymph node metastasis in the groin that remained stable for 6 months but now was growing (Fig. 19-7). His main complaint was neuropathic pain radiating into his scrotum; the pain was poorly controlled with pain

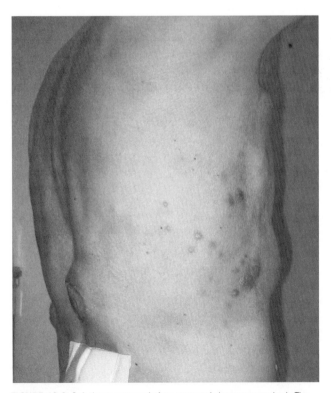

FIGURE 19-3 Soft tissue metastasis from metastatic lung cancer to back. The large metastasis on the patient's back was very painful. However, there were a number of other lesions on the patient's abdominal wall that were growing rapidly. In addition, the patient's respiratory status was poor, significantly increasing the risk of anesthesia. This patient was not offered surgical resection.

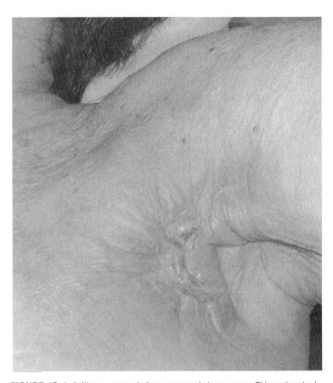

FIGURE 19-4 Axillary metastasis from metastatic lung cancer. This patient had slow growing lung cancer, whose recurrence in the lung was stable on chemotherapy. The axillary metastasis, however, was growing despite local radiation therapy, causing her pain and limiting her movement.

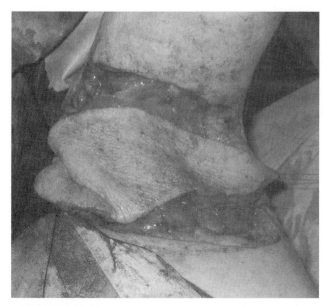

FIGURE 19-5 An axillary dissection was performed. Tumor was found close to but not involving the brachial plexus. Because the axilla had been previously radiated, the soft tissue in the area was replaced with a latissimus dorsi flap mobilized by a plastic surgeon.

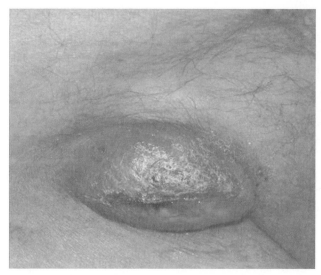

FIGURE 19-7 Groin metastasis from metastatic anal cancer. This patient has metastatic anal cancer with metastases to the lung, and this groin node, which is enlarging. His biggest complaint was neuropathic pain in his scrotum.

medication. On imaging studies, the tumor appeared to be separate from the femoral artery and vein. After careful discussion with patient and family, the patient was taken to the operating room for a resection of the groin metastasis and a lateral thigh flap for closure of the skin defect. Unfortunately, the tumor was more extensive than predicted and could not be completely resected. Although the patient's scrotal pain disappeared for several weeks, he became rapidly weaker and died within 2 months from his disease progression.

CONCLUSION

The decision to offer any surgical procedure to a patient must balance the potential benefits of the intervention with the inevitable risks of postsurgical pain and complications. This is particularly important for a patient who is suffering from a terminal illness. For a surgeon, trained to intervene, a decision to operate is often the easiest one to make. The true skill of the surgeon as physician, however, lies in the careful selection and preparation of patients who will benefit from a surgical procedure, as well as a continued commitment to the care of patients for whom surgery is not selected. The question that must be answered is not "Can this operation be done?" but rather "Should this operation be done for this patient at this time?"

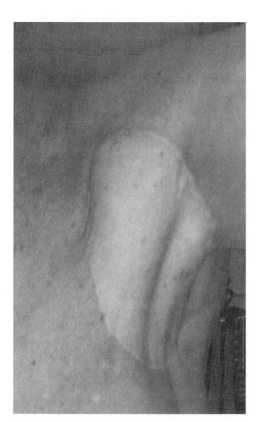

FIGURE 19-6 The axilla 1 year after an axillary dissection. Skin was removed along with the tumor and replaced with a latissimus dorsi flap from the back. She has no pain in her arm and she is able to play golf. Her lung lesions are growing, however, and her chemotherapy has been changed.

REFERENCES

1. Friel JP, ed. *Dorland's Illustrated Medical Dictionary*. 26th ed. Philadelphia: W.B. Saunders; 1985.
2. Easson AM, Asch M, Swallow CJ. Palliative general surgical procedures. *Surg Onc Clin N Am*. 2001;10:161–184.
3. McCahill LE, Krouse RS, Chu DZ, et al. Decision making in palliative surgery. *J Am Coll Surg*. 2002;195:411–422.
4. International Association for the Study of Pain. Classification of chronic pain. *Pain*. 1986(Suppl. 3):51.
5. Finlayson CA, Eisenberg BL. Palliative pelvic exenteration: patient selection and results. *Oncology (Williston Park)*. 1996;10:479–484.
6. Krouse RS, McCahill LE, Easson AM, et al. When the sun can set on an unoperated bowel obstruction: management of malignant bowel obstruction. *J Am Coll Surg*. 2002;195:117–128.

7. Pollak JS, Burdge CM, Rosenblatt M, et al. Treatment of malignant pleural effusions with tunneled long-term drainage catheters. *J Vasc Interv Radiol.* 2001;12:201–208.

8. Parsons SL, Lang MW, Steele RJ. Malignant ascites: a 2-year review from a teaching hospital. *Eur J Surg Oncol.* 1996;22:237–239.

9. Adam RA, Adam YG. Malignant ascites: past, present, and future. *J Am Coll Surg.* 2004;198:999–1011.

10. Cady B, Easson A, Aboulafia AJ, et al. Part 1: Surgical palliation of advanced illness—what's new, what's helpful. *J Am Coll Surg.* 2005;200: 115–127.

11. Mirels H. Metastatic disease in long bones: a proposed scoring system for diagnosing impending pathologic fractures. *Clin Orthop Relat Res.* 1989;249:256.

12. Damron TA, Morgan H, Prakash D, et al. Critical evaluation of Mirels' rating system for impending pathologic fractures. *Clin Orthop Relat Res.* 2003;(Suppl. 415):S201–S207.

13. Van der Linden YM, Dijkstra PD, Kroon HM, et al. Comparative analysis of risk factors for pathological fracture with femoral metastases. *J Bone Joint Surg Br.* 2004;86:566–573.

14. Wedin R, Bauer HC, Rutqvist LE. Surgical treatment for skeletal breast cancer metastases: a population-based study of 641 patients. *Cancer.* 2001;92:257–262.

15. Wedin R, Bauer HC, Wersall P. Failures after operation for skeletal metastatic lesions of long bones. *Clin Orthop Relat Res.* 1999;358:128–139.

16. Galasko CSB. Orthopedic principles and management. In: Doyle D, Hanks G, MacDonald N, eds. *Oxford Textbook of Palliative Medicine, 2nd ed.* Oxford: Oxford University Press; 1999:477.

17. Arbit E, Bilksy MH. Neurosurgical approaches in palliative care. In: Doyle D, Hanks G, MacDonald N, eds. *Oxford Textbook of Palliative Medicine, 2nd ed.* Oxford: Oxford University Press; 1999:414.

18. Arbit E, Galicich JH, Burt M, et al. Modified open thoracic rhizotomy for treatment of intractable chest wall pain of malignant etiology. *Ann Thorac Surg.* 1989;48:820–823.

19. Rozen TD. Trigeminal neuralgia and glossopharyngeal neuralgia. *Neurol Clin.* 2004;22:185–206.

20. Eisenberg E, Carr DB, Chalmers TC. Neurolytic celiac plexus block for treatment of cancer pain: a meta-analysis. *Anesth Analg.* 1995;80: 290–295.

21. Lillemoe KD, Cameron JL, Kaufman HS, et al. Chemical splanchnicectomy in patients with unresectable pancreatic cancer. A prospective randomized trial. *Ann Surg.* 1993;217:447–455.

22. Polati E, Finco G, Gottin L, et al. Prospective randomized double-blind trial of neurolytic coeliac plexus block in patients with pancreatic cancer. *Br J Surg.* 1998;85:199–201.

23. Le Pimpec Barthes F, Chapuis O, Riquet M, et al. Thoracoscopic splanchnicectomy for control of intractable pain in pancreatic cancer. *Ann Thorac Surg.* 1998;65:810–813.

24. Saenz A, Kuriansky J, Salvador L, et al. Thoracoscopic splanchnicectomy for pain control in patients with unresectable carcinoma of the pancreas. *Surg Endosc.* 2000;14:717–720.

25. Hayashi M, Taira T, Chernov M, et al. Role of pituitary radiosurgery for the management of intractable pain and potential future applications. *Stereotact Funct Neurosurg.* 2003;81:75–83.

26. Jones B, Finlay I, Ray A, et al. Is there still a role for open cordotomy in cancer pain management? *J Pain Symptom Manage.* 2003;25:179–184.

27. Taber SW, Fingar VH, Wieman TJ. Photodynamic therapy for palliation of chest wall recurrence in patients with breast cancer. *J Surg Oncol.* 1998;68(4):209.

28. Paiva MB, Blackwell KE, Saxton RE, et al. Nd:YAG laser therapy for palliation of recurrent squamous cell carcinomas in the oral cavity. *Lasers Surg Med.* 2002;31:64–69.

29. Cohen MM, Duncan PG, Tate RB. Does anesthesia contribute to operative mortality? *JAMA.* 1988;260:2859–2863.

30. Weeks JC, Cook EF, O'Day SJ, et al. Relationship between cancer patients' predictions of prognosis and their treatment preferences. *JAMA.* 1998;279:1709–1714.

31. Vigano A, Bruera E, Jhangri GS, et al. Clinical survival predictors in patients with advanced cancer. *Arch Intern Med.* 2000;160:861–868.

32. Sloan JA, Loprinzi CL, Laurine JA, et al. A simple stratification factor prognostic for survival in advanced cancer: the good/bad/uncertain index. *J Clin Oncol.* 2001;19:3539–3546.

33. Morita T, Tsunoda J, Inoue S, et al. Improved accuracy of physicians' survival prediction for terminally ill cancer patients using the Palliative Prognostic Index. *Palliat Med.* 2001;15:419–424.

34. Seidman AD, Portenoy R, Yao TJ, et al. Quality of life in phase II trials: a study of methodology and predictive value in patients with advanced breast cancer treated with paclitaxel plus granulocyte colony-stimulating factor. *J Natl Cancer Inst.* 1995;87:1316–1322.

35. Degner LF, Sloan JA. Symptom distress in newly diagnosed ambulatory cancer patients and as a predictor of survival in lung cancer. *J Pain Symptom Manage.* 1995;10:423–431.

36. Prause G, Offner A, Ratzenhofer-Komenda B, et al. Comparison of two preoperative indices to predict perioperative mortality in non-cardiac thoracic surgery. *Eur J Cardiothorac Surg.* 1997;11:670–675.

37. Fearon KC, Barber MD, Moses AG. The cancer cachexia syndrome. *Surg Oncol Clin N Am.* 2001;10:109–126.

38. Chochinov HM, Tataryn DJ, Wilson KG, et al. Prognostic awareness and the terminally ill. *Psychosomatics.* 2000;41:500–504.

Palliative Radiation Therapy Techniques

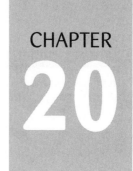

Nora Janjan, Sunil Krishnan, Prajnan Das
M. Spencer Gould, Joan Zampieri, Christopher Crane
Marc Delclos, Charles Cleeland
Stephen T. Lutz, Edward Chow

Within this decade, 11 million cases of cancer were diagnosed and 5 million people have died from cancer worldwide. Prognosis is influenced by the overall metastatic burden, and the number and location of the sites involved by disease. When metastases are found in the lung, liver, and/or central nervous system, the prognosis is especially poor.[1–10]

The demographics for cancer are changing because of effective screening procedures and are exemplified in prostate and breast cancers. Prostate cancer is the second leading cause of death from cancer among men; more than 1 million men >50 years of age in the United States die of prostate cancer.[11–13] Because of an aging population and screening, the incidence of prostate cancer is increasing significantly. However, the clinical presentation of prostate cancer has changed in the past 20 years with routine use of digital rectal examination (DRE) and prostate-specific antigen (PSA) screening. In the 1970s, only 50% of such cancers were confined to the prostate gland, and metastases were present in 30% of cases at diagnosis. When patients are referred to an urologist for symptoms, only 70% of cases have disease confined to the prostate gland. However, with routine screening using DRE and PSA, more than 90% of cases have disease confined to the gland.

The risk for the subsequent development of distant metastases is significantly lower when the primary tumor is controlled. Survival rates after an isolated recurrence of disease in prostate cancer are influenced by the initial stage of the disease and the disease-free interval from the time of initial treatment.[12–15] In greater than 70% of cases of locally recurrent prostate cancer, radiation can control symptoms that include hematuria, urinary outflow obstruction, ureteral obstruction, and lower extremity edema.[12–15] With or without local recurrence, the survival rate is most compromised by the presence of distant metastases. The survival rates at 5 years and 10 years after pelvic recurrence alone equal 50% and 22%, respectively. With distant metastases, the survival rate at 5 years is 20% and less than 5% at 10 years.[13] Pain is the presenting symptom in only 11% of newly diagnosed prostate cancer patients.[6,7,14] However, pain develops in 75% of prostate cancer patients during the course of their disease.[14] Radiographically identified bone metastases develop in 20% of patients with stage A_2 (T_{1b}) and B (T_2) disease, in 40% of patients with stage C (T_3), and in 62% of patients with stage D_1 (T_4) disease presentations.[6,13,15]

SITE-SPECIFIC PALLIATIVE RADIATION

The site and volume of tumor involvement are the most important considerations in the development of a palliative radiation treatment plan because of the radiation tolerance of adjacent normal tissues to treatment. Unlike the comprehensive radiation treatment portals used in curative therapy that include adjacent lymph node regions, palliative radiation generally only encompasses the radiographically evident tumor volume. Radiation treatment planning must minimize possible toxicities, and account for prior courses of radiation. Toxicities are reduced by limiting the volume irradiated, and through the application of dosimetric principles that reduce integral dose.

▶ Localized bone metastases

Radiation of localized bone metastases relieves symptoms and helps prevent pathologic fracture. There has been much controversy about palliative radiation schedules for localized symptomatic bone metastases. The Radiation Therapy Oncology Group (RTOG) conducted a prospective trial that included diverse treatment schedules. To account for prognosis, patients were stratified on the basis of whether they had a solitary or multiple sites of bony metastases. The initial analysis of the study concluded that low-dose, short-course treatment schedules were as effective as high-dose, protracted treatment programs.[16] For solitary bone metastases, there was no difference in the relief of pain when 20 gray (Gy) using 4 Gy fractions was compared to 40.5 Gy delivered as 2.7 Gy per fraction. In patients with multiple bone metastases, the following dose schedules were compared: 30 Gy at 3 Gy per fraction, 15 Gy given as 3 Gy per fraction, 20 Gy using 4 Gy per fraction, and 25 Gy using 5 Gy per fraction. No difference was identified in the rates of pain relief between these treatment schedules (Table 20-1). Partial relief of pain was achieved in 83%, and complete relief occurred in 53% of the patients studied. More than 50% of these patients developed recurrent pain, and 8% of patients developed a pathologic fracture rate.

In a reanalysis of the data, a different definition for complete pain relief was used and excluded the continued administration of analgesics. Using this definition, the relief of pain was significantly related to the number of fractions and the total dose of radiation that was administered.[17] Complete relief of pain was achieved in 55% of patients with solitary bone metastases who received 40.5 Gy at 2.7 Gy per fraction compared to 37% of patients who received a total dose of 20 Gy given as 4 Gy per fraction. A similar relationship was observed in the reanalysis of patients who had multiple bone metastases. Complete relief of pain was achieved in 46% of patients who received 30 Gy at 3 Gy per fraction versus 28% of patients treated to 25 Gy using 5 Gy fractions.

Table 20-1

Dose Response Evaluation from the Reanalysis of the RTOG Bone Metastases Protocol

	Dose/fx (Gy)	Total Dose(Gy)	Tumor Dose at 2 Gy/fx	CR	p Value
Solitary bone mets					p <0.0003
	2.7	40.5	42.9	55%	
	4.0	20.0	23.3	37%	
Multiple bone mets					p <0.0003
	3.0	30	32.5	46%	
	3.0	15.0	16.2	36%	
	4.0	20.0	23.3	40%	
	5.0	25.0	31.25	28%	

Note: Listed are the dose per fraction (dose/fx), total radiation dose, the radiobiological equivalent dose if administered at 2 Gy/fx, the complete response rate (CR) using the definition that excludes the use of analgesics and that accounts for retreatment.
Source: From Tong D, Gillick L, Hendrickson FR. The palliation of symptomatic osseous metastases: final results of the Study by the Radiation Therapy Oncology Group. Cancer. 1982;50:893–899.

Table 20-2

Percentage of Patients Who Responded to Radiation Relative to Time, Designated in Weeks after Completion of Radiation Therapy

Total Dose (Gy)	Dose per Fraction (Gy)	Tumor Dose at 2 Gy/fx	<2	Weeks 2–4	Post 4–12	XRT 12–20
Solitary mets						
40.5	2.7	42.9	7%	29%	53%	77%
20.0	4	23.3	16%	50%	66%	82%
Multiple mets						
30.0	3	32.5	19%	48%	73%	84%
15.0	3	16.2	34%	70%	84%	93%
20.0	4	23.3	28%	53%	75%	88%
25.0	5	31.25	22%	41%	72%	80%

Note: This prospective trial, conducted by the RTOG, randomized radiation dose and number of fractions and stratified the randomization on the basis of solitary or multiple bone metastases. Also listed is the radiobiological equivalent dose if administered at 2 Gy per fraction.
Source: From Serafini AN, Houston SJ, Resche I, et al. Palliation of pain associated with metastatic bone cancer using samarium-153 lexidronam: a double-blind placebo-controlled clinical trial. J Clin Oncol. 1998;16:1574–1581; Rogers CL, Speiser BL, Ram PC, et al. Efficacy and toxicity of intravenous strontium-89 for symptomatic osseous metastases. J Brachytherapy Int. 1998;14:133–142.

Three important issues are identified from this RTOG experience. First, the results of the reanalysis demonstrate the importance of carefully defining what represents a response to therapy. Second, this revised definition of response showed that the total radiation dose did influence the degree to which pain was relieved.[16,17] Third, the RTOG experience identified the amount of time that was needed to experience relief of pain after irradiation for bone metastases (Table 20-2). It is important to note that only 50% of the patients who were going to respond had relief of symptoms at 2–4 weeks after radiation.[16,17] This finding underscores the need for continued analgesic support after completing radiation therapy. It consistently required 12–20 weeks after irradiation to accomplish the maximal level of relief. That period of time may reflect the time needed for reossification.

Radiographic evidence of recalcification is observed in about 25% of cases, and 70% of the time recalcification is seen within 6 months of completing radiation and other palliative therapies.[18–20] Therefore, it is critical to determine the time and parameters of response. Pretreatment characteristics can also influence the level of response. Neuropathic pain is a significant clinical variable that reduces the response to palliative radiation.[21–23]

The parameters of response to palliative treatment also are multifactorial. In one study, 49 patients, with an ECOG score of 1 received palliative radiation therapy (20 Gy in 5 fractions) and were evaluated every 2 weeks for 2 months. Treatment was most commonly administered to the pelvis (43%) and lumbar spine (17%), and 16% of the group had more than one site irradiated. The majority of patients had improvements in their pain scores.[24] Four weeks after completing radiation, 37% of patients were taking more analgesics than at baseline (flare reaction), but analgesic requirements subsequently declined in most patients. By week four, 63% were more active, and 83% had functional improvement by week eight. Quality of life improved in 42% by week four and was stable or improved in all patients by week eight. Overall response to palliative radiation for bone metastases equaled 67%, with 37% having a partial response and 30% having a complete response at 12 weeks.[25] But when the pain scores were integrated with the analgesic requirements, the overall response rate declined to 45%. Because most patients have multiple sites of metastatic disease, a decline in analgesic requirements does not represent a good index of response to localized radiation.

At consultation, the pain levels among 518 patients were classified as moderate in 31% and severe in 45%, but 34% of these patients had no analgesics or only codeine was prescribed for their pain.[26] However, 87% of 2132 bone metastases patients, and 71% of patients without bone metastases received opioids at some point during their final year of life. Corresponding figures for the use of long-acting opioids were 53% and 24%. Long-acting opioids were used for more than 25% of the days in the outpatient setting of patients with bone metastases during their last year of life.[27] In comparison, patients without bone metastases only used long-acting opioids for 14% of the days they lived in the outpatient setting. However, during the last month of life, 61% of bone metastases patients and 29% of patients with metastatic cancer to sites other than bone needed long-acting analgesics.

Therefore, functional parameters may prove more reliable than analgesic dose in evaluating response to palliative therapy. An international consensus on palliative radiotherapy endpoints for future clinical trials has been developed. Issues addressed involved the definition of pain relief relative to continued analgesic use, time to and duration of response, the need for reirradiation, and the validity and reliability of instruments used to assess symptoms.[28] Research is needed to determine the accuracy of pain reports from caregivers, what constitutes a partial response, better methods of predicting survival, and cost-effectiveness of treatment.

▶ Single fraction radiation

A single large radiation fraction is as effective in relieving pain as other radiation schedules that have more treatments. In more than 10 prospective randomized trials conducted in Europe, no difference was reported either in how quickly symptoms resolved or in the duration of pain relief when a single dose of radiation was compared to a radiation schedule with multiple radiation fractions.[29–45] In each case, symptom relief lasted 3 months in 70% of patients, 6 months in 37%, and 12 months in 20% of cases. Like the RTOG study, approximately 69% responded at 4 weeks, and response rates leveled off, totaling 80% at 8 weeks. Complete response rates after a single 8 Gy fraction totaled 15% at 2 weeks, 23% at 4 weeks, 28% at 8 weeks, and 39% at 12 weeks postirradiation. Because survival is determined by the location and number of sites of metastatic disease rather than the number of radiation fractions used for a localized area of disease, overall survival rates for a single fraction of radiation are equivalent to a course of palliative radiation with multiple fractions.

A meta-analysis of 18 prospective randomized trials evaluated three approaches to palliative radiation dose schedules. These three approaches to palliative radiation dose schedules included different doses of single-fraction radiation therapy. Comparisons among single-fraction versus multiple-fraction radiotherapy versus comparisons of different doses of multiple-fraction radiotherapy showed no difference in response rates based on radiotherapy dose given.[33] The median period of pain relief ranged between 11 and 24 weeks, and no difference was found in the 1–4 week median time to pain relief. There was a significant difference between remineralization of lytic lesions at 6 months follow-up, which was 173% after 30 Gy in 10 fractions compared to 120% after a single 8 Gy fraction, but the pretreatment and posttreatment risk of pathologic fracture was not determined.[45] Factors found retrospectively that influenced the use of a single versus multiple radiation fractions for bone metastases included patient's age, performance status, anatomic site, and year of radiation therapy.[44]

The RTOG also conducted a prospective randomized trial consisting of 949 breast and prostate cancer patients comparing 30 Gy in 10 fractions to a single 8 Gy fraction for bone metastases. The pretreatment characteristics of the 847 evaluable patients were equally balanced between treatment arms, including 56% having a weight-bearing painful site, 72% having severe pain, 27% who were receiving bisphosphonates, and 57% with a solitary painful site. Acute toxicity was mild, with a total of only 2 patients experiencing a grade-4 toxicity and 24 with a grade-3 toxicity.[43] But, there was significantly more grade-2 to grade-4 toxicity, 17% versus 10%, in the 30 Gy arm. Median survival was 9 months with 41% of patients alive at 1 year. No difference was observed in pain relief at 3 months. The rates of complete pain relief and partial pain relief were 15% and 50% for the 8 Gy arm, and 18% and 48% for the 30 Gy arm. At 3 months, one-third of patients no longer required analgesics.

A shorter radiation schedule, like a single fraction, is advantageous for patients with poor prognostic factors. First, it is easier for patients with a poor Karnofsky Performance Status score to complete therapy. Second, response and survival rates are equal for single and multifraction therapy at 3 months because median survival is less than 6 months among patients with poor prognostic factors and average around 24 months among patients with metastatic disease.[33,34,37,38,40,41,44] This is an important consideration when the number of weeks of survival is evaluated relative to the number of weeks of palliative treatment. Third, the option of retreatment after a single fraction of radiation may also provide an advantage for patients with good prognostic factors as a means to periodically reduce tumor burden and control symptoms in noncritical anatomic sites. Fourth, a single fraction of radiation is more cost-effective. The cost of radiation therapy is reduced by 41% with the use of a single fraction of radiation therapy compared to a 10-fraction course of palliative radiation. The cost of radiation therapy is less expensive than the continued cost of analgesics.[46] An analysis of a Dutch prospective study showed cost benefit for a single fraction of radiation versus multiple radiation fractions, even when retreatment is included in the single fraction arm, versus continued use of analgesics.[40,41]

Metastatic cancer is now being treated as a chronic disease. Treatment is given to prevent or relieve symptoms of the disease. None of the radiation schedules used for palliation eradicates the disease, and symptoms will recur with regrowth of the tumor. Reirradiation for persistent or recurrent pain is often precluded when higher radiation doses are administered, but reirradiation is possible after a single fraction of radiation.[29,30,32,47,48] Reirradiation was necessary in 25% of patients who received a single 8 Gy radiation fraction, but all of these patients were reported to respond to the second dose of radiation. When a single fraction of 4 Gy was compared to a single 8 Gy fraction, the rate of response was slightly lower and fewer acute radiation reactions were noted, but a greater proportion of patients required reirradiation.[31] With reirradiation, the overall rate of response was equivalent for 8 Gy and 4 Gy fractions. A single fraction of radiation can then be repeatedly used to suppress symptoms when they recur.

The projected length of survival is the critical issue for radiation dose selected and for establishing the schedule of palliative radiation. In one study, only 12 of 245 patients were alive at the time of analysis, with approximately 50% alive at 6 months, 25% at 1 year, 8% at 2 years, and 3% at 3 years after palliative radiation. For breast cancer patients, the survival rates at these time points after palliative radiation were 60%, 44%, 20%, and 7%, respectively. For prostate cancer patients, the survival rates were 60% at 6 months, 24% at 1 year, and no patients survived at 2 years.[49] In the RTOG trial, the median survival for solitary bone metastases was 36 weeks and 24 weeks for multiple bone metastases.[16,17] The RTOG study also demonstrated that the level of pain correlated with prognosis among patients with multiple bone metastases. This survival difference may be an important observation because unrelieved pain and the resultant sequelae of immobility may contribute to mortality as well as morbidity.

The influence of improved control of pain on overall survival was demonstrated in a prospective randomized trial among 202 patients with intractable pain. Improved pain control was achieved in 85% of patients with intrathecal analgesics compared to 71% with optimized medical management.[50] Significantly less toxicity due to analgesic therapy occurred with intrathecal analgesics; compared to baseline, the toxicity rate decreased by 50% with intrathecal analgesics versus 17% for medical management. Intrathecal analgesics also were associated with decreases in fatigue and depression. With comparable stages of disease in the two groups, the overall survival at 6 months was 54% with intrathecal analgesics compared to 37% with optimized medical management. While performance status has long been associated with prognosis, this is one of the first studies to demonstrate how medical intervention to improve the performance status impacts survival.

For patients with metastatic disease, time is critical. The time under radiation needs to be considered as the opportunity cost of palliative treatment.[51] If the median survival of a patient with bone metastases is 6 months (180 days), the patient will spend 0.6% of remaining survival time under radiation treatment when a single fraction of radiation is given. If 10 radiation fractions are given, 8% of the remaining survival time will be expended, and if 20 fractions are prescribed 16% of the remaining survival time will be consumed by radiation therapy. Even if retreatment with a second single fraction is required, the patient will continue to spend about 1% of the survival time under radiation therapy. For lung cancer patients with a 3-month survival rate, 1% of the remaining time is spent with a single fraction of radiation compared to 16% if 10 fractions are given, or 30% if 20 fractions are prescribed.

Acute radiation toxicities are a function of the dose per fraction, total dose, and the area and volume of tissue irradiated. If mucosal surfaces like the upper aerodigestive tract, bowel, and bladder can be excluded from the radiation portals, acute radiation side effects can be significantly reduced whether a single or multiple fractions are prescribed. A more protracted course of radiation is still used for patients with good prognostic factors who require treatment of the spine and other critical sites.[37,44,52–58] But, for most patients who receive palliative radiation, a single fraction of radiation provides an efficient and effective therapeutic option.

▶ Pathologic fracture

The most significant morbidity of bone metastases relates to pathologic fracture and spinal cord compression. Pain that persists or that recurs after palliative radiation should be evaluated to exclude progression of disease, possible extension of disease outside the radiation portal that results in referred pain, and bone fracture. Reduced cortical strength can result in compression, stress, or microfractures associated with reduced cortical strength. Plain radiographs have a 91% concordance rate in detecting posttreatment disease progression and fractures compared to the 57% specificity rate of bone scans performed after radiotherapy.[19]

Pathologic fractures occur in about 20% of patients with bone metastases.[59–66] More than 80% of pathologic fractures occur in breast (50%), kidney, lung, and thyroid cancers. Proximal long bones are more commonly involved than distal bones. Consequently, pathologic fractures occur 50% of the time in the femur and 15% in the humerus (Fig. 20-1). The femoral neck and head are the most frequent locations for pathologic fracture because of the propensity for metastases to involve proximal bones and the stress of weight placed on this part of the femur. Patients with bone scan evidence of metastases in the femur or humerus at the time of diagnosis of bone metastases are significantly more likely to fracture these bones compared to other patients with bone metastases.[65] Pathologic fracture occurred in 1 of 8 patients with bone scan evidence of humeral disease

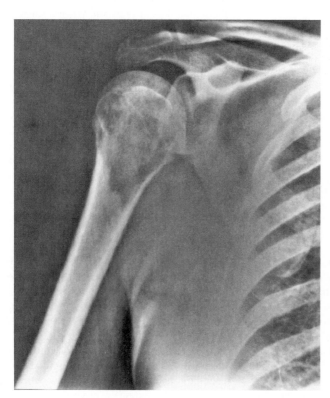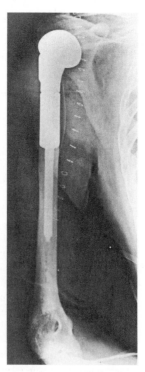

FIGURE 20-1 (A) An extensive lytic lesion in the proximal humerus; (B) prophylactic internal fixation was performed to prevent pathologic fracture. This patient, who complained primarily of pain in the hip, would have been placed on crutches to reduce stress on the involved femur. A bone scan and x-rays, obtained to exclude other sites of metastatic involvement, identified this lesion in the humerus. The humerus would have certainly fractured if all the patient's weight had been displaced to the upper extremities with crutches.

compared to 1 in 35 patients without humeral involvement at diagnosis of bone metastases. Presence of an abnormality on plain x-ray and bone scan did not place the patient at greater risk for fracture.

Approximately 20% of metastatic lesions in long bones develop a pathologic fracture that requires surgical intervention. Patients with pathologic fracture due to bone metastases have clinical outcomes following surgical repair that are comparable to patients sustaining a traumatic fracture.[59,61,62] Prognosis is generally poor if hypercalcemia is present and if parenteral narcotics are required to control pain from other sites of bone metastases; in these cases, the decision for surgical intervention should be based on the severity of and the symptoms associated with the fracture.[59,61,62] As shown in Fig. 20-2, postoperative radiation is often given after surgical fixation of a pathologic fracture to reduce the risk of progressive disease in the bone that could result in instability of the internal fixation.[61]

A retrospective analysis of 859 patients was performed that divided patients into 4 groups based on extent of disease at the time of diagnosis of bone metastases. These groups included bone metastases only, bone and soft tissue disease, bone and pleuropulmonary disease, and bone and liver disease. Survival from diagnosis of bone-only metastases was the longest of any group; the shortest survival was 5.5 months for patients with liver and bone metastases.[65] The time to vertebral fracture was the shortest for the bone-only metastases group, but there was no difference in the time to pathologic long-bone fractures. Because of an extended survival, most fractures occurred in the bone-only metastases group (17%) compared to a 5% risk for pathologic long-bone fracture in the bone and liver metastases group.

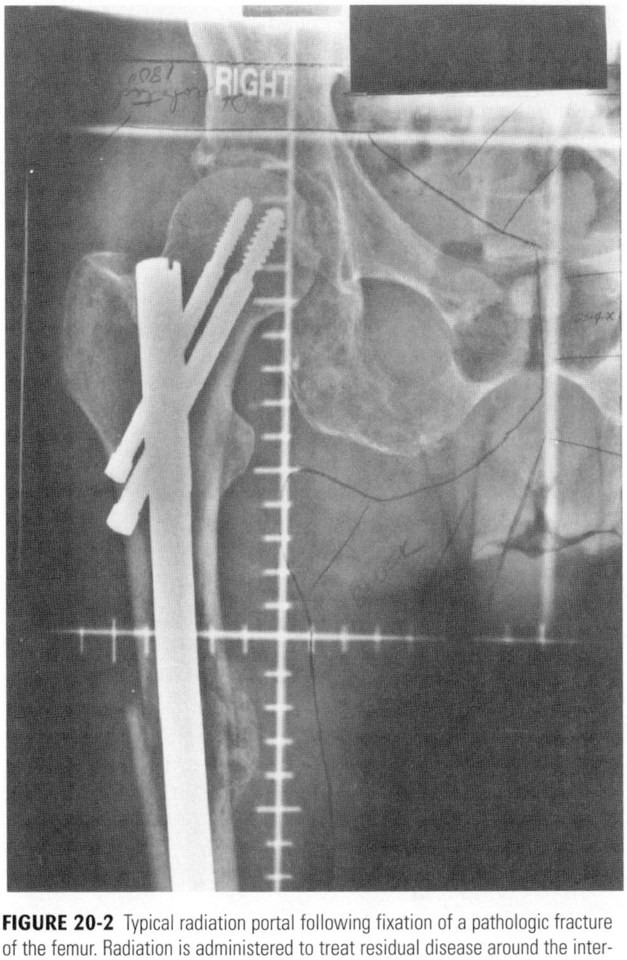

Treatment of pathologic fracture or impending fracture depends on the bone involved and the clinical status of the patient. Indications for surgical intervention of pathologic fracture or impending fracture include these factors:[67] an expected survival of more than 6 weeks;[68] an ability to accomplish internal stability of the fracture site;[69] no coexistent medical conditions that preclude early mobilization;[70] metastases involving weight-bearing bones;[71] and lytic lesions more than 2–3 cm in size or metastases that destroy more than 50% of the cortex.[59,63,64] It is unclear whether osteolytic metastases are more likely to fracture than osteoblastic lesions because osteoblastic lesions, by definition, have an osteolytic component so that new bone can be formed.

The cost of treatment for 2 years was evaluated among 28 prostate cancer patients with bone metastases in the Netherlands who were receiving hormonal therapy. Approximately one skeletal-related event occurred per patient per year totaling 54 events.[66] External beam radiation was administered 33 times, and 21 patients were treated with radiopharmaceuticals. Eight patients were hospitalized—four for spinal cord compression and four for pathologic fracture. The average cost of care for patients with prostate cancer metastatic to bone was £13,051 per patient and about half of this cost was due to the treatment of skeletal-related events.

▶ Spinal cord compression

Pain is the initial symptom in approximately 90% of patients with spinal cord compression, and the development of spinal cord compression is associated with a poor overall prognosis. Paraparesis or paraplegia occur in more than 60% of these patients, sensory loss is noted in 70%–80%, and 14%–77% have bladder and/or bowel disturbances.[47,72–100] The extent of the epidural mass influences prognosis because a complete spinal block results in greater residual neurologic impairment than a partial block. The time from the original diagnosis to the development of metastatic spinal disease averages 32 months, and the average time is reported to be 27 months from diagnosis of skeletal metastases to spinal cord compression. Median survival among patients with spinal cord compression ranges between 3 and 7 months with a 36% probability of a 1-year survival. For specific types of cancer, the mean survival time is 14 months for breast cancer, 12 months for prostate cancer, 6 months for malignant melanoma, and 3 months for lung cancer once epidural spinal cord compression is diagnosed.[57,60] The vertebral column is involved by metastatic tumor in 40% of patients who die of cancer. Approximately 70% of vertebral metastases involve the thoracic spine, 20% the lumbosacral region, and 10% the cervical spine. When a tumor registry of 121,435 patients was analyzed, the cumulative probability of at least one episode of spinal cord compression occurring in the last 5 years of life was 2.5%.[89] The diagnosis of spinal cord compression was associated with a doubling of the time spent in hospital in the last year of life.

Weakness can signal the rapid progression of symptoms and 30% of patients with weakness become paraplegic within 1 week. Rapid development of weakness, defined as occurring in less than 2 months, is seen most commonly in lung cancer whereas breast and prostate cancers can progress more slowly. Neurologic deficits can develop within a few hours in as many as 20% of patients with spinal cord compression.[25,57,75,90,91] The rate of development of motor symptoms correlates with therapeutic improvement.[90,91] Motor function

FIGURE 20-2 Typical radiation portal following fixation of a pathologic fracture of the femur. Radiation is administered to treat residual disease around the internal fixation device, pubis, and acetabulum.

improved among 86% of patients who had a >14-day time to development of symptoms. Only 29% improved when motor deficits developed over 8–14 days before the diagnosis of spinal cord compression. Improvements occurred in only 10% of patients if motor deficits developed between 1 and 7 days. The severity of weakness at presentation is the most significant factor for recovery of function.[90,91] Ninety percent of patients who are ambulatory at presentation will be ambulatory after treatment. Only 13% of paraplegic patients regain function, particularly if paraplegia is present for more than 24 hours before the initiation of therapy. More than 30% of patients who develop spinal cord compression are alive 1 year later and 50% of these patients remain ambulatory with appropriate therapy.

Among 153 consecutive cases of spinal cord compression in one study, 37% of patients had breast cancer, 28% had prostate cancer, 18% had lung cancer, and 17% had other solid tumors. The time between primary tumor diagnosis and development of spinal cord compression was dependent on tumor type, with the shortest time associated with lung cancer and the longest time for breast cancer. Lung cancer patients had the most severe functional deficit with more than 50% being totally paralyzed. Breast cancer patients were ambulatory 59% of the time. More severe disturbances in gait occurred when the time between the interval from the diagnosis of the primary tumor and spinal cord compression was short. Total blockage of the spinal cord occurred in 54% of patients, and 46% had partial blockage.[93] Total paralysis was present in 43 patients, 31 could move their legs but could not walk, 19 were able to walk with assistance, and 60 could walk unassisted. Sensory examination of the legs was normal in 34, slight disturbances were present in 84, and total lack of pain perception occurred in 35 patients. After radiation, 40 were totally paralyzed, 20 could move their legs without being able to walk, 17 were able to walk with assistance, and 76 had unassisted gait. The median survival time was 3.4 months. Survival depended upon time from primary tumor diagnosis, and ambulatory function at diagnosis and after treatment.

Pain can be present for months to days before neurologic dysfunction evolves. Unlike degenerative joint disease, which occurs primarily in the low cervical and low lumbar regions, pain due to epidural spinal cord compression can occur anywhere in the spinal axis, and is aggravated by recumbency. Any cancer patient with back pain, especially with known metastatic involvement of the vertebral bodies, should be suspected of having spinal cord compression. The risk of spinal cord compression exceeds 60% among patients with back pain and plain film evidence of vertebral collapse due to metastatic cancer.[52–58,73–78] Epidural spinal cord disease is documented in 17% of asymptomatic patients who have an abnormal bone scan but normal plain films. When vertebral metastases are present both on bone scan and plain film, 47% of asymptomatic patients have epidural disease.[75] Magnetic resonance imaging (MRI) to rule out spinal cord compression should be performed in symptomatic patients with osteoblastic changes on plain film even if the vertebral contour and bone scan are normal (Fig. 20-3).

Radiographic determination of the involved spinal levels is critical to radiation treatment planning. Clinical determination of the location of epidural spinal cord compression is incorrect in 33% of cases.[52,53,57] Plain film radiographs show involvement of more than one spinal level in about one-third of patients. If the results of MRI, tomographic studies, and surgical findings are included, more than 85% of patients will have multiple sites of vertebral involvement.[52–58,74,75,77,88,96] Bone scans fail to detect bone metastases 13% of the time.[88] In one study when there was evidence of spinal metastases

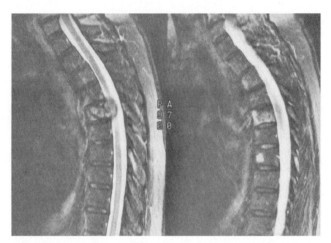

FIGURE 20-3 Magnetic resonance imaging of the spine demonstrating epidural spinal cord compression.

on bone scan, 49% had more extensive disease on MRI.[88] While spinal cord compression is caused by soft tissue epidural metastases in 75% of cases, the remaining 25% of cases are caused by bone collapse.[87] Computed tomography (CT) finds metastases in the posterior portion of the vertebral body, and that destruction of the pedicles occurs only in combination with involvement of the vertebral body.[77] With plain x-rays, the destruction of the pedicles is the most common finding that identifies spine metastases. Osteoblastic bony expansion, typically seen in both prostate and breast cancers, can result in spinal cord compromise as well as osteolytic vertebral compression fractures (Fig. 20-4).[76,87] MRI findings correlated with stage of multiple myeloma, the β_2 microglobulin level, the type of chain, and the response to therapy.[96]

Treatment of spinal cord compression includes emergent corticosteroids, radiotherapy, and/or neurosurgical intervention. Radiotherapy is the treatment of choice for most cases of spinal cord compression

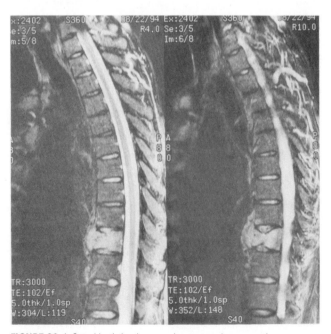

FIGURE 20-4 Osteoblastic involvement, demonstrated on magnetic resonance imaging of the spine, associated with vertebral collapse with breast cancer.

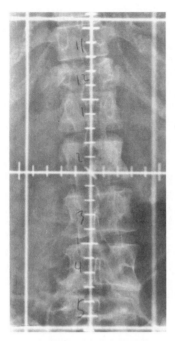

FIGURE 20-5 Typical radiation portal to treat disease involvement in the vertebral bodies and epidural region.

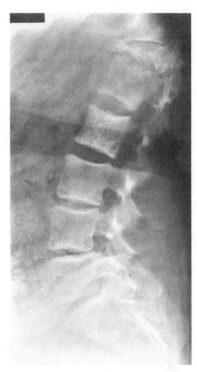

FIGURE 20-6 Compression fraction of the twelfth thoracic vertebral body following an initial pain-free interval after palliative radiation. Vertebral weakness with rapid tumor regression resulting in the compression fracture, which caused recurrent back pain due to spinal instability.

and is a radiotherapeutic emergency (Fig. 20-5). Functional outcome depends upon the level of symptoms at the time radiation is administered.[47,52–58,74,75,94] In these cases, 73% of patients have pain relief following treatment. Among 108 breast cancer patients, the mean time to pain relief was 35 days. Recurrent symptoms at a different spinal levels occurred in more than 75% of patients and within 6 months of the initial treatment.[94]

A statistically significant improvement in functional outcome occurs when laminectomy and radiotherapy are used to treat epidural spinal cord compression compared to either modality alone for selected clinical presentations. Laminectomy has been recommended to promptly reduce tumor volume in an attempt to relieve compression and injury of the spinal cord and provide stabilization to the spinal axis. The rate of tumor regression following radiotherapy is too slow in these cases to effect recovery of lost neurologic function, and radiation therapy cannot relieve compression of the spinal column due to vertebral collapse. After radiation alone to treat a partial spinal cord block, 64% of patients regain ambulation, 33% have normalization of sphincter tone, 72% are pain free, and median survival is 9 months.[54,56,58,74,75,92] With a complete spinal cord block, only 27% demonstrate improved motor function and 42% continue to have pain after radiation alone. In paraparetic patients who undergo laminectomy and radiation, 82% regain the ability to walk, 68% have improved sphincter function, and 88% have relief of pain.

Laminectomy is indicated for rapid neurologic deterioration, tumor progression in a previously irradiated area, stabilization of the spine, paraplegic patients with limited disease and good probability of survival, and to establish a diagnosis.[52,53,55,56,58,78] Adjuvant radiotherapy is often given to treat microscopic residual disease after neurosurgical intervention.[52,53,55,56,58,75,78] Surgical restoration of the vertebral alignment may be required due to neurologic compromise and pain caused by progressive vertebral collapse. Vertebral collapse may occur due to cancer or vertebral instability after cancer therapy

(Fig. 20-6). Appropriate diagnostic studies and intervention should be pursued with persistent pain because the neurologic compromise and pain from vertebral instability can be as devastating as that with epidural spinal cord metastases.[56,78]

Radiation tolerance of the spinal cord

The potential for the development of radiation myelitis with total radiation doses that exceed 40 Gy at 2 Gy per fraction is the limiting factor in treating large tumor burdens near or involving the spinal canal. Furthermore, the length of spinal cord that needs to be irradiated significantly affects its radiation tolerance.[81–83,95,97] Persistent pain after radiotherapy for vertebral metastases should be investigated to exclude the possibility of progressive disease in or outside the radiation portal, or mechanical spinal instability because of a vertebral compression fracture. Changes seen in the bone marrow on MRI after palliative radiotherapy initially include decreased cellularity, edema, and hemorrhage followed by fatty replacement and fibrosis. These well-defined changes on MRI after radiotherapy can be distinguished from those seen with progressive disease.[77,84,85]

Histopathologic changes experimentally observed after fractionated irradiation of the spinal cord include white matter necrosis, massive hemorrhage, and segmental parenchymal atrophy that are consistently associated with abnormal neurologic signs.[83] Other pathologic responses involve focal fiber loss and white matter vacuolation. Two separate mechanisms of radiation injury can occur and result from white matter damage and vasculopathies. White matter damage is associated with diffuse demyelination and swollen axons that can be focally necrotic with an associated glial reaction. Experimentally, vascular damage has been shown to be age-dependent, and can result in hemorrhage, telangiectasia, and vascular necrosis.[81–83] Low doses of radiation have been shown to interfere with the formation of syringomyelia and glial scarring, which facilitates the recovery of paraplegic animals.[97]

Experimentally, six major types of injury have been shown to result from radiation to the spinal column. Five of these occur in the spinal cord and one in the dorsal root ganglia. The most severe spinal lesions, all of which are due to vascular damage and result in neurologic dysfunction, include white matter necrosis, hemorrhage, and segmental parenchymal atrophy. The two less severe spinal lesions are focal fiber loss and scattered white matter vacuolation caused by damage to glial cells, axons, and/or the vasculature; these less severe sequelae are seen with lower total doses of radiation and are less likely to result in neurologic dysfunction. In dorsal root ganglia, radiation damage includes intracytoplasmic vacuoles and loss of neurons and satellite cells that could affect sensory function. These findings are distinct from the demyelination of the posterior columns associated with the self-limiting Lhermitte's syndrome.[82] Meningeal thickening and fibrosis can also be observed after radiation, but the clinical significance of this is unknown. Ependymal and nerve root damage from radiation are rare.

Clinical and experimental experiences have failed to demonstrate any difference in radiosensitivity among different segments of the spinal cord.[81] The risk of radiation myelitis in the cervico-thoracic spine is less than 5% when 6000 centigray (cGy) is administered at 172 cGy per fraction, or when 5000 cGy is given with daily fractions of 200 cGy per fraction. Especially among patients who have received chemotherapy or need to have a significant length of spinal cord irradiated, the total dose to the spinal cord is generally limited to 4000 cGy administered at 200 cGy per fraction to minimize any risk of irreversible radiation injury to the spinal cord. A steep curve based on total radiation dose predicts the risk of developing radiation myelopathy; a small increase in total radiation dose can result in a large increased risk for radiation myelopathy.[81,83] Retreatment of a previously irradiated segment of spinal cord results in high risk for radiation-induced myelopathy because other neurologic pathways cannot compensate for an injury to a specific level of the spinal cord. Experimental data also have demonstrated that the time course and extent of long-term recovery from radiation are dependent on the specific type and age of involved tissue.

The radiation tolerance of the spinal cord can be compromised by prior injury. Difficulty arises in separating pathologic from radiotherapeutic injury as the origin of spinal cord compression. Vasogenic edema of the spinal cord and nerve roots can be caused by compression injury. Metastatic epidural compression results in vasogenic spinal cord edema, venous hemorrhage, loss of myelin, and ischemia. Vasogenic edema results in an increased synthesis of prostaglandin E_2 that can be inhibited by steroids or nonsteroidal antiinflammatory agents. Other consequences of pathologic compression include hemorrhage, loss of myelin, and ischemia.[81–83]

Surgery often is the only available option for therapy because previously administered radiation may preclude further radiotherapy in the region of malignant spinal cord compression. This is often the case in lung cancer because metastases are located in the thoracic spine in more than 70% of cases, and many of these patients have received mediastinal irradiation.[80] Early involvement by the radiotherapist in the management of patients with suspected spinal cord involvement is important to allow time to obtain prior radiotherapy records and determine if further irradiation is possible and to expedite the clinical decision-making process. Reirradiation has been performed among selected patients with cumulative radiation doses

of 68 Gy.[98,99] Using stereotactic conformal radiotherapy and intensity modulated radiation therapy (IMRT) to total doses of 39 Gy, reirradiation resulted in 95% local control at 12 months follow-up reported in one study.[98] Fifty percent of patients had neurologic improvement, and 13 of 16 patients had relief of pain. No significant late toxicity was reported.

Based on clinical and radiographic evidence, leptomeningeal carcinomatosis must also be considered in diagnostic evaluation. Leptomeningeal carcinomatosis occurs more commonly than expected. For example, only 50% of breast cancer patients with leptomeningeal carcinomatosis are diagnosed before death.[57,58,75,86,100] The need to perform a lumbar puncture is a relative barrier to the diagnosis. At least three cerebrospinal fluid (CSF) samples are necessary to cytologically exclude the diagnosis of leptomeningeal disease because in 10%–40% of patients, the initial CSF sample fails to document tumor cells.[100] MRI can identify leptomeningeal disease among patients with normal CSF cytology, and is sensitive and specific in locating regions of nodular leptomeningeal involvement. Except in the case of nodular leptomeningeal involvement where localized radiotherapy can be of benefit as an adjuvant, intrathecal chemotherapy is generally the treatment of choice.[86]

▶ Treatment of diffuse bone metastases

Systemic radionuclides and bisphosphonates have been used in patients with disseminated bone metastases. Both approaches are useful in augmenting the therapeutic effect of localized radiation and in preventing asymptomatic bony lesions from progressing. Although usually not a significant consideration in localized irradiation, adequate bone marrow reserve is required for systemic radionuclides. Bone marrow scans can be performed to determine the volume of functioning marrow and assess the feasibility of delivering radionuclides.[101–118]

Radiopharmaceuticals

The most commonly used radiopharmaceutical in the treatment of bone metastases is Strontium-89. Many reports indicate effective palliation of pain lasting more than 6 months in 60%–80% of patients with breast and prostate cancers.[101–105,107,108,115,119] Improvements in functional status and quality of life have been observed, and about 20% of patients have complete resolution of pain. Pain control has been reported to be superior among patients with disseminated prostate cancer treated both with Strontium-89 and local radiotherapy compared to localized irradiation alone. Experience from clinical trials has shown that Strontium-89 is an effective therapy that is easily administered in an outpatient setting. An important contraindication to the use of radiopharmaceuticals is when epidural disease is associated with vertebral metastases because the activity of radiopharmaceuticals is limited to bone and disease outside the bone is untreated.

Strontium-89 combines with the calcium component of hydroxyapatite in osteoblastic lesions. Because the activity of Strontium-89 is limited to bone, there are no systemic toxicities. Myelotoxicity, resulting in a 25% decline of initial platelet and white blood cell counts, is usually transient and represents the only significant toxicity associated with Strontium-89.[109,119] Marrow suppression caused by radioisotopes is due either to penetrating gamma-radiation or a radioisotope with a long half-life. Even though Strontium-89 emits a beta particle with low penetrance and low energy (1.46 MeV), myelosuppression can occur. Radiation doses to metastatic bony lesions with Strontium-89 can range from 3 Gy to more than 300 Gy. The radiation dose absorbed by the bone marrow is 2–50 times less than the dose administered by Strontium-89 to the osteoblastic lesion. The half-life of Strontium-89 in normal bone is about 14 days and its half-life in the diseased bone is 51 days. Hematotoxicity is more pronounced in patients with pretreatment platelet counts of $\leq 60 \times 10^3$, white blood counts of $\leq 2.5 \times 10^3$, or $\geq 30\%$ involvement of the red marrow-bearing bone.[109,116,119] Compromise of the red marrow-bearing bone can also be a consequence of tumor or prior radiation and chemotherapy.

Response to Strontium-89 therapy has been subjectively and objectively documented. Subjective response, manifested as symptomatic improvement, was reported by more than 80% of prostate cancer patients using a validated survey. Objective evidence of response was documented by reductions in alkaline and acid phosphatase levels that were also associated with a decreased uptake in metastatic lesions observed on sequential bone scans.[101–105,107,108,115,119]

Prior therapies for prostate cancer, including local radiation therapy and systemic chemotherapy or hormone therapy, do not influence toxicity or affect clinical response to Strontium-89. Administered as an adjuvant to localized external beam radiotherapy in metastatic prostate cancer, Strontium-89 has been shown to improve pain relief and delay progression of disease in prospective randomized clinical trials. Almost twice as many patients treated with Strontium-89 were reported to be pain free at 3 months in follow-up compared to patients treated with localized external beam radiation. Analgesics were no longer required by 17% of patients treated with Strontium-89, whereas only 2% of the patients treated with localized radiotherapy alone were able to discontinue analgesic use. Quality-of-life assessments demonstrated increased physical activity along with improved pain relief after Strontium-89 was administered in conjunction with localized external beam radiation therapy. Cost-benefit analysis has also suggested an advantage to the administration of Strontium-89 with reductions in costs of hospitalization for tertiary care.[101,102,110,119]

Several other radiopharmaceuticals are available for clinical application, including Samarium-153, Gallium Nitrate, Phosphorus-32, and Rhenium-186.[104,106,109,111–113,115,116] The therapeutic mechanism of action relates to the physical and biologic half-life in the bony lesion, the mean energy, and the delivered dose of the radiopharmaceutical. Table 20-3 summarizes some of the physical characteristics and clinical data of various radionuclides. Phosphorus-32 and Strontium-89 emit pure beta rays (little penetration in tissue), whereas Rhenium-186 and Samarium-153 emit both beta rays and relatively high-energy gamma-ray photons that penetrate tissue for some distance (103–159 KeV).

Because Samarium-153 has a gamma-ray component, it is possible to directly image the distribution of the radiation dose. The scans after injection of Samarium-153 are comparable to diagnostic scans obtained with Technitium-99m. The mean skeletal uptake is more than 50% of the dose.[104,106,109,111–113] Nonskeletal sites receive negligible radiation doses and complete clearance of radiation not absorbed by the radiation occurs within 6–8 hours of administration. In a double-blind, placebo-controlled clinical trial,[104] Samarium-153 was shown to be an effective agent in palliating painful bone metastases in breast cancer patients. Pain relief occurred within 1 week and lasted at least 16 weeks after administration. Approximately 65% of patients responded within the first 4 weeks and 43% had relief of pain for at least 16 weeks duration. No significant bone marrow toxicities have been observed. Recommended doses range between 1.0 and 1.5 mCi/kg. In more than one-third of patients, multiple administrations are possible.

Table 20-3

Characteristics of Isotopes used in Brachytherapy

Isotope	Energy	Half-Life
Radium	2.29 MeV	1620 years
Cesium-137	0.662 MeV	30 years
Cobalt-60	1.17 MeV	5 years
Iridium-192	0.34 MeV	75 days
Iodine-125	30 KeV	60 days
Gold-198	0.412 MeV	2.7 days
Strontium-90	2.2 MeV (beta)	28 years

Note: All of these are gamma-emitting isotopes except Strontium-90 which emits beta particles. Beta radiation penetrates tissue poorly, as evidenced by a half value layer of 1 mm in tissue and the fact that only 3% of the dose is measured at a distance of 5 mm from the surface of the source. Strontium-90 is generally used in the eye to treat pterygia. Iodine-125 is characterized as a weak gamma-emitting isotope (average energy of 30 KeV or 0.03 MeV) used in permanent implants. Cesium-137 is generally used in intracavitary implants in gynecologic malignancies and Iridium-192 is used for interstitial implants. The term mg Radium equivalent relates to the amount (millicuries) of the isotope that would be necessary to deliver the same amount of radiation as 1 mg of Radium, which continues to represent the standard in brachytherapy.

Sequential x-rays and bone scans after hormonal and radiopharmaceutical therapy for breast and prostate cancers demonstrate a response.[19,20] Approximately one-third of patients demonstrate evidence of increased pain and increased tracer uptake on bone scans (flare) obtained 8–16 weeks after treatment. Of these patients with a flare response on bone scan, 72% experience a response to the treatment. In comparison, only 36% have pain relief when a limited-to-no flare response is observed.

Despite this experience, recent trials using Strontium-89 have failed to demonstrate significant benefit. One study evaluating 95 patients used physician-assessed subjective progression at 3 months and showed no improvement. However, 50% of the patients had significant relief of pain at 3 months, and 34% had improved social function.[117] Furthermore, Strontium-89 administration resulted in highly significant reductions in serum alkaline phosphatase, reaching a nadir at 3 months. No reductions in PSA levels occurred and Strontium-89 did not improve survival. Improved progression-free survival occurred in a subgroup, having the characteristics of prostate cancer, with few bone scan-detected metastases and low alkaline phosphatase levels. However, Strontium-89 did not incur benefit among 203 prostate cancer patients when the parameters of pain relief, biochemical reduction, or treatment toxicity were considered in a recent EORTC study.[118]

▶ Visceral metastases

The symptoms caused by visceral metastases result in bleeding, obstruction, edema, and pain. Palliative radiation can relieve these symptoms in about 70% of cases. Radiation therapy treatment planning is especially important to exclude mucosal surfaces and reduce treatment-related toxicity. Minimizing treatment-related toxicities in symptomatic and often frail patients referred for palliative radiation is critical.

This is especially important when mucosal surfaces of the head and neck region, and the esophagus are included in the radiation portal. Among the most radiosensitive visceral structures are the small bowel, stomach, lung, and skin. Radiation toxicities resulting from the small bowel include diarrhea. Nausea and vomiting can result when the stomach is in the radiation portal. Radiation pneumonitis, manifested by cough and scarring of the lung, can occur, especially when large volumes of lung are in the treatment field. Dry and moist desquamation can be painful and lead to a secondary infection.

Lung

Locally advanced primary or metastatic involvement of the lung often requires palliative intervention because cure is possible in only a few of these cases. A variety of symptoms, some of them emergent, can manifest due to tumor involvement of the lung.[120] Pain can result from tumor invasion of the ribs and nerve roots of the chest wall. Vertebral involvement can be associated with spinal cord compression. Obstructive pneumonitis and hemoptysis can result from bronchial obstruction. Mediastinal infiltration can cause superior vena cava syndrome. All of these clinical presentations can be palliated with external beam radiation that encompasses the disease that is evident on diagnostic images and that treats pain referred along involved nerve roots.

Radiation schedules that administer 20 Gy in 5 fractions or 30 Gy in 10 fractions over 2 weeks are typically prescribed to sites that have not previously been irradiated. If the area has been previously irradiated, techniques that exclude critical anatomic structures like the spinal cord are applied. Other approaches can be used when the symptomatic site is well localized and accessible. Brachytherapy, which applies radioactive sources next to tumors, can be used to treat bronchial obstruction and bleeding by placing a radioactive source directly against the tumor under bronchoscopic guidance. In these cases, large doses of radiation can be delivered over a few minutes by a high-dose rate brachytherapy unit.

Abdomen

Various clinical presentations require palliative management for tumors involving the gastrointestinal region. Recurrent rectal cancer is the most common, but pain associated with the infiltration and biliary obstruction caused by pancreatic cancer often requires palliative therapy. Nausea and vomiting due to obstruction at many locations along the gastrointestinal tract may require surgical decompression if other less invasive approaches are not successful. Metastases from gastrointestinal malignancies can occur in any location, become symptomatic, and require palliative care.

The most common presenting symptoms of gastric and esophageal cancers are upper abdominal discomfort, weakness from anemia, weight loss, and hematemesis. Exophytic tumors can cause significant bleeding. Infiltrative tumors can invade the celiac plexus and cause severe back pain like that observed with pancreatic cancer. Tumor infiltration resulting in linitis plastica is associated with an extremely poor prognosis. Epigastric pain from gastric cancer can also result from acid secretion. Early satiety, hematemesis, and melena occur less commonly. Obstructing lesions in either the antrum or cardia can cause vomiting or dysphagia, respectively. Several series indicate that 50%–75% of patients experience improvement of bleeding, gastric outlet obstruction, and pain.

Treatment-related side effects are known, and medications should be prophylactically administered. The importance of aggressive supportive care in the setting of a multidisciplinary care team cannot be overemphasized. This is illustrated by the Gastrointestinal Tumor Study Group (GITSG) experience. Even though the chemoradiation group eventually had a better outcome, 6 of 45 patients in that group died because of sepsis or nutritional inadequacy. Prior to initiation of chemoradiation of gastric cancer, laparoscopic placement of a jejunostomy feeding tube may be necessary to support the extended need for nutrition and hydration. Prophylactic antiemetic therapy, like that given with administration of systemic therapy, should be given prior to and during the course of radiation and chemotherapy as needed. A proton pump inhibitor and/or H-2 blocker, or other antiemetics are also recommended during the course of chemoradiation.

The most common presenting symptoms of pancreatic cancer are jaundice, weight loss due to anorexia and exocrine insufficiency, and abdominal pain. Jaundice is usually a presenting symptom in pancreatic head lesions. Pain occurs more commonly among lesions arising in the body or tail of the pancreas. Direct extension of tumor to the first and second celiac ganglia posteriorly leads to characteristic sharp pain, which is perceived as back pain. Pain is a symptom of locally advanced disease. It is typically described as sharp and knife-like located in the midepigastric region with radiation to the back and is often a clinical indicator of unresectable disease.

The dose-limiting structures surrounding the pancreas include the stomach, duodenum, small bowel, kidneys, spinal cord, and liver. Despite the generally poor overall prognosis with pancreatic cancer, most treatment programs for pancreatic cancer administer radiation over 4–6 weeks to deliver 45–60 Gy. However, at M. D. Anderson Cancer Center, we found no survival advantage to the use of higher doses of radiation in the definitive treatment of pancreatic cancer. Routinely, 30 Gy, administered in 10 radiation fractions, is given and is well tolerated both for definitive and palliative therapy. Furthermore, this fractionation schedule limits the time under treatment, which is of particular importance in the palliative setting. In our experience with preoperative chemoradiation and pancreaticoduodenectomy using 50.4 Gy and rapid-fractionation chemoradiation totaling 30 Gy, and pancreaticoduodenectomy plus postoperative adjuvant chemoradiation totaling 50.4 Gy with 5-fluorouracil (5FU), it was found that no patient who received preoperative chemoradiation experienced a delay in surgery because of chemoradiation toxicity.[120] In contrast to the rapid fractionation group treated to 30 Gy over 2 weeks, hospitalization due to acute gastrointestinal toxicity was required by one-third of the preoperative patients who received 50.4 Gy over 5.5 weeks. Also, 24% of patients did not receive intended postoperative chemoradiation because of delayed recovery following pancreaticoduodenectomy.

Pelvis

Hemorrhage and visceral, lymphovascular and nerve root obstruction present most commonly with locally advanced or metastatic disease in the pelvis. Treatment may require emergent radiotherapeutic and/or surgical interventions. Hemorrhage is commonly associated with tumors involving the rectum and genitourinary tracts, like the cervix or bladder. As with tumors in the lung, radiation therapy is an effective means of stopping active bleeding. Colorectal cancers are often diagnosed among patients with unexplained bleeding. Obstruction by colorectal tumors may require stent placement to maintain the integrity of the visceral lumen while administering radiation.[176] Occasionally, a diverting colostomy will be required to bypass intestinal obstruction or fistula formation.

Because rectal tumors are generally locally advanced, preoperative radiation is given in 25 treatments over 5–6 weeks if no or limited metastatic disease is evident; this is intended to stop bleeding, render the patient operable, and provide a chance for cure. Radiation schedules at M. D. Anderson Cancer Center have included 35 Gy per 14 fractions, 30 Gy per 10 fractions, and 30 Gy per 6 fractions given twice weekly for 3 weeks.[121] In our experience, a diverting colostomy was required by 16% of patients prior to irradiation. No significant treatment-related toxicities were observed. Whether administered as conventional or hypofractionated radiation with infusional 5FU, symptoms from the primary tumor resolved in 94% of cases. The endoscopic complete response rate was 36%. Twenty-five patients underwent primary tumor resection. Although the 2-year survival was greater in the group that underwent resection (46% vs. 11%), the colostomy-free survival was greater in the unresected group (79% vs. 51%). Durable control of pelvic symptoms was not significantly different and was 81% for palliative chemoradiation and 91% for preoperative chemoradiation. Predictors for a worse prognosis included pelvic pain at presentation, biologic equivalent dose at 2 Gy per fraction of <35 Gy, and poor tumor differentiation.[122] Among patients with locally advanced rectal cancer who also had liver metastases at presentation, the median survival was 17 months when treated with palliative radiation and chemotherapy.

The influence of tumor factors on response to therapy and survival was also demonstrated at the Princess Margaret Hospital.[123] The most frequent palliative radiation schedule for locally advanced rectal cancer administered 50 Gy in 20 fractions in 4 weeks using a four-field technique. The 5-year survival was directly dependent on the extent of the tumor; 48% with mobile, 27% with partially fixed, and only 4% of patients with fixed tumors were alive at 5 years. Tumor extent also predicted response to radiation; 50% of mobile, 30% of partially fixed, and only 9% of fixed tumors achieved a complete clinical response to radiation. The rate of tumor regression was slow; only 60% achieved a complete response by 4 months and 9 months were required by 90% of those who had a complete response. Of the complete responders, approximately 50% of the mobile and partially fixed and over 70% of the fixed tumors developed progressive disease. Salvage surgery to relieve symptoms was accomplished without significant complication in more than 90% of patients who developed progressive or recurrent disease.

Tumors involving the cervix can hemorrhage and require emergent radiotherapeutic intervention. Superficial x-rays are applied directly to the bleeding cervix through a cone so that the bleeding site is treated without compromising later radiation of other pelvic structures.[120] Usually radiation doses between 5 and 10 Gy are administered in one to three applications of cone therapy. Brachytherapy also can be used to treat gynecologic tumors, especially in the vagina, cervix, and endometrium.

Bladder cancers or tumors that secondarily invade the bladder can also result in significant bleeding that can be palliated by external beam radiation. Urinary obstruction commonly occurs with locally advanced pelvic cancers, especially prostate and cervical cancers. Occasionally, placement of a urinary stent or urostomy/nephrostomy is required until sufficient tumor regression can be accomplished by radiation to reestablish integrity of the urinary tract.[120] As with the bowel and gynecologic tracts, a vesical fistula, resulting from either the tumor itself or from tumor regression, remains a concern.

The pelvic lymph nodes and major blood vessels may become obstructed by tumor. This most frequently is seen when tumor arises in pelvic structures, but can also occur with pelvic metastases from breast and other cancers. Lymphovascular obstruction results in painful edema that is refractory to diuretic and other therapies. When severe, fluid and electrolyte imbalances can occur. Pelvic radiation can relieve lymphovascular obstruction through tumor regression.

Pelvic tumors can also invade the sacral plexus and result in intractable pain. Tumor can tract along nerve roots and can be associated with bony invasion of the sacrum. Pain due to visceral and/or lymphovascular obstruction often responds more rapidly to palliative radiation than the neuropathic pain seen with sacral plexus involvement. Other radiotherapeutic approaches, like brachytherapy, are extremely limited for when the cancer persists or recurs after external beam radiation. Interventional pain management techniques are frequently required to control pain associated with sacral plexus involvement.

Skin and subcutaneous tissues

Tumors can cause ulceration of the skin and subcutaneous tissues that are often painful and distressing due to constant drainage. Representing a source for the development of sepsis in immunocompromised patients, localized radiation can be applied to destroy tumor and allow reepithelialization of the skin. Radiation that treats only the skin and subcutaneous tissues (electron beam therapy) is generally used to avoid radiation side effects to underlying uninvolved normal structures. Although 10 radiation treatments are usually given, the course of radiation can be abbreviated further, ranging from 1 to 5 days. Occasionally these lesions are treated with brachytherapy. The radioactive sources can be placed in a mold that sits on top of the tumor and delivers treatment over a few minutes (high-dose rate) or a few days (low-dose rate).

▶ Brain metastases

Radiation is used to relieve the symptoms of headache, seizure, nausea/vomiting, and neurologic dysfunction associated with brain metastases. Surgery, either alone or in combination with radiation, is often performed when a solitary brain metastasis is present, if the patient's performance status is good and if the cancer burden is otherwise limited.[124] Radiation is generally given over 2–3 weeks with daily fractions of 2.5–3 Gy per day; total radiation doses range from 25 Gy after resection to 30 Gy with unresectable disease and a poor prognosis.

PALLIATIVE RADIATION TECHNIQUES

Pain, bleeding, and obstruction are the most common symptoms relieved by palliative radiation. Combined clinical, prognostic, and therapeutic factors must be considered to determine the optimal treatment approach. Depending on prognostic factors and known treatment-related side effects, palliative treatment can range from the use of surgery, radiation, and chemotherapy or a single therapeutic modality alone, such as radiation therapy.

Radiotherapy techniques vary considerably depending upon which adjacent normal structures are involved. Basic to an understanding of applied techniques and potential morbidity during a course of radiation are the following principles.[125] Radiation therapy is delivered in units designated as the *gray*. Relating this to the previously used term *rad*, equivalent doses can be expressed as 1 gray (Gy), 100 centigray (cGy), and 100 rad; 1 rad equals 1 cGy.

Radiation can be delivered by either *external beam therapy* (linear accelerators, Cobalt-60 units) or *brachytherapy* using radioactive isotopes applied directly to the region impinged upon by tumor. External beam therapy is administered as a prescribed number of daily fractions over several weeks, whereas brachytherapy is a continuous application of radiation to the tumor bed ranging from a number of minutes to days. Various radiation energies and biologic characteristics are now available to help localize treatment to areas at risk while sparing uninvolved normal tissues.

▶ External beam irradiation

Photons are included within the classification of external beam radiation, which are penetrating forms of radiation. *Electrons*, also included, deliver treatment to superficial areas. Other specialized types of external radiation beams are available at only a few centers. These include *proton beam therapy* (administering radiation with high precision to well-defined small areas of tumor involvement like pituitary or midbrain lesions) and *neutrons* (used by a few centers to treat bulky unresectable or recurrent tumors).

The concept of integral dose relates to the amount of radiation deposited to uninvolved normal tissues located between the skin surface and tumor; the goal in any radiation plan is to minimize integral dose by selecting the appropriate beam energy (Table 20-4). The *D*max radiation dose is the depth at which 100% of the prescribed radiation is deposited. Higher energy photon radiation, like 18 meV photons, reduces integral dose because it deposits more radiation to deeper structures while delivering relatively little radiation to superficial tissues.

Multiple radiation portals, each of which is treated daily, are also routinely used in radiotherapy to reduce integral dose. Table 20-5 demonstrates an example of the impact on integral radiation dose when 200 cGy are prescribed at a depth of 10 cm from a 6 meV linear accelerator. When only the anterior radiation portal is used to deliver radiation in the example, the integral dose is high because more superficial tissues receive an almost 50% greater dose than the prescribed radiation dose at the site of the tumor located 10 cm below the skin surface; at 1.5 cm from the skin surface the daily radiation dose is 294 cGy per fraction and the total dose is 5880 cGy compared to the 200 cGy per fraction and total radiation dose of 4000 cGy at the tumor. Radiation tolerance is based primarily on the

daily radiation dose; as the daily radiation dose increases, the total radiation dose that can be delivered to normal tissues decreases. Because of this, treatment with an anterior field alone would result in significant side effects due to the high integral dose. It is important to realize that giving the first half of the radiation course from the anterior (AP) field alone, and the second half of the radiation course from the posterior (PA) field alone would not reduce radiation side effects. Although the total radiation dose would be even greater using an AP field during the first half and a PA field during the last half of a radiation dose, side effects still may be severe because of the high daily (integral) dose of radiation.

When the radiation is delivered each day from an AP and PA radiation portal, the radiation dose given in the portal is the sum of the radiation dose from each field (Fig. 20-7). The integral dose in the case presented decreases significantly with AP and PA treatment fields because the daily radiation dose throughout the treatment field is within 6% (with a daily dose of 211 cGy per fraction at 16.5 cm below the anterior skin surface) of the prescribed dose of 200 cGy per fraction (Fig. 20-8). Likewise, the maximum total radiation dose in the field is 4220 cGy, just 220 cGy more than the prescribed radiation dose at the tumor (Fig. 20-9). Newer treatment approaches, like conformal radiation therapy, exploit this relationship by treating as many as eight different radiation fields each day. Reducing integral dose is a principal concept of radiation treatment planning because it allows higher radiation doses to be delivered to the tumor and less radiation to the surrounding normal tissues.

External beam irradiation is administered from specialized machines, which emit gamma rays from a housed isotope (Cobalt-60) or x-rays (linear accelerators), which are more than 1000 times as powerful as those used in diagnostic radiology, that are generated by electricity. The availability of higher energy radiation beams and the development of various different radiation energies were critical to the advancement of radiation therapy. These advancements allowed more precise deposition of radiation in the area of the tumor while sparing surrounding uninvolved normal tissues.

Placing this in perspective, the first machines used in radiation therapy emitted *orthovoltage* radiation. In contrast to the 18 MeV linear accelerators currently available, the low radiation energy of orthovoltage radiation ranges between 125 and 250 KeV (Fig. 20-10). Orthovoltage is generally delivered in one or two fractions through a cone that is directly applied to the tumor. Orthovoltage has limited applications, but it continues to be highly effective in reducing bleeding from rectal and cervical cancers. Protracted courses with orthovoltage radiation, however, resulted in late radiation complications that included osteonecrosis. Osteonecrosis developed because of the increased absorption of low-energy radiation by tissues that have a high atomic number, like the bone. This characteristic allows the differentiation to be drawn between bones and soft tissues in diagnostic radiology, but the radiation doses used in the treatment of cancer are several magnitudes greater than those used for diagnostic purposes. The increased absorption of radiation in bone or other tissues with a high atomic number does not, however, occur in current megavoltage radiation beams because of the higher energies used (Fig. 20-11).

A wide variety of photon energies are available. This allows selective administration of treatment to the tumor and minimizes radiation to uninvolved tissues. As a standard, available photon beam energies range from Cobalt-60 to 22 MeV photons. Cobalt-60 delivers 100% of the prescribed radiation dose, indicated as the maximum radiation dose (*D*max), 0.5 cm below the skin surface. 6 MeV x-rays from a linear accelerator have a D_{max} of 1.5 cm, and 18 MeV

Table 20-4

The Concept of Integral Dose is Demonstrated by the Following Radiation Dose Distributions for Three Different Energies Including Cobalt-60, and 6 and 18 MV photons

	Cobalt-60	6 MV	18 MV
Skin Surface			
0.5 cm	100%	30%	25%
1.0 cm	98%	90%	50%
1.5 cm	95%	100%	90%
2.0 cm	93%	98%	96%
2.5 cm	90%	97%	98%
3.0 cm	88%	95%	98%
3.5 cm	85%	92%	100%
5.0 cm	80%	88%	96%
10 cm	55%	68%	80%

Note: D_{max}, the maximum dose, refers to the depth at which 100% of the prescribed dose is located below the skin surface. The greater the *D*max, the greater the skin sparing associated with less of an integral dose.

Table 20-5

The Impact on Integral Radiation Dose When 200 cGy are Prescribed at Midline (10 cm Depth; Patient Diameter is 20 cm) from an 6 meV Linear Accelerator

Radiation dose = 200 cGy at 10 cm depth; percentage depth dose = 68%.
Radiation dose at 1.5 cm (D_{max} or 100%) is the radiation dose Rx'ed/0.68
Radiation dose at other depths is the D_{max} dose × % isodose (see Table 20-4)

Distance from Skin Surface	6 MeV Photons
0.5 cm	30%
1.0 cm	90%
1.5 cm	100%
2.0 cm	98%
2.5 cm	97%
3.0 cm	95%
3.5 cm	92%
5.0 cm	88%
10 cm	68%
15.0 cm	51%
16.5 cm	48%
17.5 cm	44%
18.5 cm	42%
19.5 cm	40%

Single Anterior Radiation Field Delivering 200 cGy at Midline (10 cm)

Depth from Anterior Skin Surface	Dose from AP	Total Dose × 20 Fractions
0.5 cm	88 cGy (294 × 0.30)	1760 cGy (88 × 20)
1.5 cm	294 cGy (200/0.68)	5880 cGy (294 × 20)
2.5 cm	285 cGy (294 × 0.97)	5700 cGy (285 × 20)
3.5 cm	279 cGy (294 × 0.92)	5580 cGy (279 × 20)
5.0 cm	259 cGy (294 × 0.88)	5180 cGy (259 × 20)
10 cm	200 cGy (294 × 0.68)	4000 cGy (200 × 20)
15 cm	150 cGy (294 × 0.51)	3000 cGy (165 × 20)
16.5 cm	141 cGy (294 × 0.48)	2820 cGy (144 × 20)
17.5 cm	129 cGy (294 × 0.44)	2580 cGy (129 × 20)
18.5 cm	123 cGy (294 × 0.42)	2460 cGy (126 × 20)
19.5 cm	118 cGy (294 × 0.40)	2360 cGy (118 × 20)

Parallel Opposed (AP and PA) Radiation Fields Treated Each Day Delivering 200 cGy at Midline (10 cm)

Depth from Anterior Skin Surface	Dose from AP	Dose from PA	Total Dose per Fraction (AP + PA)	Total Dose × 20 Fractions (AP + PA)
0.5 cm	44 cGy (147 × 0.30)	59 cGy (147 × 0.40)	103 cGy	2060 cGy
1.5 cm	147 cGy (100/0.68)	62 cGy (147 × 0.42)	209 cGy	4180 cGy
2.5 cm	143 cGy (147 × 0.97)	65 cGy (147 × 0.44)	208 cGy	4160 cGy
3.5 cm	140 cGy (147 × 0.92)	71 cGy (147 × 0.48)	211 cGy	4220 cGy
5.0 cm	129 cGy (147 × 0.88)	75 cGy (147 × 0.51)	204 cGy	4080 cGy
10.0 cm	100 cGy (147 × 0.68)	100 cGy (147 × 0.68)	200 cGy	4000 cGy
15.0 cm	75 cGy (147 × 0.51)	129 cGy (147 × 0.88)	204 cGy	4080 cGy
16.5 cm	71 cGy (147 × 0.48)	140 cGy (147 × 0.92)	211 cGy	4220 cGy
17.5 cm	65 cGy (147 × 0.44)	143 cGy (147 × 0.97)	208 cGy	4160 cGy
18.5 cm	62 cGy (147 × 0.42)	147 cGy (100/0.68)	209 cGy	4180 cGy
19.5 cm	59 cGy (147 × 0.40)	44 cGy (147 × 0.30)	103 cGy	2060 cGy

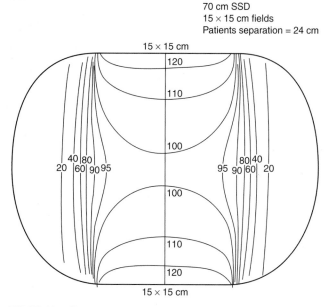

Colbalt-60
70 cm SSD
15 × 15 cm fields
Patients separation = 24 cm

FIGURE 20-7 The radiation isodose distribution for a 15 cm × 15 cm radiation field using anterior and posterior (AP and PA) parallel opposed portals with Cobalt-60. In this case, the patient has a 24 cm diameter. Each number represents a percentage of the prescribed radiation dose. If 200 cGy was prescribed to the 100% isodose line, then 240 cGy would be delivered to the 120% isodose line near the skin surface and only 180 cGy would be given at the edge of the radiation field at the 90% isodose line. The edges of the field receive less radiation dose because there is opportunity for radiation dose contributed by interactions with adjacent radiated tissue at the blocked edge than in the middle of the field.

photons have a D_{max} of 3.5 cm below the skin. Tissues 0.5 cm below the skin surface treated with 18 MeV photons receive only 30% of the prescribed radiation dose. This demonstrates the relationship in radiation physics that there is more sparing of superficial structures (skin and subcutaneous tissues) from radiation with higher photon energies even though the beam penetrates deeply into the tissue.

Electron beam radiation is an important therapeutic option in the treatment of superficial tumors. The penetration of the beam can be

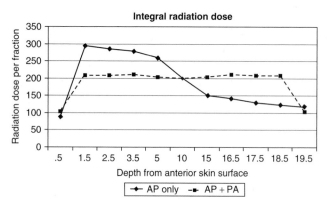

FIGURE 20-8 Graphic comparison of the integral dose, defined as the radiation dose deposited between the skin surface and the tumor. In this case, the tumor is 10 cm below the skin surface. If radiation were only given from the anterior treatment portal, the radiation dose to the skin would result in complications because of the high radiation dose per fraction as well as the high total dose of radiation.

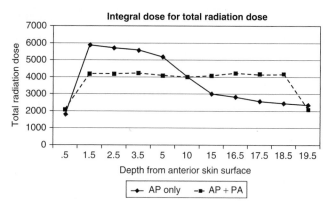

FIGURE 20-9 Graphic comparison of the total radiation dose given when a single anterior radiation field is used instead of parallel opposed radiation fields (AP and PA fields) treated every day. With the AP field alone, the skin would receive 30% more radiation than the parallel opposed treatment approach to achieve the same radiation dose at the tumor.

approximated by dividing the energy by different numerical factors. For example, 80% of the radiation dose from a 9 MeV electron beam is deposited within 3 cm of the surface (9 divided by 3), whereas essentially all of the radiation is given within 4.5 cm of the skin (9 divided by 2) with no radiation penetrating beyond that depth. Different electron beam energies are available to allow precise localization of the radiation to superficial lesions while sparing underlying critical structures. Electron beam radiation is routinely used in head and neck cancer to treat the posterior cervical lymph nodes while avoiding treatment of the underlying spinal cord.

Proton beam therapy and "radiosurgery" are more limited in application and availability; however, the underlying concept is to precisely deposit a large amount of radiation to a well-defined volume of tumor while sparing intervening tissues. The precision of proton beam therapy is to the level of the millimeter, requiring exact mapping of the tumor volume and potential microscopic areas of involvement. An additional advantage of proton irradiation is the improvement of relative biologic effectiveness of this type of radiation because of the characteristic Bragg-Peak distribution of radiation within a narrow volume of tissue (Fig. 20-12). Chordomas and localized intracranial tumors, especially around the optic chiasm, have been treated with proton irradiation. Because of its precision, research is ongoing to define further applications for proton therapy, especially in pediatric tumors and previously irradiated recurrent tumors.

Neutron radiation is primarily used among patients who have undergone previous aggressive cancer therapy resulting in the presence of resistant clonogens, or for patients with large tumor burdens. Neutron radiation is more efficient than photons at killing tumor cells because neutron radiation is less dependent on oxygen radicals to cause irreversible radiation damage. The radiobiologic effectiveness (RBE), which describes the relative efficiency of different radiation beams in terms of a ratio of doses to produce the same level of cellular damage, is less for neutron radiation. A single fraction of neutron radiation has an RBE of 1.5, compared to an RBE of 3.0 for photons.[126] This characteristic reflects a reduced initial shoulder of radiation resistance on the cell survival curve and the decreased influence of oxygen on radiosensitivity with neutron irradiation (Fig. 20-13). All solid tumors greater than 180 micron in size contain hypoxic cells. Although promising in preclinical evaluation and for treating unresectable tumors, only a few centers continue to have neutrons.

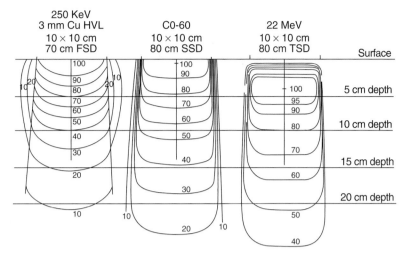

FIGURE 20-10 Demonstrates the different radiation isodose distributions for 10 cm × 10 cm radiation fields. The three beams compared include orthovoltage radiation with a 250 KeV radiation beam (*left*), a Cobalt-60 unit (*middle*), and a 22 MeV linear accelerator (*right*). The 250 KeV unit has no skin sparing and little depth of penetration of the radiation beam. The Cobalt-60 unit is ideal to treat head and neck cancers so that adequate radiation is given to superficial lymph nodes and scars in the postoperative setting. Because the diameter of the head and neck region is limited, a highly penetrating photon beam is not advisable. 22 MeV photons are ideal for deep-seated tumor like in the pelvis and abdomen because of skin sparring and deep penetration of the photon beams.

Because radiation therapy is frequently used to palliate localized sites of disease, many radiotherapeutic options are needed for tumors that cause localized symptoms. The clinical status of the patient is accounted for in the treatment setup and in the number of radiation treatments that are prescribed. The radiation dose-fractionation schedule and technique also considers the site and volume irradiated, and the integration of other therapies. Conformal external beam radiation and IMRT, intraoperative radiation therapy (IORT), brachytherapy, and endocavitary therapy are techniques that can better localize radiation dose and reduce side effects, especially in a previously irradiated area.

▶ Reirradiation

Issues regarding reirradiation are especially important in palliative therapy. Experimental data suggest that acute responding tissues

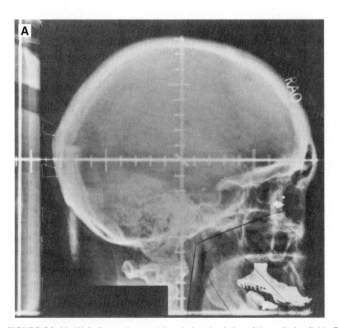

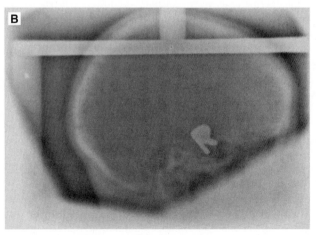

FIGURE 20-11 (A) A diagnostic x-ray taken during simulation of the radiation fields. There is a significant difference in the contrast between the bones and the soft tissues due to the low energy of the photons used in diagnostic x-rays. Because calcium has a high atomic number, this results in the bones absorbing a dose of radiation that is about three times more than the radiation dose absorbed by the soft tissues (photoelectric effect). (B) An image taken during a radiation treatment. Because of the high energy of the radiation photons used during radiation therapy, the contrast between the bones and soft tissues is less apparent. Because the energy of the radiation is so high, the bones and soft tissues absorb about the same dose of radiation (Compton Effect).

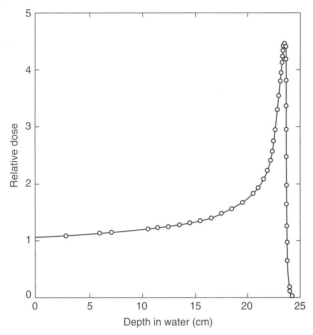

FIGURE 20-12 The Bragg-Peak effect in radiation associated with proton radiation. Only the designated tumor area received radiation and the surrounding normal tissues are spared radiation. Although currently used to treat intracranial tumors and pediatric cases, proton radiation may have application in palliative care for the retreatment of tumors.

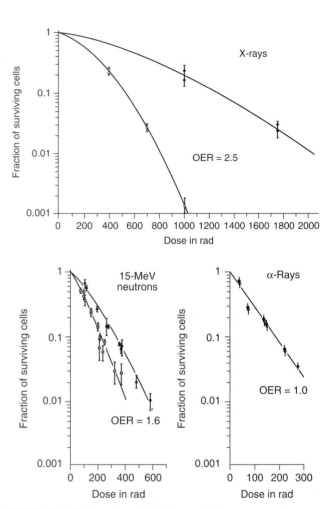

FIGURE 20-13 The dependence of radiation sensitivity on oxygen tension; (B) the radiobiologic effectiveness (RBE) of photon and neutron radiation. Because neutron radiation is less dependent on oxygen, tumors are more sensitive to neutron radiation. Neutron radiation has been used in palliative care to treat recurrent or unresectable tumors.

recover from radiation injury in a few months and can tolerate additional radiation therapy. However, there is considerable variability in recovery from radiation among late reacting tissues.[127] This recovery depends on the technique used, the organ irradiated, the volume irradiated, the initial total dose of radiation, the radiation dose given with each fraction, and the time interval between the initial and second courses of radiation.[128]

Correlating with existing clinical experience, limited toxicities occur with reirradiation when there is careful attention paid to treatment techniques and radiobiologic factors. Radiotherapeutic techniques that localize the radiation dose to the recurrent tumor and limit the dose to the surrounding normal tissues allow the reirradiation of recurrent tumors. Other techniques include conformal external beam radiation and IMRT, IORT, brachytherapy, and endocavitary radiation.[129–135]

Conformal radiation therapy/intensity-modulated radiation therapy

Conformal radiation techniques precisely localize the radiation dose using external beam radiation from a linear accelerator. Because very low doses of radiation are given through a number of beams, no one area of normal tissues receives a significant dose of radiation. The tumor, however, is given the sum of the radiation from the beams and receives a high dose of radiation. This technique has allowed high doses of radiation to be given, and has allowed for reirradiation of normal tissues without significant side effects.

IMRT is a form of conformal external beam radiation that even more precisely administers radiation. It is possible to deliver different doses of radiation to specific areas in a single radiation fraction. For example, with IMRT the center of the tumor may receive 2.20 Gy with each radiation treatment to a total dose of 66 Gy over

30 fractions in 6 weeks, whereas the periphery of the tumor may receive 2.0 Gy with each radiation treatment to a total dose of 60 Gy. At the same time, the normal tissues within 2 cm of the tumor (clinical tumor volume used to account for possible microscopic tumor extension) may receive 1.8 Gy with each radiation treatment to a total dose of 54 Gy. IMRT provides the radiobiologic advantage of giving a high daily dose of radiation localized within a tumor while concomitantly delivering a well-tolerated lower daily dose of radiation to the surrounding tissues. Localizing high daily and total doses of radiation in the tumor, IMRT is able to kill more cancer cells with higher radiation doses without harming the surrounding tissues. Any shape or configuration of radiation dose, like an hourglass, can be designed with IMRT. Because of these factors, this radiotherapeutic tool is extremely helpful for delivering high radiation doses to inoperable tumors over a shorter period of time, and in treating tumors that recur in a previously irradiated field.

Intraoperative radiation therapy

IORT has also been used as a supplement to external beam radiation or as the only therapy when further external beam radiation is not possible. Intraoperative radiation therapy administers radiation totaling 10–20 Gy in a single fraction to a localized region during the surgical procedure. Adjacent tissues, like the bowel, receive no radiation because they are displaced from the radiation field.[132–135] External beam radiation is generally used with IORT because it penetrates only the first few centimeters of tissue. Studies have demonstrated that IORT significantly improves the control of symptoms and the tumor, but the level of success depends upon the volume of residual tumor treated.

Brachytherapy and endocavitary radiation

Brachytherapy involves placing radioactive sources within a tumor bed and is another means of administering well-localized radiotherapy to limit the dose to adjacent uninvolved structures. Uninterrupted radiation is delivered precisely to the tumor bed over a determined number of minutes to hours. Brachytherapy has been used as definitive treatment for localized disease, as a boost in conjunction with external beam irradiation, and for the treatment of disease recurring in a previously irradiated area.

Practical advantages of brachytherapy include reduced overall treatment time and sparing of uninvolved surrounding structures that also allows reirradiation. The theoretical advantages of brachytherapy also include the direct placement of radiation in the operative bed that is at risk for microscopic residual disease, relative sparing of adjacent normal tissues, and better oxygenation of the surgical bed. Because brachytherapy localizes the radiation dose within a 3 cm radius of the catheters, considerably less normal tissue is irradiated with brachytherapy compared to external beam radiotherapy (Fig. 20-14). Reirradiation is then possible because the radiation from brachytherapy is well localized and does not injure surrounding previously irradiated tissues.[129–131] The localization of radiation dose with brachytherapy is based on the inverse-square law wherein the radiation dose rapidly decreases as the distance increases from the radiation source (Fig. 20-15). For example, only one-fourth the radiation dose is given to tissues that are located 2 cm away from the radiation source. Tissue hypoxia significantly reduces radiosensitivity; with brachytherapy, radiation is administered before hypoxic scar tissue develops in the wound. The inverse

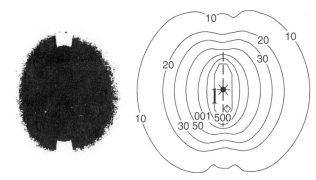

FIGURE 20-15 The emitted radioactivity and the radiation dose distribution from a radioactive source. Because the radiation is so localized and placed adjacent to or within tumors, high radiation doses can be administered even in cases of reirradiation.

square law and tissue hypoxia are critical to limiting the radiation dose needed for reirradiation of recurrent tumors. Like IMRT, the inverse square law allows for higher doses of radiation to be given directly to the tumor, while limiting the radiation dose to the surrounding tissues.

Brachytherapy sources can be placed either temporarily or permanently within the tumor. There are a wide variety of brachytherapy sources and strengths that can be used (Table 20-3). Low-dose rate brachytherapy places a lower energy radiation source either adjacent to (temporary implant) or inside tumors (permanent implant). Temporary implants sit within a site, much like a drain, generally for 2–5 days and can deliver 20–50 Gy during that time frame. Sources commonly used for low-dose rate brachytherapy include Iridium-192 for temporary implants, and Iodine-125 and Gold-198 for permanent implants.

High-dose rate brachytherapy places an intense radioactive radiation source adjacent to a tumor for a few minutes. High-dose rate brachytherapy is often used to treat tumors involving the biliary tract, esophagus, cervix, and bronchus. A number of reports show that dysphagia and bronchial obstruction relief ranges between 70% and 85% in the treatment of esophageal cancer. A combination of a short course of external beam radiation (30 Gy in 10 fractions) plus high-dose rate brachytherapy used as a localized radiation boost relieves dysphagia or bronchial obstruction for several months.[129–131] Relative contraindications to performing brachytherapy for esophageal cancer include a tumor length of 10 cm or more, extension to the gastroesophageal junction or cardia, skip lesions, extensive extraesophageal spread of disease, macroscopic regional adenopathy, tracheoesophageal fistula, cervical esophageal involvement, or stenosis that cannot be bypassed.

Brachytherapy and endocavitary radiation can be used alone, or more commonly, in conjunction with external beam radiation for pelvic tumors. Administering highly localized doses of radiation, brachytherapy can provide high doses of radiation directly to well-defined volumes to palliate bleeding and obstructive symptoms. Most often, these approaches are used among patients who are unable or unwilling to undergo surgical resection.

PALLIATIVE RADIATION TREATMENT SCHEDULES

Despite the wide variety of available treatment approaches, external beam radiation remains the most common application of radiotherapy. The administration of external beam irradiation is analogous to

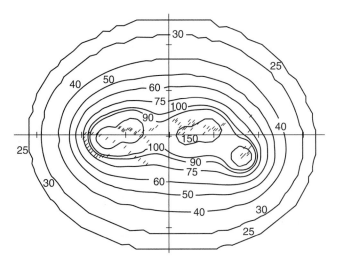

FIGURE 20-14 An isodose plan for brachytherapy in a tumor bed. The small dashes represent radiation seeds. Notice that within 2 cm on the X-axis, only 70% of the prescribed radiation dose is given and on the Y-axis, the tissues receive only 30% of the prescribed radiation dose.

the prescription of medications based upon pharmacologic principles of dosing. A balance is required between the dose required to kill the tumor and the radiation dose tolerated by the normal tissues; this is similar to the limitations imposed by renal tolerance to certain classes of antibiotics or by bone marrow and gastrointestinal tolerance to chemotherapy.

The concept of fractionated radiation allows treatment of the cancer while not exceeding the tolerance of the surrounding normal tissues. The four "Rs" of radiation biology are repair of sublethal damage, reoxygenation, repopulation, and reassortment of cells within the cell cycle.[126] These four factors are key to deciding the radiation schedule to optimize tumor regression while minimizing effects to normal tissues.

With fractionated radiation normal tissues are able to *repair* sublethal radiation effects between treatments. With large daily doses of radiation, a large number of tumor cells are killed, but repair of normal tissues is lower (Fig. 20-16). Because normal tissues are unable to repair the radiation damage of large daily doses of radiation, the total radiation dose that can be given is also much lower.[126]

Equivalent normal tissue effects can be achieved using various radiation treatment schedules. The following clinical radiation schedules are used to treat spine metastases: 2000 cGy is delivered in 5 fractions, 3000 cGy is administered in 10 fractions, 3500 cGy in 14 fractions, or 4000 cGy in 20 fractions. The late radiation effects on the spinal cord would be equal to giving 2800 cGy, 3600 cGy, and 3900 cGy, respectively, at 200 cGy per fraction. This shows that as the radiation dose per fraction increases, the late radiation toxicities biologically exceed the total radiation dose administered. This effect is more exaggerated as the radiation dose per fraction increases from the standard 200 cGy per fraction.[136] Relating back to the example of integral dose in Table 20-5, administration of 5880 cGy at 294 cGy per fraction would result in severe long-term radiation effects because this would be biologically equal to a total radiation dose of 7200 cGy at 200 cGy per fraction to a large area of small bowel.[137]

The total dose of radiation necessary to eradicate a tumor is a function of the volume of disease and the number of tumor cells killed with each radiation fraction. The tumor volume is the sum of viable and nonviable cells. In most tumors, the potential number of tumor cells is directly proportional to the tumor volume. In some tumors, like soft tissue sarcomas, there is a large necrotic fraction and the rate of cell loss and removal of dead tumor cells from the tumor volume is low. The viable cells may be less responsive to radiation because of the low oxygen tension in the nearby necrotic region. The radiosensitivity of cells also varies during the cell cycle. Cells are most resistant to radiation when they are in the late S-phase, and in the late G1/G0 phase. Radiation resistance results from either rapidly proliferating tumors that spend most of their time in S-phase or a slowly proliferating tumor where many cells are in G1/G0.

Less total radiation dose is required to control microscopic residual disease than bulk disease. For example, the 2-year rate of local control following irradiation alone in the treatment of cervical node metastases in head and neck cancer is directly related to the node diameter and total dose. Using 200 cGy per daily fraction of radiation, more than 95% of patients with only microscopic residual cancer achieve tumor control, and more than 85% of patients with lymph node diameters of less than 2 cm in size are controlled with a median dose of 6600 cGy. But, only 69% of nodes measuring between 2.5 and 3.0 cm are controlled after 6900 cGy and 59% of nodes larger than 3.5 cm are controlled after 7000 cGy. Large tumors have a large hypoxic fraction of cells.[126] Hypoxic cells are relatively resistant to radiation effects; it takes three times the dose of radiation to control hypoxic tumors as it does well-oxygenated tumors (Fig. 20-10). With fractionated radiation, hypoxic areas are able to reoxygenate to some degree during the course of treatment.

Additionally, tumor cells and normal tissues vary widely in their tolerance to radiation because of cellular repopulation. Radiation doses need to be high enough to kill tumor cells but low enough to

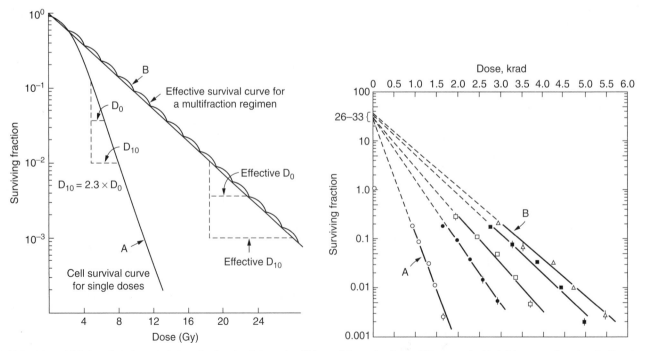

FIGURE 20-16 (A) Cell survival after a single large fraction of radiation and multiple small doses of radiation; (B) because of sublethal damage and repair, a significantly greater total dose of radiation is needed to achieve tumor control when multiple radiation fractions are used.

Table 20-6A

Comparison of Radiation Dose and Fraction Schedules

	Conventional	Hyperfractionation	Accelerated	Hypofractionation
Intent	Curative	Curative	Curative	Palliative
# fractions per day	1	2 (↑)	▶ 1/day for the first 3 to 4 weeks of XRT (↔) ▶ Then 2/day (large field + boost field around the tumor) for the last 1 to 2 weeks of XRT (↑)	1 (↔)
# fractions	25–30	60–70 (↑)	30–35 (↑)	1–15 (↓)
Dose per fraction	1.8–2 Gy	1.2 Gy BID (↓)	▶ 1.8–2 Gy to a large field (↔) ▶ 1.5 Gy to a boost field (↔)	8 Gy (1 fraction) to 2.5 Gy (15 fractions) (↑)
# weeks	5–6	7–9 (↑)	5–6 (↔)	1–3 (↓)
Total Radiation Dose	45–60 Gy	70–84 Gy (↑)	52–65 Gy (↑)	8–35 Gy (↓)

Note: Arrows represent a comparison to conventional fractionation.

allow normal tissues to repair and repopulate. Very low doses of radiation have limited acute effects on normal tissues. No inflammation of the skin or mucosa occurs when the radiation dose is less than 2000 cGy when given in 200 cGy fractions over 2 weeks. But this total dose of radiation is not sufficient to permanently kill tumor cells due to repopulation of the tumor cells. In the past, a course of radiation was interrupted after 2 weeks of treatment to minimize the side effects of treatment. These so-called "split courses of radiation" that allowed repair and repopulation of normal tissues and improved tolerance to radiation have been abandoned because tumor control rates were compromised by tumor repopulation during the interruption in treatment.[138,139] In fact, tumor repopulation was found during radiobiologic evaluations to be accelerated after 2 weeks of radiation because of tumor reoxygenation.

Tolerance to radiation also depends on the type of tissue treated. There are two types of normal tissues. *Acute reacting tissues*, which are rapidly proliferating tissues like mucosal surfaces, usually develop an inflammatory radiation reaction during the course of treatment. *Late reacting tissues*, which do not proliferate, like brain, liver, and muscle, generally do not develop a significant inflammatory reaction during the radiation course. Acute radiation reactions do not predict the extent of late radiation effects. Scar tissue is the most common form of late radiation effect. These effects are similar to those seen in wound healing. The alpha-beta ratio is a calculation that relates to the ability of normal tissues to repair the damage caused by radiation.[126] With low daily doses of radiation over several weeks, more acute radiation effects are seen during the course of radiation. When high daily doses of radiation are given over a short period of time, the most significant radiation side effects occur months to years after the radiation is completed.

Relating normal tissue tolerance to a 5% risk of a treatment-related complication at 5 years, the tolerance doses (TD 5/5) of each organ have been reported by a National Cancer Institute Task Force.[51] Radiation tolerance is a function of the type and volume of tissue irradiated. The TD 5/5 ranges from 1000 cGy for the eye, 1750 cGy for the lung, 4500 cGy for the brain, and 7000 cGy for the larynx when the entire organ is treated. When only one-third of the organ is irradiated, these values equal 4500 cGy for the lung, 6000 cGy for the brain, and 7900 cGy for the larynx.

With palliative radiation, shorter external beam radiation schedules are generally used that administer a higher radiation dose with each radiation fraction. This is known as *hypofractionation* (Tables 20-6A and B). Tumor cell kill is proportional to the radiation dose that is administered. Therefore, symptomatic relief is more quickly achieved because of the large number of tumor cells that are killed in a short period of time with large daily doses of radiation.

A shorter course of therapy also has a significant impact on quality of life. This short course of treatment not only provides more prompt relief of tumor-related symptoms, but it limits the amount of time needed for the patient to come back and forth for radiation treatments. This is particularly important because the median survival is less than 6 months among patients with poor prognostic factors. However, higher radiation doses, that provide more durable pain relief, are considered warranted for patients with good prognostic factors who require treatment over the spine and other critical sites.

In contrast to the low daily radiation doses (1.8–2 Gy) given with each treatment during conventional radiation schedules to total

Table 20-6B

The Relative Relationships of Radiation Dose per Fraction and Total Dose in a Variety of Radiation Schedules

	Total Dose		
	Number of Fractions		
LOW			HIGH
Hypofractionation	Conventional Fractionation	Hyperfractionation	Accelerated Fractionation
20–30 Gy	50–60 Gy	70–80 Gy	55–65 Gy
5–10 fractions	25–30 fractions	60–70 fractions	28–35 fractions
1–2 weeks	5–6 weeks	7–8 weeks	5–6 weeks

Note: When a high dose of radiation is given per fraction, the total dose must be low and given in a small number of fractions.

radiation doses of 50–60 Gy over 5–6 weeks, large daily radiation fractions are given with hypofractionated radiation schedules used for palliative radiation. Because of normal tissue tolerance to radiation, the total radiation dose that can be administered is low when high doses of radiation are given with each daily fraction. Hypofractionated radiation schedules can range from 2.5 Gy per fraction administered over 3 weeks for a total radiation dose of 35 Gy to a single 8 Gy dose of radiation.[140,141] Most frequently, 30 Gy is administered in 10 fractions over 2 weeks. The radiation schedule selected depends on the radiation tolerance of the tissues in the field and the patient's prognosis.

Various other radiation schedules have been developed that administer very high total doses of radiation, but use small daily doses, given twice a day, in an attempt to improve local regional control of the tumor. This approach is now also being used in palliative radiation, especially in cases of reirradiation, because the radiation effects to normal tissues are reduced. As shown in Tables 20-6A and B, hyperfractionated radiation administers two small radiation doses each day, usually 120 cGy per fraction, with a 6-hour separation between doses to allow normal tissues to repair the effects of radiation between doses.[126,140,141] Studies have shown that the 6-hour separation is critical because it takes 6 hours to complete repair of radiation effects in normal tissues. If the radiation doses were given less than 6 hours apart, the late radiation effects would be more significant. The total radiation doses with hyperfractionation for curative radiation range from 70 Gy to more than 80 Gy. These hyperfractionated radiation doses result in late normal tissue effects that are equivalent to a total radiation dose of 58–68 Gy with a conventional radiation schedule that uses one daily fraction of 180–200 cGy. Although the total radiation doses with hyperfractionation in the palliative setting are generally lower, the most significant advantage is reduction in the development of late side effects to normal tissues, such as small bowel injury.

Loosely defined, any course of radiation that relieves symptoms is palliative treatment. More commonly, palliative radiation is designated for patients with incurable disease due to extensive local tumor infiltration and/or metastatic disease. Short courses of radiation are used in these cases. However, symptomatic patients with an extensive primary tumor, but who do not have distant metastases or have limited metastatic disease, may have a prolonged survival. Therefore, the radiation schedule that is used to relieve symptoms must be indexed to the types of tissues treated, the potential for tumor resection, and/or overall prognosis.

▶ Therapeutic recommendations

Radiation remains an important modality in palliative care. A number of clinical, prognostic, and therapeutic factors must be considered to determine the most optimal treatment regimen in palliative radiotherapy. Adequate management of cancer-related pain is important both during and after completing palliative irradiation. Efficient and effective palliative treatment is imperative for locally advanced and metastatic cancer in order to relieve symptoms, improve function, and minimize disease-related morbidity.

Symptoms that persist after palliative radiation should be evaluated to exclude progression of disease in the treated area, possible extension of disease outside the radiation portal, or treatment-related side effects. For example, reduced cortical strength after treatment of bone metastases can result in compression, stress fractures, or microfractures.

More specific criteria need to be delineated for prognosis to determine the appropriate treatment regimen for metastases. A staging system within the category of metastatic disease should incorporate the performance status, type and extent of bone and visceral involvement, time to disease progression, the primary tumor site, and account for prior failed therapies. Therefore, the responses to and outcomes after radiation therapy must be specifically defined relative to the irradiated and unirradiated sites of disease, and the other antineoplastic and supportive care therapies administered.

Radiation therapy is an important means of treating localized symptoms related to tumor involvement by providing a wide range of therapeutic options. Radiobiologic principles, the radiation tolerance of adjacent normal tissues, and the patient's clinical condition influence the selection of radiation technique, dose, and fraction size. Validated symptom assessment tools, analgesic use, prognostic factors, and radiobiologic principles should be applied to deliver the most efficient and efficacious treatment schedule in accordance with the specific clinical presentation.

Palliative irradiation should be integrated within a multidisciplinary therapeutic approach because of the need to treat associated symptoms and other underlying medical problems. Antineoplastic therapy can provide tumor regression, relief of cancer-related symptoms, and maintain functional integrity. Control of cancer-related pain with the use of analgesics is imperative to allow comfort during and while awaiting response to radiation and other therapies. Pain represents a sensitive measure of disease activity. Close follow-up should be performed to ensure control of cancer and treatment-related pain, and to assess progressive or recurrent disease.

REFERENCES

1. Chang VT, Thaler HT, Polyak TA, et al. Quality of life and survival: the role of multidimensional symptom assessment. *Cancer.* 1998;83:173–179.
2. Greenwald HP, Bonica JJ, Bergner M. The prevalence of pain in four cancers. *Cancer.* 1987;60:2563–2569.
3. Sherry MM, Greco FA, Johnson DH, Hainsworth JD. Breast cancer with skeletal metastases at initial diagnosis. Distinctive clinical characteristics and favorable prognosis. *Cancer.* 1986;58:178–182.
4. Jacobson AF. Musculoskeletal pain as an indicator of occult malignancy. Yield of bone scintigraphy. *Arch Intern Med.* 1997;157:105–109.
5. Abbas F, Scardino PT. The natural history of clinical prostate carcinoma. *Cancer.* 1997;80:827–833.
6. Borre M, Nerstrom B, Overgaard J. The natural history of prostate carcinoma based on a Danish population treated with no intent to cure. *Cancer.* 1997;80:917–928.
7. Vuorinen E. Pain as an early symptom in cancer. *Clin J Pain.* 1993;9:272–278.
8. Reuben DB, Mor V, Hiris J. Clinical symptoms and length of survival in patients with terminal cancer. *Arch Intern Med.* 1988;148:1586–1591.
9. Portenoy RK, Miransky J, Thaler HT, et al. Pain in ambulatory patients with lung or colon cancer. Prevalence, characteristics, and effect. *Cancer.* 1992;70:1616–1624.
10. Fielding LP, Henson DE. Multiple prognostic factors and outcome analysis in patients with cancer. Communication from the American Joint Committee on Cancer. *Cancer.* 1993;71:2426–2429.
11. Pienta KJ, Esper PS. Risk factors for prostate cancer. *Ann Intern Med.* 1993;118:793–803.
12. Perez CA, Cosmatos D, Garcia DM, Eisbruch A, Poulter CA. Irradiation in relapsing carcinoma of the prostate. *Cancer.* 1993;71:1110–1122.
13. Lai PP, Perez CA, Lockett MA. Prognostic significance of pelvic recurrence and distant metastasis in prostate carcinoma following definitive radiotherapy. *Int J Radiat Oncol Biol Phys.* 1992;24:423–430.
14. Chisolm GD, Rana A, Howard GCW. Management options for painful carcinoma of the prostate. *Semin Oncol.* 1993;20:34–37.
15. Yamashita K, Denno K, Ueda T, et al. Prognostic significance of bone metastases in patients with metastatic prostate cancer. *Cancer.* 1993;71:1297–1302.

16. Tong D, Gillick L, Hendrickson FR. The palliation of symptomatic osseous metastases: final results of the Study by the Radiation Therapy Oncology Group. *Cancer.* 1982;50:893–899.

17. Blitzer PH. Reanalysis of the RTOG study of the palliation of symptomatic osseous metastasis. *Cancer.* 1985;55:1468–1472.

18. Ford HT, Yarnold JR. Radiation therapy—pain relief and recalcification. In: Stoll BA, Parbhoo S, eds. *Bone Metastases: Monitoring and Treatment.* New York: Raven Press; 1983:343–354.

19. Hortobagyi GN, Libshitz HI, Seabold JE. Osseous metastases of breast cancer. Clinical, biochemical, radiographic, and scintigraphic evaluation of response to therapy. *Cancer.* 1984;53:577–582.

20. Vogel CL, Schoenfelder J, Shemano I, et al. Worsening bone scan in the evaluation of antitumor response during hormonal therapy of breast cancer. *J Clin Oncol.* 1995;13:1123–1128.

21. Rutten EHJM, Crul BJP, van der Toorn PPG, et al. Pain characteristics help to predict the analgesic efficacy of radiotherapy for the treatment of cancer pain. *Pain.* 1997;69:131–135.

22. Kelly JB, Payne R. Pain syndromes in the cancer patient. *Neurol Clin.* 1991;9:937–953.

23. Portenoy RK. Cancer pain management. *Semin Oncol.* 1993;20:19–35.

24. Wilson PC, et al. Palliative radiation for bone metastases—does pain response reflect full clinical benefit? *Int J Radiat Oncol Biol Phys.* 2002;54:309.

25. Chow E, Wong R, Hruby G, et al. Prospective patient-based assessment of effectiveness of palliative radiotherapy for bone metastases. *Radiother Oncol.* 2001;61:77–82.

26. Yau V, Chow E, Davis L, et al. Pain management in cancer patients with bone metastases remains a challenge. *J Pain Symptom Manage.* 2004;27:1–3.

27. Berger A, Dukes E., Smith M, et al. Use of oral and transdermal opioids among patients with metastatic cancer during the last year of life. *J Pain Symptom Manage.* 2003;26:723–730.

28. Chow E, Wu J, Hoskin P, et al. International consensus on palliative radiotherapy endpoints for future clinical trials in bone metastases. *Radiother Oncol.* 2002;64:275–280.

29. Barak F, Werner A, Walach N, et al. The palliative efficacy of a single high dose of radiation in treatment of symptomatic osseous metastases. *Int J Radiat Oncol Biol Phys.* 1987;13:1233–1235.

30. Cole DJ. A randomized trial of a single treatment versus conventional fractionation in the palliative radiotherapy of painful bone metastases. *Clin Oncol (R Coll Radiol).* 1989;1:59–62.

31. Hoskin PJ. Werner A, Walach N, et al. A prospective randomized trial of 4 Gy or 8 Gy single doses in the treatment of metastatic bone pain. *Radiother Oncol.* 1992;23:74–78.

32. Price P, Hoskin PJ, Easton D, et al. Prospective randomized trial of single and multifraction radiotherapy schedules in the treatment of painful bony metastases. *Radiother Oncol.* 1986;6:247–255.

33. Wu JS, Wong R, Johnston M, et al. Meta-analysis of dose-fractionation radiotherapy trials for the palliation of painful bone metastases. *Int J Radiat Oncol Biol Phys.* 2003;55:594–605.

34. Kal HB. Single fraction radiotherapy is as effective as multiple fractions for palliating painful bone metastases. *Cancer Treat Rev.* 2003;29:345–347.

35. Jeremic B. Single fraction external beam radiation therapy in the treatment of localized metastatic bone pain. A review. *J Pain Symptom Manage.* 2001;22:1048–1058.

36. Fiorica F. Short fractionation radiotherapy versus multiple factionated radiotherapy in patients with bone metastases: a meta-analysis of randomized clinical trials. *Int J Radiat Oncol Biol Phys.* 2003;57:S446.

37. Chow E, Lutz S, Beyene J. A single fraction for all, or an argument for fractionation tailored to fit the needs of each individual patient with bone metastases? *Int J Radiat Oncol Biol Phys.* 2003;55:565–567.

38. Sze WM, Shelley MD, Helds I, et al. Palliation of metastatic bone pain: single fraction versus multifraction radiotherapy—a systematic review of randomized trials. *Clin Oncol (R Coll Radiol).* 2003;15:345–352.

39. Yarnold JR, Party BPTW. 8 Gy single fraction radiotherapy for the treatment of metastatic skeletal pain: randomized comparison with a multifraction schedule over 12 months of patient follow up. *Radiother Oncol.* 1999;52:111–121.

40. Steenland E, Leer J, van Houwelingen H, et al. The effect of a single fraction compared to multiple fractions on painful bone metastases: a global analysis of the Dutch Bone Metastasis Study. *Radiother Oncol.* 1999;52:101–109.

41. van den Hout WB, Van der Linden YM, Steenland E, et al. Single- versus multiple-fraction radiotherapy in patients with painful bone metastases: cost-utility analysis based on a randomized trial. *J Natl Cancer Inst.* 2003;95:222–229.

42. McQuay HJ, Collins SL, Carroll D, Moore RA. Radiotherapy for the palliation of painful bone metastases. *Cochrane Database Syst Rev.* 2000: CD001793.

43. Haartsell WF, et al. Phase III randomized trial of 8 Gy in 1 fraction vs. 30 Gy in 10 fractions for palliation of painful bone metastases: preliminary results of RTOG 97-14. *Int J Radiat Oncol Biol Phys.* 2003;57:S124.

44. Haddad P, Wong RKS, Pond GR, et al. Factors influencing the use of single vs multiple fractions of palliative radiotherapy for bone metastases: a 5-year review. *Clin Oncol (R Coll Radiol).* 2005;17:430–434.

45. Koswig S, Budach V. Remineralization and pain relief in bone metastases after after different radiotherapy fractions (10 times 3 Gy vs. 1 time 8 Gy). A prospective study. *Strahlenther Onkol.* 1999;175:500–508.

46. Macklis RM, Cornelli H, Lasher J. Brief courses of palliative radiotherapy for metastatic bone pain: a pilot cost-minimization comparison with narcotic analgesics. *Am J Clin Oncol.* 1998;21:617–622.

47. Hoskin PJ, Grover A, Bhana R. Metastatic spinal cord compression: radiotherapy outcome and dose fractionation. *Radiother Oncol.* 2003;68:175–180.

48. van der Linden YM, Lok J, Steenland E, et al. Re-irradiation of painful bone metastases. A further analysis of the Dutch Bone Metastasis Study. *Int J Radiat Oncol Biol Phys.* 2003;57:S222.

49. Gaze MN, Kelly CG, Kerr GR, et al. Pain relief and quality of life following radiotherapy for bone metastases: a randomized trial of two fractionation schedules. *Radiother Oncol.* 1997;45:109–116.

50. Smith TJ, Staats PS, Deer T, et al. Randomized clinical trial of an implantable drug delivery system compared with comprehensive medical management for refractory cancer pain: impact on pain, drug-related toxicity, and survival. *J Clin Oncol.* 2002;20:4040–4049.

51. Chow E, Coia L, Wu J, et al. This house believes that multiple-fraction radiotherapy is a barrier to referral for palliative radiotherapy for bone metastases. *Curr Oncol.* 2002;9:60–66.

52. Byrne TN. Spinal cord compression from epidural metastases. *N Engl J Med.* 1992;327:614–619.

53. Grant R, Papadopoulos SM, Greenberg HS. Metastatic epidural spinal cord compression. *Neurol Clin.* 1991;9:825–841.

54. Maranzano E, Latini P, Checcaglini F, et al. Radiation therapy in metastatic spinal cord compression. A prospective analysis of 105 consecutive patients. *Cancer.* 1991;67:1311–1317.

55. Janjan NA. Radiotherapeutic management of spinal metastases. *J Pain Symptom Manage.* 1996;1:47–56.

56. Loblaw DA, Laperriere NJ. Emergency treatment of malignant extradural spinal cord compression: an evidence-based guideline. *J Clin Oncol.* 1998;16:1613–1624.

57. Boogerd W, van der Sande JJ. Diagnosis and treatment of spinal cord compression in malignant disease. *Cancer Treat Rev.* 1993;19: 129–150.

58. Boogerd W. Central nervous system metastasis in breast cancer. *Radiother Oncol.* 1996;40:5–22.

59. Bunting RW, Boublik M, Blevins FT, et al. Functional outcome of pathologic fracture secondary to malignant disease in a rehabilitation hospital. *Cancer.* 1992;69:98–102.

60. Paterson AH. Bone metastases in breast cancer, prostate cancer and myeloma. *Bone.* 1987;8(Suppl. 1):S17–S22.

61. Townsend PW, Smalley SR, Cozad SC, et al. Role of postoperative radiation therapy after stabilization of fractures caused by metastatic disease. *Int J Radiat Oncol Biol Phys.* 1995;31:43–49.

62. Heisterberg L, Johansen TS. Treatment of pathological fractures. *Acta Orthop Scand.* 1979;50:787–790.

63. Fidler M. Incidence of fracture through metastases in long bones. *Acta Orthop Scand.* 1981;52:623–627.

64. Oda MA, Schurman DJ. Monitoring of pathologic fracture. In: Stoll BA, Parbhoo S, eds. *Bone Metastases: Monitoring and Treatment.* New York: Raven; 1983:271–288.

65. Plunkett TA, Smith P, Rubens RD. Risk of complications from bone metastases in breast cancer. implications for management. *Eur J Cancer.* 2000;36:476–482.

66. Groot MT, Boeken Kruger CG, Pelger RC, et al. Costs of prostate cancer, metastatic to the bone, in the Netherlands. *Eur Urol.* 2003;43:226–232.

67. Cleeland CS, Gonin R, Hatfield AK, et al. Pain and its treatment in outpatients with metastatic cancer. *N Engl J Med.* 1994;330:592–596.

68. Jacox AK, Carr DB, Payne R. *Management of Cancer Pain. Clinical Practice Guideline No. 9.* Rockville, MD: Agency for Health Care Policy and Research; 1994. AHCPR publication no. 94-0592.

69. Jacox A, Carr DB, Payne R. New clinical-practice guidelines for the management of pain in patients with cancer. *N Engl J Med.* 1994;330: 651–655.

70. Brescia FJ, Portenoy RK, Ryan M, et al. Pain, opioid use, and survival in hospitalized patients with advanced cancer. *J Clin Oncol.* 1992;10: 149–155.

71. Porzsolt F. Goals of palliative cancer therapy: scope of the problem. *Cancer Treat Rev.* 1993;19(Suppl. A):3–14.

72. Bates T, Yarnold JR, Blitzer P, et al. Bone metastasis consensus statement. *Int J Radiat Oncol Biol Phys.* 1992;23:215–216.

73. Bates T. A review of local radiotherapy in the treatment of bone metastases and cord compression. *Int J Radiat Oncol Biol Phys.* 1992;23: 217–221.

74. Turner S, Marosszeky B, Timms I, et al. Malignant spinal cord compression: a prospective evaluation. *Int J Radiat Oncol Biol Phys.* 1993;26:141–146.

75. Boogerd W, van der Sande JJ, Kroger R. Early diagnosis and treatment of spinal epidural metastasis in breast cancer: a prospective study. *J Neurol Neurosurg Psychiatry.* 1992;55:1188–1193.

76. Wada E, Yamamoto T, Furuno M, et al. Spinal cord compression secondary to osteoblastic metastasis. *Spine.* 1993;18:1380–1381.

77. Algra PR, Hermans JJ, Valk J, et al. Do metastases in vertebrae begin in the body or the pedicles? Imaging study in 45 patients. *AJR Am J Roentgenol.* 1992;158:1275–1279.

78. Landmann C, Hunig R, Gratzl O. The role of laminectomy in the combined treatment of metastatic spinal cord compression. *Int J Radiat Oncol Biol Phys.* 1992;24:627–631.

79. Kim RY, Smith JW, Spencer S, et al. Malignant epidural spinal cord compression associated with a paravertebral mass: its radiotherapeutic outcome on radiosensitivity. *Int J Radiat Oncol Biol Phys.* 1993;27:1079–1083.

80. Bach F, Agerlin N, Sorensen JB, et al. Metastatic spinal cord compression secondary to lung cancer. *J Clin Oncol.* 1992;10:1781–1787.

81. Jeremic B, Djuric L, Mijatovic L. Incidence of radiation myelitis of the cervical spinal cord at doses of 5500 cGy or greater. *Cancer.* 1991;68:2138–2141.

82. Wen PY, Blanchard KL, Block CC, et al. Development of Lhermitte's sign after bone marrow transplantation. *Cancer.* 1992;69:2262–2266.

83. Powers BE, Thames HD, Gillette SM, et al. Volume effects in the irradiated canine spinal cord: do they exist when the probability of injury is low? *Radiother Oncol.* 1998;46:297–306.

84. Sugimura H, Kisanuki A, Tamura S, et al. Magnetic resonance imaging of bone marrow changes after irradiation. *Invest Radiol.* 1994;29:35–41.

85. Yankelevitz DF, Henschke CI, Knapp PH, et al. Effect of radiation therapy on thoracic and lumbar bone marrow: evaluation with MR imaging. *AJR Am J Roentgenol.* 1991;157:87–92.

86. Russi EG, Pergolizzi S, Gaeta M, et al. Palliative-radiotherapy in lumbosacral carcinomatous neuropathy. *Radiother Oncol.* 1993;26: 172–173.

87. Saarto T, Janes R, Tenhunen M, et al. Palliative radiotherapy in the treatment of skeletal metastases. *Eur J Pain.* 2002;6:323–330.

88. Altehoefer C, Ghanem N, Hogerle S, et al. Comparative detectability of bone metastases and impact on therapy of magnetic resonance imaging and bone scintigraphy in patients with breast cancer. *Eur J Radiol.* 2001;40:16–23.

89. Loblaw DA, Laperriere NJ, Mackillop WJ. A population-based study of malignant spinal cord compression in Ontario. *Clin Oncol (R Coll Radiol).* 2003;15:211–217.

90. Rades D, Heidenreich F, Karstens JH. Final results of a prospective study of the prognostic value of the time to develop motor deficits before irradiation in metastatic spinal cord compression. *Int J Radiat Oncol Biol Phys.* 2002;53:975–979.

91. Rades D, Blach M, Bremer M, et al. Prognostic significance of the time of developing motor deficits before radiation therapy in metastatic spinal cord compression: one-year results of a prospective trial. *Int J Radiat Oncol Biol Phys.* 2000;48:1403–1408.

92. Hatrick NC, Lucas JD, Timothy AR, et al. The surgical treatment of metastatic disease of the spine. *Radiother Oncol.* 2000;56:335–339.

93. Helweg-Larsen S, Sorensen PS, Kreiner S. Prognostic factors in metastatic spinal cord compression: a prospective study using multivariate analysis of variables influencing survival and gait function in 153 patients. *Int J Radiat Oncol Biol Phys.* 2000;46:1163–1169.

94. Prie L, Lagarde P, Palussiere J, et al. [Radiotherapy of spinal metastases in breast cancer. Apropos of a series of 108 patients]. *Cancer Radiother.* 1997;1:234–239.

95. Maranzano E, Bellavita R, Floridi P, et al. Radiation-induced myelopathy in long-term surviving metastatic spinal cord compression patients after hypofractionated radiotherapy: a clinical and magnetic resonance imaging analysis. *Radiother Oncol.* 2001;60:281–288.

96. Moineuse C, et al. Magnetic resonance imaging findings in multiple myeloma: descriptive and predictive value. *Joint Bone Spine.* 2001;68: 334–344.

97. Ridet JL, Pencalet P, Belcram M, et al. Effects of spinal cord X-irradiation on the recovery of paraplegic rats. *Exp Neurol.* 2000;161:1–14.

98. Milker-Zabel S, Zabel A, Thilmann C, et al. Clinical results of retreatment of vertebral bone metastases by stereotactic conformal radiotherapy and intensity-modulated radiotherapy. *Int J Radiat Oncol Biol Phys.* 2003;55:162–167.

99. Grosu AL, Andratschke N, Nieder C, Molls M. Retreatment of the spinal cord with palliative radiotherapy. *Int J Radiat Oncol Biol Phys.* 2002;52:1288–1292.

100. Bach F, Bjerregaard B, Soletormos G, et al. Diagnostic value of cerebrospinal fluid cytology in comparison with tumor marker activity in central nervous system metastases secondary to breast cancer. *Cancer.* 1993;72:2376–2382.

101. Porter AT, McEwan AJ, Powe JE, et al. Results of a randomized phase-III trial to evaluate the efficacy of strontium-89 adjuvant to local field external beam irradiation in the management of endocrine resistant metastatic prostate cancer. *Int J Radiat Oncol Biol Phys.* 1993;25:805–813.

102. Porter AT, McEwan AJ. Strontium-89 as an adjuvant to external beam radiation improves pain relief and delays disease progression in advanced prostate cancer: results of a randomized controlled trial. *Semin Oncol.* 1993;20:38–43.

103. Robinson RG, Preston DF, Schiefelbein M, et al. Strontium 89 therapy for the palliation of pain due to osseous metastases. *JAMA.* 1995;274:420–424.

104. Serafini AN, Houston SJ, Resche I, et al. Palliation of pain associated with metastatic bone cancer using samarium-153 lexidronam: a double-blind placebo-controlled clinical trial. *J Clin Oncol.* 1998;16:1574–1581.

105. Rogers CL, Speiser BL, Ram PC, et al. Efficacy and toxicity of intravenous strontium-89 for symptomatic osseous metastases. *J Brachytherapy Int.* 1998;14:133–142.

106. de Klerk JM, Zonnenberg BA, van het Schip AD, et al. Dose escalation study of rhenium-186 hydroxyethylidene diphosphonate in patients with metastatic prostate cancer. *Eur J Nucl Med.* 1994;21:1114–1120.

107. Sciuto R, Maini CL, Tofani A, et al. Radiosensitization with low-dose carboplatin enhances pain palliation in radioisotope therapy with strontium-89. *Nucl Med Commun.* 1996;17:799–804.

108. Bolger JJ, Dearnaley DP, Kirk D, et al. Strontium-89 (Metastron) versus external beam radiotherapy in patients with painful bone metastases secondary to prostatic cancer: preliminary report of a multicenter trial. UK Metastron Investigators Group. *Semin Oncol.* 1993;20:32–33.

109. Bayouth JE, Macey DJ, Kasi PL, Fossell FU, et al. Dosimetry and toxicity of samarium-153-EDTMP administered for bone pain due to skeletal metastases. *J Nucl Med.* 1994;35:63–69.

110. McEwan AJ, Amyotte GA, McGowan DG, et al. A retrospective analysis of the cost effectiveness of treatment with Metastron in patients with prostate cancer metastatic to bone. *Eur Urol.* 1994;26(Suppl. 1):26–31.

111. Alberts AS, Smit BJ, Louw WK, et al. Dose response relationship and multiple dose efficacy and toxicity of samarium-153-EDTMP in metastatic cancer to bone. *Radiother Oncol.* 1997;43:175–179.

112. Franzius C, Schuck A, Bielack SS. High-dose samarium-153 ethylene diamine tetramethylene phosphonate: low toxicity of skeletal irradiation in patients with osteosarcoma and bone metastases. *J Clin Oncol.* 2002;20:1953–1954.

113. Anderson PM, Wiseman GA, Dispenzeri A, et al. High-dose samarium-153 ethylene diamine tetramethylene phosphonate: low toxicity of skeletal irradiation in patients with osteosarcoma and bone metastases. *J Clin Oncol.* 2002;20:189–196.

114. Windsor PM. Predictors of response to strontium-89 (Metastron) in skeletal metastases from prostate cancer: report of a single centre's 10-year experience. *Clin Oncol (R Coll Radiol).* 2001;13:219–227.

115. Holmes RA. Radiopharmaceuticals in clinical trials. *Semin Oncol.* 1993;20:22–26.

116. Eary JF, Collins C, Stabin M, et al. Samarium-153-EDTMP biodistribution and dosimetry estimation. *J Nucl Med.* 1993;34:1031–1036.

117. Smeland S, Erikstein B, Aas M, et al. Role of strontium-89 as adjuvant to palliative external beam radiotherapy is questionable: results of a double-blind randomized study. *Int J Radiat Oncol Biol Phys.* 2003;56:1397–1404.

118. Oosterhof GO, Roberts JT, de Reijke TM, et al. Strontium(89) chloride versus palliative local field radiotherapy in patients with hormonal escaped prostate cancer: a phase III study of the European Organization for Research and Treatment of Cancer, Genitourinary Group. *Eur Urol.* 2003;44:519–526.

119. Porter AT, Ben-Josef E. Strontium 89 in the treatment of bony metastases. *Important Adv Oncol.* 1995:87–94.

120. Kagan AR. Palliation of visceral recurrences and metastases. In: Perez CA, Brady LW, eds. *Principles and Practice of Radiation Oncology.* Philadelphia: Lippincott Raven; 1998:2219–2226.

121. Janjan NA, Breslin T, Lenzi R, et al. Avoidance of colostomy placement in advanced colorectal cancer with twice weekly hypofractionated radiation plus continuous infusion 5-fluorouracil. *J Pain Symptom Manage.* 2000;20:266–272.

122. Crane CH, Janjan NA, Abbruzzese JL, et al. Effective pelvic symptom control using initial chemoradiation without colostomy in metastatic rectal cancer. *Int J Radiat Oncol Biol Phys.* 2001;49:107–116.

123. Brierley JD, Cummings BJ, Wong CS, et al. Adenocarcinoma of the rectum treated by radical external radiation therapy. *Int J Radiat Oncol Biol Phys.* 1995;31:255–259.

124. Kagan AR. Palliation of brain and spinal cord metastases. In: Perez CA, Brady LW, eds. *Principles and Practice of Radiation Oncology.* Philadelphia: Lippincott Raven; 1998:2187–2198.

125. Kahn FM. Dose Distribution and Scatter Analysis. In: *The Physics of Radiation Therapy.* Baltimore: Williams & Wilkins; 2003.

126. Hall E. Dose response relationships for normal tissues. In: *Radiobiiology for the Radiologist.* Philadelphia: JB Lippincott; 1994:45–75.

127. Nieder C, Milas L, Ang KK. Tissue tolerance to reirradiation. *Semin Radiat Oncol.* 2000;10:200–209.

128. Morris DE. Clinical experience with retreatment for palliation. *Semin Radiat Oncol.* 2000;10:210–221.

129. Shasha D, Harrison LB. The role of brachytherapy for palliation. *Semin Radiat Oncol.* 2000;10:222–239.

130. Erickson B, Janjan NA, Wilson JF. Brachytherapy: more versatile, more important for local control. *Intern Med.* 1993;14:33–46.

131. Janjan NA, et al. Control of unresectable recurrent anorectal cancer with Au198 seed implantation. *J Brachyther Int.* 1999;15:115–129.

132. Bussieres E, Gilly FN, Rouanet P, et al. Recurrences of rectal cancers: results of a multimodal approach with intraoperative radiation therapy. French Group of IORT. Intraoperative Radiation Therapy. *Int J Radiat Oncol Biol Phys.* 1996;34:49–56.

133. Martinez-Monge R, Nag S, Martin EW. Three different intraoperative radiation modalities (electron beam, high-dose-rate brachytherapy, and iodine-125 brachytherapy) in the adjuvant treatment of patients with recurrent colorectal adenocarcinoma. *Cancer.* 1999;86:236–247.

134. Mohiuddin M, Regine WF, Stevens J, et al. Combined intraoperative radiation and perioperative chemotherapy for unresectable cancers of the pancreas. *J Clin Oncol.* 1995;13:2764–2768.

135. Mohiuddin M, Marks GM, Lingareddy V, Marks J. Curative surgical resection following reirradiation for recurrent rectal cancer. *Int J Radiat Oncol Biol Phys.* 1997;39:643–649.

136. Barton M. Tables of equivalent dose in 2 Gy fractions: a simple application of the linear quadratic formula. *Int J Radiat Oncol Biol Phys.* 1995;31:371–378.

137. Minsky BD, Conti JA, Huang Y, et al. Relationship of acute gastrointestinal toxicity and the volume of irradiated small bowel in patients receiving combined modality therapy for rectal cancer. *J Clin Oncol.* 1995;13:1409–1416.

138. Cox JD, Pajak TF, Marcial VA, et al. Interruptions adversely affect local control and survival with hyperfractionated radiation therapy of carcinomas of the upper respiratory and digestive tracts. New evidence for accelerated proliferation from Radiation Therapy Oncology Group Protocol 8313. *Cancer.* 1992;69:2744–2748.

139. Cox JD, Pajak TF, Asbell SA, et al. Interruptions of high-dose radiation therapy decrease long-term survival of favorable patients with unresectable non-small cell carcinoma of the lung: analysis of 1244 cases from 3 Radiation Therapy Oncology Group (RTOG) trials. *Int J Radiat Oncol Biol Phys.* 1993;27:493–498.

140. Cox JD. Fractionation: a paradigm for clinical research in radiation oncology. *Int J Radiat Oncol Biol Phys.* 1987;13:1271–1281.

141. Cox JD. Large-dose fractionation (hypofractionation). *Cancer.* 1985;55:2105–2111.

PART

5

APPENDICES

The M. D. Anderson Approach to Cancer Pain

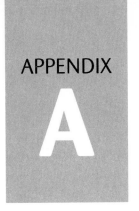

Tarun Jolly
Madhuri Are
Allen W. Burton

INTRODUCTION

Cancer pain remains a problem in spite of immense efforts aimed at protocol-based treatment regimens, education campaigns, and growing research.[1,2] Many entities have developed cancer pain treatment guidelines.[3] Unfortunately, implementation of these strategies is difficult. In a recent survey of cancer patient charts chosen at random at five different institutions, only 57% of outpatients and 53% of inpatients had pain documented in accordance with Joint Commission on Accreditation of Healthcare Organizations (JCAHO) standards that included adequate assessment, treatment, and/or follow-up pertaining to their pain.[4]

The University of Texas M. D. Anderson Cancer Center is an institution optimally suited to dealing with cancer pain. More than 70,000 patients will receive treatment for their cancer this year at M. D. Anderson, with more than 25,000 of those patients being new to the hospital.[5] The author's cancer pain service will see more than 10,000 of these patients and will apply a combination of pain management strategies, including nonpharmacologic methods, pharmacotherapy, nerve blocks, implants, and other procedural pain management approaches. Two other M. D. Anderson services, the postoperative pain service and the palliative care department, also provide specialized pain care. Additionally, institutional educational efforts, including a pain care task force in 2002, have been set in place to make pain assessment and treatment an institution-wide mandate, with specialty consultation reserved for problematic situations.

TREATMENT ALGORITHMS

Our approach to the cancer pain patient begins with a comprehensive initial assessment (Fig. A-1). We attempt to address the pain in the context of the patient's cancer diagnosis. For example, the patient may be receiving treatment for the cancer that may alter the pain (radiation, chemotherapy, or surgical resection). An initial determination is made about whether the patient's pain can be controlled using modalities such as physical therapy, coping strategies, exercise, or over-the-counter analgesics. For the patient who presents with severe pain due to significant tumor burden or who has failed treatment with the above-noted therapies, we proceed to administer opioid analgesics. An appropriate regimen of long-acting/short-acting opioids +/− adjuvant medications is chosen for the patient and is guided by the type of pain process with which they present. If during

the reassessment, the patient complains of continued pain or intolerable side effects, switching opioids (opioid rotation) is attempted in addition to treating the patient's side effects.

As often is the case with cancer pain, opioids alone may not adequately address the pain or side effects may vitiate employing opioid management alone. Current pain management protocols allow for a supplementation of analgesics with interventions that can be used therapeutically as well as diagnostically. After a patient has failed more conservative therapies, an interdisciplinary approach utilizing opioids, surgical, and minimally invasive interventional modalities should be considered.[6] Interventions currently being done by pain management specialists span a broad range, from standard epidural steroid injections to surgically implanted devices such as intrathecal drug delivery systems or spinal cord stimulators.[7]

Our approach to interventions is summarized in Fig. A-2. Prior to considering any interventional procedure for a patient, it must be verified that the patient will be an appropriate surgical candidate. This involves ensuring that the patient does not have a coagulopathy, an active infection, significant psychopathology, or be seeking secondary gains from the intervention, and finally that the patient is in agreement with the treatment plan. Once this has been verified, our approach is outlined in Fig. A-2. Guidelines have been written to outline such an approach in the chronic spinal pain population.[8]

If the patient complains of diffuse pain, then he or she will most likely be considered for an intrathecal implantable device. Indications that deserve consideration for this therapy include diffuse cancer pain, spinal fractures with diffuse pain, axial somatic pain syndromes, failed back syndrome, complex regional pain syndrome, and arachnoiditis.[9] After the patient is properly screened, an intrathecal trial is scheduled as outlined in Ref. 9. Once the decision is made to implant an infusion pump, care must be taken to adhere to strict surgical guidelines for sterility and wound care to ensure continued proper functioning of the device.

If the pain is primarily myofascial in origin, our approach involves physical therapy, alone or in combination with trigger point injections and/or botulinum toxin injections. A treatment modality gaining popularity is radiofrequency ablation. This is a procedure that can be applied for nerve lesioning. The duration of effect varies, lasting anywhere from 1 week to 1 year. Specific application includes lesioning of median branches supplying facets, the thoracic dorsal root ganglion for postthoracotomy pain, or even peripheral nerves if the pain distribution can be localized to its distribution. For the terminal cancer pain patient a more permanent method of neurolysis using alcohol or neurosurgical cordotomy may also be considered.

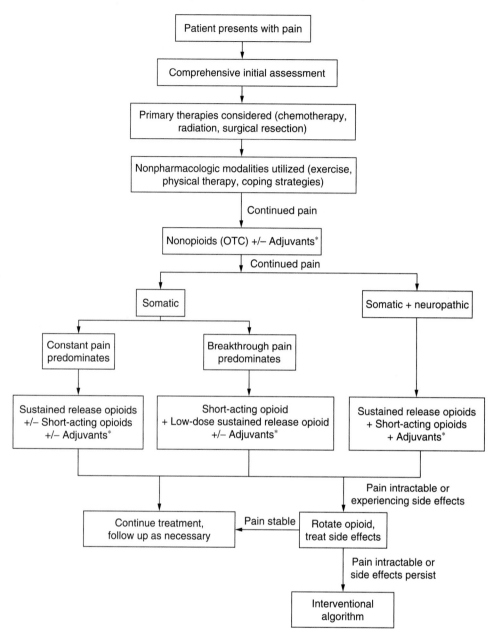

FIGURE A-1 The M. D. Anderson approach to cancer pain (conservative algorithm).

The last leg of the interventional algorithm may also be one of the most comprehensive. Ninety percent of adults experience low back pain during their lifetime. In patients under the age of 45, low back pain results in more disability than any other health problem, and overall is second only to the common cold in incidence.[10] At M. D. Anderson we begin by obtaining spinal imaging, usually a magnetic resonance imaging (MRI) study with contrast. This allows us to rule out metastatic carcinoma before considering the other more common sources of back pain, including facet arthropathy, a herniated or degenerated disc, vertebral body compression fracture, spinal/foraminal stenosis, or other sources.

If the patient fails conservative measures for his or her spinal pain, including physiotherapy and antiinflammatory agents, spinal diagnostic/therapeutic procedures can be considered. Although spinal pain is outside of the scope of cancer pain, due to the ubiquitous nature of back pain an overview has been provided here and in Fig. A-2. Spinal pain can be generated in the disc, nerve roots, zygapophyseal (facet) joints, the vertebral bodies, the surrounding soft tissues, or referred from the viscera. Numerous diagnostic and therapeutic pain procedures can be entertained depending on the nature of the spinal pain and its responsiveness to conservative treatments. Our general nonmalignant spinal pain algorithm is outlined in Fig. A-2.

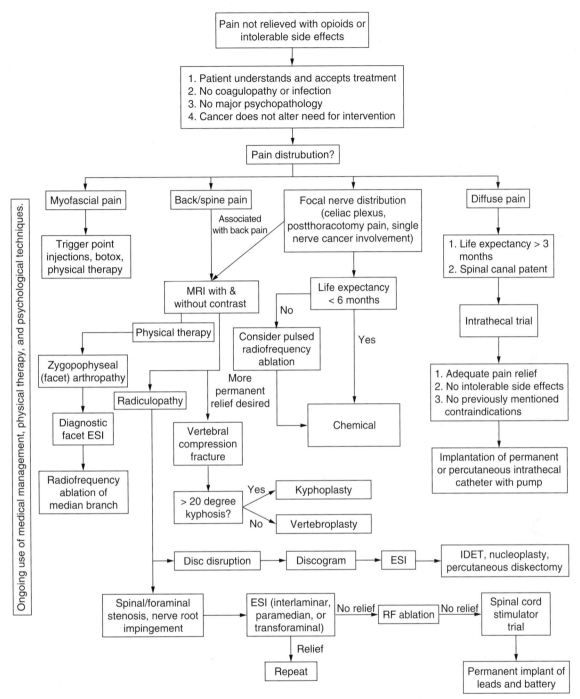

FIGURE A-2 The M. D. Anderson approach to cancer pain (interventional algorithm).

CONCLUSION

At M. D. Anderson, we believe a balanced treatment plan is necessary for the management of cancer pain. Interventions, when used in the appropriate setting, afford the pain management specialist a way to supplement the analgesic effect of opioids, thereby allowing an increase in activity level and downward dose titration and reduction of side effects.

REFERENCES

1. Daut RL, Cleeland CS. The prevalence and severity of pain in cancer. *Cancer.* 1982;50:1913–1918.
2. Foley KM. Treatment of cancer-related pain. *J Natl Cancer Inst Monogr.* 2004;(32):103–104.
3. Benedetti C, Brock C, Cleeland C, et al. National Comprehensive Cancer Network. Practice guidelines for cancer pain. *Oncology.* 2000;14:135–150.
4. Cohen MZ, Easley MK, Ellis C, et al. Cancer pain management and the JCAHO's pain standards: an institutional challenge. *J Pain Symptom Manage.* 2003;25:519–527.

5. Institutional Data for the University of Texas M. D. Anderson. http://www.mdanderson.org/About_MDA/Who_We_Are/display.cfm?id=29E3FCE1-2828-11D5-811100508B603A14&method=displayFull, accessed: December 23, 2005 at 9:30 AM.

6. Cahana A, Mavrocordatos P, Van Gessel E, et al. The role of interventional pain management in chronic pain. *J Anesth.* 2004;18:29–35.

7. Breivik H. The future role of the anesthesiologist in pain management. *Acta Anaesthesiol Scand.* 2005;49:922–926.

8. Boswell, MV, Shah RV, Everett CR, et al. Interventional techniques in the management of chronic spinal pain: Evidence-based practice guidelines. *Pain Physician.* 2005;8:1–47.

9. Burton AW, Rajagopal A, Shah HN, et al. Epidural and iintrathecal analgesia is effective in treating refractory cancer pain. *Pain Med.* 2004;5:239–247.

10. Andersson GB. Epidemiological features of low back pain. *Lancet.* 1999;354:581–585.

Troubleshooting Intrathecal Infusion Pumps

APPENDIX

B

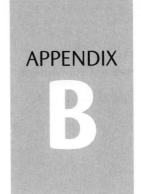

Tarun Jolly

Madhuri Are

Allen W. Burton

As the fields of pain medicine and palliative care continue to evolve, advanced technologies are being used more frequently. The use of the implanted intrathecal pain pump (ITP) is increasing so that it is prudent for the supportive care practitioner to establish a comfort zone for its use in the care of patients requiring palliative care and care for cancer pain.

COMMON ADVERSE EVENTS

Many adverse events can contribute to problems with an ITP. Broadly, these problems can be divided into device-related or drug-related problems. Table B-1 presents a summary of these problems.

Meticulous sterile technique should be maintained when implanting and refilling the pump. To avoid infection, several recommendations, largely based on cerebrospinal fluid (CSF) shunt data, have been made for the perioperative care of patients undergoing implantation. The reader is referred to this excellent reference for more details.[3] In general, infections are rare, but should be treated aggressively to avoid possible evolution into meningitis.

INTRATHECAL CATHETER TIP GRANULOMA

A catheter tip granuloma is a sterile mass at the catheter tip. Such masses are a rare but increasingly noted clinical phenomenon with the escalation of chronically ongoing pain pump management. This phenomenon has been a topic of discussion at numerous consensus meetings. The clinical manifestation of this mass is a gradual loss of pain relief and/or new back pain (occasionally with neurologic deficit) in a patient with an indwelling ITP, especially a pump with a high concentration of morphine (>25 mg/mL). Diagnosis of this mass is made with a contrast magnetic resonance imaging (MRI) to evaluate the catheter tip. Management is conservative, and entails decreasing or stopping IT infusion and observation except in cases of neurologic deficit. For a complete discussion, please see Refs 4 and 5.

AN APPROACH TO TROUBLESHOOTING AN IMPLANTED INTRATHECAL PUMP

The basic approach in evaluating a patient with an ITP includes the tenets of good medical practice. A thorough evaluation of the patient, including a complete history and focused examination, is mandatory. If the patient appears to be having analgesic or pump-related issues

such as underdosing/withdrawal or overdosing, a first step should focus on identifying possible life-threatening issues (see Fig. B-1).

If an excessive amount of medication has been delivered, begin basic life support including advanced cardiac life support (ACLS) protocols (including airway patency, adequate ventilation, and circulation) plus administration of naloxone (0.4–2 mg). Either a programming device or a pacemaker magnet (readily available in emergency rooms [ERs] and emergency medical service [EMS] units) can be used to shut off the pump, which will stop the infusion. See Fig. B-2 for further details, which should include toxicology testing to rule out oral medication overdose. Note, with a nonprogrammable pump (which usually delivers a fixed amount between 0.5 and 1.0 cc³ per day), the only way to "shut off" the infusion is to empty the pump reservoir.

Approaching a dosage insufficiency mandates a similar approach, with attention first directed toward issues endangering the health of the patient. Initially, the patient should be assessed neurologically to ensure that a granuloma has not formed (manifesting as a spinal cord compression), and that nerve root irritation due to a spinal catheter problem or new progressive spinal disease is not present.[4] Next, adequate medication delivery should be confirmed by interrogating the device, confirming proper programming. The drug, concentration, flow rate, and reservoir volume should each be verified. A determination should then be made as to whether the pump is delivering the programmed dose by administering a bolus equivalent to 20%–30% of the total daily dose. Bolus dosing via nonprogrammable pumps must be done manually via needle access into a specific pump port, and the exact procedure varies depending on pump type. If the patient feels relief, or at the very least demonstrates some response, it is likely that the pump is functioning properly. Pain relief at this new, higher dose is suggestive of tolerance, new pain sites, or worsening primary disease (as is often the case in cancer pain) and is similar to dose finding with oral medications. Depending on the amount of analgesia obtained with the bolus dose, the daily dose should be modified accordingly. In the event that the bolus did not elicit a response in the patient, the ITP-catheter system requires diagnostic troubleshooting.[5] Plain radiographs of the pump, including the catheter (usually an abdominal film AP and LAT), will help rule out catheter migration, a sheared catheter, or catheter kinks. A normal appearing catheter should be assessed with a dye injection to rule out a catheter disconnect, occlusion, or leak. In the event of a catheter problem, a catheter revision should be done. Finally, if no other defects are found, one must consider pump mechanism or battery failure (batteries usually last

Table B-1

Complications of Intrathecal Infusion Pumps

Systemic	Pump/Pocket	Catheter	Programming
Infection	Pump rotation/flip	Dislodged from pump	Rate error
Meningitis	Hematoma/seroma	Migration	Wrong dose/drug
Epidural abscess	Reservoir empty	Kink	Telemetry failure
Local wound	Rotor failure	Cut during placement	
Wound dehiscence	Depleted battery	Sheared catheter	
CSF leakage/hygroma		Occlusion	
Nerve irritation		Granuloma	
Postdural puncture			
Headache			

Source: Modified from Prager JP. Neuraxial medication delivery. The development and maturity of a concept for treating chronic pain of spinal origin. *Spine.* 2002;27:2593–2605; Burton AW, Conroy B, Garcia E, et al. Illicit substance abuse via an implanted intrathecal pump. *Anesthesiology.* 1998;89:1264–1267.

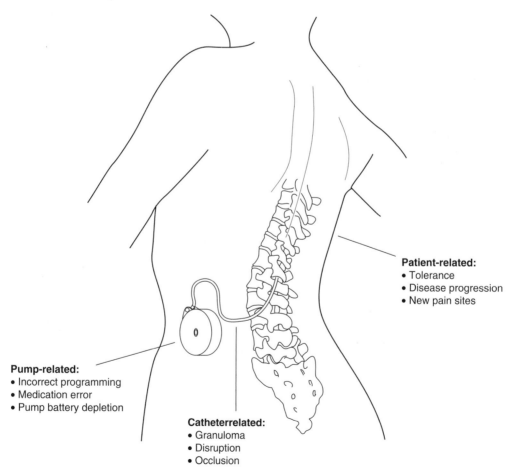

FIGURE B-1 Troubleshooting programmble intrathecal pumps.

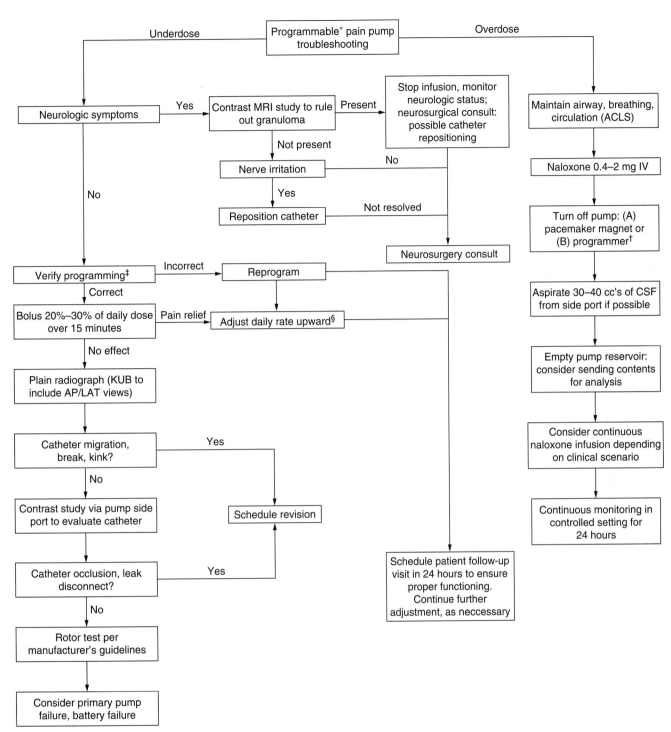

FIGURE B-2 Troubleshooting with an inthrathecal pump.

* For nonprogrammable pumps, eliminate all steps involving programming (i.e., the pump infusion, usually fixed 0.5–1.0 mL per day can only be stopped by emptying the reservoir of medication). Bolus dosing via nonprogrammable pumps must be done manually via needle access into a specific pump port; the exact procedure varies depending on pump type.

† Pump should be restarted as soon as possible following acute event (normal saline) to prevent internal catheter kink by stopped rotor.

‡ On/Off, Medication, Rate, Reservoir Volume, double check pharmacy records of last medication infused into pump if available.

§ Consider tolerance, new pain sites, worsening disease (work-up disease as necessary).

more than 5 years). In either case, removal of the device with subsequent reimplantation of a new device is required.

REFERENCES

1. Prager JP. Neuraxial medication delivery. The development and maturity of a concept for treating chronic pain of spinal origin. *Spine.* 2002;27:2593–2605.
2. Burton AW, Conroy B, Garcia E, et al. Illicit substance abuse via an implanted intrathecal pump. *Anesthesiology.* 1998;89:1264–1267.
3. Follett KA, Boortz-Marx RL, Drake JM, et al. Prevention and management of intrathecal drug delivery and spinal cord stimulation system infections. *Anesthesiology.* 2004;100:1582–1594.
4. Coffey RJ, Burchiel K. Inflammatory mass lesions associated with intrathecal drug infusion catheters: report and observations on 41 Patients. *Neurosurgery.* 2002;50:78–86.
5. Hassenbusch S, Burchiel K, Coffey RJ, et al. Management of intrathecal catheter-tip inflammatory masses: a consensus statement. *Pain Med.* 2002;3:313–323.

Practical Options for Distress Screening

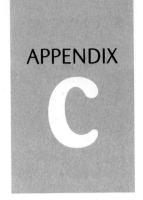

APPENDIX C

Debra Sivesind

Patient comfort and level of function are pressing concerns for clinicians as patients survive longer and have chronic symptom problems or persisting pain. There are several different things to consider when cancer-related pain is assessed. Pain intensity, duration, relief, and interference with daily functioning are important considerations. Other variables that make up a multidimensional picture may interfere with the patient's ability to cope. These factors affect the patient's overall experience of distress and include emotional, social, and spiritual concerns.

Screening for distress has several pitfalls. Not only is it subjective but patients may be reluctant to disclose their distress and clinicians may be too busy to notice subclinical levels of distress. Two methods of measuring distress include a clinical interview and the use of written tools/questionnaires. An assessment is not complete without a face-to-face interview by an experienced clinician that can provide invaluable nonverbal and behavioral information. Using the combination of a clinical interview and reliable written assessment tools provides the most comprehensive information for distress screening.

Several assessment tools have been developed to measure multidimensional distress and are available in the literature and online. More recently, the National Comprehensive Cancer Network (NCCN) and the American Cancer Society (ACS) have developed a distress measure for patients and clinicians available on the Web sites www.cancer.org or www.nccn.org. The unique quality of these guidelines provides a practical method of screening for distress. These tools are not only written in understandable language for patients but can also assist clinicians in addressing the most objective and up-to-date areas for distress screening.

For clinicians who are screening distress it is important to determine the level and nature of the distress and these guidelines do both. The degree of distress is measured on a continuum. Normal levels of distress could be described as expected feelings of sadness or fear. More severe problems that can become disabling are described as depression, anxiety, panic, social isolation, and existential and spiritual crisis. The NCCN tool uses a subjective distress measure that is analogous to a thermometer reading. A 0–10 range is used where 0 is no distress and 10 is extreme distress. Scores rated at 5 or above are considered moderate to severe distress and may benefit from intervention. The nature of the distress is determined with a problem list, including practical problems (like housing or child care), family problems, emotional problems, spiritual or religious concerns, and physical problems (Table C-1).

Table C-1

Screening Tool for Measuring Distress (the Nature of Distress)

Indicate if any of the following has been a cause of distress in the past week, including today. Mark NO or YES for each item.

Practical Problems	Physical Problems
Housing	Pain
Insurance	Nausea
Work/school	Fatigue
Transportation	Sleep
Child care	Getting around
	Bathing/dressing
Family Problems	Breathing
Dealing with partner	Mouth sores
Dealing with children	Eating
Spiritual/Religious	Indigestion
Concerns	Constipation
Relating to God	Diarrhea
Loss of faith	Changes in urination
	Fevers
	Skin dry/itchy
	Nose dry/congested
	Tingling in hands/feet
	Feeling swollen
	Sexual

Source: Modified with permission from National Comprehensive Cancer Network. Distress: Treatment Guidelines for Patients. Version 1/July 2004, pp. 6–8. Available at: www.nccn.org. (Accessed January 31, 2005).

The NCCN guidelines also include a list of "red flags" to help determine whether distress is normal or becoming serious followed by a list of past vulnerabilities that may make coping difficult (Table C-2).

Another list provided by the NCCN in their guidelines reflects key times that a patient may be more prone to distress symptoms (Table C-3).

Table C-2

"Red Flags" (That Distress is Becoming Excessive)

- ▶ Feeling overwhelmed by fear to the point of panic or an overpowering sense of dread
- ▶ Feeling so sad that you feel you cannot go through treatment
- ▶ Unusual irritability and anger
- ▶ Inability to cope with pain, fatigue, and nausea
- ▶ Poor concentration, having "fuzzy thinking," and sudden memory problems
- ▶ Having a very difficult time making any decisions
- ▶ Feeling despair and hopelessness—wondering if there is any point in going on
- ▶ Constant thoughts about cancer and/or death
- ▶ Trouble sleeping (less than 4 hours)
- ▶ Trouble eating (a noticeable decrease in appetite, or no appetite, for a period of weeks)
- ▶ Family conflicts and issues that seem impossible to resolve
- ▶ Questioning your faith and religious beliefs that once gave you comfort
- ▶ Feeling worthless and useless
- ▶ Things from the past that may make you or your family more vulnerable to distress
- ▶ Having a relative who died as a result of cancer
- ▶ Having a recent loss of someone close to you
- ▶ Having depression or suicidal thoughts in the past
- ▶ Reliving a painful event from your past that seems unrelated to the current situation
- ▶ Having had thought of harming yourself or someone else

Source: Modified with permission from National Comprehensive Cancer Network. Distress: Treatment Guidelines for Patients. Version 1/July 2004, pp. 6–8. Available at: www.nccn.org. (Accessed January 31, 2005).

Table C-3

Periods of Increased Vulnerability

- ▶ Finding a suspicious symptom
- ▶ During work-up
- ▶ Finding out the diagnosis
- ▶ Awaiting treatment
- ▶ Change in treatment modality
- ▶ End of treatment
- ▶ Discharge from hospital following treatment
- ▶ Stresses of survivorship
- ▶ Medical follow-up and surveillance
- ▶ Treatment failure
- ▶ Recurrence/progression
- ▶ Advanced cancer
- ▶ End of life

Source: Modified with permission from National Comprehensive Cancer Network. Distress: Clinical Practice Guidelines in Oncology. Version 1/2005, pp. DIS–5B. Available at: www.nccn.org. (Accessed January 31, 2005).

These aids for screening distress can assist the clinician in formulating a comprehensive treatment plan. A face-to-face clinical interview by an experienced clinician is also an integral part of collecting screening information.

REFERENCES

1. National Comprehensive Cancer Network. Distress: Treatment Guidelines for Patients. Version 1/July 2004, pp. 6–8. Available at: www.nccn.org. (Accessed January 31, 2005).
2. National Comprehensive Cancer Network. Distress: Clinical Practice Guidelines in Oncology. Version 1/2005, pp. DIS–5B. Available at: www.nccn.org. (Accessed January 31, 2005).

Dosing Strategies for Oral Methadone

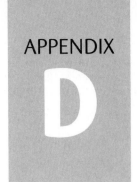

Michael J. Fisch

Oral methadone is a unique analgesic. On the one hand, it is an opioid analgesic, which appears to have similar efficacy to other opioids when dosed appropriately. It also has other properties that may contribute to analgesic efficacy, including (1) antagonistic activity at the *N*-methyl-*D*-aspartate receptors (NMDA) and (2) inhibition of norepinephrine and serotonin reuptake. Methadone has the advantage of extremely low cost (often 10–30-fold less expensive than other strong opioids), and lack of known active metabolites. Because of its long and unpredictable half-life and relatively unknown equianalgesic dose compared with other opioids, methadone was generally used by pain specialists with experience in its use. Since the mid-1990s, however, the utility of this agent in cancer pain has become more widely appreciated, with numerous publications in pain and palliative care journals as well as clinical oncology journals. The methadone preparation widely used in the United States is a racemic mix of the *d*-isomer and *l*-isomer of methadone. The *d*-isomer has antagonist activity at the NMDA receptor and animal data as well as anecdotal and retrospective reports suggest that this produces clinically relevant benefits in the control of neuropathic pain and minimizes opioid tolerance. However, adequately sized, prospective data are lacking in the cancer pain population. Thus, it is no surprise that the use of methadone as well as specific dosing strategies remains variable and somewhat controversial.

Pain specialists at M. D. Anderson Cancer Center are often contacted by telephone or e-mail for advice regarding methadone and how to prescribe it in outpatient settings (particularly hospice settings). Similarly, there is no consensus among specialists at M. D. Anderson about how this should be done. However, because I am one of the physicians who is frequently consulted about its use, I will share my advice about methadone dosing, as well as some references that can be used as guides.

STARTING METHADONE AS THE FIRST-LINE (INITIAL) OPIOID ANALGESIC

▶ Basic principles

- ▸ Think of methadone as a "long-acting" opioid, just as you would think of a sustained-release preparation of morphine or oxycodone.
- ▸ Use a "typical" short-acting opioid for breakthrough pain or incidental pain (rather than using methadone).

- ▸ Manage opioid side effects aggressively and monitor the patient carefully, just as you would if you were starting any other strong opioid.
- ▸ Oral methadone can be given as a tablet, and tablets can be cut in half or crushed or prescribed as an elixir (usually as 1 mg/cc concentration).
- ▸ After 3–5 days, titrate methadone as you would any other long-acting opioid to achieve optimum pain control.

▶ Dosing

Most patients: 5 mg twice daily for 2 or 3 days, then increase to 5 mg three times daily

Frail or elderly patients: 2.5 mg qhs on day 1, then 2.5 mg BID for 2–3 days, then 2.5 mg TID

SWITCHING TO METHADONE FROM MORPHINE OR OTHER OPIOIDS

Opioid switching (also called "opioid rotation") is intended to improve analgesia and/or reduce opioid side effects when the existing opioid regimen is producing unsatisfactory results. There is no gold standard or evidence-based criteria for exactly when this ought to be done or exactly how to do it. There is no question, however, that it is a useful technique to have in one's toolbox of maneuvers for the cancer pain patient. Some experts use methadone as the "first switch" opioid. That is, methadone is the drug they like to switch to when medical pain management needs improvement. For other experts, methadone is used as a second or subsequent opioid. The methods that are used for switching to methadone employ either an "ad libitum" technique, a "fixed-dose ratio" technique, or a "sliding-dose ratio." The ad libitum approach calls for the previous dose to be discontinued and a single fixed dose of methadone to be given at the start, calculated using an equianalgesic dose ratio of morphine to methadone of 10:1 (i.e., morphine 10 mg being roughly equivalent to 1 mg of methadone). No more than but up to 50 mg of methadone is given per dose. After the initial single priming dose, the same dose is administered every 3 hours as needed. The clinician observes the patient and when the demand for rescue doses reduces or stabilizes (usually on day 4–7), the daily requirement is calculated and the dose is given every 8–12 hours. In contrast, the fixed-dose ratio technique involves an immediate switch using an equianalgesic dose ratio of morphine to methadone of 5:1 (i.e., morphine 5 mg being roughly equivalent to 1 mg of methadone). It has been shown that stable methadone concentrations are reached within two days of using this fixed ratio.

I favor the sliding-dose ratio approach, which involves rapid switching and a dosing scheme for the switch that is based upon the morphine equivalent daily dose (MEDD) of the currently used opioid (the drug that you are switching from). The principle distinction from the fixed-dose ratio technique is to use a table to determine the dose ratio, rather than using a fixed 5:1 ratio.

HOW TO CALCULATE THE MEDD OF AN OPIOID REGIMEN

The first step for the switch to methadone based on this sliding dose ratio technique is to determine the oral MEDD of the current regimen. The method resembles calculating a currency exchange to the U.S. dollar before making a trade, if your understanding of the proper pricing is based in dollars. Here, we want to know the value of the current regimen in "morphine dollars." The exchange rates that are used vary to some extent among experts. Once again, this reflects the paucity of data by which to base these judgments. Table D-1 reflects the standards used at M. D. Anderson Cancer Center.

▶ Examples of calculations of morphine-equivalent doses

- ▶ A 4 mg tablet of hydromorphone equals 20 mg of oral morphine
- ▶ A 40 mg dose of oxycodone (immediate or sustained-release) equals 60 mg of oral morphine
- ▶ A 1 mg/h basal infusion of intravenous hydromorphone (24 mg/day) equals 240 mg of oral morphine
- ▶ A 75 mcg fentanyl patch equals 150 mg of oral morphine

USING THE MEDD TO CHOOSE THE DAILY DOSE OF METHADONE

Once the MEDD of the existing regimen has been calculated, Table D-2 is used to calculate the daily methadone dose to be given. The table is not meant to be precise, but it puts the dosing into a conservative and acceptable range from which proper assessment and dose titration can be applied to maximize pain relief with acceptable side effects. The daily dose is usually administered in 2 or 3 doses given 8–12 hours apart. The exact dose and schedule used is often influenced by the pill size. Thus, if a patient is calculated to receive approximately 24 mg/day of methadone, the actual dosing might be 10 mg in the morning, 5 mg in the afternoon, and 10 mg at bedtime.

▶ Examples of opioid rotations to methadone

- ▶ If a patient is using a 100 mcg fentanyl patch and is receiving intravenous morphine doses of 10 mg four times daily, then the MEDD is $(100 \times 2) + (40 \times 3) = 320$ mg/day. The table suggests that a dose of 300 mg should be divided by 10 to obtain the daily methadone dose. This patient can have the fentanyl patch removed and begin oral methadone at a dose of 10 mg three times daily. An appropriate breakthrough pain regimen would be about 10% of the MEDD given as a short-acting opioid. This patient could receive oral morphine at 30 mg every 4 hours for breakthrough pain.
- ▶ If a patient is receiving sustained-release oxycodone at 40 mg twice daily and immediate-release oxycodone at 10 mg four times daily (a total of 80 + 40 = 120 mg) and is experiencing inadequate pain relief, an appropriate switch to methadone would be based on the MEDD of $(120 \times 1.5) = 180$ mg/day. The table suggests that 180/6 = 30 mg/day of methadone. Methadone could then be prescribed at a dose of 10 mg TID.

▶ How to convert to methadone from very large MEDD doses

There are precious little data concerning how to safely and effectively switch from very large opioid doses to methadone. As such, each of these cases should be handled individually rather than by using a fixed-dose conversion table. Some points to keep in mind for managing patients on very large opioid doses (>400 mg/day) include:

- ▶ Some of these patients will not have improved with incremental dose escalations, and thus the appropriate new dose of methadone or another opioid may be much, much lower than any table would predict.

Table D-1
Calculating the Oral Morphine Equivalent Dose

Starting from This Opioid	Multiply by This Number to Calculate the Oral Morphine Equivalent Dose (mg)
Oral agents	
Hydromorphone	5
Oxycodone	1.5
Hydrocodone	0.5
Intravenous agents	
Morphine	3
Hydromorphone	10
Transdermal agents	
Fentanyl patch (micrograms)	2

Table D-2
Calculating the Target Daily Methadone Dose

Oral Morphine Equivalent Daily Dose (MEDD) of the Current Opioid (mg)	Divide by This Number to Calculate the Target Daily Methadone Dose (mg)
30–99	4
100–180	6
181–240	8
250–300	10

▶ Some of these patients will have developed paradoxical increases in pain during the opioid dose escalations due to hyperalgesia related to opioid neurotoxicity. Once again, the appropriate dose of methadone may be quite low (<30 mg/day).

▶ A strategy that may be used involves incremental removal of 300 mg of morphine equivalents at a time and adding 30 mg/day of methadone to the existing regimen, and repeating this approach every 2–3 days while undertaking punctilious daily assessments.

    ▶ Example: A patient taking 200 mg of sustained-release morphine three times daily and 20 mg of hydromorphone eight times daily has an MEDD of 1400 mg/day. Such a patient may have the sustained-release morphine reduced to 100 mg three times daily (a 300 mg/day reduction) and start methadone 10 mg three times daily. On day 3, the hydromorphone may be reduced to 20 mg taken only five times daily (another 300 mg/day reduction in oral morphine equivalents), while the methadone would be increased to 20 mg three times daily (another 30 mg/day methadone added).

DRUG INTERACTIONS AND PRECAUTIONS

Methadone is metabolized primarily by the hepatic cytochrome-P450-system isoenzyme CYP3A4, and to a lesser extent, by isoenzyme CYP2D6. Drugs that inhibit CYP3A4 cause the methadone levels to drift upward, and drugs that induce the metabolism of CYP3A4 will cause the methadone levels to drift downward. Important drugs to consider when prescribing methadone are summarized in Table D-3.

Methadone is one of a long list of medications that can cause prolongation of the Q-T interval and torsades de pointes ventricular tachycardia. This is caused by inhibition of the rapid component of the delayed rectifier potassium ion current. Other common drugs that share this attribute include haloperidol, chlorpromazine, clarithromycin, pentamidine, and others. The level of risk associated with these drugs is low, and depends on the dose and the population being treated. Oral methadone can be safely administered in the low doses (<100 mg/day) that are generally prescribed for the treatment of cancer pain, and routine electrocardiograms are not performed at our institution when prescribing oral methadone. Caution should be taken when prescribing methadone to certain patients who may be at higher risk of Q-T prolongation, as summarized below.

▶ Conditions associated with higher risk of torsades de pointes with high dose methadone

▶ Elderly women with advanced heart failure

▶ Severe metabolic disarray (particularly hypokalemia)

▶ Family history of sudden death

▶ Cocaine abuse

▶ Use of the cardiac drugs amiodarone or quinidine

▶ Concomitant use of drugs that cause methadone levels to rise

    ▶ Ciprofloxacin

    ▶ Ketoconazole, itraconazole, fluconazole

    ▶ Erythromycin, clarithromycin, doxycycline

    ▶ Grapefruit juice

    ▶ HIV protease inhibitors

    ▶ Nefazodone

▶ Use of intravenous methadone

Intravenous methadone is considered equivalent to one-half of the calculated dose of oral methadone. Thus, if a patient is taking oral methadone at 10 mg TID, and the patient is hospitalized and cannot take the pills, an appropriate intravenous methadone dose would be 5 mg IV every 8 hours. A special consideration with the use of IV methadone is the fact that some commercial solutions contain methadone preserved with chlorobutanol. Chlorobutanol is associated with its own, independent effects on the heart and the Q-T interval. For this reason, hospitalized patients receiving methadone are monitored carefully for control of their electrolytes, and routine electrocardiograms before and 24 hours after starting IV methadone (or making significant dose adjustments) may be prudent.

SELECTED REFERENCES FOR FURTHER READING

1. Alfort DP, Compton P, Samet JH. Acute pain management for patients receiving maintenance methadone or buprenorphine therapy. *Ann Intern Med.* 2006;144:127–134.

2. Bruera E, Palmer JL, Bosnjak S, et al. Methadone versus morphine as a first-line strong opioid for cancer pain: a randomized, double-blind study. *J Clin Oncol.* 2004;22:185–192.

3. Bruera E, Sweeney C. Methadone use in cancer patients with pain: a review. *J Palliat Med.* 2002;5:127–138.

4. Indelicato RA, Portenoy RK. Opioid rotation in the management of refractory cancer pain. *J Clin Oncol.* 2002;20:348–352.

5. Manfredi PL, Houde RW. Prescribing methadone, a unique analgesic. *J Support Oncol.* 2003;1:216–220.

6. Mercadante S, Ferrera P, Villari P, et al. Rapid switching between transdermal fentanyl and methadone in cancer patients. *J Clin Oncol.* 2005;23:5229–5234.

7. Mercadante S, Casuccio A, Fulfaro F, et al. Switching from morphine to methadone to improve analgesia and tolerability in cancer patients: a prospective study. *J Clinl Oncol.* 2001;19:2898–2904.

8. Mercadante S, Fulfaro F, Dabbene M. Methadone in treatment of tenesmus not responding to morphine escalation. *Support Care Cancer.* 2001;9:129–130.

9. Mercadante S, Casuccio A, Agnello A, et al. Methadone response in advanced cancer patients with pain followed at home. *J Pain Symptom Manage.* 1999;18:188–192.

Table D-3

Drugs Affecting Methadone Dose Levels

Drugs Causing Methadone Levels to Drift Upward (Higher Effects)	Drugs Causing Methadone Levels to Drift Downward (Lower Effects)
Ciprofloxacin	Rifampin
Ketoconazole, itraconazole, fluconazole	Phenytoin
Erythromycin, clarithromycin, doxycycline	Corticosteroids
Grapefruit juice	Carbamazepine
HIV protease inhibitors	St. John's wort
Imatinib	
Nefazodone	

10. Mercadante S, Casuccio A, Calderone L. Rapid switching from morphine to methadone in cancer patients with poor response to morphine. *J Clin Oncol.* 1999;17:3307–3312.

11. Mercadante S, Casuccio A, Agnello A, et al. Morphine versus methadone in the pain treatment of advanced-cancer patients followed up at home. *J Clin Oncol.* 1998;16:3656–3661.

12. Mercadante S, Casuccio A, Calderone L. Rapid switching from morphine to methadone in cancer patients with poor response to morphine. *J Clin Oncol.* 1999;17:3307–3312.

13. Morley JS, Watt JW, Wells JC, et al. Methadone in pain uncontrolled by morphine. *Lancet.* 1993;342:1243.

14. Nauck F, Ostgathe C, Dickerson ED. A German model for methadone conversion. *Am Hosp Palliat Care.* 2001;18:200–202.

15. Reddy S, Fisch M, Bruera E. Oral methadone for cancer pain: no indication of Q-T interval prolongation or torsades de pointes. *J Pain Symptom Manage.* 2004;28:301–303.

16. Ripamonti C, De Conno F, Groff L, et al. Equianalgesic dose/ratio between methadone and other opioid agonists in cancer pain: comparison of two clinical experiences. *Ann Oncol.* 1998;9:79–83.

17. Ripamonti C, Groff L, Brunelli C, et al. Switching from morphine to oral methadone in treating cancer pain: what is the equianalgesic dose ratio? *J Clin Oncol.* 1998;16:3216–3221.

18. Roden DM. Drug-induced prolongation of the Q-T interval. *N Engl J Med.* 2004;350:1013–1022.

19. Ripamonti C, Zecca E, Brunelli C, et al. Rectal methadone in cancer patients with pain. A preliminary clinical and pharmacokinetic study. *Ann Oncol.* 1995;6:841–843.

20. Soares LG. Methadone for cancer pain: what have we learned from clinical studies? *Am J Hosp Palliat Care.* 2005;22:223–227.

21. Ventafridda V, Ripamonti C, Bianchi M, et al. A randomized study on oral administration of morphine and methadone in the treatment of cancer pain. *J Pain Symptom Manage.* 1986;1:203–207.

INDEX

Page numbers followed by *f* or *t* indicate figures or tables, respectively.